Edmund's
Food Ratings
for Dieters

Publisher
Peter Steinlauf

Editor-in-Chief
Michael G. Samet, Ph.D.
Consumer Psychologist

Nutrition Editor
Joanne Larsen, M.S., R.D.
Registered Dietitian

Nutrition Database
Hopkins Technology

Information Technology
Haim Hirsch
Debra Katzir

PREFACE

Michael G. Samet, Ph.D.

This food rating book is designed as a decision guide for people who enjoy eating, but who also want to shed extra pounds or control their weight. Since so many people fall into this category, we have chosen to present standard nutritional data and a new system of easy-to-use ratings for many of the foods most commonly eaten in our culture. Because of their differences in origin, composition, and preparation, these foods vary significantly in how relatively *good* or *bad* they are for you and your diet — all, of course, depending on your personal health status and your weight loss or maintenance goals.

For this guide, a multi-attribute approach was taken to develop a set of unique scientifically-based ratings that address the interplay of several food factors including caloric and fat content, dietary fiber, vitamin and mineral percentages, and the degree to which a food is filling and energizing. By computing and displaying these ratings and an overall rating for each food, our goal was to offer a new and simple way for you to identify and compare specific nutritious foods that can make your weight loss or maintenance program easier. In fact, the results of some of the better food choices may surprise you and many nutrition experts as well.

This book is a creative product of the information age. The 900 common foods rated here have been selected and analyzed from a nutrition database containing nearly 40,000 foods, which has been developed and maintained by Hopkins Technology — a Minnesota company that has produced and marketed state-of-the-art health and nutrition software for consumers since 1986 (see pages 460-462). The expertise, dedicated efforts, and pioneering contributions of Carol and Philip Dunn, the founders of Hopkins Technology, are evident throughout the pages of this book.

In all our guide books, Edmund's strives to provide accurate data and valuable information to enable you to make wiser and better consumer decisions. In this regard, any comments or suggestions you have about the food ratings within this book are welcome by mail [or e-mail].

Edmund Publications Corporation
300 N. Sepulveda Blvd., Suite 2050
El Segundo, CA 90245
[e-mail: Edmund@enews.com]

Good luck in your daily selections of the best and healthiest food alternatives for you, and for your diet — if you're on one.

FOOD RATINGS FOR DIETERS

TABLE OF CONTENTS

ISBN: 0-312-91978-6
ISSN: 1079-1493

Edmund Publications Corporation
300 Sepulveda Blvd., Suite 2050
El Segundo, CA 90245

Edmund's books are available at special quantity discounts when purchased in bulk by corporations, organizations, and other special interest groups. Custom covers and/or customized copy on available pages may also be prepared to fit particular needs.

NOTE: All information and ratings published herein are based on the editors' interpretations and analyses of data available from sources which, in the editors' opinions, are considered reliable. Under no circumstances should the reader assume that the information presented in this book is official or final; the information is subject to change at any time. All ratings are represented as approximations only, and the use or application of the food ratings, nutritional data and values, and any other information presented within this book are not the responsibility of the publisher.

Michael G. Samet, Ph.D. and Joanne Larsen, M.S., R.D.

Dieters often ask: "What can I eat?" "What are the most nutritious diet foods?" "What should I avoid more, calories or grams of fat?" "Which low calorie foods provide the most energy, fiber, vitamins, and minerals?" "Which good-for-my-diet foods are most filling?" "What should I eat once I go off my diet?" To help dieters and everyone else answer these questions and make healthy food choices, this book of food ratings has been prepared. Our goal is to provide new information that will give you more choices and control over what you eat. Use this guide as a companion while grocery shopping, or when eating out, or at home.

The more you know about your body and the basics of weight control, the more you can take advantage of the food ratings in this guide. You should know your desired weight, and develop a practical plan and realistic schedule for achieving it. For example, depending on how active you are, you need to take in about 10 calories per day for every pound of your target weight (e.g., about 1350 calories for 135 pounds). And keep in mind that 3500 excess calories are equivalent to one pound of body weight. Furthermore, you'll want to know the role that fat, carbohydrates, fiber, vitamins, and minerals play in your diet and health maintenance plan. Whatever your level of nutritional knowledge, the ratings in this book will make it easy for you to evaluate food in light of your weight control goals.

By customizing your eating plan, you will quickly appreciate that the word "diet" simply means "the foods you eat", and not that you have to eat less or deny yourself good tasting, satisfying, nutritional portions of food.

Foods Selected for Evaluation

This book describes, analyzes, and rates 900 representative foods commonly eaten within our culture, and drawn from the comprehensive database maintained by the United States Department of Agriculture (USDA). The selected foods range from beverages and snacks, to soups and entrees, to bakery items and desserts, and to everything in between. Complete meals and sandwiches (many of them of the fast food variety) are evaluated, as well as traditional components of meals such as bread, salad, sauce, fruit, vegetables, and fish. Both unprocessed, uncooked foods are listed, along with processed, cooked, brand name, and ready-to-eat foods like dry cereals and frozen dinners.

Whenever possible, different versions of the same foods are included for comparison, such as meat versus vegetarian substitutes, dairy versus tofu equivalents, and foods low in calories and fat versus alternatives that are not.

The food evaluations are presented alphabetically two to a page, on pages 10 through 459. The identical half-page format is used for each evaluation, headed at the top by the name of the food printed in white letters on a black bar. Most of the food names are generic (e.g., croissant, apple juice, almond chicken), but many brand names are also listed (especially for cereals, e.g., Cheerios). After the food name, modifiers usually appear to qualify the particular content of the food (e.g. *pizza, cheese* or *stew, vegetarian*) or how it is prepared (e.g., *egg, white only, cooked*, or *cauliflower, cooked without added fat)*.

Serving Size. The all-important serving size appears to the left under each food name. The serving size (which is the exact amount of the food to which the nutritional data and ratings apply) is provided as a physical measure (e.g., piece or slice with or without dimensions in inches) or volume (e.g., cup, tablespoon), as well as a weight in ounces in parentheses. For beverages, the measure given is also weight in ounces and not fluid ounces. Supplied by the USDA database, the serving sizes represent common, practical portions that an average person would (or should) consume at a meal or snack. Whenever possible, an attempt was made to select food options to be compared (e.g., vegetarian versus meat meals) on the basis of their having more or less equivalent serving sizes.

Food Categories

To the right of the serving size for each food rated, a food category name appears within the rating form. These familiar categories were created to help you make comparisons and decisions among similar foods. The 900 common representative foods were classified into 21 food categories - based on the what, when, and how of practical food groups. The table on the next page lists the food categories in alphabetical order, together with statistics on their constituent foods including the number of foods represented, their average serving-size weight, and their average calories and range of calories.

Food Category	Number of Foods	Average Serving Weight (oz)	Average Calories	Calorie Range
Bakery	54	1.2	118	29 - 266
Beverage	33	9.1	107	2 - 360
Bread	43	1.2	95	45 - 217
Breakfast	30	3.5	210	17 - 600
Cereal	49	2.4	177	56 - 541
Cheese	13	1.9	84	23 - 216
Dessert	89	4.5	267	17 - 544
Entree	165	7.4	313	37 - 1476
Fat & Oil	32	0.8	82	12 - 492
Fish	39	3.5	192	25 - 521
Fruit	34	5.4	124	17 - 435
Meat	38	2.4	158	16 - 359
Poultry	15	2.9	174	40 - 416
Salad	25	5.7	238	9 - 550
Sandwich	39	4.9	347	140 - 729
Sauce	9	5.1	177	10 - 598
Shellfish	13	3.4	139	37 - 258
Snack	44	1.2	147	9 - 701
Soup	37	8.8	139	17 - 275
Sweets	3	0.6	35	6 - 49
Vegetable	96	5.0	124	1 - 483

Food and Nutrient Data

In two columns on the top portion of the rating form (page 10), the nutrient data are presented based on the serving size listed for the food. All the source data were taken without modification from the USDA database. The arrangement of the data here is consistent, to the extent possible, with the order on the new food labels required by the Nutrition Labeling and Education Act. The computation of percent Daily Value (%DV) for each nutrient is based on available data and recommendations supplied by the Food and Drug Administration (FDA). The %DVs are based on the requirements of most healthy individuals who eat an average of about 2,000 calories per day.

The first food item listed on the rating form is the number of calories, followed in parentheses by the caloric density or number of calories per ounce. The next listing is the number of fat calories, followed in parentheses by the percentage of fat calories (from all fats) relative to total calories. Next appear the amounts in grams (g) for total fat, saturated fat, polyunsaturated fat, and monounsaturated fat; for both total and saturated fat, the computed %DV for the food is also given in parentheses. The last three data items presented in the left column are cholesterol, sodium, and potassium content, all measured in milligrams (mg) and all accompanied by their %DV in parentheses.

At the top of the right column are listed the grams (g) of carbohydrate, dietary fiber, and protein; the sugar level of a food is included in the grams of carbohydrate. Next comes Vitamin A (in International Units - IU), followed by the milligram (mg) levels of Vitamin C, calcium, and iron. Finally, amounts are given for folate (also known as folic acid or folacin) in micrograms (mcg), and beta carotene in Retinol Equivalents (RE). For each food element in the right column except beta carotene, the %DV is listed in parentheses.

Food Ratings

Because of their complexity, it's hard to compare the nutritional content and impact of foods without a calculator (or better, a computer) and a degree in nutrition, even with the summary information provided on the new food labels. To allow you to make quick and meaningful comparisons among foods yourself, Edmund's has developed a unique rating system involving seven factors that affect weight control in most people. For each separate factor, a numerical rating was computed (by a scientifically-based weighted algorithm applied to the food's nutritional parameters) on a 1 to 10 interval scale with 10 the best, 1 the worst, and a rating of 5 to 6 on average. The individual factor ratings outlined below were then weighted and combined into a single overall rating for the food.

The <u>Weight Loss</u> rating is computed from total calories (adjusted for average number of calories within the food category), total fat, and alcohol content. The lower the relative content of calories, fat, and alcohol, the higher the rating. Foods with higher ratings (e.g., fruits and vegetables) are better for weight loss than foods with lower ratings (e.g., salad dressing and nuts).

The <u>LowCal Density</u> rating is derived from the inverse of calories per ounce. The lower the density of calories in the measured serving, the higher the rating. Ideally, the best foods for dieters are those that offer fewer calories in bigger portions (e.g., a 9 oz beef stew entree - 20 cal/oz) rather than more calories in smaller portions (e.g., a 5.6 oz fish and chips entree - 58 cal/oz).

The <u>Filling</u> rating is computed from the levels of carbohydrates and fiber relative to calories. The more the carbohydrate and fiber, the more filling and satisfying the food is at meal time, and the higher its rating. As examples, some cereals and dried cooked beans (legumes) rate high in filling, whereas cheese and chicken by themselves rate low in filling.

The Energizing rating is based on the amount of carbohydrates, including sugar, found in the food. The more carbohydrate content in the food, the more mental and physical energy to be derived, and the greater the rating. Foods like potatoes, beans, cake and some cereals rate high in energizing, whereas most meats, cheeses and vegetables rate low in energizing.

The Fiber rating is based on the relative amount of dietary fiber found in the food. The higher the grams of dietary fiber, the higher the fiber rating. High fiber foods are generally more filling. Furthermore, appropriate levels of daily fiber intake are important for the digestive tract of dieters. Foods high in fiber are fruits, vegetables, and grains (rice). Many foods contain little or no fiber at all, such as meats, cheeses and fish.

The Vitamins rating reflects both the number of vitamins (including A, C, folate, B6, B12, E, thiamin, riboflavin and niacin) contained in the food and the %DV contributed by each vitamin. The higher the total vitamin content, the higher the rating. Since you may eat fewer foods when dieting, it's wise to include high vitamin foods in your selections. The foods with the highest level of vitamins are enriched cereals and green or orange vegetables and fruits.

The Minerals rating reflects both the number of minerals (including calcium, iron, phosphorus, magnesium and zinc) contained in the food and the %DV contributed by each mineral. The higher the total mineral content, the higher the rating. To maintain an adequate level of overall nutrition when dieting, it is important that you also pad your eating plan with high mineral-rated foods. The foods with the highest mineral content are entrees with beans, cheese or shellfish, and enriched cereals.

The Overall rating is computed by an exclusive combination formula that weights the relative contributions (to the overall rating) of the seven rating factors, such that the level of importance (weight) is highest for Weight Loss and LowCal Density, mid-level for Filling, and lowest for Energizing, Fiber, Vitamins and Minerals. Of course, when comparing two or more foods, readers with specific preferences or needs for specific rating factors can develop and apply (to the individual ratings) their own personalized weighting scheme.

The ratings outlined above are displayed on the rating page in a set of bar graphs presented below the nutritional data for the food. The actual rounded-off numerical rating for each factor is shown in the rightmost shaded rectangle of the respective extended bar. The density or number of shaded rectangles in the rating matrix gives a quick indication of how good or bad a food is rated. The more the gray space (more rectangles), the better the ratings; the more the white space (fewer rectangles), the worse the ratings.

The food ratings allow you to make thousands of meaningful comparisons within and between foods, with respect to both the overall ratings and the seven individual rating factors. As examples, consider the following. By looking at page 102, note the rating benefits of *Cauliflower, cooked without added fat* (Overall=9) over *Cauliflower, batter-dipped and fried (Overall=4)*. Or, compare almost equivalent size portions of *Beef Stew, potatoes, vegetables and gravy* (page 35) with *Beef Stroganoff with noodles* (page 36). Which of these two entrees would you choose? Finally, if you had your heart set on a frozen lasagna meal, you could compare ratings for the Healthy Choice (page 255), Weight Watchers (page 255), and Le Menu (page 257) varieties.

Food Rankings. An index to all 900 foods described and rated in this book appears on pages 463 to 480. Within each food category (sequenced alphabetically from Bakery to Vegetable), the foods are listed in order of the <u>rank</u> of their overall rating from best to worst; the closer the food is to the top of the category list, the higher its rating and rank. Provided next to each food are the overall rating and the page number on which the food is rated. In the ranked index, the overall rating is listed to one decimal place (e.g., 7.7 for *tea*), whereas on the food rating page it is rounded off to the nearest whole number(e.g., 8 for *tea*). The food rankings in the index offer a handy reference to help you quickly choose the best (or avoid the worst) foods within each food category. For example, within Bakery (page 463), note that a *fig bar cookie* (4.4) or an *oatmeal raisin cookie* (3.6) rate higher overall than a *dietetic chocolate chip cookie* (3.1). Or, if you look in the Snack category (pages 476-477), observe that soft or hard pretzels (4.8 and 4.2, respectively) are better overall choices than any of the chips (3.4 and lower).

Abbreviation Key

approx	approximately	mg	milligrams
bbq	barbeque	mix	mixture
cal	calorie	mono	monounsaturated fat
choc	chocolate	oz	ounces
dia	diameter	poly	polyunsaturated fat
DV %	percent Daily Value	RE	Retinol Equivalents
fl	fluid	sub	submarine
g	grams	tbsp	tablespoon
IU	International Units	tsp	teaspoon
mcg	micrograms	veg	vegetable

Conversion Table

1 gram fat x 9 calories = fat calories	1 gram = .035 ounces
1 gram carbohydrate x 4 calories = carbohydrate calories	1 ounce = 28.35 grams
1 gram protein x 4 calories = protein calories	1 cup = 8 fluid ounces
1 Retinol Unit = 5 International Units	1 teaspoon = 5 grams
1 gram = 1,000 milligrams = 1,000,000 micrograms	1 tablespoon = 3 teaspoons
	16 tablespoons = 1 cup

ABALONE, COOKED

Serving: 1 piece (3.04 oz)　　　　　　　　　**Shellfish**

Calories	128	(41.9 cal/oz)	Carbohydrate	6.29 g	(2% DV)
Fat Calories	31	(24% fat)	Dietary Fiber	0 g	(0% DV)
Total Fat	3.4 g	(5% DV)	Protein	17 g	(34% DV)
Saturated Fat	.85 g	(4% DV)	Vitamin A	135.2 IU	(3% DV)
Poly Fat	.85 g		Vitamin C	3.4 mg	(6% DV)
Mono Fat	.85 g		Calcium	32.3 mg	(3% DV)
Cholesterol	84.2 mg	(28% DV)	Iron	3.2 mg	(18% DV)
Sodium	561 mg	(23% DV)	Folate	17 mcg	(1% DV)
Potassium	253.3 mg	(7% DV)	Beta Carotene	2.6 RE	

Ratings	Worst	Bad		Average	Good	Best
Weight Loss				6		
LowCal Density				6		
Filling		3				
Energizing			4			
Fiber	1					
Vitamins				5		
Minerals				6		
Overall				5		

ABALONE, FLOURED OR BREADED & FRIED

Serving: 1 piece (3.04 oz)　　　　　　　　　**Shellfish**

Calories	162	(53.1 cal/oz)	Carbohydrate	9.44 g	(3% DV)
Fat Calories	54	(33% fat)	Dietary Fiber	0 g	(0% DV)
Total Fat	5.95 g	(9% DV)	Protein	17 g	(34% DV)
Saturated Fat	1.7 g	(8% DV)	Vitamin A	4.3 IU	(0% DV)
Poly Fat	1.7 g		Vitamin C	1.7 mg	(3% DV)
Mono Fat	2.55 g		Calcium	30.6 mg	(3% DV)
Cholesterol	80.8 mg	(27% DV)	Iron	3.2 mg	(18% DV)
Sodium	503.2 mg	(21% DV)	Folate	17 mcg	(1% DV)
Potassium	241.4 mg	(7% DV)	Beta Carotene	0 RE	

Ratings	Worst	Bad		Average	Good	Best
Weight Loss				5		
LowCal Density				6		
Filling		3				
Energizing			4			
Fiber	1					
Vitamins				5		
Minerals				6		
Overall				5		

ALFALFA SPROUTS, RAW

Serving: 1 cup (1.18 oz)

Vegetable

Calories	10	(8.1 cal/oz)	Carbohydrate	1.25 g	(0% DV)
Fat Calories	3	(31% fat)	Dietary Fiber	.99 g	(4% DV)
Total Fat	.33 g	(1% DV)	Protein	1.32 g	(3% DV)
Saturated Fat	0 g	(0% DV)	VItamin A	51.2 IU	(1% DV)
Poly Fat	0 g		Vitamin C	2.6 mg	(4% DV)
Mono Fat	0 g		Calcium	10.6 mg	(1% DV)
Cholesterol	0 mg	(0% DV)	Iron	.3 mg	(2% DV)
Sodium	2 mg	(0% DV)	Folate	1.3 mcg	(3% DV)
Potassium	26.1 mg	(1% DV)	Beta Carotene	5.3 RE	

Ratings	Worst	Bad	Average	Good	Best
Weight Loss					9
LowCal Density					9
Filling			4		
Energizing		2			
Fiber			4		
Vitamins		3			
Minerals		3			
Overall				7	

ALL-BRAN

Serving: 1 cup (2.18 oz)

Cereal

Calories	152	(69.7 cal/oz)	Carbohydrate	45.38 g	(15% DV)
Fat Calories	11	(7% fat)	Dietary Fiber	21.35 g	(85% DV)
Total Fat	1.22 g	(2% DV)	Protein	8.54 g	(17% DV)
Saturated Fat	0 g	(0% DV)	VItamin A	1613.5 IU	(32% DV)
Poly Fat	.61 g		Vitamin C	32.3 mg	(54% DV)
Mono Fat	0 g		Calcium	49.4 mg	(5% DV)
Cholesterol	0 mg	(0% DV)	Iron	9.7 mg	(54% DV)
Sodium	688.1 mg	(29% DV)	Folate	8.5 mcg	(54% DV)
Potassium	752.7 mg	(22% DV)	Beta Carotene	0 RE	

Ratings	Worst	Bad	Average	Good	Best
Weight Loss				8	
LowCal Density		4			
Filling			6		
Energizing				9	
Fiber					10
Vitamins					10
Minerals					10
Overall				7	

ALMOND CHICKEN

Serving: 1 cup (8.64 oz)

Entree

Calories	273	(31.7 cal/oz)	Carbohydrate	18.39 g	(6% DV)
Fat Calories	131	(48% fat)	Dietary Fiber	4.84 g	(19% DV)
Total Fat	14.52 g	(22% DV)	Protein	19.36 g	(39% DV)
Saturated Fat	2.42 g	(12% DV)	Vitamin A	738.1 IU	(15% DV)
Poly Fat	4.84 g		Vitamin C	9.7 mg	(16% DV)
Mono Fat	4.84 g		Calcium	79.9 mg	(8% DV)
Cholesterol	33.9 mg	(11% DV)	Iron	2 mg	(11% DV)
Sodium	614.7 mg	(26% DV)	Folate	19.4 mcg	(8% DV)
Potassium	551.8 mg	(16% DV)	Beta Carotene	72.6 RE	

Ratings	Worst	Bad	Average	Good	Best
Weight Loss			5		
LowCal Density				7	
Filling			6		
Energizing			6		
Fiber					9
Vitamins				7	
Minerals				7	
Overall			6		

ALMONDS, ROASTED

Serving: 22 whole kernels (1 oz)

Snack

Calories	173	(173 cal/oz)	Carbohydrate	4.45 g	(1% DV)
Fat Calories	146	(84% fat)	Dietary Fiber	3.08 g	(12% DV)
Total Fat	16.24 g	(25% DV)	Protein	5.6 g	(11% DV)
Saturated Fat	1.4 g	(7% DV)	Vitamin A	0 IU	(0% DV)
Poly Fat	3.36 g		Vitamin C	.3 mg	(0% DV)
Mono Fat	10.36 g		Calcium	65.5 mg	(7% DV)
Cholesterol	0 mg	(0% DV)	Iron	1.1 mg	(6% DV)
Sodium	218.1 mg	(9% DV)	Folate	5.6 mcg	(4% DV)
Potassium	191.2 mg	(5% DV)	Beta Carotene	0 RE	

Ratings	Worst	Bad	Average	Good	Best
Weight Loss	2				
LowCal Density	1				
Filling	2				
Energizing		3			
Fiber					8
Vitamins			4		
Minerals			6		
Overall		3			

ALPHA-BITS

Serving: 1 cup (1.21 oz)   **Cereal**

Calories	133	(110.1 cal/oz)	Carbohydrate	29.44 g	(10% DV)
Fat Calories	6	(5% fat)	Dietary Fiber	1.02 g	(4% DV)
Total Fat	.68 g	(1% DV)	Protein	2.72 g	(5% DV)
Saturated Fat	0 g	(0% DV)	Vitamin A	1499.1 IU	(30% DV)
Poly Fat	.34 g		Vitamin C	0 mg	(0% DV)
Mono Fat	.34 g		Calcium	9.9 mg	(1% DV)
Cholesterol	0 mg	(0% DV)	Iron	3.2 mg	(18% DV)
Sodium	215.9 mg	(9% DV)	Folate	2.7 mcg	(30% DV)
Potassium	66 mg	(2% DV)	Beta Carotene	0 RE	

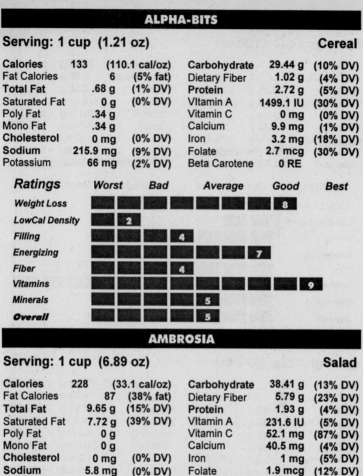

Ratings — Worst / Bad / Average / Good / Best

- Weight Loss: 8
- LowCal Density: 2
- Filling: 4
- Energizing: 7
- Fiber: 4
- Vitamins: 9
- Minerals: 5
- Overall: 5

AMBROSIA

Serving: 1 cup (6.89 oz)   **Salad**

Calories	228	(33.1 cal/oz)	Carbohydrate	38.41 g	(13% DV)
Fat Calories	87	(38% fat)	Dietary Fiber	5.79 g	(23% DV)
Total Fat	9.65 g	(15% DV)	Protein	1.93 g	(4% DV)
Saturated Fat	7.72 g	(39% DV)	Vitamin A	231.6 IU	(5% DV)
Poly Fat	0 g		Vitamin C	52.1 mg	(87% DV)
Mono Fat	0 g		Calcium	40.5 mg	(4% DV)
Cholesterol	0 mg	(0% DV)	Iron	1 mg	(5% DV)
Sodium	5.8 mg	(0% DV)	Folate	1.9 mcg	(12% DV)
Potassium	550.1 mg	(16% DV)	Beta Carotene	23.2 RE	

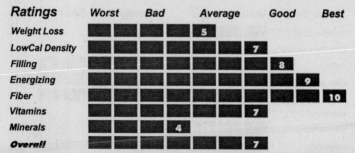

Ratings — Worst / Bad / Average / Good / Best

- Weight Loss: 5
- LowCal Density: 7
- Filling: 8
- Energizing: 9
- Fiber: 10
- Vitamins: 7
- Minerals: 4
- Overall: 7

APPLE CINNAMON CHEERIOS

Serving: 1 cup (1.36 oz)   **Cereal**

Calories	147	(108.4 cal/oz)	Carbohydrate	29.49 g	(10% DV)
Fat Calories	24	(16% fat)	Dietary Fiber	2.66 g	(11% DV)
Total Fat	2.66 g	(4% DV)	Protein	2.66 g	(5% DV)
Saturated Fat	.38 g	(2% DV)	VItamin A	1675.4 IU	(34% DV)
Poly Fat	1.14 g		Vitamin C	20.1 mg	(34% DV)
Mono Fat	1.14 g		Calcium	53.6 mg	(5% DV)
Cholesterol	0 mg	(0% DV)	Iron	6 mg	(34% DV)
Sodium	228 mg	(10% DV)	Folate	2.7 mcg	(34% DV)
Potassium	100.7 mg	(3% DV)	Beta Carotene	0 RE	

Ratings	Worst	Bad	Average	Good	Best
Weight Loss				7	
LowCal Density	2				
Filling		4			
Energizing				7	
Fiber				7	
Vitamins					10
Minerals			6		
Overall			5		

APPLE CRISP

Serving: 1 cup (8.79 oz)   **Dessert**

Calories	401	(45.6 cal/oz)	Carbohydrate	79.21 g	(26% DV)
Fat Calories	89	(22% fat)	Dietary Fiber	4.92 g	(20% DV)
Total Fat	9.84 g	(15% DV)	Protein	4.92 g	(10% DV)
Saturated Fat	2.46 g	(12% DV)	VItamin A	410.8 IU	(8% DV)
Poly Fat	2.46 g		Vitamin C	4.9 mg	(8% DV)
Mono Fat	2.46 g		Calcium	71.3 mg	(7% DV)
Cholesterol	0 mg	(0% DV)	Iron	1.8 mg	(10% DV)
Sodium	450.2 mg	(19% DV)	Folate	4.9 mcg	(3% DV)
Potassium	236.2 mg	(7% DV)	Beta Carotene	12.3 RE	

Ratings	Worst	Bad	Average	Good	Best
Weight Loss		4			
LowCal Density			6		
Filling				9	
Energizing					10
Fiber				9	
Vitamins			5		
Minerals			5		
Overall			6		

APPLE JACKS

Serving: 1 cup (1 oz)   **Cereal**

Calories	108	(108.4 cal/oz)	Carbohydrate	25.4 g	(8% DV)
Fat Calories	3	(2% fat)	Dietary Fiber	.56 g	(2% DV)
Total Fat	.28 g	(0% DV)	Protein	1.4 g	(3% DV)
Saturated Fat	0 g	(0% DV)	VItamin A	740.6 IU	(15% DV)
Poly Fat	0 g		Vitamin C	14.8 mg	(25% DV)
Mono Fat	0 g		Calcium	3.1 mg	(0% DV)
Cholesterol	0 mg	(0% DV)	Iron	4.5 mg	(25% DV)
Sodium	123.2 mg	(5% DV)	Folate	1.4 mcg	(25% DV)
Potassium	22.7 mg	(1% DV)	Beta Carotene	0 RE	

Ratings	Worst	Bad	Average	Good	Best
Weight Loss					9
LowCal Density	2				
Filling		4			
Energizing			6		
Fiber		3			
Vitamins					9
Minerals			6		
Overall			5		

APPLE JUICE

Serving: 1 cup (8.86 oz)   **Beverage**

Calories	117	(13.2 cal/oz)	Carbohydrate	29.02 g	(10% DV)
Fat Calories	0	(0% fat)	Dietary Fiber	0 g	(0% DV)
Total Fat	0 g	(0% DV)	Protein	0 g	(0% DV)
Saturated Fat	0 g	(0% DV)	VItamin A	2.5 IU	(0% DV)
Poly Fat	0 g		Vitamin C	2.5 mg	(4% DV)
Mono Fat	0 g		Calcium	17.4 mg	(2% DV)
Cholesterol	0 mg	(0% DV)	Iron	.9 mg	(5% DV)
Sodium	7.4 mg	(0% DV)	Folate	0 mcg	(0% DV)
Potassium	295.1 mg	(8% DV)	Beta Carotene	0 RE	

Ratings	Worst	Bad	Average	Good	Best
Weight Loss			7		
LowCal Density				9	
Filling					10
Energizing			7		
Fiber	1				
Vitamins		3			
Minerals		3			
Overall			7		

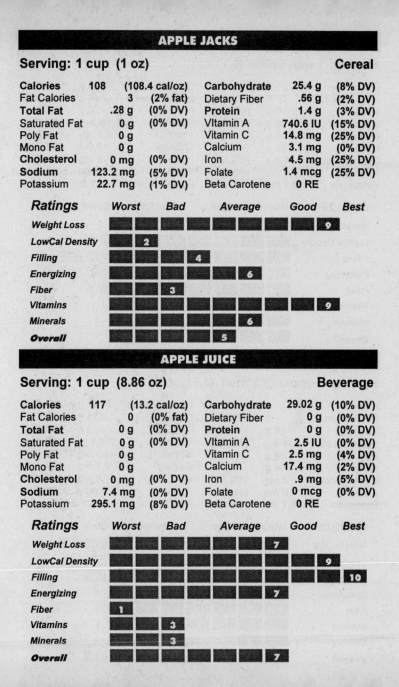

APPLE, BAKED WITH SUGAR

Serving: 1 with liquid (6.11 oz)   **Fruit**

Calories	164	(26.9 cal/oz)	Carbohydrate	42.24 g	(14% DV)
Fat Calories	0	(0% fat)	Dietary Fiber	3.42 g	(14% DV)
Total Fat	0 g	(0% DV)	Protein	0 g	(0% DV)
Saturated Fat	0 g	(0% DV)	Vitamin A	75.2 IU	(2% DV)
Poly Fat	0 g		Vitamin C	6.8 mg	(11% DV)
Mono Fat	0 g		Calcium	12 mg	(1% DV)
Cholesterol	0 mg	(0% DV)	Iron	.3 mg	(2% DV)
Sodium	0 mg	(0% DV)	Folate	0 mcg	(1% DV)
Potassium	172.7 mg	(5% DV)	Beta Carotene	6.8 RE	

Ratings	Worst	Bad	Average	Good	Best
Weight Loss				7	
LowCal Density				8	
Filling					9
Energizing					9
Fiber				8	
Vitamins		4			
Minerals	2				
Overall				7	

APPLE, RAW

Serving: 1 apple (2¾" dia) (4.93 oz)   **Fruit**

Calories	81	(16.5 cal/oz)	Carbohydrate	21.11 g	(7% DV)
Fat Calories	0	(0% fat)	Dietary Fiber	2.76 g	(11% DV)
Total Fat	0 g	(0% DV)	Protein	0 g	(0% DV)
Saturated Fat	0 g	(0% DV)	Vitamin A	73.1 IU	(1% DV)
Poly Fat	0 g		Vitamin C	8.3 mg	(14% DV)
Mono Fat	0 g		Calcium	9.7 mg	(1% DV)
Cholesterol	0 mg	(0% DV)	Iron	.3 mg	(1% DV)
Sodium	0 mg	(0% DV)	Folate	0 mcg	(1% DV)
Potassium	158.7 mg	(5% DV)	Beta Carotene	6.9 RE	

Ratings	Worst	Bad	Average	Good	Best
Weight Loss				9	
LowCal Density				9	
Filling				8	
Energizing			6		
Fiber				7	
Vitamins		4			
Minerals	2				
Overall				8	

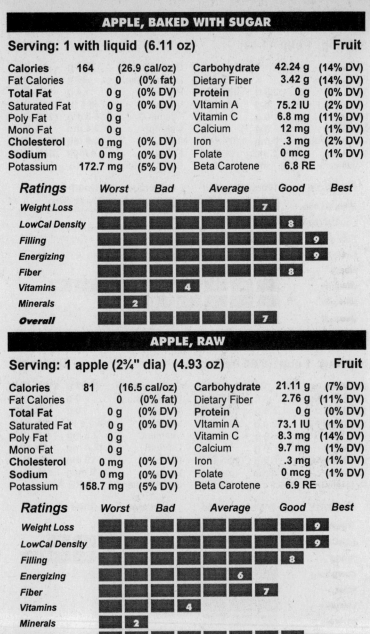

APPLESAUCE, STEWED APPLES WITH SUGAR

Serving: 1 cup (9.11 oz)   Fruit

Calories	194	(21.3 cal/oz)	Carbohydrate	50.75 g	(17% DV)
Fat Calories	0	(0% fat)	Dietary Fiber	2.55 g	(10% DV)
Total Fat	0 g	(0% DV)	Protein	0 g	(0% DV)
Saturated Fat	0 g	(0% DV)	Vitamin A	28.1 IU	(1% DV)
Poly Fat	0 g		Vitamin C	5.1 mg	(8% DV)
Mono Fat	0 g		Calcium	10.2 mg	(1% DV)
Cholesterol	0 mg	(0% DV)	Iron	.9 mg	(5% DV)
Sodium	7.7 mg	(0% DV)	Folate	0 mcg	(1% DV)
Potassium	155.6 mg	(4% DV)	Beta Carotene	2.6 RE	

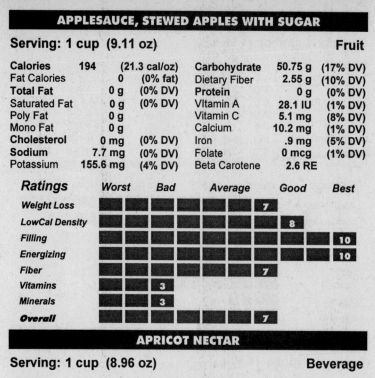

Ratings	Worst	Bad	Average	Good	Best
Weight Loss				7	
LowCal Density				8	
Filling					10
Energizing					10
Fiber				7	
Vitamins		3			
Minerals		3			
Overall				7	

APRICOT NECTAR

Serving: 1 cup (8.96 oz)   Beverage

Calories	141	(15.7 cal/oz)	Carbohydrate	36.14 g	(12% DV)
Fat Calories	0	(0% fat)	Dietary Fiber	2.51 g	(10% DV)
Total Fat	0 g	(0% DV)	Protein	0 g	(0% DV)
Saturated Fat	0 g	(0% DV)	Vitamin A	3303.2 IU	(66% DV)
Poly Fat	0 g		Vitamin C	2.5 mg	(4% DV)
Mono Fat	0 g		Calcium	17.6 mg	(2% DV)
Cholesterol	0 mg	(0% DV)	Iron	1 mg	(5% DV)
Sodium	7.5 mg	(0% DV)	Folate	0 mcg	(1% DV)
Potassium	286.1 mg	(8% DV)	Beta Carotene	331.3 RE	

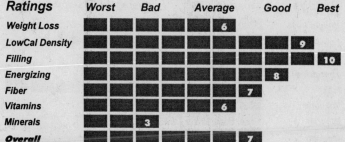

Ratings	Worst	Bad	Average	Good	Best
Weight Loss			6		
LowCal Density				9	
Filling					10
Energizing				8	
Fiber			7		
Vitamins			6		
Minerals		3			
Overall				7	

APRICOT, RAW

Serving: 1 apricot (1.25 oz)   **Fruit**

Calories	17	(13.4 cal/oz)	Carbohydrate	3.89 g	(1% DV)
Fat Calories	0	(0% fat)	Dietary Fiber	.7 g	(3% DV)
Total Fat	0 g	(0% DV)	Protein	.35 g	(1% DV)
Saturated Fat	0 g	(0% DV)	Vitamin A	914.2 IU	(18% DV)
Poly Fat	0 g		Vitamin C	3.5 mg	(6% DV)
Mono Fat	0 g		Calcium	4.9 mg	(0% DV)
Cholesterol	0 mg	(0% DV)	Iron	.2 mg	(1% DV)
Sodium	.4 mg	(0% DV)	Folate	.4 mcg	(1% DV)
Potassium	103.6 mg	(3% DV)	Beta Carotene	91.4 RE	

Ratings	Worst	Bad	Average	Good	Best
Weight Loss					10
LowCal Density					9
Filling		4			
Energizing		3			
Fiber		3			
Vitamins		4			
Minerals	2				
Overall				7	

ARTICHOKE, GLOBE, COOKED WITH FAT

Serving: 1 globe (4.46 oz)   **Vegetable**

Calories	126	(28.3 cal/oz)	Carbohydrate	12.88 g	(4% DV)
Fat Calories	68	(53% fat)	Dietary Fiber	6.25 g	(25% DV)
Total Fat	7.5 g	(12% DV)	Protein	3.75 g	(8% DV)
Saturated Fat	1.25 g	(6% DV)	Vitamin A	607.5 IU	(12% DV)
Poly Fat	2.5 g		Vitamin C	11.3 mg	(19% DV)
Mono Fat	3.75 g		Calcium	55 mg	(6% DV)
Cholesterol	0 mg	(0% DV)	Iron	1.5 mg	(8% DV)
Sodium	461.3 mg	(19% DV)	Folate	3.8 mcg	(15% DV)
Potassium	410 mg	(12% DV)	Beta Carotene	28.8 RE	

Ratings	Worst	Bad	Average	Good	Best
Weight Loss	3				
LowCal Density				8	
Filling			6		
Energizing			5		
Fiber					10
Vitamins			5		
Minerals			5		
Overall			6		

18   **Edmund's Food Ratings**

ASPARAGUS SOUP, CREAM OF, PREPARED WITH MILK

Serving: 1 cup (8.86 oz)   **Soup**

Calories	161	(18.2 cal/oz)	Carbohydrate	16.37 g	(5% DV)
Fat Calories	67	(42% fat)	Dietary Fiber	0 g	(0% DV)
Total Fat	7.44 g	(11% DV)	Protein	7.44 g	(15% DV)
Saturated Fat	2.48 g	(12% DV)	Vitamin A	600.2 IU	(12% DV)
Poly Fat	2.48 g		Vitamin C	5 mg	(8% DV)
Mono Fat	2.48 g		Calcium	173.6 mg	(17% DV)
Cholesterol	22.3 mg	(7% DV)	Iron	.9 mg	(5% DV)
Sodium	1041.6 mg	(43% DV)	Folate	7.4 mcg	(7% DV)
Potassium	359.6 mg	(10% DV)	Beta Carotene	44.6 RE	

Ratings	Worst	Bad	Average	Good	Best
Weight Loss			4		
LowCal Density				8	
Filling			6		
Energizing			5		
Fiber	1				
Vitamins			5		
Minerals			6		
Overall			6		

ASPARAGUS, COOKED WITHOUT ADDED FAT

Serving: 1 cup (6.43 oz)   **Vegetable**

Calories	43	(6.7 cal/oz)	Carbohydrate	7.56 g	(3% DV)
Fat Calories	0	(0% fat)	Dietary Fiber	3.6 g	(14% DV)
Total Fat	0 g	(0% DV)	Protein	5.4 g	(11% DV)
Saturated Fat	0 g	(0% DV)	Vitamin A	964.8 IU	(19% DV)
Poly Fat	0 g		Vitamin C	19.8 mg	(33% DV)
Mono Fat	0 g		Calcium	36 mg	(4% DV)
Cholesterol	0 mg	(0% DV)	Iron	1.3 mg	(7% DV)
Sodium	435.6 mg	(18% DV)	Folate	5.4 mcg	(65% DV)
Potassium	286.2 mg	(8% DV)	Beta Carotene	149.4 RE	

Ratings	Worst	Bad	Average	Good	Best
Weight Loss				9	
LowCal Density					10
Filling				9	
Energizing			4		
Fiber				8	
Vitamins				8	
Minerals			5		
Overall				9	

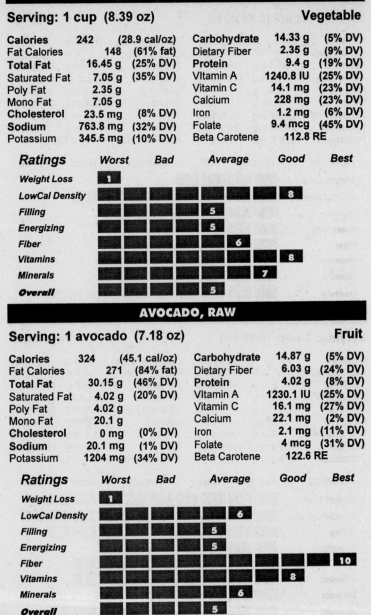

ASPARAGUS, CREAMED OR WITH CHEESE SAUCE

Serving: 1 cup (8.39 oz)   **Vegetable**

Calories	242	(28.9 cal/oz)	Carbohydrate	14.33 g	(5% DV)
Fat Calories	148	(61% fat)	Dietary Fiber	2.35 g	(9% DV)
Total Fat	16.45 g	(25% DV)	Protein	9.4 g	(19% DV)
Saturated Fat	7.05 g	(35% DV)	Vitamin A	1240.8 IU	(25% DV)
Poly Fat	2.35 g		Vitamin C	14.1 mg	(23% DV)
Mono Fat	7.05 g		Calcium	228 mg	(23% DV)
Cholesterol	23.5 mg	(8% DV)	Iron	1.2 mg	(6% DV)
Sodium	763.8 mg	(32% DV)	Folate	9.4 mcg	(45% DV)
Potassium	345.5 mg	(10% DV)	Beta Carotene	112.8 RE	

Ratings	Worst	Bad	Average	Good	Best
Weight Loss	1				
LowCal Density					8
Filling			5		
Energizing			5		
Fiber			6		
Vitamins					8
Minerals				7	
Overall			5		

AVOCADO, RAW

Serving: 1 avocado (7.18 oz)   **Fruit**

Calories	324	(45.1 cal/oz)	Carbohydrate	14.87 g	(5% DV)
Fat Calories	271	(84% fat)	Dietary Fiber	6.03 g	(24% DV)
Total Fat	30.15 g	(46% DV)	Protein	4.02 g	(8% DV)
Saturated Fat	4.02 g	(20% DV)	Vitamin A	1230.1 IU	(25% DV)
Poly Fat	4.02 g		Vitamin C	16.1 mg	(27% DV)
Mono Fat	20.1 g		Calcium	22.1 mg	(2% DV)
Cholesterol	0 mg	(0% DV)	Iron	2.1 mg	(11% DV)
Sodium	20.1 mg	(1% DV)	Folate	4 mcg	(31% DV)
Potassium	1204 mg	(34% DV)	Beta Carotene	122.6 RE	

Ratings	Worst	Bad	Average	Good	Best
Weight Loss	1				
LowCal Density				6	
Filling			5		
Energizing			5		
Fiber					10
Vitamins					8
Minerals				6	
Overall			5		

BACON, LETTUCE, & TOMATO SANDWICH WITH SPREAD

Serving: 1 sandwich (5.86 oz)   Sandwich

Calories	338	(57.7 cal/oz)	Carbohydrate	30.18 g	(10% DV)
Fat Calories	177	(52% fat)	Dietary Fiber	1.64 g	(7% DV)
Total Fat	19.68 g	(30% DV)	Protein	11.48 g	(23% DV)
Saturated Fat	4.92 g	(25% DV)	Vitamin A	534.6 IU	(11% DV)
Poly Fat	6.56 g		Vitamin C	21.3 mg	(36% DV)
Mono Fat	8.2 g		Calcium	70.5 mg	(7% DV)
Cholesterol	23 mg	(8% DV)	Iron	2.3 mg	(13% DV)
Sodium	808.5 mg	(34% DV)	Folate	11.5 mcg	(9% DV)
Potassium	341.1 mg	(10% DV)	Beta Carotene	50.8 RE	

Ratings	Worst	Bad	Average	Good	Best
Weight Loss			4		
LowCal Density			5		
Filling			5		
Energizing				7	
Fiber			5		
Vitamins				7	
Minerals			6		
Overall			5		

BACON, MEATLESS, VEGETARIAN

Serving: 1 strip (.18 oz)   Meat

Calories	16	(86.1 cal/oz)	Carbohydrate	.32 g	(0% DV)
Fat Calories	14	(87% fat)	Dietary Fiber	.2 g	(1% DV)
Total Fat	1.5 g	(2% DV)	Protein	.55 g	(1% DV)
Saturated Fat	.25 g	(1% DV)	Vitamin A	4.4 IU	(0% DV)
Poly Fat	.75 g		Vitamin C	0 mg	(0% DV)
Mono Fat	.35 g		Calcium	1.2 mg	(0% DV)
Cholesterol	0 mg	(0% DV)	Iron	.1 mg	(1% DV)
Sodium	73.3 mg	(3% DV)	Folate	.6 mcg	(1% DV)
Potassium	8.5 mg	(0% DV)	Beta Carotene	.5 RE	

Ratings	Worst	Bad	Average	Good	Best
Weight Loss			5		
LowCal Density		3			
Filling	1				
Energizing		2			
Fiber		2			
Vitamins			3		
Minerals		2			
Overall			3		

BAGEL, MULTIGRAIN, WITH RAISINS

Serving: 1 bagel (3" dia) (1.96 oz)   **Bread**

Calories	145	(74.1 cal/oz)	Carbohydrate	30.53 g	(10% DV)
Fat Calories	5	(3% fat)	Dietary Fiber	3.85 g	(15% DV)
Total Fat	.55 g	(1% DV)	Protein	6.05 g	(12% DV)
Saturated Fat	0 g	(0% DV)	Vitamin A	1.7 IU	(0% DV)
Poly Fat	0 g		Vitamin C	0 mg	(0% DV)
Mono Fat	0 g		Calcium	20.4 mg	(2% DV)
Cholesterol	0 mg	(0% DV)	Iron	1.7 mg	(9% DV)
Sodium	218.4 mg	(9% DV)	Folate	6.1 mcg	(9% DV)
Potassium	228.8 mg	(7% DV)	Beta Carotene	0 RE	

Ratings	Worst	Bad	Average	Good	Best
Weight Loss			5		
LowCal Density		4			
Filling			5		
Energizing				7	
Fiber					9
Vitamins		4			
Minerals			5		
Overall			5		

BAGEL, PUMPERNICKEL

Serving: 1 bagel (3" dia) (1.96 oz)   **Bread**

Calories	153	(78.3 cal/oz)	Carbohydrate	31.46 g	(10% DV)
Fat Calories	5	(3% fat)	Dietary Fiber	2.75 g	(11% DV)
Total Fat	.55 g	(1% DV)	Protein	4.95 g	(10% DV)
Saturated Fat	0 g	(0% DV)	Vitamin A	.6 IU	(0% DV)
Poly Fat	.55 g		Vitamin C	0 mg	(0% DV)
Mono Fat	0 g		Calcium	9.9 mg	(1% DV)
Cholesterol	0 mg	(0% DV)	Iron	1.7 mg	(9% DV)
Sodium	272.3 mg	(11% DV)	Folate	5 mcg	(9% DV)
Potassium	83.6 mg	(2% DV)	Beta Carotene	0 RE	

Ratings	Worst	Bad	Average	Good	Best
Weight Loss			5		
LowCal Density		4			
Filling			5		
Energizing				8	
Fiber				7	
Vitamins			5		
Minerals		4			
Overall			5		

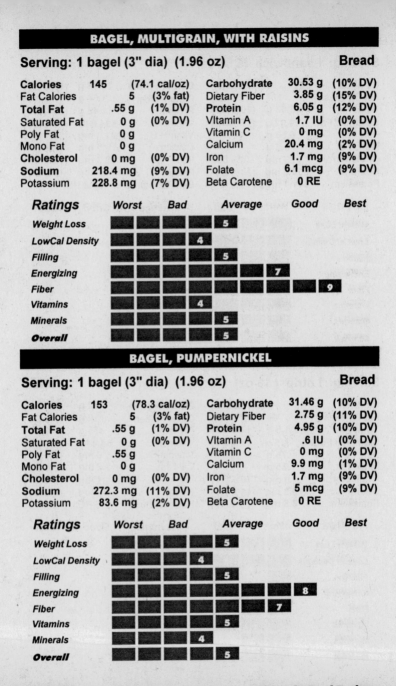

BAGEL, WHEAT

Serving: 1 bagel (3" dia) (1.96 oz)   **Bread**

Calories	153	(78.3 cal/oz)	Carbohydrate	31.41 g	(10% DV)
Fat Calories	5	(3% fat)	Dietary Fiber	2.75 g	(11% DV)
Total Fat	.55 g	(1% DV)	Protein	5.5 g	(11% DV)
Saturated Fat	0 g	(0% DV)	VItamin A	0 IU	(0% DV)
Poly Fat	.55 g		Vitamin C	0 mg	(0% DV)
Mono Fat	0 g		Calcium	10.5 mg	(1% DV)
Cholesterol	0 mg	(0% DV)	Iron	1.9 mg	(11% DV)
Sodium	265.7 mg	(11% DV)	Folate	5.5 mcg	(9% DV)
Potassium	105.1 mg	(3% DV)	Beta Carotene	0 RE	

Ratings	Worst	Bad	Average	Good	Best
Weight Loss			5		
LowCal Density		4			
Filling			5		
Energizing				8	
Fiber				7	
Vitamins			5		
Minerals			5		
Overall			5		

BAGEL, WHOLE WHEAT, 100%

Serving: 1 bagel (3" dia) (1.96 oz)   **Bread**

Calories	145	(74.1 cal/oz)	Carbohydrate	31.08 g	(10% DV)
Fat Calories	5	(3% fat)	Dietary Fiber	5.5 g	(22% DV)
Total Fat	.55 g	(1% DV)	Protein	6.05 g	(12% DV)
Saturated Fat	0 g	(0% DV)	VItamin A	0 IU	(0% DV)
Poly Fat	.55 g		Vitamin C	0 mg	(0% DV)
Mono Fat	0 g		Calcium	16 mg	(2% DV)
Cholesterol	0 mg	(0% DV)	Iron	1.8 mg	(10% DV)
Sodium	270.6 mg	(11% DV)	Folate	6.1 mcg	(10% DV)
Potassium	189.8 mg	(5% DV)	Beta Carotene	0 RE	

Ratings	Worst	Bad	Average	Good	Best
Weight Loss			5		
LowCal Density		4			
Filling			5		
Energizing				8	
Fiber					9
Vitamins		4			
Minerals			6		
Overall			5		

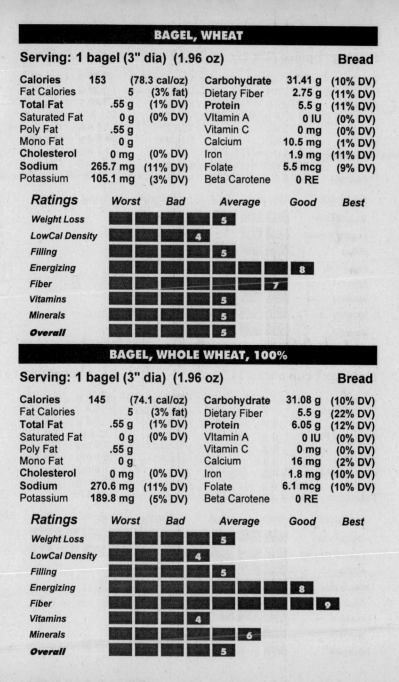

BAKLAVA

Serving: 1 piece (2"x 2"x 1½") (2.79 oz) Dessert

Calories	333	(119.4 cal/oz)	Carbohydrate	29.09 g	(10% DV)
Fat Calories	204	(61% fat)	Dietary Fiber	1.56 g	(6% DV)
Total Fat	22.62 g	(35% DV)	Protein	5.46 g	(11% DV)
Saturated Fat	9.36 g	(47% DV)	VItamin A	511.7 IU	(10% DV)
Poly Fat	3.9 g		Vitamin C	1.6 mg	(3% DV)
Mono Fat	8.58 g		Calcium	33.5 mg	(3% DV)
Cholesterol	35.1 mg	(12% DV)	Iron	1.7 mg	(9% DV)
Sodium	290.9 mg	(12% DV)	Folate	5.5 mcg	(2% DV)
Potassium	139.6 mg	(4% DV)	Beta Carotene	14.8 RE	

Ratings	Worst	Bad	Average	Good	Best
Weight Loss		3			
LowCal Density	2				
Filling		4			
Energizing				7	
Fiber			5		
Vitamins			5		
Minerals			5		
Overall		4			

BAMBOO SHOOTS, COOKED WITHOUT ADDED FAT

Serving: 1 cup slices (4.29 oz) Vegetable

Calories	34	(7.8 cal/oz)	Carbohydrate	6.36 g	(2% DV)
Fat Calories	0	(0% fat)	Dietary Fiber	1.2 g	(5% DV)
Total Fat	0 g	(0% DV)	Protein	3.6 g	(7% DV)
Saturated Fat	0 g	(0% DV)	VItamin A	21.6 IU	(0% DV)
Poly Fat	0 g		Vitamin C	3.6 mg	(6% DV)
Mono Fat	0 g		Calcium	15.6 mg	(2% DV)
Cholesterol	0 mg	(0% DV)	Iron	.6 mg	(3% DV)
Sodium	290.4 mg	(12% DV)	Folate	3.6 mcg	(2% DV)
Potassium	590.4 mg	(17% DV)	Beta Carotene	2.4 RE	

Ratings	Worst	Bad	Average	Good	Best
Weight Loss					10
LowCal Density					10
Filling			6		
Energizing		4			
Fiber			5		
Vitamins		4			
Minerals		4			
Overall				8	

BANANA, RAW

Serving: 1 banana (8¾" long) (4.07 oz)   **Fruit**

Calories	105	(25.8 cal/oz)	Carbohydrate	26.68 g	(9% DV)
Fat Calories		0	(0% fat)	Dietary Fiber	2.28 g	(9% DV)
Total Fat	0 g	(0% DV)	Protein	1.14 g	(2% DV)
Saturated Fat	0 g	(0% DV)	VItamin A	92.3 IU	(2% DV)
Poly Fat	0 g		Vitamin C	10.3 mg	(17% DV)
Mono Fat	0 g		Calcium	6.8 mg	(1% DV)
Cholesterol	0 mg	(0% DV)	Iron	.4 mg	(2% DV)
Sodium	1.1 mg	(0% DV)	Folate	1.1 mcg	(5% DV)
Potassium	451.4 mg	(13% DV)	Beta Carotene	9.1 RE	

Ratings

	Worst	Bad	Average	Good	Best
Weight Loss					9
LowCal Density				8	
Filling				7	
Energizing				7	
Fiber			6		
Vitamins			6		
Minerals	3				
Overall				7	

BASIC 4

Serving: 1 cup (1.75 oz)   **Cereal**

Calories	173	(98.8 cal/oz)	Carbohydrate	37.24 g	(12% DV)
Fat Calories	22	(13% fat)	Dietary Fiber	2.45 g	(10% DV)
Total Fat	2.45 g	(4% DV)	Protein	3.92 g	(8% DV)
Saturated Fat	.49 g	(2% DV)	VItamin A	1661.6 IU	(33% DV)
Poly Fat	.98 g		Vitamin C	20.1 mg	(33% DV)
Mono Fat	.98 g		Calcium	266.1 mg	(27% DV)
Cholesterol	0 mg	(0% DV)	Iron	6 mg	(33% DV)
Sodium	305.8 mg	(13% DV)	Folate	3.9 mcg	(33% DV)
Potassium	146 mg	(4% DV)	Beta Carotene	0 RE	

Ratings

	Worst	Bad	Average	Good	Best
Weight Loss				7	
LowCal Density		3			
Filling			5		
Energizing				8	
Fiber				7	
Vitamins					10
Minerals				8	
Overall			6		

BEAN CURD (TOFU)

Serving: 1 piece (2½"x 2¾"x 1") (4.29 oz)   **Vegetable**

Calories	91	(21.3 cal/oz)	Carbohydrate	2.28 g	(1% DV)
Fat Calories	54	(59% fat)	Dietary Fiber	1.2 g	(5% DV)
Total Fat	6 g	(9% DV)	Protein	9.6 g	(19% DV)
Saturated Fat	1.2 g	(6% DV)	VItamin A	102 IU	(2% DV)
Poly Fat	3.6 g		Vitamin C	0 mg	(0% DV)
Mono Fat	1.2 g		Calcium	126 mg	(13% DV)
Cholesterol	0 mg	(0% DV)	Iron	6.4 mg	(36% DV)
Sodium	8.4 mg	(0% DV)	Folate	9.6 mcg	(4% DV)
Potassium	145.2 mg	(4% DV)	Beta Carotene	10.8 RE	

Ratings	Worst	Bad	Average	Good	Best
Weight Loss		4			
LowCal Density				8	
Filling	3				
Energizing	3				
Fiber			5		
Vitamins	3				
Minerals				8	
Overall			5		

BEAN DIP, MADE WITH REFRIED BEANS

Serving: 1 cup (9.36 oz)   **Snack**

Calories	364	(38.9 cal/oz)	Carbohydrate	47.16 g	(16% DV)
Fat Calories	118	(32% fat)	Dietary Fiber	18.34 g	(73% DV)
Total Fat	13.1 g	(20% DV)	Protein	15.72 g	(31% DV)
Saturated Fat	2.62 g	(13% DV)	VItamin A	1412.2 IU	(28% DV)
Poly Fat	7.86 g		Vitamin C	36.7 mg	(61% DV)
Mono Fat	2.62 g		Calcium	86.5 mg	(9% DV)
Cholesterol	0 mg	(0% DV)	Iron	3.8 mg	(21% DV)
Sodium	3057.5 mg	(127% DV)	Folate	15.7 mcg	(46% DV)
Potassium	770.3 mg	(22% DV)	Beta Carotene	141.5 RE	

Ratings	Worst	Bad	Average	Good	Best
Weight Loss	2				
LowCal Density				7	
Filling					9
Energizing					9
Fiber					10
Vitamins					9
Minerals				8	
Overall			6		

BEAN SALAD, YELLOW AND/OR GREEN STRING BEANS

Serving: 1 cup (5.36 oz)

Salad

Calories	140	(26 cal/oz)	Carbohydrate	13.5 g	(4% DV)
Fat Calories	81	(58% fat)	Dietary Fiber	3 g	(12% DV)
Total Fat	9 g	(14% DV)	Protein	4.5 g	(9% DV)
Saturated Fat	1.5 g	(8% DV)	VItamin A	198 IU	(4% DV)
Poly Fat	4.5 g		Vitamin C	4.5 mg	(8% DV)
Mono Fat	1.5 g		Calcium	36 mg	(4% DV)
Cholesterol	0 mg	(0% DV)	Iron	1.4 mg	(8% DV)
Sodium	514.5 mg	(21% DV)	Folate	4.5 mcg	(13% DV)
Potassium	225 mg	(6% DV)	Beta Carotene	18 RE	

Ratings	Worst	Bad	Average	Good	Best
Weight Loss			5		
LowCal Density				8	
Filling			5		
Energizing			5		
Fiber				8	
Vitamins		4			
Minerals		4			
Overall			6		

BEAN SPROUTS, RAW (SOYBEAN OR MUNG)

Serving: 1 cup (3.71 oz)

Vegetable

Calories	31	(8.4 cal/oz)	Carbohydrate	6.14 g	(2% DV)
Fat Calories	0	(0% fat)	Dietary Fiber	1.04 g	(4% DV)
Total Fat	0 g	(0% DV)	Protein	3.12 g	(6% DV)
Saturated Fat	0 g	(0% DV)	VItamin A	21.8 IU	(0% DV)
Poly Fat	0 g		Vitamin C	13.5 mg	(23% DV)
Mono Fat	0 g		Calcium	13.5 mg	(1% DV)
Cholesterol	0 mg	(0% DV)	Iron	1 mg	(5% DV)
Sodium	6.2 mg	(0% DV)	Folate	3.1 mcg	(16% DV)
Potassium	155 mg	(4% DV)	Beta Carotene	2.1 RE	

Ratings	Worst	Bad	Average	Good	Best
Weight Loss					10
LowCal Density				9	
Filling			6		
Energizing		4			
Fiber		4			
Vitamins			5		
Minerals		4			
Overall				8	

BEAN WITH BACON OR PORK SOUP

Serving: 1 cup (9.04 oz)   **Soup**

Calories	172	(19 cal/oz)	Carbohydrate	22.77 g	(8% DV)
Fat Calories	46	(26% fat)	Dietary Fiber	7.59 g	(30% DV)
Total Fat	5.06 g	(8% DV)	Protein	7.59 g	(15% DV)
Saturated Fat	2.53 g	(13% DV)	Vitamin A	888 IU	(18% DV)
Poly Fat	2.53 g		Vitamin C	2.5 mg	(4% DV)
Mono Fat	2.53 g		Calcium	81 mg	(8% DV)
Cholesterol	2.5 mg	(1% DV)	Iron	2.1 mg	(11% DV)
Sodium	951.3 mg	(40% DV)	Folate	7.6 mcg	(8% DV)
Potassium	402.3 mg	(11% DV)	Beta Carotene	88.6 RE	

Ratings	Worst	Bad	Average	Good	Best
Weight Loss			5		
LowCal Density				8	
Filling				9	
Energizing			6		
Fiber					10
Vitamins			5		
Minerals			6		
Overall				7	

BEANS & FRANKS, FROZEN MEAL

Serving: 1 meal (12.14 oz)   **Entree**

Calories	527	(43.4 cal/oz)	Carbohydrate	73.44 g	(24% DV)
Fat Calories	184	(35% fat)	Dietary Fiber	6.8 g	(27% DV)
Total Fat	20.4 g	(31% DV)	Protein	17 g	(34% DV)
Saturated Fat	6.8 g	(34% DV)	Vitamin A	333.2 IU	(7% DV)
Poly Fat	3.4 g		Vitamin C	17 mg	(28% DV)
Mono Fat	6.8 g		Calcium	78.2 mg	(8% DV)
Cholesterol	61.2 mg	(20% DV)	Iron	3.4 mg	(19% DV)
Sodium	1207 mg	(50% DV)	Folate	17 mcg	(21% DV)
Potassium	782 mg	(22% DV)	Beta Carotene	27.2 RE	

Ratings	Worst	Bad	Average	Good	Best
Weight Loss	3				
LowCal Density			6		
Filling				9	
Energizing					10
Fiber					10
Vitamins			7		
Minerals				8	
Overall			6		

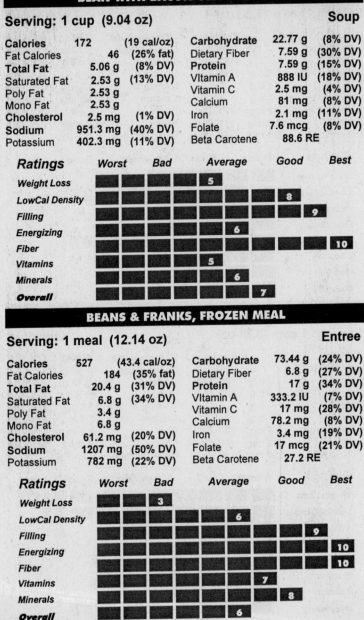

Edmund's Food Ratings

BEEF BURGUNDY

Serving: 1 cup (8.71 oz)   **Entree**

Calories	285	(32.8 cal/oz)	Carbohydrate	9.76 g	(3% DV)
Fat Calories	110	(38% fat)	Dietary Fiber	2.44 g	(10% DV)
Total Fat	12.2 g	(19% DV)	Protein	34.16 g	(68% DV)
Saturated Fat	2.44 g	(12% DV)	Vitamin A	58.6 IU	(1% DV)
Poly Fat	2.44 g		Vitamin C	4.9 mg	(8% DV)
Mono Fat	4.88 g		Calcium	31.7 mg	(3% DV)
Cholesterol	90.3 mg	(30% DV)	Iron	4.9 mg	(27% DV)
Sodium	109.8 mg	(5% DV)	Folate	34.2 mcg	(6% DV)
Potassium	834.5 mg	(24% DV)	Beta Carotene	4.9 RE	

Ratings	Worst	Bad	Average	Good	Best
Weight Loss			5		
LowCal Density				7	
Filling		4			
Energizing		4			
Fiber				7	
Vitamins			5		
Minerals					9
Overall			6		

BEEF CHOW MEIN OR CHOP SUEY WITH NOODLES

Serving: 1 cup (7.86 oz)   **Entree**

Calories	425	(54 cal/oz)	Carbohydrate	31.24 g	(10% DV)
Fat Calories	218	(51% fat)	Dietary Fiber	4.4 g	(18% DV)
Total Fat	24.2 g	(37% DV)	Protein	22 g	(44% DV)
Saturated Fat	4.4 g	(22% DV)	Vitamin A	631.4 IU	(13% DV)
Poly Fat	8.8 g		Vitamin C	19.8 mg	(33% DV)
Mono Fat	8.8 g		Calcium	39.6 mg	(4% DV)
Cholesterol	46.2 mg	(15% DV)	Iron	4.2 mg	(23% DV)
Sodium	818.4 mg	(34% DV)	Folate	22 mcg	(11% DV)
Potassium	514.8 mg	(15% DV)	Beta Carotene	28.6 RE	

Ratings	Worst	Bad	Average	Good	Best
Weight Loss	3				
LowCal Density			6		
Filling			6		
Energizing				8	
Fiber					9
Vitamins			7		
Minerals				8	
Overall			6		

Serving: 1 cup (8.43 oz)   **Entree**

Calories	437	(51.8 cal/oz)	Carbohydrate	12.98 g	(4% DV)
Fat Calories	276	(63% fat)	Dietary Fiber	2.36 g	(9% DV)
Total Fat	30.68 g	(47% DV)	Protein	25.96 g	(52% DV)
Saturated Fat	7.08 g	(35% DV)	VItamin A	2487.4 IU	(50% DV)
Poly Fat	9.44 g		Vitamin C	23.6 mg	(39% DV)
Mono Fat	14.16 g		Calcium	44.8 mg	(4% DV)
Cholesterol	68.4 mg	(23% DV)	Iron	4.5 mg	(25% DV)
Sodium	1324 mg	(55% DV)	Folate	26 mcg	(5% DV)
Potassium	972.3 mg	(28% DV)	Beta Carotene	146.3 RE	

Ratings	Worst	Bad	Average	Good	Best
Weight Loss	2				
LowCal Density				6	
Filling			4		
Energizing			5		
Fiber				6	
Vitamins					9
Minerals					9
Overall			5		

Serving: 1 frozen meal (15.18 oz)   **Entree**

Calories	633	(41.7 cal/oz)	Carbohydrate	67.57 g	(23% DV)
Fat Calories	268	(42% fat)	Dietary Fiber	8.5 g	(34% DV)
Total Fat	29.75 g	(46% DV)	Protein	21.25 g	(42% DV)
Saturated Fat	8.5 g	(42% DV)	VItamin A	382.5 IU	(8% DV)
Poly Fat	8.5 g		Vitamin C	4.3 mg	(7% DV)
Mono Fat	12.75 g		Calcium	182.8 mg	(18% DV)
Cholesterol	38.3 mg	(13% DV)	Iron	5.5 mg	(31% DV)
Sodium	1691.5 mg	(70% DV)	Folate	21.3 mcg	(32% DV)
Potassium	569.5 mg	(16% DV)	Beta Carotene	21.3 RE	

Ratings	Worst	Bad	Average	Good	Best
Weight Loss	2				
LowCal Density				6	
Filling				9	
Energizing					10
Fiber					10
Vitamins			7		
Minerals				9	
Overall			6		

BEEF GOULASH WITH NOODLES

Serving: 1 cup (8.89 oz)   **Entree**

Calories	341	(38.4 cal/oz)	Carbohydrate	23.41 g	(8% DV)
Fat Calories	134	(39% fat)	Dietary Fiber	2.49 g	(10% DV)
Total Fat	14.94 g	(23% DV)	Protein	29.88 g	(60% DV)
Saturated Fat	2.49 g	(12% DV)	Vitamin A	440.7 IU	(9% DV)
Poly Fat	4.98 g		Vitamin C	7.5 mg	(12% DV)
Mono Fat	4.98 g		Calcium	24.9 mg	(2% DV)
Cholesterol	89.6 mg	(30% DV)	Iron	4.1 mg	(22% DV)
Sodium	455.7 mg	(19% DV)	Folate	29.9 mcg	(6% DV)
Potassium	587.6 mg	(17% DV)	Beta Carotene	42.3 RE	

Ratings	Worst	Bad	Average	Good	Best
Weight Loss			5		
LowCal Density				7	
Filling			6		
Energizing			6		
Fiber				7	
Vitamins			6		
Minerals				8	
Overall			6		

BEEF LIVER, FRIED OR BROILED, NO COATING

Serving: 1 slice (3.04 oz)   **Meat**

Calories	184	(60.7 cal/oz)	Carbohydrate	6.72 g	(2% DV)
Fat Calories	61	(33% fat)	Dietary Fiber	0 g	(0% DV)
Total Fat	6.8 g	(10% DV)	Protein	22.95 g	(46% DV)
Saturated Fat	2.55 g	(13% DV)	Vitamin A	30689.3 IU	(614% DV)
Poly Fat	1.7 g		Vitamin C	19.6 mg	(33% DV)
Mono Fat	1.7 g		Calcium	9.4 mg	(1% DV)
Cholesterol	409.7 mg	(137% DV)	Iron	5.3 mg	(30% DV)
Sodium	90.1 mg	(4% DV)	Folate	23 mcg	(47% DV)
Potassium	309.4 mg	(9% DV)	Beta Carotene	79.1 RE	

Ratings	Worst	Bad	Average	Good	Best
Weight Loss			5		
LowCal Density			5		
Filling	2				
Energizing		4			
Fiber	1				
Vitamins					10
Minerals					9
Overall			5		

BEEF ROLLS, STUFFED WITH VEGETABLES OR MEAT

Serving: 1 beef roll (4.79 oz)   **Entree**

Calories	308	(64.3 cal/oz)	Carbohydrate	8.71 g	(3% DV)
Fat Calories	169	(55% fat)	Dietary Fiber	1.34 g	(5% DV)
Total Fat	18.76 g	(29% DV)	Protein	25.46 g	(51% DV)
Saturated Fat	6.7 g	(34% DV)	VItamin A	3591.2 IU	(72% DV)
Poly Fat	1.34 g		Vitamin C	2.7 mg	(4% DV)
Mono Fat	8.04 g		Calcium	17.4 mg	(2% DV)
Cholesterol	79.1 mg	(26% DV)	Iron	2.9 mg	(16% DV)
Sodium	483.7 mg	(20% DV)	Folate	25.5 mcg	(4% DV)
Potassium	466.3 mg	(13% DV)	Beta Carotene	359.1 RE	

Ratings	Worst	Bad	Average	Good	Best
Weight Loss			4		
LowCal Density			5		
Filling		3			
Energizing			4		
Fiber			5		
Vitamins					7
Minerals					7
Overall			5		

BEEF SAUSAGE, BROWN & SERVE, LINKS, COOKED

Serving: 1 link, cooked (.46 oz)   **Breakfast**

Calories	41	(89 cal/oz)	Carbohydrate	.23 g	(0% DV)
Fat Calories	34	(83% fat)	Dietary Fiber	0 g	(0% DV)
Total Fat	3.77 g	(6% DV)	Protein	1.56 g	(3% DV)
Saturated Fat	1.56 g	(8% DV)	VItamin A	0 IU	(0% DV)
Poly Fat	.13 g		Vitamin C	3.1 mg	(5% DV)
Mono Fat	1.82 g		Calcium	2.6 mg	(0% DV)
Cholesterol	7.9 mg	(3% DV)	Iron	.2 mg	(1% DV)
Sodium	133.4 mg	(6% DV)	Folate	1.6 mcg	(0% DV)
Potassium	21.6 mg	(1% DV)	Beta Carotene	0 RE	

Ratings	Worst	Bad	Average	Good	Best
Weight Loss			4		
LowCal Density		3			
Filling	1				
Energizing	2				
Fiber	1				
Vitamins	2				
Minerals	2				
Overall		3			

BEEF SHISHKABOB WITH VEGETABLES (NO POTATOES)

Serving: 1 shishkabob (7.21 oz)   **Entree**

Calories	168	(23.3 cal/oz)	Carbohydrate	10.5 g	(4% DV)
Fat Calories	36	(22% fat)	Dietary Fiber	2.02 g	(8% DV)
Total Fat	4.04 g	(6% DV)	Protein	20.2 g	(40% DV)
Saturated Fat	2.02 g	(10% DV)	Vitamin A	537.3 IU	(11% DV)
Poly Fat	0 g		Vitamin C	28.3 mg	(47% DV)
Mono Fat	2.02 g		Calcium	22.2 mg	(2% DV)
Cholesterol	50.5 mg	(17% DV)	Iron	2.4 mg	(13% DV)
Sodium	448.4 mg	(19% DV)	Folate	20.2 mcg	(7% DV)
Potassium	593.9 mg	(17% DV)	Beta Carotene	52.5 RE	

Ratings	Worst	Bad	Average	Good	Best
Weight Loss				8	
LowCal Density				8	
Filling			5		
Energizing		4			
Fiber			6		
Vitamins				7	
Minerals				7	
Overall				7	

BEEF SHORT RIBS, BONELESS, BBQ SAUCE, POTATOES

Serving: 1 meal (10.64 oz)   **Entree**

Calories	387	(36.4 cal/oz)	Carbohydrate	29.5 g	(10% DV)
Fat Calories	161	(42% fat)	Dietary Fiber	2.98 g	(12% DV)
Total Fat	17.88 g	(28% DV)	Protein	26.82 g	(54% DV)
Saturated Fat	8.94 g	(45% DV)	Vitamin A	1174.1 IU	(23% DV)
Poly Fat	0 g		Vitamin C	17.9 mg	(30% DV)
Mono Fat	5.96 g		Calcium	62.6 mg	(6% DV)
Cholesterol	77.5 mg	(26% DV)	Iron	4.5 mg	(25% DV)
Sodium	578.1 mg	(24% DV)	Folate	26.8 mcg	(10% DV)
Potassium	840.4 mg	(24% DV)	Beta Carotene	110.3 RE	

Ratings	Worst	Bad	Average	Good	Best
Weight Loss		4			
LowCal Density				7	
Filling			6		
Energizing				7	
Fiber				8	
Vitamins				7	
Minerals					9
Overall			6		

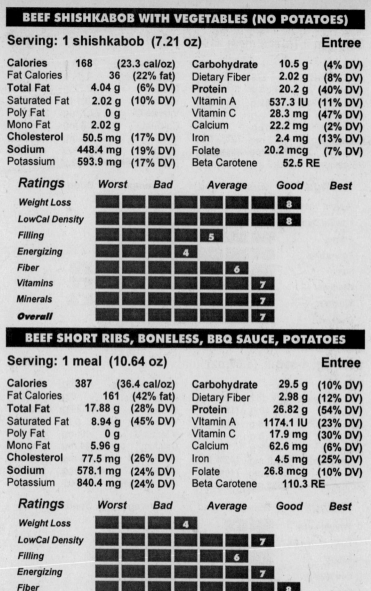

BEEF SIRLOIN TIPS, GRAVY, POTATO, VEGETABLE

Serving: 1 frozen meal (10.14 oz)   Entree

Calories	344	(33.9 cal/oz)	Carbohydrate	21.58 g	(7% DV)
Fat Calories	179	(52% fat)	Dietary Fiber	2.84 g	(11% DV)
Total Fat	19.88 g	(31% DV)	Protein	22.72 g	(45% DV)
Saturated Fat	8.52 g	(43% DV)	VItamin A	2323.1 IU	(46% DV)
Poly Fat	0 g		Vitamin C	22.7 mg	(38% DV)
Mono Fat	8.52 g		Calcium	31.2 mg	(3% DV)
Cholesterol	68.2 mg	(23% DV)	Iron	3.5 mg	(19% DV)
Sodium	752.6 mg	(31% DV)	Folate	22.7 mcg	(9% DV)
Potassium	772.5 mg	(22% DV)	Beta Carotene	232.9 RE	

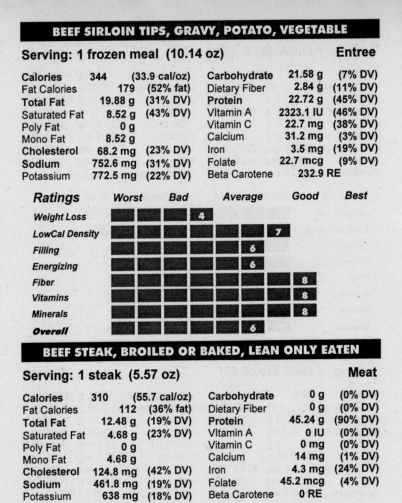

Ratings	Worst	Bad	Average	Good	Best
Weight Loss			4		
LowCal Density				7	
Filling			6		
Energizing			6		
Fiber					8
Vitamins					8
Minerals					8
Overall			6		

BEEF STEAK, BROILED OR BAKED, LEAN ONLY EATEN

Serving: 1 steak (5.57 oz)   Meat

Calories	310	(55.7 cal/oz)	Carbohydrate	0 g	(0% DV)
Fat Calories	112	(36% fat)	Dietary Fiber	0 g	(0% DV)
Total Fat	12.48 g	(19% DV)	Protein	45.24 g	(90% DV)
Saturated Fat	4.68 g	(23% DV)	VItamin A	0 IU	(0% DV)
Poly Fat	0 g		Vitamin C	0 mg	(0% DV)
Mono Fat	4.68 g		Calcium	14 mg	(1% DV)
Cholesterol	124.8 mg	(42% DV)	Iron	4.3 mg	(24% DV)
Sodium	461.8 mg	(19% DV)	Folate	45.2 mcg	(4% DV)
Potassium	638 mg	(18% DV)	Beta Carotene	0 RE	

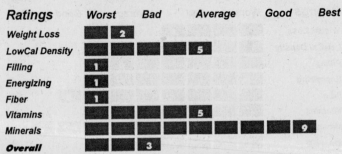

Ratings	Worst	Bad	Average	Good	Best
Weight Loss	2				
LowCal Density			5		
Filling	1				
Energizing	1				
Fiber	1				
Vitamins			5		
Minerals					9
Overall		3			

BEEF STEAK, FRIED, LEAN ONLY EATEN

Serving: 1 steak (5.57 oz)   **Meat**

Calories	359	(64.4 cal/oz)	Carbohydrate	0 g	(0% DV)
Fat Calories	140	(39% fat)	Dietary Fiber	0 g	(0% DV)
Total Fat	15.6 g	(24% DV)	Protein	53.04 g	(106% DV)
Saturated Fat	4.68 g	(23% DV)	Vltamin A	0 IU	(0% DV)
Poly Fat	1.56 g		Vitamin C	0 mg	(0% DV)
Mono Fat	6.24 g		Calcium	12.5 mg	(1% DV)
Cholesterol	151.3 mg	(50% DV)	Iron	5.4 mg	(30% DV)
Sodium	474.2 mg	(20% DV)	Folate	53 mcg	(5% DV)
Potassium	762.8 mg	(22% DV)	Beta Carotene	0 RE	

Ratings	Worst	Bad	Average	Good	Best
Weight Loss	2				
LowCal Density			5		
Filling	1				
Energizing	1				
Fiber	1				
Vitamins				8	
Minerals					9
Overall		4			

BEEF STEW, POTATOES, VEGETABLES & GRAVY

Serving: 1 cup (9 oz)   **Entree**

Calories	176	(19.6 cal/oz)	Carbohydrate	18.14 g	(6% DV)
Fat Calories	23	(13% fat)	Dietary Fiber	2.52 g	(10% DV)
Total Fat	2.52 g	(4% DV)	Protein	17.64 g	(35% DV)
Saturated Fat	2.52 g	(13% DV)	Vltamin A	5014.8 IU	(100% DV)
Poly Fat	0 g		Vitamin C	12.6 mg	(21% DV)
Mono Fat	2.52 g		Calcium	22.7 mg	(2% DV)
Cholesterol	40.3 mg	(13% DV)	Iron	2.6 mg	(14% DV)
Sodium	526.7 mg	(22% DV)	Folate	17.6 mcg	(6% DV)
Potassium	645.1 mg	(18% DV)	Beta Carotene	501.5 RE	

Ratings	Worst	Bad	Average	Good	Best
Weight Loss				8	
LowCal Density				8	
Filling			7		
Energizing			6		
Fiber			7		
Vitamins					9
Minerals			7		
Overall				8	

BEEF STROGANOFF WITH NOODLES

Serving: 1 cup (9.14 oz) — Entree

Calories	343	(37.5 cal/oz)	Carbohydrate	20.74 g	(7% DV)
Fat Calories	184	(54% fat)	Dietary Fiber	2.56 g	(10% DV)
Total Fat	20.48 g	(32% DV)	Protein	20.48 g	(41% DV)
Saturated Fat	7.68 g	(38% DV)	Vitamin A	294.4 IU	(6% DV)
Poly Fat	5.12 g		Vitamin C	2.6 mg	(4% DV)
Mono Fat	5.12 g		Calcium	69.1 mg	(7% DV)
Cholesterol	74.2 mg	(25% DV)	Iron	3.3 mg	(18% DV)
Sodium	453.1 mg	(19% DV)	Folate	20.5 mcg	(4% DV)
Potassium	455.7 mg	(13% DV)	Beta Carotene	7.7 RE	

Ratings	Worst	Bad	Average	Good	Best
Weight Loss			4		
LowCal Density				7	
Filling			5		
Energizing			6		
Fiber				7	
Vitamins			5		
Minerals				7	
Overall			6		

BEEF VEGETABLE SOUP WITH POTATO, STEW TYPE

Serving: 1 cup (8.57 oz) — Soup

Calories	170	(19.9 cal/oz)	Carbohydrate	19.68 g	(7% DV)
Fat Calories	43	(25% fat)	Dietary Fiber	2.4 g	(10% DV)
Total Fat	4.8 g	(7% DV)	Protein	12 g	(24% DV)
Saturated Fat	2.4 g	(12% DV)	Vitamin A	2611.2 IU	(52% DV)
Poly Fat	0 g		Vitamin C	7.2 mg	(12% DV)
Mono Fat	2.4 g		Calcium	31.2 mg	(3% DV)
Cholesterol	14.4 mg	(5% DV)	Iron	2.3 mg	(13% DV)
Sodium	866.4 mg	(36% DV)	Folate	12 mcg	(4% DV)
Potassium	336 mg	(10% DV)	Beta Carotene	261.6 RE	

Ratings	Worst	Bad	Average	Good	Best
Weight Loss			5		
LowCal Density				8	
Filling				7	
Energizing			6		
Fiber				7	
Vitamins			6		
Minerals			5		
Overall			6		

Edmund's Food Ratings

BEEF, BROTH, BOUILLON, OR CONSOMME

Serving: 1 cup (8.57 oz)   **Soup**

Calories	17	(2 cal/oz)	Carbohydrate	0 g	(0% DV)
Fat Calories	0	(0% fat)	Dietary Fiber	0 g	(0% DV)
Total Fat	0 g	(0% DV)	Protein	2.4 g	(5% DV)
Saturated Fat	0 g	(0% DV)	VItamin A	0 IU	(0% DV)
Poly Fat	0 g		Vitamin C	0 mg	(0% DV)
Mono Fat	0 g		Calcium	14.4 mg	(1% DV)
Cholesterol	0 mg	(0% DV)	Iron	.4 mg	(2% DV)
Sodium	782.4 mg	(33% DV)	Folate	2.4 mcg	(1% DV)
Potassium	129.6 mg	(4% DV)	Beta Carotene	0 RE	

Ratings	Worst	Bad	Average	Good	Best
Weight Loss					10
LowCal Density					10
Filling	1				
Energizing	1				
Fiber	1				
Vitamins		3			
Minerals		3			
Overall				6	

BEEF, GRAVY, VEGETABLE, DESSERT

Serving: 1 frozen meal (11.64 oz)   **Entree**

Calories	375	(32.2 cal/oz)	Carbohydrate	36.84 g	(12% DV)
Fat Calories	117	(31% fat)	Dietary Fiber	3.26 g	(13% DV)
Total Fat	13.04 g	(20% DV)	Protein	29.34 g	(59% DV)
Saturated Fat	3.26 g	(16% DV)	VItamin A	577 IU	(12% DV)
Poly Fat	3.26 g		Vitamin C	9.8 mg	(16% DV)
Mono Fat	6.52 g		Calcium	32.6 mg	(3% DV)
Cholesterol	78.2 mg	(26% DV)	Iron	3.7 mg	(20% DV)
Sodium	1294.2 mg	(54% DV)	Folate	29.3 mcg	(12% DV)
Potassium	687.9 mg	(20% DV)	Beta Carotene	35.9 RE	

Ratings	Worst	Bad	Average	Good	Best
Weight Loss			5		
LowCal Density				7	
Filling				7	
Energizing				8	
Fiber				8	
Vitamins				7	
Minerals				8	
Overall				7	

BEEF, GROUND, REGULAR, COOKED

Serving: 1 patty (3.04 oz)   **Meat**

Calories	243	(80 cal/oz)	Carbohydrate	0 g	(0% DV)
Fat Calories	153	(63% fat)	Dietary Fiber	0 g	(0% DV)
Total Fat	17 g	(26% DV)	Protein	20.4 g	(41% DV)
Saturated Fat	6.8 g	(34% DV)	VItamin A	0 IU	(0% DV)
Poly Fat	.85 g		Vitamin C	0 mg	(0% DV)
Mono Fat	7.65 g		Calcium	9.4 mg	(1% DV)
Cholesterol	75.7 mg	(25% DV)	Iron	2.1 mg	(11% DV)
Sodium	396.1 mg	(17% DV)	Folate	20.4 mcg	(2% DV)
Potassium	245.7 mg	(7% DV)	Beta Carotene	0 RE	

Ratings	Worst	Bad	Average	Good	Best
Weight Loss	2				
LowCal Density			4		
Filling	1				
Energizing	1				
Fiber	1				
Vitamins			4		
Minerals				6	
Overall		3			

BEEF, NOODLES, & VEGETABLES

Serving: 1 cup (5.79 oz)   **Entree**

Calories	203	(35 cal/oz)	Carbohydrate	18.14 g	(6% DV)
Fat Calories	44	(22% fat)	Dietary Fiber	3.24 g	(13% DV)
Total Fat	4.86 g	(7% DV)	Protein	19.44 g	(39% DV)
Saturated Fat	1.62 g	(8% DV)	VItamin A	4341.6 IU	(87% DV)
Poly Fat	0 g		Vitamin C	4.9 mg	(8% DV)
Mono Fat	1.62 g		Calcium	27.5 mg	(3% DV)
Cholesterol	64.8 mg	(22% DV)	Iron	3.1 mg	(17% DV)
Sodium	455.2 mg	(19% DV)	Folate	19.4 mcg	(6% DV)
Potassium	280.3 mg	(8% DV)	Beta Carotene	432.5 RE	

Ratings	Worst	Bad	Average	Good	Best
Weight Loss				7	
LowCal Density				7	
Filling			5		
Energizing			6		
Fiber					8
Vitamins					8
Minerals				7	
Overall				7	

BEEF, ORIENTAL STYLE, VEGETABLE, RICE

Serving: 1 Lean Cuisine frozen meal (8.75 oz)   Entree

Calories	289	(33 cal/oz)	Carbohydrate	34.79 g	(12% DV)
Fat Calories	66	(23% fat)	Dietary Fiber	2.45 g	(10% DV)
Total Fat	7.35 g	(11% DV)	Protein	22.05 g	(44% DV)
Saturated Fat	2.45 g	(12% DV)	Vitamin A	3623.6 IU	(72% DV)
Poly Fat	0 g		Vitamin C	7.4 mg	(12% DV)
Mono Fat	2.45 g		Calcium	36.8 mg	(4% DV)
Cholesterol	53.9 mg	(18% DV)	Iron	3.7 mg	(20% DV)
Sodium	1220.1 mg	(51% DV)	Folate	22.1 mcg	(7% DV)
Potassium	306.3 mg	(9% DV)	Beta Carotene	362.6 RE	

Ratings	Worst	Bad	Average	Good	Best
Weight Loss			6		
LowCal Density			7		
Filling			7		
Energizing				8	
Fiber			7		
Vitamins				8	
Minerals				8	
Overall			7		

BEEF, ORIENTAL STYLE, VEGETABLE, RICE, & FRUIT

Serving: 1 Healthy Choice meal (11.11 oz)   Entree

Calories	305	(27.4 cal/oz)	Carbohydrate	36.7 g	(12% DV)
Fat Calories	56	(18% fat)	Dietary Fiber	3.11 g	(12% DV)
Total Fat	6.22 g	(10% DV)	Protein	24.88 g	(50% DV)
Saturated Fat	3.11 g	(16% DV)	Vitamin A	1390.2 IU	(28% DV)
Poly Fat	0 g		Vitamin C	62.2 mg	(104% DV)
Mono Fat	3.11 g		Calcium	77.8 mg	(8% DV)
Cholesterol	56 mg	(19% DV)	Iron	3.4 mg	(19% DV)
Sodium	615.8 mg	(26% DV)	Folate	24.9 mcg	(9% DV)
Potassium	600.2 mg	(17% DV)	Beta Carotene	133.7 RE	

Ratings	Worst	Bad	Average	Good	Best
Weight Loss			6		
LowCal Density				8	
Filling				8	
Energizing				8	
Fiber				8	
Vitamins					9
Minerals				8	
Overall				8	

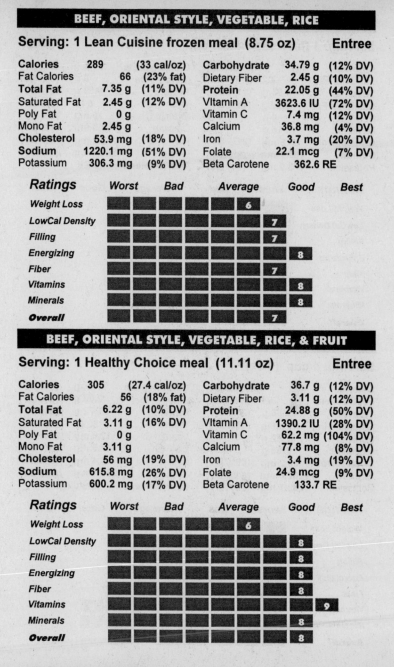

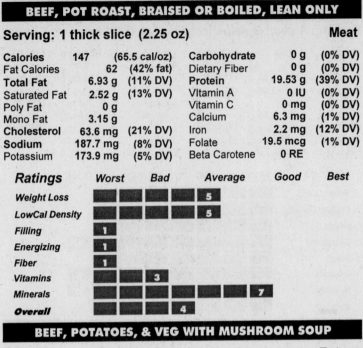

BEEF, POT ROAST, BRAISED OR BOILED, LEAN ONLY

Serving: 1 thick slice (2.25 oz)   Meat

Calories	147	(65.5 cal/oz)	Carbohydrate	0 g	(0% DV)
Fat Calories	62	(42% fat)	Dietary Fiber	0 g	(0% DV)
Total Fat	6.93 g	(11% DV)	Protein	19.53 g	(39% DV)
Saturated Fat	2.52 g	(13% DV)	Vitamin A	0 IU	(0% DV)
Poly Fat	0 g		Vitamin C	0 mg	(0% DV)
Mono Fat	3.15 g		Calcium	6.3 mg	(1% DV)
Cholesterol	63.6 mg	(21% DV)	Iron	2.2 mg	(12% DV)
Sodium	187.7 mg	(8% DV)	Folate	19.5 mcg	(1% DV)
Potassium	173.9 mg	(5% DV)	Beta Carotene	0 RE	

Ratings	Worst	Bad	Average	Good	Best
Weight Loss			5		
LowCal Density			5		
Filling	1				
Energizing	1				
Fiber	1				
Vitamins		3			
Minerals					7
Overall			4		

BEEF, POTATOES, & VEG WITH MUSHROOM SOUP

Serving: 1 cup (9 oz)   Entree

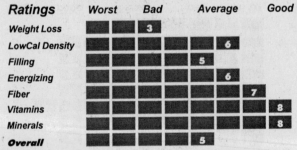

Calories	403	(44.8 cal/oz)	Carbohydrate	21.67 g	(7% DV)
Fat Calories	204	(51% fat)	Dietary Fiber	2.52 g	(10% DV)
Total Fat	22.68 g	(35% DV)	Protein	27.72 g	(55% DV)
Saturated Fat	7.56 g	(38% DV)	Vitamin A	4163 IU	(83% DV)
Poly Fat	2.52 g		Vitamin C	12.6 mg	(21% DV)
Mono Fat	7.56 g		Calcium	47.9 mg	(5% DV)
Cholesterol	88.2 mg	(29% DV)	Iron	3.4 mg	(19% DV)
Sodium	1267.6 mg	(53% DV)	Folate	27.7 mcg	(6% DV)
Potassium	783.7 mg	(22% DV)	Beta Carotene	415.8 RE	

Ratings	Worst	Bad	Average	Good	Best
Weight Loss		3			
LowCal Density				6	
Filling			5		
Energizing				6	
Fiber				7	
Vitamins					8
Minerals					8
Overall			5		

BEEF, RICE, & VEGETABLES

Serving: 1 cup (5.79 oz)   Entree

Calories	201	(34.7 cal/oz)	Carbohydrate	21.55 g	(7% DV)
Fat Calories	44	(22% fat)	Dietary Fiber	1.62 g	(6% DV)
Total Fat	4.86 g	(7% DV)	Protein	17.82 g	(36% DV)
Saturated Fat	1.62 g	(8% DV)	VItamin A	4020.8 IU	(80% DV)
Poly Fat	0 g		Vitamin C	4.9 mg	(8% DV)
Mono Fat	1.62 g		Calcium	25.9 mg	(3% DV)
Cholesterol	45.4 mg	(15% DV)	Iron	2.8 mg	(15% DV)
Sodium	421.2 mg	(18% DV)	Folate	17.8 mcg	(5% DV)
Potassium	270.5 mg	(8% DV)	Beta Carotene	401.8 RE	

Ratings

	Worst	Bad	Average	Good	Best
Weight Loss				7	
LowCal Density				7	
Filling			6		
Energizing			6		
Fiber			5		
Vitamins					8
Minerals				7	
Overall				7	

BEET SOUP (BORSCHT)

Serving: 1 cup (8.75 oz)   Soup

Calories	74	(8.4 cal/oz)	Carbohydrate	6.62 g	(2% DV)
Fat Calories	44	(60% fat)	Dietary Fiber	2.45 g	(10% DV)
Total Fat	4.9 g	(8% DV)	Protein	2.45 g	(5% DV)
Saturated Fat	2.45 g	(12% DV)	VItamin A	169.1 IU	(3% DV)
Poly Fat	0 g		Vitamin C	9.8 mg	(16% DV)
Mono Fat	0 g		Calcium	46.6 mg	(5% DV)
Cholesterol	7.4 mg	(2% DV)	Iron	.7 mg	(4% DV)
Sodium	497.4 mg	(21% DV)	Folate	2.5 mcg	(9% DV)
Potassium	313.6 mg	(9% DV)	Beta Carotene	7.4 RE	

Ratings

	Worst	Bad	Average	Good	Best
Weight Loss			5		
LowCal Density					9
Filling			7		
Energizing		4			
Fiber			7		
Vitamins		4			
Minerals		4			
Overall			6		

BEETS WITH HARVARD SAUCE

Serving: 1 cup (8.79 oz) — Vegetable

Calories	271	(30.8 cal/oz)	Carbohydrate	50.68 g	(17% DV)
Fat Calories	66	(25% fat)	Dietary Fiber	2.46 g	(10% DV)
Total Fat	7.38 g	(11% DV)	Protein	2.46 g	(5% DV)
Saturated Fat	2.46 g	(12% DV)	VItamin A	425.6 IU	(9% DV)
Poly Fat	2.46 g		Vitamin C	9.8 mg	(16% DV)
Mono Fat	2.46 g		Calcium	24.6 mg	(2% DV)
Cholesterol	0 mg	(0% DV)	Iron	1.3 mg	(7% DV)
Sodium	573.2 mg	(24% DV)	Folate	2.5 mcg	(23% DV)
Potassium	575.6 mg	(16% DV)	Beta Carotene	9.8 RE	

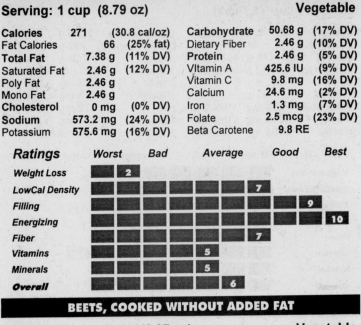

Ratings	Worst	Bad	Average	Good	Best
Weight Loss	2				
LowCal Density				7	
Filling					9
Energizing					10
Fiber				7	
Vitamins			5		
Minerals			5		
Overall				6	

BEETS, COOKED WITHOUT ADDED FAT

Serving: 1 cup, slices (6.07 oz) — Vegetable

Calories	53	(8.7 cal/oz)	Carbohydrate	11.39 g	(4% DV)
Fat Calories	0	(0% fat)	Dietary Fiber	3.4 g	(14% DV)
Total Fat	0 g	(0% DV)	Protein	1.7 g	(3% DV)
Saturated Fat	0 g	(0% DV)	VItamin A	22.1 IU	(0% DV)
Poly Fat	0 g		Vitamin C	8.5 mg	(14% DV)
Mono Fat	0 g		Calcium	18.7 mg	(2% DV)
Cholesterol	0 mg	(0% DV)	Iron	1.1 mg	(6% DV)
Sodium	476 mg	(20% DV)	Folate	1.7 mcg	(23% DV)
Potassium	527 mg	(15% DV)	Beta Carotene	1.7 RE	

Ratings	Worst	Bad	Average	Good	Best
Weight Loss				9	
LowCal Density				9	
Filling				9	
Energizing			5		
Fiber				8	
Vitamins			5		
Minerals			5		
Overall				8	

BEETS, PICKLED

Serving: 1 cup, slices (6.04 oz)   **Vegetable**

Calories	85	(14 cal/oz)	Carbohydrate	19.94 g	(7% DV)
Fat Calories	0	(0% fat)	Dietary Fiber	1.69 g	(7% DV)
Total Fat	0 g	(0% DV)	Protein	1.69 g	(3% DV)
Saturated Fat	0 g	(0% DV)	VItamin A	16.9 IU	(0% DV)
Poly Fat	0 g		Vitamin C	5.1 mg	(8% DV)
Mono Fat	0 g		Calcium	16.9 mg	(2% DV)
Cholesterol	0 mg	(0% DV)	Iron	.9 mg	(5% DV)
Sodium	417.4 mg	(17% DV)	Folate	1.7 mcg	(14% DV)
Potassium	422.5 mg	(12% DV)	Beta Carotene	1.7 RE	

Ratings	Worst	Bad	Average	Good	Best
Weight Loss					9
LowCal Density					9
Filling				8	
Energizing			6		
Fiber		5			
Vitamins	4				
Minerals	4				
Overall				8	

BERNAISE SAUCE

Serving: 1 tbsp (.57 oz)   **Sauce**

Calories	59	(102.9 cal/oz)	Carbohydrate	.3 g	(0% DV)
Fat Calories	56	(95% fat)	Dietary Fiber	0 g	(0% DV)
Total Fat	6.2 g	(10% DV)	Protein	.64 g	(1% DV)
Saturated Fat	3.5 g	(18% DV)	VItamin A	265.2 IU	(5% DV)
Poly Fat	.32 g		Vitamin C	.6 mg	(1% DV)
Mono Fat	1.91 g		Calcium	8.1 mg	(1% DV)
Cholesterol	60.9 mg	(20% DV)	Iron	.2 mg	(1% DV)
Sodium	82.4 mg	(3% DV)	Folate	.6 mcg	(2% DV)
Potassium	12.4 mg	(0% DV)	Beta Carotene	5.6 RE	

Ratings	Worst	Bad	Average	Good	Best
Weight Loss		3			
LowCal Density	2				
Filling	1				
Energizing	2				
Fiber	1				
Vitamins		3			
Minerals	2				
Overall	2				

BISCUIT, BAKING POWDER OR BUTTERMILK, FROM MIX

Serving: 1 medium (2" dia) (1.07 oz) — Bakery

Calories	105	(97.9 cal/oz)	Carbohydrate	16.38 g	(5% DV)
Fat Calories	30	(28% fat)	Dietary Fiber	.3 g	(1% DV)
Total Fat	3.3 g	(5% DV)	Protein	2.1 g	(4% DV)
Saturated Fat	.9 g	(5% DV)	Vitamin A	13.8 IU	(0% DV)
Poly Fat	.3 g		Vitamin C	0 mg	(0% DV)
Mono Fat	1.8 g		Calcium	60.6 mg	(6% DV)
Cholesterol	1.8 mg	(1% DV)	Iron	.8 mg	(4% DV)
Sodium	296.7 mg	(12% DV)	Folate	2.1 mcg	(0% DV)
Potassium	35.1 mg	(1% DV)	Beta Carotene	.3 RE	

Ratings	Worst	Bad	Average	Good	Best
Weight Loss				6	
LowCal Density	3				
Filling	3				
Energizing			5		
Fiber	2				
Vitamins	3				
Minerals	4				
Overall	4				

BISCUIT, CHEESE

Serving: 1 biscuit (2" dia) (1.07 oz) — Bakery

Calories	115	(107.7 cal/oz)	Carbohydrate	11.79 g	(4% DV)
Fat Calories	57	(49% fat)	Dietary Fiber	.3 g	(1% DV)
Total Fat	6.3 g	(10% DV)	Protein	3 g	(6% DV)
Saturated Fat	2.1 g	(11% DV)	Vitamin A	72 IU	(1% DV)
Poly Fat	1.2 g		Vitamin C	0 mg	(0% DV)
Mono Fat	2.4 g		Calcium	79.8 mg	(8% DV)
Cholesterol	6 mg	(2% DV)	Iron	.7 mg	(4% DV)
Sodium	196.8 mg	(8% DV)	Folate	3 mcg	(1% DV)
Potassium	41.4 mg	(1% DV)	Beta Carotene	2.1 RE	

Ratings	Worst	Bad	Average	Good	Best
Weight Loss		4			
LowCal Density	2				
Filling	2				
Energizing			5		
Fiber	2				
Vitamins	3				
Minerals		4			
Overall	3				

BLACK BEAN SOUP

Serving: 1 cup (8.82 oz)   Soup

Calories	116	(13.2 cal/oz)	Carbohydrate	19.76 g	(7% DV)
Fat Calories	22	(19% fat)	Dietary Fiber	4.94 g	(20% DV)
Total Fat	2.47 g	(4% DV)	Protein	4.94 g	(10% DV)
Saturated Fat	0 g	(0% DV)	Vitamin A	506.4 IU	(10% DV)
Poly Fat	0 g		Vitamin C	0 mg	(0% DV)
Mono Fat	0 g		Calcium	44.5 mg	(4% DV)
Cholesterol	0 mg	(0% DV)	Iron	2.2 mg	(12% DV)
Sodium	1198 mg	(50% DV)	Folate	4.9 mcg	(6% DV)
Potassium	274.2 mg	(8% DV)	Beta Carotene	49.4 RE	

Ratings	Worst	Bad	Average	Good	Best
Weight Loss				7	
LowCal Density					9
Filling					10
Energizing			6		
Fiber					9
Vitamins		4			
Minerals		5			
Overall				8	

BLACK, BROWN, OR BAYO BEANS, DRY, NO ADDED FAT

Serving: 1 cup, cooked (6.14 oz)   Vegetable

Calories	198	(32.2 cal/oz)	Carbohydrate	36.12 g	(12% DV)
Fat Calories	0	(0% fat)	Dietary Fiber	8.6 g	(34% DV)
Total Fat	0 g	(0% DV)	Protein	12.04 g	(24% DV)
Saturated Fat	0 g	(0% DV)	Vitamin A	8.6 IU	(0% DV)
Poly Fat	0 g		Vitamin C	0 mg	(0% DV)
Mono Fat	0 g		Calcium	67.1 mg	(7% DV)
Cholesterol	0 mg	(0% DV)	Iron	2.5 mg	(14% DV)
Sodium	366.4 mg	(15% DV)	Folate	12 mcg	(32% DV)
Potassium	643.3 mg	(18% DV)	Beta Carotene	1.7 RE	

Ratings	Worst	Bad	Average	Good	Best
Weight Loss		5			
LowCal Density				7	
Filling				8	
Energizing				8	
Fiber					10
Vitamins		5			
Minerals				7	
Overall				7	

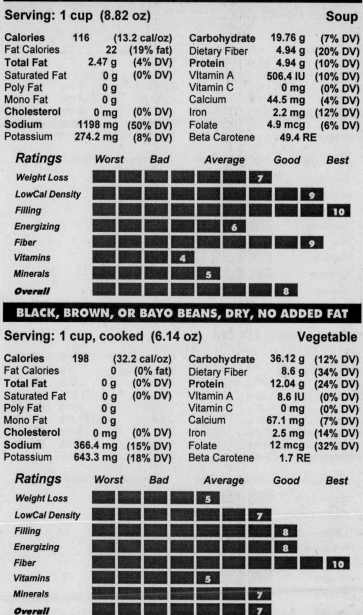

BLINTZ, CHEESE-FILLED

Serving: 1 blintz (2.5 oz)   Dessert

Calories	138	(55.2 cal/oz)	Carbohydrate	13.79 g	(5% DV)
Fat Calories	57	(41% fat)	Dietary Fiber	0 g	(0% DV)
Total Fat	6.3 g	(10% DV)	Protein	7 g	(14% DV)
Saturated Fat	2.1 g	(11% DV)	Vitamin A	298.2 IU	(6% DV)
Poly Fat	1.4 g		Vitamin C	0 mg	(0% DV)
Mono Fat	2.1 g		Calcium	55.3 mg	(6% DV)
Cholesterol	69.3 mg	(23% DV)	Iron	.7 mg	(4% DV)
Sodium	294.7 mg	(12% DV)	Folate	7 mcg	(3% DV)
Potassium	74.9 mg	(2% DV)	Beta Carotene	4.2 RE	

Ratings	Worst	Bad	Average	Good	Best
Weight Loss					6
LowCal Density			5		
Filling		4			
Energizing			5		
Fiber	1				
Vitamins	3				
Minerals		4			
Overall			5		

BLUE OR ROQUEFORT CHEESE DRESSING

Serving: 1 tbsp (.55 oz)   Fat & Oil

Calories	77	(140.2 cal/oz)	Carbohydrate	1.13 g	(0% DV)
Fat Calories	72	(93% fat)	Dietary Fiber	0 g	(0% DV)
Total Fat	7.96 g	(12% DV)	Protein	.77 g	(2% DV)
Saturated Fat	1.53 g	(8% DV)	Vitamin A	32.1 IU	(1% DV)
Poly Fat	4.28 g		Vitamin C	.3 mg	(1% DV)
Mono Fat	1.84 g		Calcium	12.4 mg	(1% DV)
Cholesterol	2.6 mg	(1% DV)	Iron	0 mg	(0% DV)
Sodium	167.4 mg	(7% DV)	Folate	.8 mcg	(0% DV)
Potassium	5.7 mg	(0% DV)	Beta Carotene	0 RE	

Ratings	Worst	Bad	Average	Good	Best
Weight Loss	2				
LowCal Density	1				
Filling	1				
Energizing	2				
Fiber	1				
Vitamins	2				
Minerals	2				
Overall	2				

BLUE OR ROQUEFORT CHEESE DRESSING, LOW-CALORIE

Serving: 1 tbsp (.55 oz)   **Fat & Oil**

Calories	15	(27.5 cal/oz)	Carbohydrate	.38 g	(0% DV)
Fat Calories	10	(64% fat)	Dietary Fiber	0 g	(0% DV)
Total Fat	1.07 g	(2% DV)	Protein	.77 g	(2% DV)
Saturated Fat	.15 g	(1% DV)	Vitamin A	2 IU	(0% DV)
Poly Fat	.46 g		Vitamin C	0 mg	(0% DV)
Mono Fat	.46 g		Calcium	13.6 mg	(1% DV)
Cholesterol	.2 mg	(0% DV)	Iron	.1 mg	(0% DV)
Sodium	183.6 mg	(8% DV)	Folate	.8 mcg	(0% DV)
Potassium	.8 mg	(0% DV)	Beta Carotene	0 RE	

Ratings	Worst	Bad	Average	Good	Best
Weight Loss			6		
LowCal Density				8	
Filling	1				
Energizing	2				
Fiber	1				
Vitamins	2				
Minerals	2				
Overall			5		

BLUEBERRIES, RAW

Serving: 1 cup (5.18 oz)   **Fruit**

Calories	81	(15.7 cal/oz)	Carbohydrate	20.44 g	(7% DV)
Fat Calories	0	(0% fat)	Dietary Fiber	2.9 g	(12% DV)
Total Fat	0 g	(0% DV)	Protein	1.45 g	(3% DV)
Saturated Fat	0 g	(0% DV)	Vitamin A	145 IU	(3% DV)
Poly Fat	0 g		Vitamin C	18.9 mg	(31% DV)
Mono Fat	0 g		Calcium	8.7 mg	(1% DV)
Cholesterol	0 mg	(0% DV)	Iron	.3 mg	(1% DV)
Sodium	8.7 mg	(0% DV)	Folate	1.5 mcg	(2% DV)
Potassium	129.1 mg	(4% DV)	Beta Carotene	14.5 RE	

Ratings	Worst	Bad	Average	Good	Best
Weight Loss				9	
LowCal Density				9	
Filling				8	
Energizing			6		
Fiber				8	
Vitamins			5		
Minerals	2				
Overall				8	

BOLOGNA SANDWICH, WITH SPREAD

Serving: 1 sandwich (2.96 oz)　　　　　　**Sandwich**

Calories	257	(86.9 cal/oz)	Carbohydrate	25.56 g	(9% DV)
Fat Calories	127	(49% fat)	Dietary Fiber	.83 g	(3% DV)
Total Fat	14.11 g	(22% DV)	Protein	7.47 g	(15% DV)
Saturated Fat	4.15 g	(21% DV)	VItamin A	210 IU	(4% DV)
Poly Fat	2.49 g		Vitamin C	5.8 mg	(10% DV)
Mono Fat	5.81 g		Calcium	63.1 mg	(6% DV)
Cholesterol	15.8 mg	(5% DV)	Iron	1.9 mg	(11% DV)
Sodium	608.4 mg	(25% DV)	Folate	7.5 mcg	(5% DV)
Potassium	110.4 mg	(3% DV)	Beta Carotene	4.2 RE	

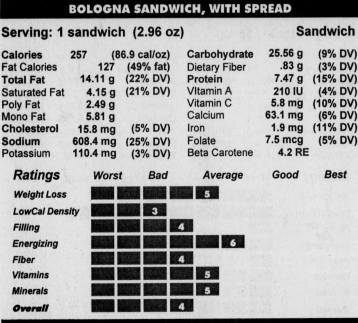

Ratings	Worst	Bad	Average	Good	Best
Weight Loss			5		
LowCal Density	3				
Filling	4				
Energizing			6		
Fiber	4				
Vitamins		5			
Minerals		5			
Overall	4				

BOLOGNA, BEEF

Serving: 1 slice (1 oz)　　　　　　**Meat**

Calories	87	(87.4 cal/oz)	Carbohydrate	.22 g	(0% DV)
Fat Calories	71	(81% fat)	Dietary Fiber	0 g	(0% DV)
Total Fat	7.84 g	(12% DV)	Protein	3.36 g	(7% DV)
Saturated Fat	3.36 g	(17% DV)	VItamin A	0 IU	(0% DV)
Poly Fat	.28 g		Vitamin C	5.9 mg	(10% DV)
Mono Fat	3.92 g		Calcium	3.4 mg	(0% DV)
Cholesterol	16.2 mg	(5% DV)	Iron	.5 mg	(3% DV)
Sodium	274.7 mg	(11% DV)	Folate	3.4 mcg	(0% DV)
Potassium	44 mg	(1% DV)	Beta Carotene	0 RE	

Ratings	Worst	Bad	Average	Good	Best
Weight Loss			4		
LowCal Density	3				
Filling	1				
Energizing	2				
Fiber	1				
Vitamins		3			
Minerals		3			
Overall	3				

BOLOGNA, TURKEY

Serving: 1 slice (1 oz)   **Meat**

Calories	56	(55.7 cal/oz)	Carbohydrate	.28 g	(0% DV)
Fat Calories	38	(68% fat)	Dietary Fiber	0 g	(0% DV)
Total Fat	4.2 g	(6% DV)	Protein	3.92 g	(8% DV)
Saturated Fat	1.4 g	(7% DV)	Vitamin A	0 IU	(0% DV)
Poly Fat	1.12 g		Vitamin C	0 mg	(0% DV)
Mono Fat	1.4 g		Calcium	23.5 mg	(2% DV)
Cholesterol	27.7 mg	(9% DV)	Iron	.4 mg	(2% DV)
Sodium	245.8 mg	(10% DV)	Folate	3.9 mcg	(0% DV)
Potassium	55.7 mg	(2% DV)	Beta Carotene	0 RE	

Ratings	Worst	Bad	Average	Good	Best
Weight Loss			5		
LowCal Density			5		
Filling	1				
Energizing	2				
Fiber	1				
Vitamins	2				
Minerals	3				
Overall	4				

BOOBERRY

Serving: 1 cup (1.18 oz)   **Cereal**

Calories	128	(108.5 cal/oz)	Carbohydrate	27.95 g	(9% DV)
Fat Calories	12	(9% fat)	Dietary Fiber	.66 g	(3% DV)
Total Fat	1.32 g	(2% DV)	Protein	1.32 g	(3% DV)
Saturated Fat	.99 g	(5% DV)	Vitamin A	1455.3 IU	(29% DV)
Poly Fat	0 g		Vitamin C	17.5 mg	(29% DV)
Mono Fat	0 g		Calcium	6.6 mg	(1% DV)
Cholesterol	0 mg	(0% DV)	Iron	5.2 mg	(29% DV)
Sodium	238.6 mg	(10% DV)	Folate	1.3 mcg	(2% DV)
Potassium	51.8 mg	(1% DV)	Beta Carotene	0 RE	

Ratings	Worst	Bad	Average	Good	Best
Weight Loss				8	
LowCal Density	2				
Filling		4			
Energizing				7	
Fiber		3			
Vitamins					9
Minerals			5		
Overall			5		

BRAN BUDS

Serving: 1 cup (3 oz)   **Cereal**

Calories	217	(72.2 cal/oz)	Carbohydrate	63.84 g	(21% DV)
Fat Calories	15	(7% fat)	Dietary Fiber	31.08 g	(124% DV)
Total Fat	1.68 g	(3% DV)	Protein	7.56 g	(15% DV)
Saturated Fat	0 g	(0% DV)	VItamin A	2221.8 IU	(44% DV)
Poly Fat	.84 g		Vitamin C	44.5 mg	(74% DV)
Mono Fat	0 g		Calcium	56.3 mg	(6% DV)
Cholesterol	0 mg	(0% DV)	Iron	13.4 mg	(74% DV)
Sodium	515.8 mg	(21% DV)	Folate	7.6 mcg	(74% DV)
Potassium	908 mg	(26% DV)	Beta Carotene	0 RE	

Ratings	Worst	Bad	Average	Good	Best
Weight Loss				6	
LowCal Density		4			
Filling				8	
Energizing					10
Fiber					10
Vitamins					10
Minerals					10
Overall				7	

BRAN FLAKES 40%

Serving: 1 cup (1.61 oz)   **Cereal**

Calories	146	(90.8 cal/oz)	Carbohydrate	35.59 g	(12% DV)
Fat Calories	8	(6% fat)	Dietary Fiber	8.55 g	(34% DV)
Total Fat	.9 g	(1% DV)	Protein	5.4 g	(11% DV)
Saturated Fat	0 g	(0% DV)	VItamin A	1719.5 IU	(34% DV)
Poly Fat	.45 g		Vitamin C	8.1 mg	(13% DV)
Mono Fat	0 g		Calcium	20.7 mg	(2% DV)
Cholesterol	0 mg	(0% DV)	Iron	16.2 mg	(90% DV)
Sodium	393.8 mg	(16% DV)	Folate	5.4 mcg	(40% DV)
Potassium	262.8 mg	(8% DV)	Beta Carotene	0 RE	

Ratings	Worst	Bad	Average	Good	Best
Weight Loss				8	
LowCal Density		3			
Filling			5		
Energizing				8	
Fiber					10
Vitamins					10
Minerals				9	
Overall			7		

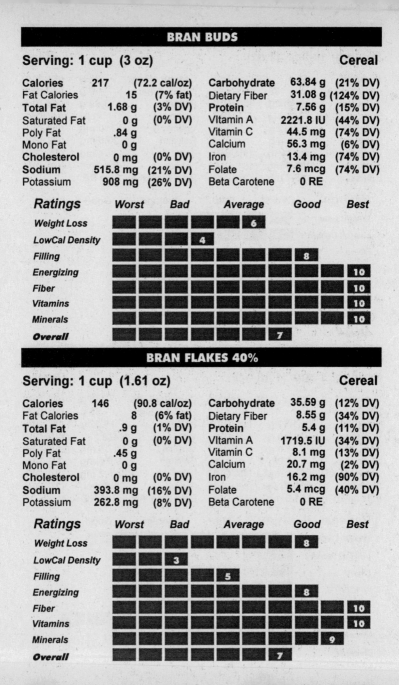

BRATWURST, COOKED

Serving: 1 link (3.04 oz)   **Meat**

Calories	256	(84.2 cal/oz)	Carbohydrate	1.78 g	(1% DV)
Fat Calories	199	(78% fat)	Dietary Fiber	0 g	(0% DV)
Total Fat	22.1 g	(34% DV)	Protein	11.9 g	(24% DV)
Saturated Fat	7.65 g	(38% DV)	VItamin A	0 IU	(0% DV)
Poly Fat	2.55 g		Vitamin C	.9 mg	(1% DV)
Mono Fat	10.2 g		Calcium	37.4 mg	(4% DV)
Cholesterol	51 mg	(17% DV)	Iron	1.1 mg	(6% DV)
Sodium	473.5 mg	(20% DV)	Folate	11.9 mcg	(0% DV)
Potassium	180.2 mg	(5% DV)	Beta Carotene	0 RE	

Ratings	Worst	Bad	Average	Good	Best
Weight Loss	2				
LowCal Density		3			
Filling	1				
Energizing		3			
Fiber	1				
Vitamins				5	
Minerals				5	
Overall		3			

BRAZIL NUTS

Serving: 5 kernels (1 oz)   **Snack**

Calories	184	(183.7 cal/oz)	Carbohydrate	3.58 g	(1% DV)
Fat Calories	166	(91% fat)	Dietary Fiber	1.68 g	(7% DV)
Total Fat	18.48 g	(28% DV)	Protein	3.92 g	(8% DV)
Saturated Fat	4.48 g	(22% DV)	VItamin A	0 IU	(0% DV)
Poly Fat	6.72 g		Vitamin C	.3 mg	(0% DV)
Mono Fat	6.44 g		Calcium	49.3 mg	(5% DV)
Cholesterol	0 mg	(0% DV)	Iron	1 mg	(5% DV)
Sodium	.6 mg	(0% DV)	Folate	3.9 mcg	(0% DV)
Potassium	168 mg	(5% DV)	Beta Carotene	0 RE	

Ratings	Worst	Bad	Average	Good	Best
Weight Loss	2				
LowCal Density	1				
Filling	1				
Energizing		3			
Fiber				5	
Vitamins			4		
Minerals					6
Overall	2				

BREAD STICKS, HARD

Serving: 1 small stick (4¼" long) (.18 oz)   **Snack**

Calories	21	(118.3 cal/oz)	Carbohydrate	3.2 g	(1% DV)
Fat Calories	6	(27% fat)	Dietary Fiber	.1 g	(0% DV)
Total Fat	.65 g	(1% DV)	Protein	.65 g	(1% DV)
Saturated Fat	.15 g	(1% DV)	VItamin A	0 IU	(0% DV)
Poly Fat	.2 g		Vitamin C	0 mg	(0% DV)
Mono Fat	.25 g		Calcium	4.1 mg	(0% DV)
Cholesterol	0 mg	(0% DV)	Iron	.2 mg	(1% DV)
Sodium	29.2 mg	(1% DV)	Folate	.7 mcg	(0% DV)
Potassium	10.8 mg	(0% DV)	Beta Carotene	0 RE	

Ratings	Worst	Bad	Average	Good	Best
Weight Loss					9
LowCal Density	2				
Filling	1				
Energizing		3			
Fiber	2				
Vitamins	2				
Minerals	2				
Overall		4			

BREAD, CINNAMON

Serving: 1 slice (.93 oz)   **Bread**

Calories	69	(74.4 cal/oz)	Carbohydrate	12.84 g	(4% DV)
Fat Calories	9	(14% fat)	Dietary Fiber	.52 g	(2% DV)
Total Fat	1.04 g	(2% DV)	Protein	2.08 g	(4% DV)
Saturated Fat	.26 g	(1% DV)	VItamin A	0 IU	(0% DV)
Poly Fat	.26 g		Vitamin C	0 mg	(0% DV)
Mono Fat	.26 g		Calcium	30.2 mg	(3% DV)
Cholesterol	.3 mg	(0% DV)	Iron	.8 mg	(4% DV)
Sodium	143.3 mg	(6% DV)	Folate	2.1 mcg	(2% DV)
Potassium	30.2 mg	(1% DV)	Beta Carotene	0 RE	

Ratings	Worst	Bad	Average	Good	Best
Weight Loss				8	
LowCal Density		4			
Filling	3				
Energizing			5		
Fiber	3				
Vitamins	3				
Minerals	3				
Overall			5		

BREAD, EGG, CHALAH

Serving: 1 slice (.82 oz)   **Bread**

Calories	75	(91.4 cal/oz)	Carbohydrate	10.99 g	(4% DV)
Fat Calories	23	(30% fat)	Dietary Fiber	.46 g	(2% DV)
Total Fat	2.53 g	(4% DV)	Protein	1.84 g	(4% DV)
Saturated Fat	.46 g	(2% DV)	Vitamin A	33.6 IU	(1% DV)
Poly Fat	1.15 g		Vitamin C	0 mg	(0% DV)
Mono Fat	.69 g		Calcium	26.5 mg	(3% DV)
Cholesterol	22.3 mg	(7% DV)	Iron	.7 mg	(4% DV)
Sodium	119.4 mg	(5% DV)	Folate	1.8 mcg	(3% DV)
Potassium	23.5 mg	(1% DV)	Beta Carotene	0 RE	

Ratings	Worst	Bad	Average	Good	Best
Weight Loss					6
LowCal Density		3			
Filling	2				
Energizing			4		
Fiber		3			
Vitamins		3			
Minerals		3			
Overall			4		

BREAD, FRENCH OR VIENNA

Serving: 1 slice (4¾"x 4"x ½") (.89 oz)   **Bread**

Calories	73	(81.5 cal/oz)	Carbohydrate	13.85 g	(5% DV)
Fat Calories	7	(9% fat)	Dietary Fiber	.75 g	(3% DV)
Total Fat	.75 g	(1% DV)	Protein	2.25 g	(4% DV)
Saturated Fat	.25 g	(1% DV)	Vitamin A	0 IU	(0% DV)
Poly Fat	.25 g		Vitamin C	0 mg	(0% DV)
Mono Fat	.25 g		Calcium	22.5 mg	(2% DV)
Cholesterol	0 mg	(0% DV)	Iron	.7 mg	(4% DV)
Sodium	145 mg	(6% DV)	Folate	2.3 mcg	(2% DV)
Potassium	22.5 mg	(1% DV)	Beta Carotene	0 RE	

Ratings	Worst	Bad	Average	Good	Best
Weight Loss					8
LowCal Density		3			
Filling		3			
Energizing			5		
Fiber		3			
Vitamins		3			
Minerals		3			
Overall			5		

BREAD, FRENCH OR VIENNA, WHOLE WHEAT, NOT 100%

Serving: 1 slice (4¾"x 4"x ½") (.89 oz)   Bread

Calories	68	(76.4 cal/oz)	Carbohydrate	13.07 g	(4% DV)
Fat Calories	7	(10% fat)	Dietary Fiber	1.25 g	(5% DV)
Total Fat	.75 g	(1% DV)	Protein	2.5 g	(5% DV)
Saturated Fat	.25 g	(1% DV)	VItamin A	.3 IU	(0% DV)
Poly Fat	.25 g		Vitamin C	0 mg	(0% DV)
Mono Fat	.25 g		Calcium	11.3 mg	(1% DV)
Cholesterol	0 mg	(0% DV)	Iron	.8 mg	(4% DV)
Sodium	122.5 mg	(5% DV)	Folate	2.5 mcg	(3% DV)
Potassium	54.5 mg	(2% DV)	Beta Carotene	0 RE	

Ratings	Worst	Bad	Average	Good	Best
Weight Loss					8
LowCal Density		4			
Filling	3				
Energizing		5			
Fiber		5			
Vitamins	3				
Minerals	3				
Overall		5			

BREAD, FRUIT & NUT

Serving: 1 slice (2 oz)   Bread

Calories	217	(108.4 cal/oz)	Carbohydrate	29.57 g	(10% DV)
Fat Calories	91	(42% fat)	Dietary Fiber	1.12 g	(4% DV)
Total Fat	10.08 g	(16% DV)	Protein	3.36 g	(7% DV)
Saturated Fat	2.24 g	(11% DV)	VItamin A	57.7 IU	(1% DV)
Poly Fat	3.36 g		Vitamin C	1.1 mg	(2% DV)
Mono Fat	3.92 g		Calcium	47 mg	(5% DV)
Cholesterol	28.6 mg	(10% DV)	Iron	1 mg	(5% DV)
Sodium	140 mg	(6% DV)	Folate	3.4 mcg	(2% DV)
Potassium	99.7 mg	(3% DV)	Beta Carotene	1.7 RE	

Ratings	Worst	Bad	Average	Good	Best
Weight Loss	2				
LowCal Density	2				
Filling		4			
Energizing			7		
Fiber		4			
Vitamins		4			
Minerals		4			
Overall	3				

54   **Edmund's Food Ratings**

BREAD, GARLIC

Serving: 1 medium slice (1.04 oz)   **Bread**

Calories	100	(96.5 cal/oz)	Carbohydrate	14.07 g	(5% DV)
Fat Calories	34	(34% fat)	Dietary Fiber	.58 g	(2% DV)
Total Fat	3.77 g	(6% DV)	Protein	2.32 g	(5% DV)
Saturated Fat	.87 g	(4% DV)	VItamin A	157.5 IU	(3% DV)
Poly Fat	1.16 g		Vitamin C	0 mg	(0% DV)
Mono Fat	1.45 g		Calcium	23.8 mg	(2% DV)
Cholesterol	0 mg	(0% DV)	Iron	.7 mg	(4% DV)
Sodium	180.4 mg	(8% DV)	Folate	2.3 mcg	(2% DV)
Potassium	27 mg	(1% DV)	Beta Carotene	3.5 RE	

Ratings	Worst	Bad	Average	Good	Best
Weight Loss				5	
LowCal Density		3			
Filling		3			
Energizing				5	
Fiber		3			
Vitamins		3			
Minerals		3			
Overall			4		

BREAD, ITALIAN, GRECIAN, ARMENIAN

Serving: 1 medium slice (.71 oz)   **Bread**

Calories	55	(78 cal/oz)	Carbohydrate	10.34 g	(3% DV)
Fat Calories	5	(10% fat)	Dietary Fiber	.6 g	(2% DV)
Total Fat	.6 g	(1% DV)	Protein	1.8 g	(4% DV)
Saturated Fat	.2 g	(1% DV)	VItamin A	0 IU	(0% DV)
Poly Fat	.4 g		Vitamin C	0 mg	(0% DV)
Mono Fat	0 g		Calcium	16 mg	(2% DV)
Cholesterol	0 mg	(0% DV)	Iron	.6 mg	(3% DV)
Sodium	117 mg	(5% DV)	Folate	1.8 mcg	(1% DV)
Potassium	14.8 mg	(0% DV)	Beta Carotene	0 RE	

Ratings	Worst	Bad	Average	Good	Best
Weight Loss					8
LowCal Density			4		
Filling	2				
Energizing			4		
Fiber		3			
Vitamins		3			
Minerals		3			
Overall				5	

BREAD, LOWFAT, 98% FAT FREE

Serving: 1 slice (.86 oz)   **Bread**

Calories	66	(77.3 cal/oz)	Carbohydrate	12.41 g	(4% DV)
Fat Calories	6	(10% fat)	Dietary Fiber	.72 g	(3% DV)
Total Fat	.72 g	(1% DV)	Protein	2.16 g	(4% DV)
Saturated Fat	.24 g	(1% DV)	VItamin A	0 IU	(0% DV)
Poly Fat	.48 g		Vitamin C	0 mg	(0% DV)
Mono Fat	0 g		Calcium	28.8 mg	(3% DV)
Cholesterol	0 mg	(0% DV)	Iron	.7 mg	(4% DV)
Sodium	140.4 mg	(6% DV)	Folate	2.2 mcg	(2% DV)
Potassium	17.8 mg	(1% DV)	Beta Carotene	0 RE	

Ratings	Worst	Bad	Average	Good	Best
Weight Loss				8	
LowCal Density		4			
Filling		3			
Energizing			5		
Fiber		3			
Vitamins		3			
Minerals		3			
Overall			5		

BREAD, MULTIGRAIN

Serving: 1 regular slice (.93 oz)   **Bread**

Calories	63	(67.7 cal/oz)	Carbohydrate	12.14 g	(4% DV)
Fat Calories	7	(11% fat)	Dietary Fiber	1.56 g	(6% DV)
Total Fat	.78 g	(1% DV)	Protein	2.34 g	(5% DV)
Saturated Fat	.26 g	(1% DV)	VItamin A	.3 IU	(0% DV)
Poly Fat	.26 g		Vitamin C	0 mg	(0% DV)
Mono Fat	.26 g		Calcium	23.7 mg	(2% DV)
Cholesterol	0 mg	(0% DV)	Iron	.7 mg	(4% DV)
Sodium	125.3 mg	(5% DV)	Folate	2.3 mcg	(3% DV)
Potassium	67.1 mg	(2% DV)	Beta Carotene	0 RE	

Ratings	Worst	Bad	Average	Good	Best
Weight Loss				8	
LowCal Density			5		
Filling		3			
Energizing			5		
Fiber			5		
Vitamins		3			
Minerals		3			
Overall			5		

BREAD, MULTIGRAIN, REDUCED CALORIE, HIGH FIBER

Serving: 1 regular slice (.93 oz)   Bread

Calories	53	(56.5 cal/oz)	Carbohydrate	11.54 g	(4% DV)
Fat Calories	5	(9% fat)	Dietary Fiber	3.12 g	(12% DV)
Total Fat	.52 g	(1% DV)	Protein	2.34 g	(5% DV)
Saturated Fat	0 g	(0% DV)	Vitamin A	0 IU	(0% DV)
Poly Fat	.26 g		Vitamin C	0 mg	(0% DV)
Mono Fat	0 g		Calcium	20.8 mg	(2% DV)
Cholesterol	2.6 mg	(1% DV)	Iron	.7 mg	(4% DV)
Sodium	132.6 mg	(6% DV)	Folate	2.3 mcg	(4% DV)
Potassium	45.2 mg	(1% DV)	Beta Carotene	0 RE	

Ratings	Worst	Bad	Average	Good	Best
Weight Loss					9
LowCal Density			5		
Filling		4			
Energizing			5		
Fiber					8
Vitamins		3			
Minerals		4			
Overall			6		

BREAD, NUT

Serving: 1 slice (1.75 oz)   Bread

Calories	169	(96.3 cal/oz)	Carbohydrate	21.66 g	(7% DV)
Fat Calories	71	(42% fat)	Dietary Fiber	.49 g	(2% DV)
Total Fat	7.84 g	(12% DV)	Protein	3.43 g	(7% DV)
Saturated Fat	1.47 g	(7% DV)	Vitamin A	66.6 IU	(1% DV)
Poly Fat	2.94 g		Vitamin C	.5 mg	(1% DV)
Mono Fat	2.45 g		Calcium	64.2 mg	(6% DV)
Cholesterol	29.4 mg	(10% DV)	Iron	.9 mg	(5% DV)
Sodium	139.2 mg	(6% DV)	Folate	3.4 mcg	(2% DV)
Potassium	74 mg	(2% DV)	Beta Carotene	1 RE	

Ratings	Worst	Bad	Average	Good	Best
Weight Loss	2				
LowCal Density		3			
Filling		4			
Energizing				6	
Fiber		3			
Vitamins		3			
Minerals		4			
Overall		3			

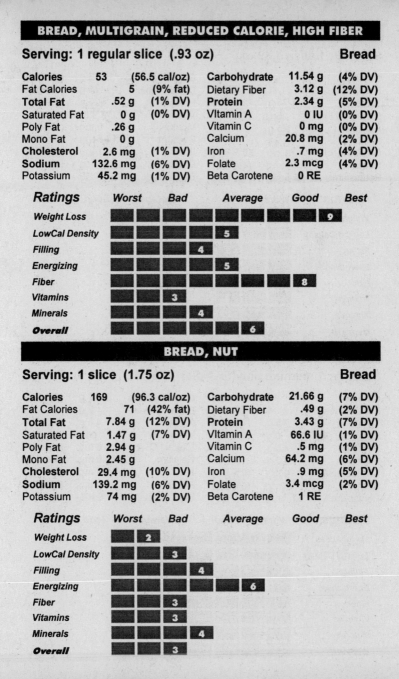

BREAD, OATMEAL

Serving: 1 slice (.89 oz)   **Bread**

Calories	66	(73.6 cal/oz)	Carbohydrate	11.42 g	(4% DV)
Fat Calories	11	(17% fat)	Dietary Fiber	.75 g	(3% DV)
Total Fat	1.25 g	(2% DV)	Protein	2.25 g	(4% DV)
Saturated Fat	.25 g	(1% DV)	Vitamin A	10.3 IU	(0% DV)
Poly Fat	.25 g		Vitamin C	0 mg	(0% DV)
Mono Fat	.5 g		Calcium	10.5 mg	(1% DV)
Cholesterol	.8 mg	(0% DV)	Iron	.7 mg	(4% DV)
Sodium	99 mg	(4% DV)	Folate	2.3 mcg	(2% DV)
Potassium	36.5 mg	(1% DV)	Beta Carotene	.3 RE	

Ratings	Worst	Bad	Average	Good	Best
Weight Loss				7	
LowCal Density		4			
Filling	3				
Energizing		5			
Fiber	3				
Vitamins	3				
Minerals	3				
Overall			5		

BREAD, PITA

Serving: 1 medium pita (5¼" dia) (1.61 oz)   **Bread**

Calories	123	(76.3 cal/oz)	Carbohydrate	24.57 g	(8% DV)
Fat Calories	4	(3% fat)	Dietary Fiber	.9 g	(4% DV)
Total Fat	.45 g	(1% DV)	Protein	4.5 g	(9% DV)
Saturated Fat	0 g	(0% DV)	Vitamin A	0 IU	(0% DV)
Poly Fat	.45 g		Vitamin C	0 mg	(0% DV)
Mono Fat	0 g		Calcium	35.6 mg	(4% DV)
Cholesterol	0 mg	(0% DV)	Iron	1.6 mg	(9% DV)
Sodium	153.9 mg	(6% DV)	Folate	4.5 mcg	(7% DV)
Potassium	52.7 mg	(2% DV)	Beta Carotene	0 RE	

Ratings	Worst	Bad	Average	Good	Best
Weight Loss			6		
LowCal Density		4			
Filling		4			
Energizing			6		
Fiber		4			
Vitamins		4			
Minerals		4			
Overall		5			

BREAD, PITA, WHEAT OR CRACKED WHEAT

Serving: 1 medium pita (5¼" dia) (1.61 oz)   **Bread**

Calories	123	(76.3 cal/oz)	Carbohydrate	25.11 g	(8% DV)
Fat Calories	4	(3% fat)	Dietary Fiber	2.7 g	(11% DV)
Total Fat	.45 g	(1% DV)	Protein	4.5 g	(9% DV)
Saturated Fat	0 g	(0% DV)	VItamin A	0 IU	(0% DV)
Poly Fat	.45 g		Vitamin C	0 mg	(0% DV)
Mono Fat	0 g		Calcium	8.6 mg	(1% DV)
Cholesterol	0 mg	(0% DV)	Iron	1.6 mg	(9% DV)
Sodium	188.6 mg	(8% DV)	Folate	4.5 mcg	(8% DV)
Potassium	96.3 mg	(3% DV)	Beta Carotene	0 RE	

Ratings	Worst	Bad	Average	Good	Best
Weight Loss				6	
LowCal Density			4		
Filling			4		
Energizing				6	
Fiber				7	
Vitamins			4		
Minerals			4		
Overall			5		

BREAD, PITA, WHOLE WHEAT, 100%

Serving: 1 medium pita (5¼" dia) (1.61 oz)   **Bread**

Calories	118	(73.5 cal/oz)	Carbohydrate	25.16 g	(8% DV)
Fat Calories	4	(3% fat)	Dietary Fiber	4.5 g	(18% DV)
Total Fat	.45 g	(1% DV)	Protein	4.95 g	(10% DV)
Saturated Fat	0 g	(0% DV)	VItamin A	0 IU	(0% DV)
Poly Fat	.45 g		Vitamin C	0 mg	(0% DV)
Mono Fat	0 g		Calcium	12.6 mg	(1% DV)
Cholesterol	0 mg	(0% DV)	Iron	1.5 mg	(8% DV)
Sodium	170.6 mg	(7% DV)	Folate	5 mcg	(8% DV)
Potassium	158.9 mg	(5% DV)	Beta Carotene	0 RE	

Ratings	Worst	Bad	Average	Good	Best
Weight Loss				6	
LowCal Density			4		
Filling			5		
Energizing				6	
Fiber					9
Vitamins			4		
Minerals			5		
Overall			5		

BREAD, POTATO

Serving: 1 regular slice (.93 oz)   **Bread**

Calories	69	(74.4 cal/oz)	Carbohydrate	12.84 g	(4% DV)
Fat Calories	9	(14% fat)	Dietary Fiber	.52 g	(2% DV)
Total Fat	1.04 g	(2% DV)	Protein	2.08 g	(4% DV)
Saturated Fat	.26 g	(1% DV)	Vitamin A	0 IU	(0% DV)
Poly Fat	.26 g		Vitamin C	0 mg	(0% DV)
Mono Fat	.26 g		Calcium	30.2 mg	(3% DV)
Cholesterol	.3 mg	(0% DV)	Iron	.8 mg	(4% DV)
Sodium	143.3 mg	(6% DV)	Folate	2.1 mcg	(2% DV)
Potassium	30.2 mg	(1% DV)	Beta Carotene	0 RE	

Ratings	Worst	Bad	Average	Good	Best
Weight Loss				8	
LowCal Density		4			
Filling	3				
Energizing			5		
Fiber	3				
Vitamins	3				
Minerals	3				
Overall			5		

BREAD, PUMPERNICKEL

Serving: 1 regular slice (.93 oz)   **Bread**

Calories	64	(69.1 cal/oz)	Carbohydrate	12.3 g	(4% DV)
Fat Calories	7	(11% fat)	Dietary Fiber	1.56 g	(6% DV)
Total Fat	.78 g	(1% DV)	Protein	2.34 g	(5% DV)
Saturated Fat	0 g	(0% DV)	Vitamin A	0 IU	(0% DV)
Poly Fat	.26 g		Vitamin C	0 mg	(0% DV)
Mono Fat	0 g		Calcium	21.8 mg	(2% DV)
Cholesterol	0 mg	(0% DV)	Iron	.8 mg	(4% DV)
Sodium	147.9 mg	(6% DV)	Folate	2.3 mcg	(1% DV)
Potassium	118 mg	(3% DV)	Beta Carotene	0 RE	

Ratings	Worst	Bad	Average	Good	Best
Weight Loss				8	
LowCal Density		4			
Filling	3				
Energizing			5		
Fiber			5		
Vitamins	3				
Minerals		4			
Overall			5		

BREAD, RAISIN

Serving: 1 regular slice (.93 oz)   **Bread**

Calories	73	(78.3 cal/oz)	Carbohydrate	13.7 g	(5% DV)
Fat Calories	9	(13% fat)	Dietary Fiber	1.04 g	(4% DV)
Total Fat	1.04 g	(2% DV)	Protein	2.08 g	(4% DV)
Saturated Fat	.26 g	(1% DV)	Vitamin A	0 IU	(0% DV)
Poly Fat	.52 g		Vitamin C	0 mg	(0% DV)
Mono Fat	.52 g		Calcium	27.3 mg	(3% DV)
Cholesterol	0 mg	(0% DV)	Iron	.8 mg	(4% DV)
Sodium	94.9 mg	(4% DV)	Folate	2.1 mcg	(2% DV)
Potassium	60.6 mg	(2% DV)	Beta Carotene	0 RE	

Ratings	Worst	Bad	Average	Good	Best
Weight Loss				8	
LowCal Density		4			
Filling		3			
Energizing			5		
Fiber		4			
Vitamins		3			
Minerals		3			
Overall			5		

BREAD, REDUCED CALORIE, HIGH FIBER, WHITE

Serving: 1 regular slice (1.04 oz)   **Bread**

Calories	59	(56.9 cal/oz)	Carbohydrate	13.14 g	(4% DV)
Fat Calories	5	(9% fat)	Dietary Fiber	2.61 g	(10% DV)
Total Fat	.58 g	(1% DV)	Protein	2.61 g	(5% DV)
Saturated Fat	.29 g	(1% DV)	Vitamin A	0 IU	(0% DV)
Poly Fat	.29 g		Vitamin C	0 mg	(0% DV)
Mono Fat	.29 g		Calcium	40.3 mg	(4% DV)
Cholesterol	0 mg	(0% DV)	Iron	.9 mg	(5% DV)
Sodium	152.5 mg	(6% DV)	Folate	2.6 mcg	(3% DV)
Potassium	50.5 mg	(1% DV)	Beta Carotene	0 RE	

Ratings	Worst	Bad	Average	Good	Best
Weight Loss				8	
LowCal Density			5		
Filling		4			
Energizing			5		
Fiber				7	
Vitamins		3			
Minerals		4			
Overall			6		

BREAD, RYE

Serving: 1 regular slice (.93 oz)   **Bread**

Calories	68	(73 cal/oz)	Carbohydrate	12.66 g	(4% DV)
Fat Calories	7	(10% fat)	Dietary Fiber	1.56 g	(6% DV)
Total Fat	.78 g	(1% DV)	Protein	2.08 g	(4% DV)
Saturated Fat	0 g	(0% DV)	Vitamin A	0 IU	(0% DV)
Poly Fat	.26 g		Vitamin C	0 mg	(0% DV)
Mono Fat	0 g		Calcium	19.5 mg	(2% DV)
Cholesterol	0 mg	(0% DV)	Iron	.7 mg	(4% DV)
Sodium	144.8 mg	(6% DV)	Folate	2.1 mcg	(3% DV)
Potassium	37.7 mg	(1% DV)	Beta Carotene	0 RE	

Ratings	Worst	Bad	Average	Good	Best
Weight Loss					8
LowCal Density		4			
Filling		3			
Energizing			5		
Fiber			5		
Vitamins		3			
Minerals		3			
Overall			5		

BREAD, RYE, REDUCED CALORIE, HIGH FIBER

Serving: 1 regular slice (.93 oz)   **Bread**

Calories	45	(48.6 cal/oz)	Carbohydrate	10.74 g	(4% DV)
Fat Calories	5	(10% fat)	Dietary Fiber	3.12 g	(12% DV)
Total Fat	.52 g	(1% DV)	Protein	2.34 g	(5% DV)
Saturated Fat	0 g	(0% DV)	Vitamin A	0 IU	(0% DV)
Poly Fat	.26 g		Vitamin C	0 mg	(0% DV)
Mono Fat	0 g		Calcium	22.6 mg	(2% DV)
Cholesterol	0 mg	(0% DV)	Iron	.8 mg	(5% DV)
Sodium	158.3 mg	(7% DV)	Folate	2.3 mcg	(4% DV)
Potassium	45.2 mg	(1% DV)	Beta Carotene	0 RE	

Ratings	Worst	Bad	Average	Good	Best
Weight Loss					9
LowCal Density			6		
Filling		4			
Energizing		4			
Fiber				8	
Vitamins		3			
Minerals		4			
Overall			6		

BREAD, SOUR DOUGH

Serving: 1 medium slice (4¾"x 4"x ½") (.89 oz)   **Bread**

Calories	73	(81.5 cal/oz)	Carbohydrate	13.85 g	(5% DV)
Fat Calories	7	(9% fat)	Dietary Fiber	.75 g	(3% DV)
Total Fat	.75 g	(1% DV)	Protein	2.25 g	(4% DV)
Saturated Fat	.25 g	(1% DV)	Vitamin A	0 IU	(0% DV)
Poly Fat	.25 g		Vitamin C	0 mg	(0% DV)
Mono Fat	.25 g		Calcium	22.5 mg	(2% DV)
Cholesterol	0 mg	(0% DV)	Iron	.7 mg	(4% DV)
Sodium	145 mg	(6% DV)	Folate	2.3 mcg	(2% DV)
Potassium	22.5 mg	(1% DV)	Beta Carotene	0 RE	

Ratings	Worst	Bad	Average	Good	Best
Weight Loss				8	
LowCal Density		3			
Filling		3			
Energizing			5		
Fiber		3			
Vitamins		3			
Minerals		3			
Overall			5		

BREAD, SOY

Serving: 1 slice (.93 oz)   **Bread**

Calories	69	(74.4 cal/oz)	Carbohydrate	11.49 g	(4% DV)
Fat Calories	9	(14% fat)	Dietary Fiber	.78 g	(3% DV)
Total Fat	1.04 g	(2% DV)	Protein	3.38 g	(7% DV)
Saturated Fat	.26 g	(1% DV)	Vitamin A	14 IU	(0% DV)
Poly Fat	.26 g		Vitamin C	0 mg	(0% DV)
Mono Fat	.26 g		Calcium	22.9 mg	(2% DV)
Cholesterol	1.3 mg	(0% DV)	Iron	.9 mg	(5% DV)
Sodium	73.8 mg	(3% DV)	Folate	3.4 mcg	(3% DV)
Potassium	109.5 mg	(3% DV)	Beta Carotene	.5 RE	

Ratings	Worst	Bad	Average	Good	Best
Weight Loss				8	
LowCal Density		4			
Filling		3			
Energizing			5		
Fiber		3			
Vitamins		3			
Minerals		4			
Overall			5		

BREAD, SPROUTED WHEAT

Serving: 1 slice (.93 oz)   **Bread**

Calories	68	(73 cal/oz)	Carbohydrate	12.48 g	(4% DV)
Fat Calories	9	(14% fat)	Dietary Fiber	1.3 g	(5% DV)
Total Fat	1.04 g	(2% DV)	Protein	2.34 g	(5% DV)
Saturated Fat	.26 g	(1% DV)	VItamin A	0 IU	(0% DV)
Poly Fat	.52 g		Vitamin C	0 mg	(0% DV)
Mono Fat	.26 g		Calcium	22.9 mg	(2% DV)
Cholesterol	0 mg	(0% DV)	Iron	.7 mg	(4% DV)
Sodium	137.5 mg	(6% DV)	Folate	2.3 mcg	(2% DV)
Potassium	34.8 mg	(1% DV)	Beta Carotene	0 RE	

Ratings	Worst	Bad	Average	Good	Best
Weight Loss				8	
LowCal Density		4			
Filling	3				
Energizing		5			
Fiber		5			
Vitamins	3				
Minerals	3				
Overall		5			

BREAD, WHEAT OR CRACKED WHEAT, REDUCED CALORIE

Serving: 1 regular slice (1 oz)   **Bread**

Calories	53	(53.5 cal/oz)	Carbohydrate	11.56 g	(4% DV)
Fat Calories	3	(5% fat)	Dietary Fiber	3.08 g	(12% DV)
Total Fat	.28 g	(0% DV)	Protein	3.08 g	(6% DV)
Saturated Fat	0 g	(0% DV)	VItamin A	0 IU	(0% DV)
Poly Fat	.28 g		Vitamin C	0 mg	(0% DV)
Mono Fat	0 g		Calcium	25.8 mg	(3% DV)
Cholesterol	0 mg	(0% DV)	Iron	1.3 mg	(7% DV)
Sodium	129.9 mg	(5% DV)	Folate	3.1 mcg	(4% DV)
Potassium	81.2 mg	(2% DV)	Beta Carotene	0 RE	

Ratings	Worst	Bad	Average	Good	Best
Weight Loss					9
LowCal Density			6		
Filling		4			
Energizing		5			
Fiber				8	
Vitamins		4			
Minerals		4			
Overall			6		

BREAD, WHITE

Serving: 1 regular slice (.93 oz)   **Bread**

Calories	69	(74.4 cal/oz)	Carbohydrate	12.84 g	(4% DV)
Fat Calories	9	(14% fat)	Dietary Fiber	.52 g	(2% DV)
Total Fat	1.04 g	(2% DV)	Protein	2.08 g	(4% DV)
Saturated Fat	.26 g	(1% DV)	VItamin A	0 IU	(0% DV)
Poly Fat	.26 g		Vitamin C	0 mg	(0% DV)
Mono Fat	.26 g		Calcium	30.2 mg	(3% DV)
Cholesterol	.3 mg	(0% DV)	Iron	.8 mg	(4% DV)
Sodium	143.3 mg	(6% DV)	Folate	2.1 mcg	(2% DV)
Potassium	30.2 mg	(1% DV)	Beta Carotene	0 RE	

Ratings	Worst	Bad	Average	Good	Best
Weight Loss					8
LowCal Density			4		
Filling		3			
Energizing			5		
Fiber		3			
Vitamins		3			
Minerals		3			
Overall			5		

BREAD, WHOLE WHEAT, 100%

Serving: 1 regular slice (.93 oz)   **Bread**

Calories	63	(68.2 cal/oz)	Carbohydrate	11.78 g	(4% DV)
Fat Calories	9	(15% fat)	Dietary Fiber	1.82 g	(7% DV)
Total Fat	1.04 g	(2% DV)	Protein	2.6 g	(5% DV)
Saturated Fat	.26 g	(1% DV)	VItamin A	0 IU	(0% DV)
Poly Fat	.26 g		Vitamin C	0 mg	(0% DV)
Mono Fat	.26 g		Calcium	25.7 mg	(3% DV)
Cholesterol	0 mg	(0% DV)	Iron	.8 mg	(4% DV)
Sodium	137 mg	(6% DV)	Folate	2.6 mcg	(4% DV)
Potassium	71 mg	(2% DV)	Beta Carotene	0 RE	

Ratings	Worst	Bad	Average	Good	Best
Weight Loss					8
LowCal Density			4		
Filling		3			
Energizing			5		
Fiber			6		
Vitamins		3			
Minerals			4		
Overall			5		

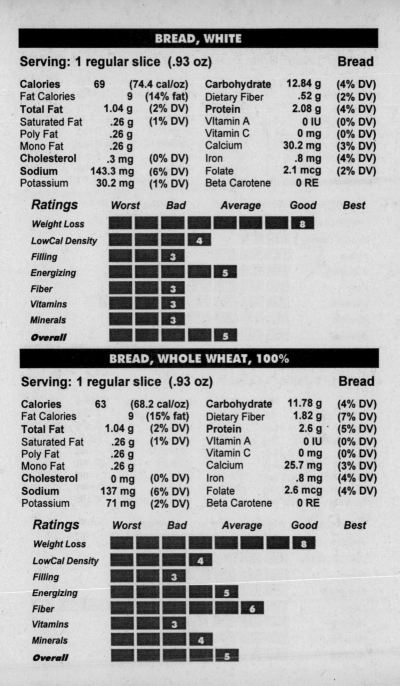

BREAKFAST BAR, CEREAL CRUST, WITH FRUIT FILLING

Serving: 1 Nutri-Grain Bar (1.32 oz)   Snack

Calories	148	(112.1 cal/oz)	Carbohydrate	23.31 g	(8% DV)
Fat Calories	53	(36% fat)	Dietary Fiber	1.11 g	(4% DV)
Total Fat	5.92 g	(9% DV)	Protein	1.85 g	(4% DV)
Saturated Fat	1.48 g	(7% DV)	Vitamin A	652.7 IU	(13% DV)
Poly Fat	.74 g		Vitamin C	0 mg	(0% DV)
Mono Fat	3.33 g		Calcium	25.5 mg	(3% DV)
Cholesterol	0 mg	(0% DV)	Iron	1.6 mg	(9% DV)
Sodium	136.9 mg	(6% DV)	Folate	1.9 mcg	(22% DV)
Potassium	62.9 mg	(2% DV)	Beta Carotene	65.1 RE	

Ratings	Worst	Bad	Average	Good	Best
Weight Loss				5	
LowCal Density	2				
Filling		3			
Energizing				6	
Fiber		4			
Vitamins					8
Minerals		4			
Overall		4			

BREAKFAST BAR, DATE, WITH YOGURT COATING

Serving: 1 Jenny's Cuisine bar (1.61 oz)   Snack

Calories	150	(93.1 cal/oz)	Carbohydrate	27.13 g	(9% DV)
Fat Calories	45	(30% fat)	Dietary Fiber	7.2 g	(29% DV)
Total Fat	4.95 g	(8% DV)	Protein	3.6 g	(7% DV)
Saturated Fat	.9 g	(5% DV)	Vitamin A	17.6 IU	(0% DV)
Poly Fat	2.25 g		Vitamin C	.5 mg	(1% DV)
Mono Fat	1.8 g		Calcium	23 mg	(2% DV)
Cholesterol	0 mg	(0% DV)	Iron	1.1 mg	(6% DV)
Sodium	5 mg	(0% DV)	Folate	3.6 mcg	(3% DV)
Potassium	198.9 mg	(6% DV)	Beta Carotene	1.4 RE	

Ratings	Worst	Bad	Average	Good	Best
Weight Loss				6	
LowCal Density		3			
Filling		4			
Energizing				7	
Fiber					10
Vitamins		4			
Minerals			5		
Overall			5		

BREAKFAST LINK, PATTIE, OR SLICE, MEATLESS

Serving: 1 link (.89 oz)   **Breakfast**

Calories	64	(71.9 cal/oz)	Carbohydrate	2.47 g	(1% DV)
Fat Calories	41	(63% fat)	Dietary Fiber	1 g	(4% DV)
Total Fat	4.5 g	(7% DV)	Protein	4.75 g	(10% DV)
Saturated Fat	.75 g	(4% DV)	Vitamin A	160 IU	(3% DV)
Poly Fat	2.25 g		Vitamin C	0 mg	(0% DV)
Mono Fat	1 g		Calcium	15.8 mg	(2% DV)
Cholesterol	0 mg	(0% DV)	Iron	.9 mg	(5% DV)
Sodium	222 mg	(9% DV)	Folate	4.8 mcg	(2% DV)
Potassium	57.8 mg	(2% DV)	Beta Carotene	16 RE	

Ratings	Worst	Bad	Average	Good	Best
Weight Loss			5		
LowCal Density		4			
Filling	2				
Energizing	3				
Fiber		4			
Vitamins			6		
Minerals		4			
Overall		4			

BREAKFAST PASTRY

Serving: 1 small (1.25 oz)   **Breakfast**

Calories	148	(118.2 cal/oz)	Carbohydrate	15.96 g	(5% DV)
Fat Calories	76	(51% fat)	Dietary Fiber	.35 g	(1% DV)
Total Fat	8.4 g	(13% DV)	Protein	2.45 g	(5% DV)
Saturated Fat	2.45 g	(12% DV)	Vitamin A	37.5 IU	(1% DV)
Poly Fat	1.05 g		Vitamin C	0 mg	(0% DV)
Mono Fat	4.2 g		Calcium	17.5 mg	(2% DV)
Cholesterol	30.1 mg	(10% DV)	Iron	.8 mg	(4% DV)
Sodium	128.1 mg	(5% DV)	Folate	2.5 mcg	(2% DV)
Potassium	39.2 mg	(1% DV)	Beta Carotene	.7 RE	

Ratings	Worst	Bad	Average	Good	Best
Weight Loss			5		
LowCal Density	2				
Filling	2				
Energizing			5		
Fiber	2				
Vitamins		3			
Minerals		3			
Overall		3			

BREAKFAST SAUSAGE, TURKEY, BULK

Serving: 1 patty (1.5 oz)   **Breakfast**

Calories	86	(57.4 cal/oz)	Carbohydrate	0 g	(0% DV)
Fat Calories	38	(44% fat)	Dietary Fiber	0 g	(0% DV)
Total Fat	4.2 g	(6% DV)	Protein	11.76 g	(24% DV)
Saturated Fat	1.26 g	(6% DV)	Vitamin A	0 IU	(0% DV)
Poly Fat	.84 g		Vitamin C	0 mg	(0% DV)
Mono Fat	1.26 g		Calcium	10.9 mg	(1% DV)
Cholesterol	34 mg	(11% DV)	Iron	.7 mg	(4% DV)
Sodium	288.5 mg	(12% DV)	Folate	11.8 mcg	(1% DV)
Potassium	115.9 mg	(3% DV)	Beta Carotene	0 RE	

Ratings	Worst	Bad	Average	Good	Best
Weight Loss					6
LowCal Density			5		
Filling	1				
Energizing	1				
Fiber	1				
Vitamins		3			
Minerals			4		
Overall			4		

BRIOCHE

Serving: 1 piece (2.75 oz)   **Bakery**

Calories	266	(96.9 cal/oz)	Carbohydrate	34.57 g	(12% DV)
Fat Calories	97	(36% fat)	Dietary Fiber	.77 g	(3% DV)
Total Fat	10.78 g	(17% DV)	Protein	7.7 g	(15% DV)
Saturated Fat	2.31 g	(12% DV)	Vitamin A	540.5 IU	(11% DV)
Poly Fat	3.08 g		Vitamin C	0 mg	(0% DV)
Mono Fat	4.62 g		Calcium	30.8 mg	(3% DV)
Cholesterol	75.5 mg	(25% DV)	Iron	2.1 mg	(11% DV)
Sodium	308 mg	(13% DV)	Folate	7.7 mcg	(7% DV)
Potassium	92.4 mg	(3% DV)	Beta Carotene	9.2 RE	

Ratings	Worst	Bad	Average	Good	Best
Weight Loss	2				
LowCal Density		3			
Filling			4		
Energizing					8
Fiber		3			
Vitamins			5		
Minerals			5		
Overall			4		

BROCCOFLOWER, COOKED WITHOUT ADDED FAT

Serving: 1 cup (2.93 oz)   Vegetable

Calories	27	(9.2 cal/oz)	Carbohydrate	5.25 g	(2% DV)
Fat Calories	0	(0% fat)	Dietary Fiber	2.46 g	(10% DV)
Total Fat	0 g	(0% DV)	Protein	2.46 g	(5% DV)
Saturated Fat	0 g	(0% DV)	Vitamin A	53.3 IU	(1% DV)
Poly Fat	0 g		Vitamin C	50 mg	(83% DV)
Mono Fat	0 g		Calcium	25.4 mg	(3% DV)
Cholesterol	0 mg	(0% DV)	Iron	.6 mg	(3% DV)
Sodium	214 mg	(9% DV)	Folate	2.5 mcg	(8% DV)
Potassium	243.5 mg	(7% DV)	Beta Carotene	4.9 RE	

Ratings	Worst	Bad	Average	Good	Best
Weight Loss					10
LowCal Density				9	
Filling			6		
Energizing		3			
Fiber				7	
Vitamins				7	
Minerals			4		
Overall				8	

BROCCOLI CHEESE SOUP, PREPARED WITH MILK

Serving: 1 cup (8.54 oz)   Soup

Calories	174	(20.4 cal/oz)	Carbohydrate	16.49 g	(5% DV)
Fat Calories	86	(49% fat)	Dietary Fiber	2.39 g	(10% DV)
Total Fat	9.56 g	(15% DV)	Protein	7.17 g	(14% DV)
Saturated Fat	4.78 g	(24% DV)	Vitamin A	1061.2 IU	(21% DV)
Poly Fat	2.39 g		Vitamin C	33.5 mg	(56% DV)
Mono Fat	2.39 g		Calcium	167.3 mg	(17% DV)
Cholesterol	16.7 mg	(6% DV)	Iron	1 mg	(5% DV)
Sodium	956 mg	(40% DV)	Folate	7.2 mcg	(7% DV)
Potassium	298.8 mg	(9% DV)	Beta Carotene	71.7 RE	

Ratings	Worst	Bad	Average	Good	Best
Weight Loss		3			
LowCal Density				8	
Filling			6		
Energizing			5		
Fiber			6		
Vitamins			7		
Minerals			6		
Overall			6		

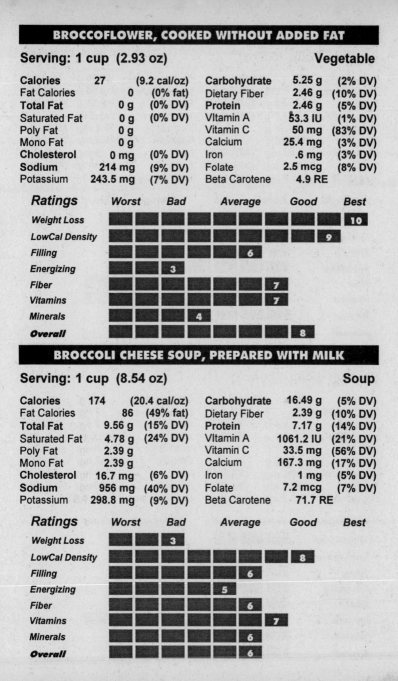

BROCCOLI SALAD, CAULIFLOWER, CHEESE, BACON BITS

Serving: 1 cup (5.5 oz)   Salad

Calories	427	(77.6 cal/oz)	Carbohydrate	16.79 g	(6% DV)
Fat Calories	333	(78% fat)	Dietary Fiber	3.08 g	(12% DV)
Total Fat	36.96 g	(57% DV)	Protein	9.24 g	(18% DV)
Saturated Fat	7.7 g	(39% DV)	Vitamin A	742.3 IU	(15% DV)
Poly Fat	16.94 g		Vitamin C	50.8 mg	(85% DV)
Mono Fat	10.78 g		Calcium	170.9 mg	(17% DV)
Cholesterol	40 mg	(13% DV)	Iron	.9 mg	(5% DV)
Sodium	492.8 mg	(21% DV)	Folate	9.2 mcg	(16% DV)
Potassium	283.4 mg	(8% DV)	Beta Carotene	49.3 RE	

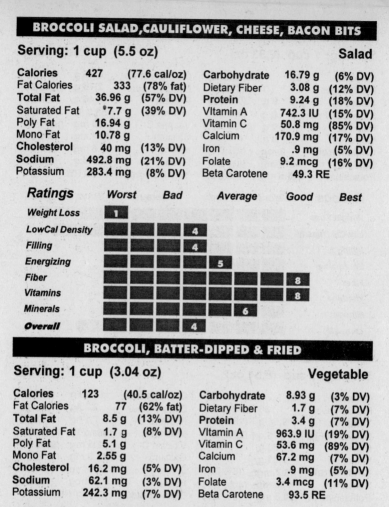

Ratings	Worst	Bad	Average	Good	Best
Weight Loss	1				
LowCal Density		4			
Filling		4			
Energizing			5		
Fiber				8	
Vitamins				8	
Minerals			6		
Overall		4			

BROCCOLI, BATTER-DIPPED & FRIED

Serving: 1 cup (3.04 oz)   Vegetable

Calories	123	(40.5 cal/oz)	Carbohydrate	8.93 g	(3% DV)
Fat Calories	77	(62% fat)	Dietary Fiber	1.7 g	(7% DV)
Total Fat	8.5 g	(13% DV)	Protein	3.4 g	(7% DV)
Saturated Fat	1.7 g	(8% DV)	Vitamin A	963.9 IU	(19% DV)
Poly Fat	5.1 g		Vitamin C	53.6 mg	(89% DV)
Mono Fat	2.55 g		Calcium	67.2 mg	(7% DV)
Cholesterol	16.2 mg	(5% DV)	Iron	.9 mg	(5% DV)
Sodium	62.1 mg	(3% DV)	Folate	3.4 mcg	(11% DV)
Potassium	242.3 mg	(7% DV)	Beta Carotene	93.5 RE	

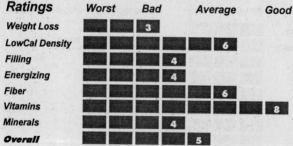

Ratings	Worst	Bad	Average	Good	Best
Weight Loss		3			
LowCal Density			6		
Filling		4			
Energizing		4			
Fiber			6		
Vitamins				8	
Minerals		4			
Overall			5		

BROCCOLI, COOKED WITHOUT ADDED FAT

Serving: 1 cup (6.57 oz)   **Vegetable**

Calories	52	(7.8 cal/oz)	Carbohydrate	9.2 g	(3% DV)
Fat Calories	0	(0% fat)	Dietary Fiber	5.52 g	(22% DV)
Total Fat	0 g	(0% DV)	Protein	5.52 g	(11% DV)
Saturated Fat	0 g	(0% DV)	Vitamin A	2539.2 IU	(51% DV)
Poly Fat	0 g		Vitamin C	136.2 mg	(227% DV)
Mono Fat	0 g		Calcium	84.6 mg	(8% DV)
Cholesterol	0 mg	(0% DV)	Iron	1.5 mg	(9% DV)
Sodium	472.9 mg	(20% DV)	Folate	5.5 mcg	(23% DV)
Potassium	533.6 mg	(15% DV)	Beta Carotene	253.9 RE	

Ratings	Worst	Bad	Average	Good	Best
Weight Loss				9	
LowCal Density					10
Filling					10
Energizing		4			
Fiber				9	
Vitamins					10
Minerals			5		
Overall				9	

BROCCOLI, COOKED, WITH CHEESE SAUCE

Serving: 1 cup (8.14 oz)   **Vegetable**

Calories	219	(26.9 cal/oz)	Carbohydrate	12.54 g	(4% DV)
Fat Calories	123	(56% fat)	Dietary Fiber	4.56 g	(18% DV)
Total Fat	13.68 g	(21% DV)	Protein	11.4 g	(23% DV)
Saturated Fat	6.84 g	(34% DV)	Vitamin A	2590.1 IU	(52% DV)
Poly Fat	2.28 g		Vitamin C	114 mg	(190% DV)
Mono Fat	4.56 g		Calcium	296.4 mg	(30% DV)
Cholesterol	29.6 mg	(10% DV)	Iron	1.5 mg	(9% DV)
Sodium	729.6 mg	(30% DV)	Folate	11.4 mcg	(21% DV)
Potassium	538.1 mg	(15% DV)	Beta Carotene	221.2 RE	

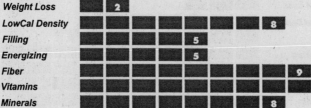

Ratings	Worst	Bad	Average	Good	Best
Weight Loss	2				
LowCal Density				8	
Filling			5		
Energizing			5		
Fiber				9	
Vitamins					10
Minerals				8	
Overall			6		

BRUSSELS SPROUTS, COOKED WITHOUT ADDED FAT

Serving: 1 cup (5.57 oz)   **Vegetable**

Calories	61	(10.9 cal/oz)	Carbohydrate	13.42 g	(4% DV)
Fat Calories	14	(23% fat)	Dietary Fiber	6.24 g	(25% DV)
Total Fat	1.56 g	(2% DV)	Protein	4.68 g	(9% DV)
Saturated Fat	0 g	(0% DV)	Vitamin A	1115.4 IU	(22% DV)
Poly Fat	0 g		Vitamin C	96.7 mg	(161% DV)
Mono Fat	0 g		Calcium	56.2 mg	(6% DV)
Cholesterol	0 mg	(0% DV)	Iron	1.9 mg	(10% DV)
Sodium	388.4 mg	(16% DV)	Folate	4.7 mcg	(23% DV)
Potassium	491.4 mg	(14% DV)	Beta Carotene	112.3 RE	

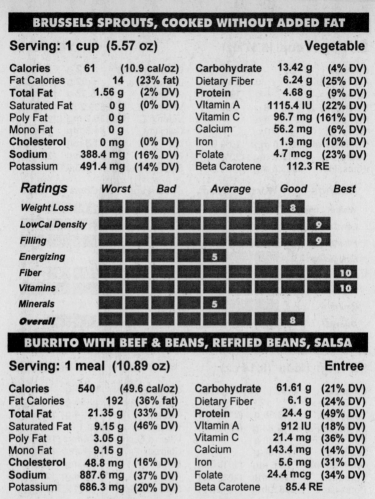

Ratings	Worst	Bad	Average	Good	Best
Weight Loss				8	
LowCal Density					9
Filling					9
Energizing			5		
Fiber					10
Vitamins					10
Minerals			5		
Overall				8	

BURRITO WITH BEEF & BEANS, REFRIED BEANS, SALSA

Serving: 1 meal (10.89 oz)   **Entree**

Calories	540	(49.6 cal/oz)	Carbohydrate	61.61 g	(21% DV)
Fat Calories	192	(36% fat)	Dietary Fiber	6.1 g	(24% DV)
Total Fat	21.35 g	(33% DV)	Protein	24.4 g	(49% DV)
Saturated Fat	9.15 g	(46% DV)	Vitamin A	912 IU	(18% DV)
Poly Fat	3.05 g		Vitamin C	21.4 mg	(36% DV)
Mono Fat	9.15 g		Calcium	143.4 mg	(14% DV)
Cholesterol	48.8 mg	(16% DV)	Iron	5.6 mg	(31% DV)
Sodium	887.6 mg	(37% DV)	Folate	24.4 mcg	(34% DV)
Potassium	686.3 mg	(20% DV)	Beta Carotene	85.4 RE	

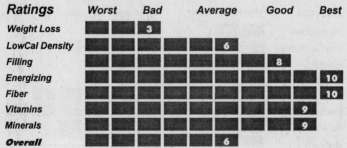

Ratings	Worst	Bad	Average	Good	Best
Weight Loss		3			
LowCal Density			6		
Filling				8	
Energizing					10
Fiber					10
Vitamins				9	
Minerals				9	
Overall			6		

BURRITO WITH CHICKEN & BEANS

Serving: 1 medium burrito (5.07 oz)   Entree

Calories	334	(65.8 cal/oz)	Carbohydrate	38.34 g	(13% DV)
Fat Calories	102	(31% fat)	Dietary Fiber	4.26 g	(17% DV)
Total Fat	11.36 g	(17% DV)	Protein	18.46 g	(37% DV)
Saturated Fat	2.84 g	(14% DV)	VItamin A	19.9 IU	(0% DV)
Poly Fat	2.84 g		Vitamin C	1.4 mg	(2% DV)
Mono Fat	4.26 g		Calcium	69.6 mg	(7% DV)
Cholesterol	36.9 mg	(12% DV)	Iron	3.2 mg	(18% DV)
Sodium	475.7 mg	(20% DV)	Folate	18.5 mcg	(22% DV)
Potassium	387.7 mg	(11% DV)	Beta Carotene	0 RE	

Ratings	Worst	Bad	Average	Good	Best
Weight Loss			5		
LowCal Density			5		
Filling			5		
Energizing					9
Fiber					9
Vitamins			6		
Minerals				7	
Overall			6		

BUTTER REPLACEMENT, FAT-FREE POWDER

Serving: 1 tbsp Molly McButter (.22 oz)   Fat & Oil

Calories	23	(103.4 cal/oz)	Carbohydrate	5.43 g	(2% DV)
Fat Calories	1	(2% fat)	Dietary Fiber	0 g	(0% DV)
Total Fat	.06 g	(0% DV)	Protein	.12 g	(0% DV)
Saturated Fat	.06 g	(0% DV)	VItamin A	0 IU	(0% DV)
Poly Fat	0 g		Vitamin C	0 mg	(0% DV)
Mono Fat	0 g		Calcium	1.4 mg	(0% DV)
Cholesterol	.1 mg	(0% DV)	Iron	.1 mg	(1% DV)
Sodium	73.2 mg	(3% DV)	Folate	.1 mcg	(0% DV)
Potassium	.1 mg	(0% DV)	Beta Carotene	0 RE	

Ratings	Worst	Bad	Average	Good	Best
Weight Loss					9
LowCal Density	2				
Filling	2				
Energizing		3			
Fiber	1				
Vitamins	1				
Minerals	2				
Overall		4			

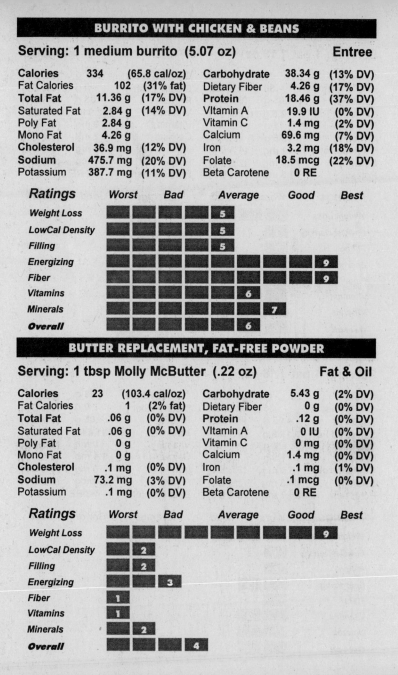

BUTTER, STICK, SALTED

Serving: 1 pat (.18 oz)   **Fat & Oil**

Calories	36	(199.2 cal/oz)	Carbohydrate	.01 g	(0% DV)
Fat Calories	36	(102% fat)	Dietary Fiber	0 g	(0% DV)
Total Fat	4.05 g	(6% DV)	Protein	.05 g	(0% DV)
Saturated Fat	2.5 g	(12% DV)	VItamin A	152.9 IU	(3% DV)
Poly Fat	.15 g		Vitamin C	0 mg	(0% DV)
Mono Fat	1.15 g		Calcium	1.2 mg	(0% DV)
Cholesterol	11 mg	(4% DV)	Iron	0 mg	(0% DV)
Sodium	41.4 mg	(2% DV)	Folate	.1 mcg	(0% DV)
Potassium	1.3 mg	(0% DV)	Beta Carotene	4.2 RE	

Ratings	Worst	Bad	Average	Good	Best
Weight Loss		3			
LowCal Density	1				
Filling	1				
Energizing	2				
Fiber	1				
Vitamins	2				
Minerals	2				
Overall	2				

BUTTER-MARGARINE BLEND

Serving: 1 pat (.18 oz)   **Fat & Oil**

Calories	36	(199.4 cal/oz)	Carbohydrate	.03 g	(0% DV)
Fat Calories	36	(102% fat)	Dietary Fiber	0 g	(0% DV)
Total Fat	4.05 g	(6% DV)	Protein	.05 g	(0% DV)
Saturated Fat	1.65 g	(8% DV)	VItamin A	181.4 IU	(4% DV)
Poly Fat	.7 g		Vitamin C	0 mg	(0% DV)
Mono Fat	1.5 g		Calcium	1.4 mg	(0% DV)
Cholesterol	5.5 mg	(2% DV)	Iron	0 mg	(0% DV)
Sodium	44.3 mg	(2% DV)	Folate	.1 mcg	(0% DV)
Potassium	1.7 mg	(0% DV)	Beta Carotene	4.3 RE	

Ratings	Worst	Bad	Average	Good	Best
Weight Loss		3			
LowCal Density	1				
Filling	1				
Energizing	2				
Fiber	1				
Vitamins	2				
Minerals	2				
Overall	2				

C.W. POST, WITH RAISINS

Serving: 1 cup (3.68 oz)   **Cereal**

Calories	446	(121.2 cal/oz)	Carbohydrate	73.95 g	(25% DV)
Fat Calories	130	(29% fat)	Dietary Fiber	5.15 g	(21% DV)
Total Fat	14.42 g	(22% DV)	Protein	9.27 g	(19% DV)
Saturated Fat	11.33 g	(57% DV)	VItamin A	4541.3 IU	(91% DV)
Poly Fat	1.03 g		Vitamin C	0 mg	(0% DV)
Mono Fat	2.06 g		Calcium	50.5 mg	(5% DV)
Cholesterol	0 mg	(0% DV)	Iron	16.4 mg	(91% DV)
Sodium	160.7 mg	(7% DV)	Folate	9.3 mcg	(91% DV)
Potassium	260.6 mg	(7% DV)	Beta Carotene	0 RE	

Ratings — Worst | Bad | Average | Good | Best

Rating	Value
Weight Loss	2
LowCal Density	2
Filling	6
Energizing	10
Fiber	9
Vitamins	10
Minerals	9
Overall	5

CABBAGE SALAD OR COLESLAW WITH APPLES, RAISINS

Serving: 1 cup (4.71 oz)   **Salad**

Calories	249	(53 cal/oz)	Carbohydrate	19.93 g	(7% DV)
Fat Calories	178	(71% fat)	Dietary Fiber	3.96 g	(16% DV)
Total Fat	19.8 g	(30% DV)	Protein	1.32 g	(3% DV)
Saturated Fat	2.64 g	(13% DV)	VItamin A	171.6 IU	(3% DV)
Poly Fat	10.56 g		Vitamin C	37 mg	(62% DV)
Mono Fat	5.28 g		Calcium	48.8 mg	(5% DV)
Cholesterol	14.5 mg	(5% DV)	Iron	.9 mg	(5% DV)
Sodium	326 mg	(14% DV)	Folate	1.3 mcg	(11% DV)
Potassium	332.6 mg	(10% DV)	Beta Carotene	10.6 RE	

Ratings — Worst | Bad | Average | Good | Best

Rating	Value
Weight Loss	3
LowCal Density	6
Filling	5
Energizing	6
Fiber	9
Vitamins	7
Minerals	4
Overall	5

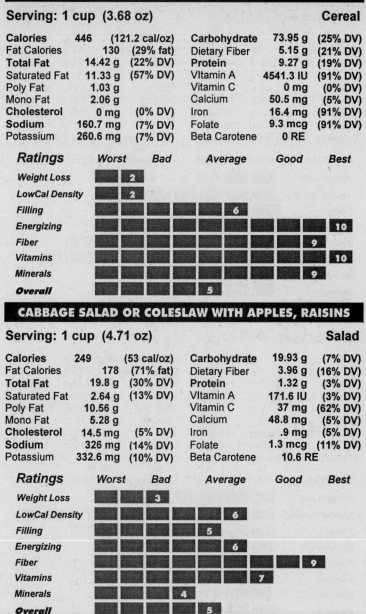

CABBAGE SALAD OR COLESLAW, WITH DRESSING

Serving: 1 cup (6.57 oz)   **Salad**

Calories	250	(38.1 cal/oz)	Carbohydrate	12.7 g	(4% DV)
Fat Calories	199	(79% fat)	Dietary Fiber	3.68 g	(15% DV)
Total Fat	22.08 g	(34% DV)	Protein	1.84 g	(4% DV)
Saturated Fat	3.68 g	(18% DV)	VItamin A	4108.7 IU	(82% DV)
Poly Fat	12.88 g		Vitamin C	55.2 mg	(92% DV)
Mono Fat	5.52 g		Calcium	68.1 mg	(7% DV)
Cholesterol	11 mg	(4% DV)	Iron	.9 mg	(5% DV)
Sodium	677.1 mg	(28% DV)	Folate	1.8 mcg	(17% DV)
Potassium	360.6 mg	(10% DV)	Beta Carotene	404.8 RE	

Ratings	Worst	Bad	Average	Good	Best
Weight Loss	2				
LowCal Density				7	
Filling			5		
Energizing			5		
Fiber				8	
Vitamins					9
Minerals		4			
Overall			5		

CABBAGE SOUP

Serving: 1 cup (8.75 oz)   **Soup**

Calories	51	(5.9 cal/oz)	Carbohydrate	5.64 g	(2% DV)
Fat Calories	22	(43% fat)	Dietary Fiber	2.45 g	(10% DV)
Total Fat	2.45 g	(4% DV)	Protein	2.45 g	(5% DV)
Saturated Fat	0 g	(0% DV)	VItamin A	147 IU	(3% DV)
Poly Fat	0 g		Vitamin C	14.7 mg	(24% DV)
Mono Fat	0 g		Calcium	34.3 mg	(3% DV)
Cholesterol	0 mg	(0% DV)	Iron	.6 mg	(3% DV)
Sodium	551.3 mg	(23% DV)	Folate	2.5 mcg	(5% DV)
Potassium	247.5 mg	(7% DV)	Beta Carotene	7.4 RE	

Ratings	Worst	Bad	Average	Good	Best
Weight Loss				7	
LowCal Density					10
Filling				8	
Energizing		3			
Fiber				7	
Vitamins			5		
Minerals		3			
Overall				7	

CABBAGE, CHINESE, COOKED WITHOUT ADDED FAT

Serving: 1 cup (6.07 oz)   **Vegetable**

Calories	24	(3.9 cal/oz)	Carbohydrate	4.25 g	(1% DV)
Fat Calories	0	(0% fat)	Dietary Fiber	1.7 g	(7% DV)
Total Fat	0 g	(0% DV)	Protein	1.7 g	(3% DV)
Saturated Fat	0 g	(0% DV)	Vitamin A	3082.1 IU	(62% DV)
Poly Fat	0 g		Vitamin C	40.8 mg	(68% DV)
Mono Fat	0 g		Calcium	141.1 mg	(14% DV)
Cholesterol	0 mg	(0% DV)	Iron	1.1 mg	(6% DV)
Sodium	428.4 mg	(18% DV)	Folate	1.7 mcg	(20% DV)
Potassium	494.7 mg	(14% DV)	Beta Carotene	307.7 RE	

Ratings	Worst	Bad	Average	Good	Best
Weight Loss					10
LowCal Density					10
Filling				8	
Energizing		3			
Fiber			6		
Vitamins				9	
Minerals			5		
Overall				9	

CABBAGE, GREEN, COOKED WITHOUT ADDED FAT

Serving: 1 cup (5.36 oz)   **Vegetable**

Calories	32	(5.9 cal/oz)	Carbohydrate	7.05 g	(2% DV)
Fat Calories	0	(0% fat)	Dietary Fiber	4.5 g	(18% DV)
Total Fat	0 g	(0% DV)	Protein	1.5 g	(3% DV)
Saturated Fat	0 g	(0% DV)	Vitamin A	127.5 IU	(3% DV)
Poly Fat	0 g		Vitamin C	36 mg	(60% DV)
Mono Fat	0 g		Calcium	49.5 mg	(5% DV)
Cholesterol	0 mg	(0% DV)	Iron	.6 mg	(3% DV)
Sodium	375 mg	(16% DV)	Folate	1.5 mcg	(8% DV)
Potassium	306 mg	(9% DV)	Beta Carotene	13.5 RE	

Ratings	Worst	Bad	Average	Good	Best
Weight Loss					10
LowCal Density					10
Filling					10
Energizing		4			
Fiber				9	
Vitamins			6		
Minerals		4			
Overall				9	

CABBAGE, RED, COOKED WITHOUT ADDED FAT

Serving: 1 cup (5.36 oz)   **Vegetable**

Calories	32	(5.9 cal/oz)	Carbohydrate	6.9 g	(2% DV)
Fat Calories	0	(0% fat)	Dietary Fiber	3 g	(12% DV)
Total Fat	0 g	(0% DV)	Protein	1.5 g	(3% DV)
Saturated Fat	0 g	(0% DV)	VItamin A	40.5 IU	(1% DV)
Poly Fat	0 g		Vitamin C	51 mg	(85% DV)
Mono Fat	0 g		Calcium	55.5 mg	(6% DV)
Cholesterol	0 mg	(0% DV)	Iron	.5 mg	(3% DV)
Sodium	358.5 mg	(15% DV)	Folate	1.5 mcg	(5% DV)
Potassium	208.5 mg	(6% DV)	Beta Carotene	4.5 RE	

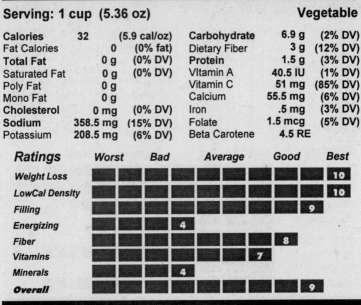

Ratings	Worst	Bad	Average	Good	Best
Weight Loss					10
LowCal Density					10
Filling				9	
Energizing		4			
Fiber				8	
Vitamins			7		
Minerals		4			
Overall				9	

CAESAR DRESSING

Serving: 1 tbsp (.53 oz)   **Fat & Oil**

Calories	78	(146.5 cal/oz)	Carbohydrate	.46 g	(0% DV)
Fat Calories	77	(99% fat)	Dietary Fiber	0 g	(0% DV)
Total Fat	8.53 g	(13% DV)	Protein	.15 g	(0% DV)
Saturated Fat	1.32 g	(7% DV)	VItamin A	3.1 IU	(0% DV)
Poly Fat	3.09 g		Vitamin C	0 mg	(0% DV)
Mono Fat	3.67 g		Calcium	3.5 mg	(0% DV)
Cholesterol	.3 mg	(0% DV)	Iron	0 mg	(0% DV)
Sodium	158.5 mg	(7% DV)	Folate	.2 mcg	(0% DV)
Potassium	4.3 mg	(0% DV)	Beta Carotene	.3 RE	

Ratings	Worst	Bad	Average	Good	Best
Weight Loss	2				
LowCal Density	1				
Filling	1				
Energizing	2				
Fiber	1				
Vitamins	2				
Minerals	2				
Overall	2				

Edmund's Food Ratings

CAESAR DRESSING, LOW-CALORIE

Serving: 1 tbsp (.54 oz)   **Fat & Oil**

Calories	17	(30.6 cal/oz)	Carbohydrate	2.79 g	(1% DV)
Fat Calories	5	(33% fat)	Dietary Fiber	0 g	(0% DV)
Total Fat	.6 g	(1% DV)	Protein	0 g	(0% DV)
Saturated Fat	.15 g	(1% DV)	VItamin A	3.2 IU	(0% DV)
Poly Fat	.3 g		Vitamin C	0 mg	(0% DV)
Mono Fat	.3 g		Calcium	3.6 mg	(0% DV)
Cholesterol	.3 mg	(0% DV)	Iron	0 mg	(0% DV)
Sodium	161.7 mg	(7% DV)	Folate	0 mcg	(0% DV)
Potassium	4.4 mg	(0% DV)	Beta Carotene	.3 RE	

Ratings	Worst	Bad	Average	Good	Best
Weight Loss				8	
LowCal Density			7		
Filling	2				
Energizing	3				
Fiber	1				
Vitamins	2				
Minerals	2				
Overall			5		

CAESAR SALAD (WITH ROMAINE)

Serving: 1 cup (3.86 oz)   **Salad**

Calories	388	(100.4 cal/oz)	Carbohydrate	10.8 g	(4% DV)
Fat Calories	311	(80% fat)	Dietary Fiber	1.08 g	(4% DV)
Total Fat	34.56 g	(53% DV)	Protein	9.72 g	(19% DV)
Saturated Fat	6.48 g	(32% DV)	VItamin A	565.9 IU	(11% DV)
Poly Fat	3.24 g		Vitamin C	8.6 mg	(14% DV)
Mono Fat	22.68 g		Calcium	166.3 mg	(17% DV)
Cholesterol	97.2 mg	(32% DV)	Iron	1.6 mg	(9% DV)
Sodium	616.7 mg	(26% DV)	Folate	9.7 mcg	(10% DV)
Potassium	160.9 mg	(5% DV)	Beta Carotene	40 RE	

Ratings	Worst	Bad	Average	Good	Best
Weight Loss	2				
LowCal Density	2				
Filling	2				
Energizing	4				
Fiber	4				
Vitamins	6				
Minerals	6				
Overall	3				

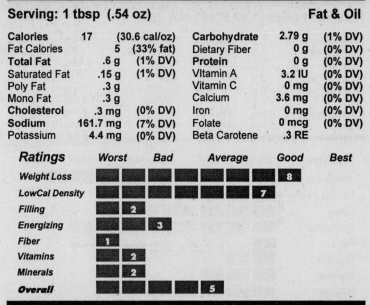

CAKE, ANGEL FOOD, WITHOUT ICING

Serving: 1 piece (1/12 of 10" dia) (2.04 oz)   Dessert

Calories	147	(71.8 cal/oz)	Carbohydrate	33.69 g	(11% DV)
Fat Calories	0	(0% fat)	Dietary Fiber	0 g	(0% DV)
Total Fat	0 g	(0% DV)	Protein	3.42 g	(7% DV)
Saturated Fat	0 g	(0% DV)	VItamin A	0 IU	(0% DV)
Poly Fat	0 g		Vitamin C	0 mg	(0% DV)
Mono Fat	0 g		Calcium	41.6 mg	(4% DV)
Cholesterol	0 mg	(0% DV)	Iron	.3 mg	(2% DV)
Sodium	73 mg	(3% DV)	Folate	3.4 mcg	(1% DV)
Potassium	42.8 mg	(1% DV)	Beta Carotene	0 RE	

Ratings	Worst	Bad	Average	Good	Best
Weight Loss					9
LowCal Density		4			
Filling			5		
Energizing				8	
Fiber	1				
Vitamins	2				
Minerals		3			
Overall			5		

CAKE, APPLESAUCE, WITHOUT ICING

Serving: 1 piece (1/12 of 10" dia) (3.11 oz)   Dessert

Calories	313	(100.7 cal/oz)	Carbohydrate	52.03 g	(17% DV)
Fat Calories	102	(33% fat)	Dietary Fiber	1.74 g	(7% DV)
Total Fat	11.31 g	(17% DV)	Protein	2.61 g	(5% DV)
Saturated Fat	2.61 g	(13% DV)	VItamin A	38.3 IU	(1% DV)
Poly Fat	2.61 g		Vitamin C	.9 mg	(1% DV)
Mono Fat	5.22 g		Calcium	17.4 mg	(2% DV)
Cholesterol	22.6 mg	(8% DV)	Iron	1.4 mg	(8% DV)
Sodium	285.4 mg	(12% DV)	Folate	2.6 mcg	(1% DV)
Potassium	145.3 mg	(4% DV)	Beta Carotene	.9 RE	

Ratings	Worst	Bad	Average	Good	Best
Weight Loss			5		
LowCal Density	2				
Filling			5		
Energizing					10
Fiber			6		
Vitamins		4			
Minerals		4			
Overall		4			

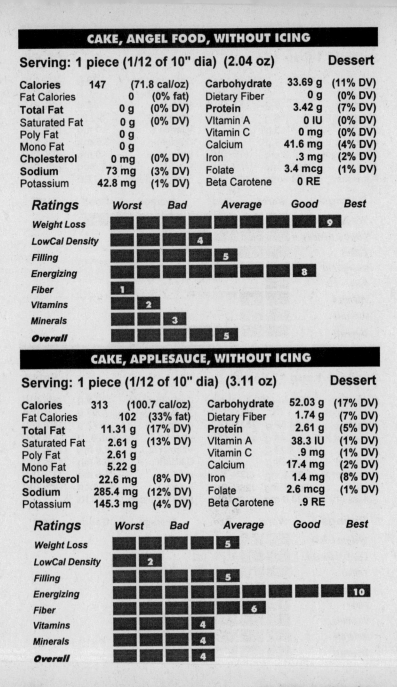

CAKE, BANANA, WITHOUT ICING

Serving: 1 piece (1/12 of 10" dia) (3.11 oz)   **Dessert**

Calories	245	(78.9 cal/oz)	Carbohydrate	43.24 g	(14% DV)
Fat Calories	63	(26% fat)	Dietary Fiber	.87 g	(3% DV)
Total Fat	6.96 g	(11% DV)	Protein	3.48 g	(7% DV)
Saturated Fat	1.74 g	(9% DV)	VItamin A	400.2 IU	(8% DV)
Poly Fat	1.74 g		Vitamin C	3.5 mg	(6% DV)
Mono Fat	3.48 g		Calcium	26.1 mg	(3% DV)
Cholesterol	29.6 mg	(10% DV)	Iron	1 mg	(5% DV)
Sodium	256.7 mg	(11% DV)	Folate	3.5 mcg	(3% DV)
Potassium	185.3 mg	(5% DV)	Beta Carotene	9.6 RE	

Ratings	Worst	Bad	Average	Good	Best
Weight Loss				6	
LowCal Density			4		
Filling			5		
Energizing					9
Fiber			4		
Vitamins			4		
Minerals			4		
Overall			5		

CAKE, BLACK FOREST (CHOCOLATE-CHERRY)

Serving: 1 piece (1/12 of 8- 9" dia) (3.82 oz)   **Dessert**

Calories	282	(73.9 cal/oz)	Carbohydrate	40.66 g	(14% DV)
Fat Calories	125	(44% fat)	Dietary Fiber	2.14 g	(9% DV)
Total Fat	13.91 g	(21% DV)	Protein	2.14 g	(4% DV)
Saturated Fat	4.28 g	(21% DV)	VItamin A	238.6 IU	(5% DV)
Poly Fat	3.21 g		Vitamin C	15 mg	(25% DV)
Mono Fat	5.35 g		Calcium	51.4 mg	(5% DV)
Cholesterol	58.9 mg	(20% DV)	Iron	1.2 mg	(7% DV)
Sodium	240.8 mg	(10% DV)	Folate	2.1 mcg	(2% DV)
Potassium	177.6 mg	(5% DV)	Beta Carotene	10.7 RE	

Ratings	Worst	Bad	Average	Good	Best
Weight Loss		4			
LowCal Density		4			
Filling			5		
Energizing					9
Fiber			6		
Vitamins			5		
Minerals			5		
Overall			5		

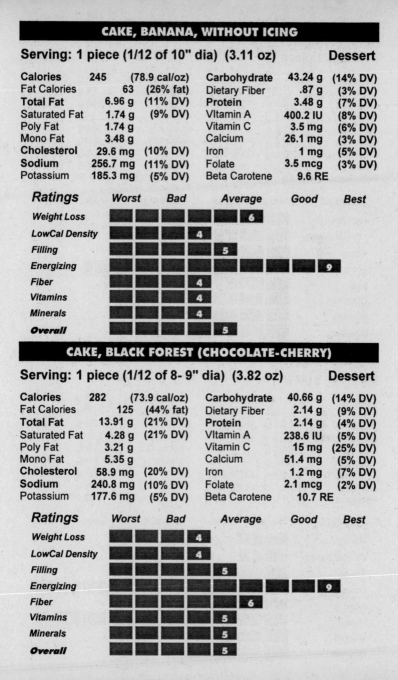

CAKE, BOSTON CREAM PIE

Serving: 1 piece (1/12 of 8" dia) (2.46 oz)   **Dessert**

Calories	225	(91.4 cal/oz)	Carbohydrate	32.36 g	(11% DV)
Fat Calories	87	(39% fat)	Dietary Fiber	.69 g	(3% DV)
Total Fat	9.66 g	(15% DV)	Protein	3.45 g	(7% DV)
Saturated Fat	3.45 g	(17% DV)	Vitamin A	107.6 IU	(2% DV)
Poly Fat	2.07 g		Vitamin C	0 mg	(0% DV)
Mono Fat	4.14 g		Calcium	62.8 mg	(6% DV)
Cholesterol	33.8 mg	(11% DV)	Iron	.9 mg	(5% DV)
Sodium	213.2 mg	(9% DV)	Folate	3.5 mcg	(2% DV)
Potassium	69 mg	(2% DV)	Beta Carotene	2.1 RE	

Ratings	Worst	Bad	Average	Good	Best	
Weight Loss						5
LowCal Density			3			
Filling				4		
Energizing						8
Fiber			3			
Vitamins			3			
Minerals				4		
Overall				4		

CAKE, CARROT, WITH ICING

Serving: 1 piece (1/12 of 8- 9" dia) (4.75 oz)   **Dessert**

Calories	544	(114.5 cal/oz)	Carbohydrate	70.49 g	(23% DV)
Fat Calories	251	(46% fat)	Dietary Fiber	1.33 g	(5% DV)
Total Fat	27.93 g	(43% DV)	Protein	5.32 g	(11% DV)
Saturated Fat	5.32 g	(27% DV)	Vitamin A	6482.4 IU	(130% DV)
Poly Fat	14.63 g		Vitamin C	1.3 mg	(2% DV)
Mono Fat	6.65 g		Calcium	29.3 mg	(3% DV)
Cholesterol	81.1 mg	(27% DV)	Iron	1.6 mg	(9% DV)
Sodium	275.3 mg	(11% DV)	Folate	5.3 mcg	(3% DV)
Potassium	131.7 mg	(4% DV)	Beta Carotene	629.1 RE	

Ratings	Worst	Bad	Average	Good	Best	
Weight Loss	2					
LowCal Density	2					
Filling			5			
Energizing						10
Fiber			5			
Vitamins						9
Minerals			4			
Overall			4			

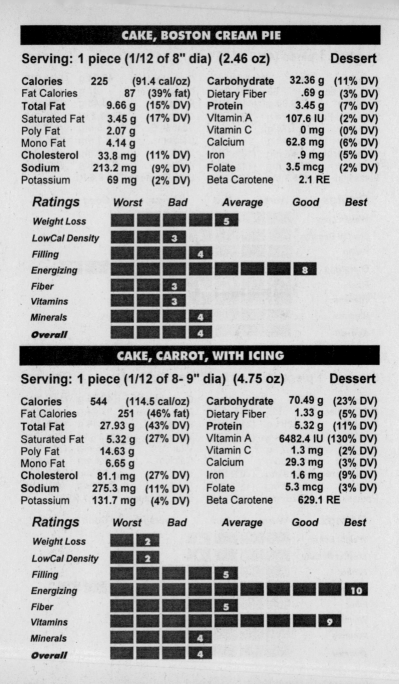

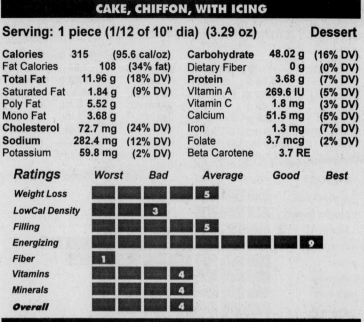

CAKE, CHIFFON, WITH ICING

Serving: 1 piece (1/12 of 10" dia) (3.29 oz)　　　**Dessert**

Calories	315	(95.6 cal/oz)	Carbohydrate	48.02 g	(16% DV)
Fat Calories	108	(34% fat)	Dietary Fiber	0 g	(0% DV)
Total Fat	11.96 g	(18% DV)	Protein	3.68 g	(7% DV)
Saturated Fat	1.84 g	(9% DV)	Vitamin A	269.6 IU	(5% DV)
Poly Fat	5.52 g		Vitamin C	1.8 mg	(3% DV)
Mono Fat	3.68 g		Calcium	51.5 mg	(5% DV)
Cholesterol	72.7 mg	(24% DV)	Iron	1.3 mg	(7% DV)
Sodium	282.4 mg	(12% DV)	Folate	3.7 mcg	(2% DV)
Potassium	59.8 mg	(2% DV)	Beta Carotene	3.7 RE	

Ratings	Worst	Bad	Average	Good	Best
Weight Loss			5		
LowCal Density		3			
Filling			5		
Energizing					9
Fiber	1				
Vitamins		4			
Minerals		4			
Overall		4			

CAKE, CHOCOLATE, DEVIL'S FOOD OR FUDGE, HOME

Serving: 1 piece (1/12 of 8- 9" dia) (3.89 oz)　　　**Dessert**

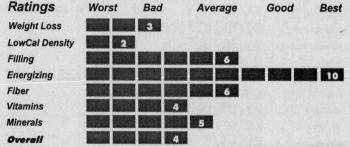

Calories	410	(105.4 cal/oz)	Carbohydrate	66.93 g	(22% DV)
Fat Calories	147	(36% fat)	Dietary Fiber	2.18 g	(9% DV)
Total Fat	16.35 g	(25% DV)	Protein	3.27 g	(7% DV)
Saturated Fat	5.45 g	(27% DV)	Vitamin A	293.2 IU	(6% DV)
Poly Fat	3.27 g		Vitamin C	0 mg	(0% DV)
Mono Fat	6.54 g		Calcium	106.8 mg	(11% DV)
Cholesterol	31.6 mg	(11% DV)	Iron	1.4 mg	(8% DV)
Sodium	296.5 mg	(12% DV)	Folate	3.3 mcg	(1% DV)
Potassium	154.8 mg	(4% DV)	Beta Carotene	5.5 RE	

Ratings	Worst	Bad	Average	Good	Best
Weight Loss		3			
LowCal Density	2				
Filling			6		
Energizing					10
Fiber			6		
Vitamins		4			
Minerals			5		
Overall		4			

CAKE, CHOCOLATE, WITH ICING, DIET

Serving: 1 individual cake (2.54 oz)   **Dessert**

Calories	216	(85 cal/oz)	Carbohydrate	39.76 g	(13% DV)
Fat Calories	51	(24% fat)	Dietary Fiber	2.84 g	(11% DV)
Total Fat	5.68 g	(9% DV)	Protein	5.68 g	(11% DV)
Saturated Fat	2.13 g	(11% DV)	Vitamin A	316.7 IU	(6% DV)
Poly Fat	1.42 g		Vitamin C	0 mg	(0% DV)
Mono Fat	2.84 g		Calcium	61.1 mg	(6% DV)
Cholesterol	34.1 mg	(11% DV)	Iron	2.1 mg	(12% DV)
Sodium	254.2 mg	(11% DV)	Folate	5.7 mcg	(3% DV)
Potassium	292.5 mg	(8% DV)	Beta Carotene	5.7 RE	

Ratings	Worst	Bad	Average	Good	Best
Weight Loss				7	
LowCal Density		3			
Filling			5		
Energizing					9
Fiber				8	
Vitamins			4		
Minerals				6	
Overall				6	

CAKE, FROZEN YOGURT & CAKE LAYER, NOT CHOCOLATE

Serving: 1 piece (1/8 cake) (5.29 oz)   **Dessert**

Calories	404	(76.4 cal/oz)	Carbohydrate	72.67 g	(24% DV)
Fat Calories	93	(23% fat)	Dietary Fiber	1.48 g	(6% DV)
Total Fat	10.36 g	(16% DV)	Protein	5.92 g	(12% DV)
Saturated Fat	2.96 g	(15% DV)	Vitamin A	140.6 IU	(3% DV)
Poly Fat	2.96 g		Vitamin C	0 mg	(0% DV)
Mono Fat	4.44 g		Calcium	170.2 mg	(17% DV)
Cholesterol	37 mg	(12% DV)	Iron	1.2 mg	(7% DV)
Sodium	432.2 mg	(18% DV)	Folate	5.9 mcg	(3% DV)
Potassium	159.8 mg	(5% DV)	Beta Carotene	1.5 RE	

Ratings	Worst	Bad	Average	Good	Best
Weight Loss		4			
LowCal Density		4			
Filling			6		
Energizing					10
Fiber			5		
Vitamins		4			
Minerals			5		
Overall			5		

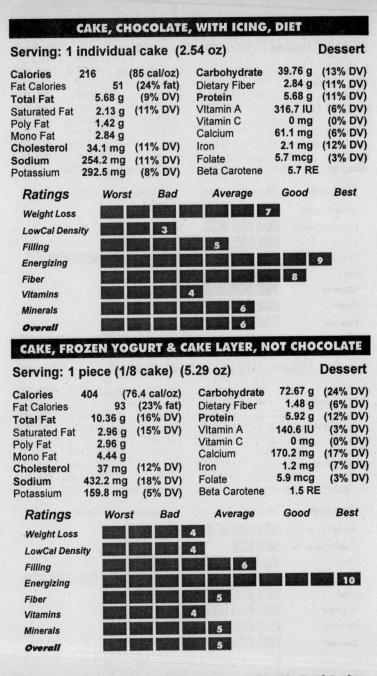

CAKE, GERMAN CHOCOLATE, WITH ICING & FILLING

Serving: 1 piece (1/12 of 8-9" dia) (3.89 oz)   **Dessert**

Calories	376	(96.7 cal/oz)	Carbohydrate	43.16 g	(14% DV)
Fat Calories	196	(52% fat)	Dietary Fiber	1.09 g	(4% DV)
Total Fat	21.8 g	(34% DV)	Protein	5.45 g	(11% DV)
Saturated Fat	6.54 g	(33% DV)	VItamin A	779.4 IU	(16% DV)
Poly Fat	5.45 g		Vitamin C	0 mg	(0% DV)
Mono Fat	8.72 g		Calcium	61 mg	(6% DV)
Cholesterol	70.9 mg	(24% DV)	Iron	1.2 mg	(7% DV)
Sodium	307.4 mg	(13% DV)	Folate	5.5 mcg	(3% DV)
Potassium	139.5 mg	(4% DV)	Beta Carotene	15.3 RE	

Ratings	Worst	Bad	Average	Good	Best
Weight Loss		3			
LowCal Density		3			
Filling			5		
Energizing					9
Fiber		4			
Vitamins			5		
Minerals			5		
Overall			4		

CAKE, GINGERBREAD, WITHOUT ICING

Serving: 1 piece (1/10 of 8" dia) (2.46 oz)   **Dessert**

Calories	216	(87.8 cal/oz)	Carbohydrate	35.19 g	(12% DV)
Fat Calories	68	(32% fat)	Dietary Fiber	.69 g	(3% DV)
Total Fat	7.59 g	(12% DV)	Protein	2.76 g	(6% DV)
Saturated Fat	2.07 g	(10% DV)	VItamin A	40.7 IU	(1% DV)
Poly Fat	2.07 g		Vitamin C	0 mg	(0% DV)
Mono Fat	3.45 g		Calcium	62.8 mg	(6% DV)
Cholesterol	26.9 mg	(9% DV)	Iron	2 mg	(11% DV)
Sodium	131.1 mg	(5% DV)	Folate	2.8 mcg	(2% DV)
Potassium	317.4 mg	(9% DV)	Beta Carotene	0 RE	

Ratings	Worst	Bad	Average	Good	Best
Weight Loss			6		
LowCal Density		3			
Filling			5		
Energizing				8	
Fiber		3			
Vitamins		4			
Minerals			5		
Overall			5		

CAKE, ICE CREAM & CAKE ROLL, CHOCOLATE

Serving: 1 cup (4.93 oz)   **Dessert**

Calories	413	(83.7 cal/oz)	Carbohydrate	55.34 g	(18% DV)
Fat Calories	186	(45% fat)	Dietary Fiber	1.38 g	(6% DV)
Total Fat	20.7 g	(32% DV)	Protein	5.52 g	(11% DV)
Saturated Fat	8.28 g	(41% DV)	Vitamin A	310.5 IU	(6% DV)
Poly Fat	2.76 g		Vitamin C	0 mg	(0% DV)
Mono Fat	6.9 g		Calcium	175.3 mg	(18% DV)
Cholesterol	63.5 mg	(21% DV)	Iron	1.9 mg	(11% DV)
Sodium	278.8 mg	(12% DV)	Folate	5.5 mcg	(2% DV)
Potassium	230.5 mg	(7% DV)	Beta Carotene	6.9 RE	

Ratings	Worst	Bad	Average	Good	Best
Weight Loss		3			
LowCal Density		3			
Filling			6		
Energizing					10
Fiber			5		
Vitamins		4			
Minerals			6		
Overall		4			

CAKE, JELLY ROLL

Serving: 1 piece (1/10 of roll) (1.82 oz)   **Dessert**

Calories	147	(80.7 cal/oz)	Carbohydrate	28.46 g	(9% DV)
Fat Calories	18	(13% fat)	Dietary Fiber	0 g	(0% DV)
Total Fat	2.04 g	(3% DV)	Protein	3.57 g	(7% DV)
Saturated Fat	.51 g	(3% DV)	Vitamin A	140.8 IU	(3% DV)
Poly Fat	.51 g		Vitamin C	1.5 mg	(3% DV)
Mono Fat	1.02 g		Calcium	12.8 mg	(1% DV)
Cholesterol	93.3 mg	(31% DV)	Iron	1 mg	(5% DV)
Sodium	89.3 mg	(4% DV)	Folate	3.6 mcg	(2% DV)
Potassium	43.4 mg	(1% DV)	Beta Carotene	0 RE	

Ratings	Worst	Bad	Average	Good	Best
Weight Loss				8	
LowCal Density		3			
Filling		4			
Energizing				7	
Fiber	1				
Vitamins		3			
Minerals		3			
Overall			5		

CAKE, LEMON, LOWFAT, WITH ICING

Serving: 1 piece (1/12 of 8- 9" dia) (3.89 oz)   **Dessert**

Calories	378	(97.2 cal/oz)	Carbohydrate	69.32 g	(23% DV)
Fat Calories	88	(23% fat)	Dietary Fiber	0 g	(0% DV)
Total Fat	9.81 g	(15% DV)	Protein	3.27 g	(7% DV)
Saturated Fat	2.18 g	(11% DV)	VItamin A	284.5 IU	(6% DV)
Poly Fat	2.18 g		Vitamin C	0 mg	(0% DV)
Mono Fat	5.45 g		Calcium	65.4 mg	(7% DV)
Cholesterol	39.2 mg	(13% DV)	Iron	.9 mg	(5% DV)
Sodium	429.5 mg	(18% DV)	Folate	3.3 mcg	(2% DV)
Potassium	48 mg	(1% DV)	Beta Carotene	4.4 RE	

Ratings	Worst	Bad	Average	Good	Best
Weight Loss			5		
LowCal Density		3			
Filling			6		
Energizing					10
Fiber	1				
Vitamins			4		
Minerals			4		
Overall			5		

CAKE, LEMON, WITH ICING

Serving: 1 piece (1/12 of 8- 9" dia) (3.89 oz)   **Dessert**

Calories	388	(99.8 cal/oz)	Carbohydrate	70.31 g	(23% DV)
Fat Calories	98	(25% fat)	Dietary Fiber	1.09 g	(4% DV)
Total Fat	10.9 g	(17% DV)	Protein	3.27 g	(7% DV)
Saturated Fat	2.18 g	(11% DV)	VItamin A	298.7 IU	(6% DV)
Poly Fat	2.18 g		Vitamin C	1.1 mg	(2% DV)
Mono Fat	5.45 g		Calcium	69.8 mg	(7% DV)
Cholesterol	33.8 mg	(11% DV)	Iron	.9 mg	(5% DV)
Sodium	248.5 mg	(10% DV)	Folate	3.3 mcg	(2% DV)
Potassium	54.5 mg	(2% DV)	Beta Carotene	5.5 RE	

Ratings	Worst	Bad	Average	Good	Best
Weight Loss		4			
LowCal Density		3			
Filling			6		
Energizing					10
Fiber		4			
Vitamins		4			
Minerals		4			
Overall		4			

CAKE, MARBLE, WITH ICING

Serving: 1 piece (1/12 of 8- 9" dia) (3.89 oz)   **Dessert**

Calories	378	(97.2 cal/oz)	Carbohydrate	64.75 g	(22% DV)
Fat Calories	118	(31% fat)	Dietary Fiber	2.18 g	(9% DV)
Total Fat	13.08 g	(20% DV)	Protein	5.45 g	(11% DV)
Saturated Fat	4.36 g	(22% DV)	Vitamin A	142.8 IU	(3% DV)
Poly Fat	2.18 g		Vitamin C	0 mg	(0% DV)
Mono Fat	5.45 g		Calcium	98.1 mg	(10% DV)
Cholesterol	43.6 mg	(15% DV)	Iron	1.8 mg	(10% DV)
Sodium	247.4 mg	(10% DV)	Folate	5.5 mcg	(3% DV)
Potassium	184.2 mg	(5% DV)	Beta Carotene	2.2 RE	

Ratings	Worst	Bad	Average	Good	Best
Weight Loss		4			
LowCal Density	3				
Filling			6		
Energizing					10
Fiber			6		
Vitamins		4			
Minerals			6		
Overall			5		

CAKE, POPPYSEED, WITHOUT ICING

Serving: 1 piece (1/12 of 10" dia) (3.21 oz)   **Dessert**

Calories	354	(110.2 cal/oz)	Carbohydrate	43.2 g	(14% DV)
Fat Calories	154	(44% fat)	Dietary Fiber	.9 g	(4% DV)
Total Fat	17.1 g	(26% DV)	Protein	6.3 g	(13% DV)
Saturated Fat	6.3 g	(31% DV)	Vitamin A	370.8 IU	(7% DV)
Poly Fat	5.4 g		Vitamin C	.9 mg	(2% DV)
Mono Fat	4.5 g		Calcium	107.1 mg	(11% DV)
Cholesterol	79.2 mg	(26% DV)	Iron	1.7 mg	(9% DV)
Sodium	251.1 mg	(10% DV)	Folate	6.3 mcg	(4% DV)
Potassium	137.7 mg	(4% DV)	Beta Carotene	7.2 RE	

Ratings	Worst	Bad	Average	Good	Best
Weight Loss		4			
LowCal Density	2				
Filling			5		
Energizing					9
Fiber		4			
Vitamins			5		
Minerals			5		
Overall		4			

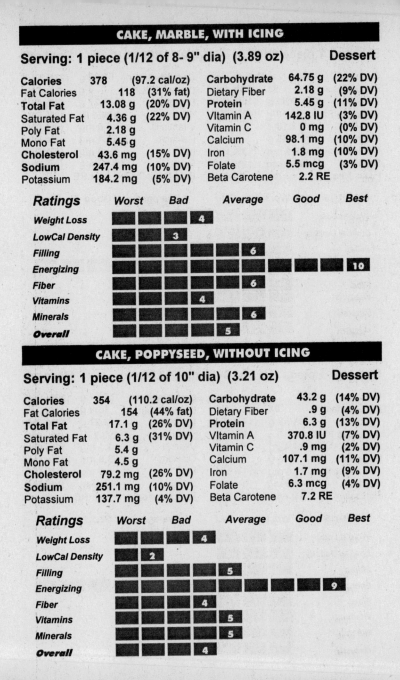

CAKE, POUND, VERY LOW FAT, NO CHOLESTEROL

Serving: 1 slice (3¼"x 2¾"x 5/8") (1 oz) **Dessert**

Calories	78	(78.1 cal/oz)	Carbohydrate	17.36 g	(6% DV)
Fat Calories	0	(0% fat)	Dietary Fiber	.28 g	(1% DV)
Total Fat	0 g	(0% DV)	Protein	1.96 g	(4% DV)
Saturated Fat	0 g	(0% DV)	Vitamin A	36.7 IU	(1% DV)
Poly Fat	0 g		Vitamin C	0 mg	(0% DV)
Mono Fat	0 g		Calcium	36.4 mg	(4% DV)
Cholesterol	.3 mg	(0% DV)	Iron	.3 mg	(2% DV)
Sodium	96.6 mg	(4% DV)	Folate	2 mcg	(1% DV)
Potassium	50.1 mg	(1% DV)	Beta Carotene	0 RE	

Ratings	Worst	Bad	Average	Good	Best
Weight Loss					10
LowCal Density			4		
Filling		3			
Energizing				6	
Fiber	2				
Vitamins	2				
Minerals		3			
Overall			5		

CAKE, POUND, WITHOUT ICING

Serving: 1 piece (1/10 of loaf) (3.25 oz) **Dessert**

Calories	349	(107.2 cal/oz)	Carbohydrate	49.23 g	(16% DV)
Fat Calories	131	(38% fat)	Dietary Fiber	.91 g	(4% DV)
Total Fat	14.56 g	(22% DV)	Protein	6.37 g	(13% DV)
Saturated Fat	3.64 g	(18% DV)	Vitamin A	766.2 IU	(15% DV)
Poly Fat	3.64 g		Vitamin C	0 mg	(0% DV)
Mono Fat	6.37 g		Calcium	51.9 mg	(5% DV)
Cholesterol	116.5 mg	(39% DV)	Iron	2.4 mg	(13% DV)
Sodium	267.5 mg	(11% DV)	Folate	6.4 mcg	(3% DV)
Potassium	79.2 mg	(2% DV)	Beta Carotene	12.7 RE	

Ratings	Worst	Bad	Average	Good	Best
Weight Loss		4			
LowCal Density	2				
Filling			5		
Energizing					9
Fiber		4			
Vitamins			5		
Minerals			5		
Overall		4			

CAKE, SHORTCAKE, BISCUIT TYPE, WITH FRUIT

Serving: 1 biscuit (2" dia) (2.32 oz)   **Dessert**

Calories	146	(63 cal/oz)	Carbohydrate	22.94 g	(8% DV)
Fat Calories	47	(32% fat)	Dietary Fiber	1.3 g	(5% DV)
Total Fat	5.2 g	(8% DV)	Protein	2.6 g	(5% DV)
Saturated Fat	1.3 g	(7% DV)	Vitamin A	34.5 IU	(1% DV)
Poly Fat	1.3 g		Vitamin C	14.3 mg	(24% DV)
Mono Fat	2.6 g		Calcium	70.2 mg	(7% DV)
Cholesterol	0 mg	(0% DV)	Iron	1 mg	(6% DV)
Sodium	167.1 mg	(7% DV)	Folate	2.6 mcg	(2% DV)
Potassium	74.8 mg	(2% DV)	Beta Carotene	.7 RE	

Ratings	Worst	Bad	Average	Good	Best
Weight Loss					7
LowCal Density			5		
Filling		4			
Energizing				6	
Fiber			5		
Vitamins			5		
Minerals		4			
Overall			5		

CAKE, SHORTCAKE, WHIPPED TOPPING & FRUIT, DIET

Serving: 1 individual (3.04 oz)   **Dessert**

Calories	161	(52.8 cal/oz)	Carbohydrate	29.5 g	(10% DV)
Fat Calories	38	(24% fat)	Dietary Fiber	.85 g	(3% DV)
Total Fat	4.25 g	(7% DV)	Protein	2.55 g	(5% DV)
Saturated Fat	1.7 g	(8% DV)	Vitamin A	23.8 IU	(0% DV)
Poly Fat	1.7 g		Vitamin C	13.6 mg	(23% DV)
Mono Fat	.85 g		Calcium	75.7 mg	(8% DV)
Cholesterol	8.5 mg	(3% DV)	Iron	1.1 mg	(6% DV)
Sodium	119.9 mg	(5% DV)	Folate	2.6 mcg	(3% DV)
Potassium	208.3 mg	(6% DV)	Beta Carotene	1.7 RE	

Ratings	Worst	Bad	Average	Good	Best
Weight Loss				7	
LowCal Density				6	
Filling			5		
Energizing				7	
Fiber		4			
Vitamins			5		
Minerals		4			
Overall				6	

CAKE, SPICE, WITH ICING

Serving: 1 piece (1/12 of 8-9" dia) (3.89 oz)   **Dessert**

Calories	374	(96.1 cal/oz)	Carbohydrate	65.18 g	(22% DV)
Fat Calories	98	(26% fat)	Dietary Fiber	1.09 g	(4% DV)
Total Fat	10.9 g	(17% DV)	Protein	4.36 g	(9% DV)
Saturated Fat	4.36 g	(22% DV)	VItamin A	143.9 IU	(3% DV)
Poly Fat	1.09 g		Vitamin C	0 mg	(0% DV)
Mono Fat	5.45 g		Calcium	77.4 mg	(8% DV)
Cholesterol	48 mg	(16% DV)	Iron	1.6 mg	(9% DV)
Sodium	270.3 mg	(11% DV)	Folate	4.4 mcg	(2% DV)
Potassium	150.4 mg	(4% DV)	Beta Carotene	1.1 RE	

Ratings	Worst	Bad	Average	Good	Best
Weight Loss			5		
LowCal Density		3			
Filling			6		
Energizing					10
Fiber		4			
Vitamins		4			
Minerals			5		
Overall			5		

CAKE, TORTE

Serving: 1 piece (1/12 of torte) (2.71 oz)   **Dessert**

Calories	223	(82.5 cal/oz)	Carbohydrate	28.8 g	(10% DV)
Fat Calories	103	(46% fat)	Dietary Fiber	.76 g	(3% DV)
Total Fat	11.4 g	(18% DV)	Protein	3.04 g	(6% DV)
Saturated Fat	4.56 g	(23% DV)	VItamin A	530.5 IU	(11% DV)
Poly Fat	2.28 g		Vitamin C	2.3 mg	(4% DV)
Mono Fat	4.56 g		Calcium	26.6 mg	(3% DV)
Cholesterol	66.9 mg	(22% DV)	Iron	.9 mg	(5% DV)
Sodium	145.2 mg	(6% DV)	Folate	3 mcg	(2% DV)
Potassium	63.1 mg	(2% DV)	Beta Carotene	9.9 RE	

Ratings	Worst	Bad	Average	Good	Best
Weight Loss			5		
LowCal Density		3			
Filling		4			
Energizing				7	
Fiber		3			
Vitamins		4			
Minerals		3			
Overall		4			

CAKE, UPSIDE DOWN (ALL FRUITS)

Serving: 1 piece (1/12 of 8" square) (2.93 oz)   **Dessert**

Calories	253	(86.5 cal/oz)	Carbohydrate	40.18 g	(13% DV)
Fat Calories	89	(35% fat)	Dietary Fiber	.82 g	(3% DV)
Total Fat	9.84 g	(15% DV)	Protein	2.46 g	(5% DV)
Saturated Fat	2.46 g	(12% DV)	VItamin A	308.3 IU	(6% DV)
Poly Fat	2.46 g		Vitamin C	3.3 mg	(5% DV)
Mono Fat	4.92 g		Calcium	61.5 mg	(6% DV)
Cholesterol	23.8 mg	(8% DV)	Iron	1 mg	(5% DV)
Sodium	202.5 mg	(8% DV)	Folate	2.5 mcg	(1% DV)
Potassium	106.6 mg	(3% DV)	Beta Carotene	5.7 RE	

Ratings	Worst	Bad	Average	Good	Best
Weight Loss			5		
LowCal Density		3			
Filling			5		
Energizing					9
Fiber		4			
Vitamins		4			
Minerals		4			
Overall			5		

CAKE, WHITE, EGGLESS, LOWFAT

Serving: 1 piece (1/10 of 8-9" dia) (1.75 oz)   **Dessert**

Calories	166	(94.6 cal/oz)	Carbohydrate	31.21 g	(10% DV)
Fat Calories	35	(21% fat)	Dietary Fiber	.49 g	(2% DV)
Total Fat	3.92 g	(6% DV)	Protein	2.45 g	(5% DV)
Saturated Fat	.49 g	(2% DV)	VItamin A	33.3 IU	(1% DV)
Poly Fat	1.96 g		Vitamin C	0 mg	(0% DV)
Mono Fat	.98 g		Calcium	60.8 mg	(6% DV)
Cholesterol	1 mg	(0% DV)	Iron	.8 mg	(4% DV)
Sodium	163.7 mg	(7% DV)	Folate	2.5 mcg	(1% DV)
Potassium	44.1 mg	(1% DV)	Beta Carotene	.5 RE	

Ratings	Worst	Bad	Average	Good	Best
Weight Loss				8	
LowCal Density		3			
Filling			4		
Energizing				8	
Fiber		3			
Vitamins		3			
Minerals		4			
Overall			5		

CAKE, WHITE, STANDARD-TYPE MIX

Serving: 1 piece (1/10 of 8-9" dia) (2.36 oz)   **Dessert**

Calories	247	(104.6 cal/oz)	Carbohydrate	46.2 g	(15% DV)
Fat Calories	59	(24% fat)	Dietary Fiber	.66 g	(3% DV)
Total Fat	6.6 g	(10% DV)	Protein	1.98 g	(4% DV)
Saturated Fat	1.98 g	(10% DV)	VItamin A	163 IU	(3% DV)
Poly Fat	1.32 g		Vitamin C	0 mg	(0% DV)
Mono Fat	2.64 g		Calcium	48.8 mg	(5% DV)
Cholesterol	0 mg	(0% DV)	Iron	.8 mg	(4% DV)
Sodium	150.5 mg	(6% DV)	Folate	2 mcg	(0% DV)
Potassium	71.9 mg	(2% DV)	Beta Carotene	3.3 RE	

Ratings	Worst	Bad	Average	Good	Best
Weight Loss			6		
LowCal Density	2				
Filling			5		
Energizing					9
Fiber		3			
Vitamins		3			
Minerals		4			
Overall		4			

CAKE, YELLOW, STANDARD-TYPE MIX

Serving: 1 piece (1/10 of 8-9" dia) (2.36 oz)   **Dessert**

Calories	234	(99 cal/oz)	Carbohydrate	42.24 g	(14% DV)
Fat Calories	65	(28% fat)	Dietary Fiber	.66 g	(3% DV)
Total Fat	7.26 g	(11% DV)	Protein	1.98 g	(4% DV)
Saturated Fat	1.98 g	(10% DV)	VItamin A	178.9 IU	(4% DV)
Poly Fat	1.32 g		Vitamin C	0 mg	(0% DV)
Mono Fat	3.3 g		Calcium	44.9 mg	(4% DV)
Cholesterol	19.8 mg	(7% DV)	Iron	.7 mg	(4% DV)
Sodium	172.9 mg	(7% DV)	Folate	2 mcg	(1% DV)
Potassium	66.7 mg	(2% DV)	Beta Carotene	3.3 RE	

Ratings	Worst	Bad	Average	Good	Best
Weight Loss			6		
LowCal Density		3			
Filling			5		
Energizing					9
Fiber		3			
Vitamins		3			
Minerals		4			
Overall			5		

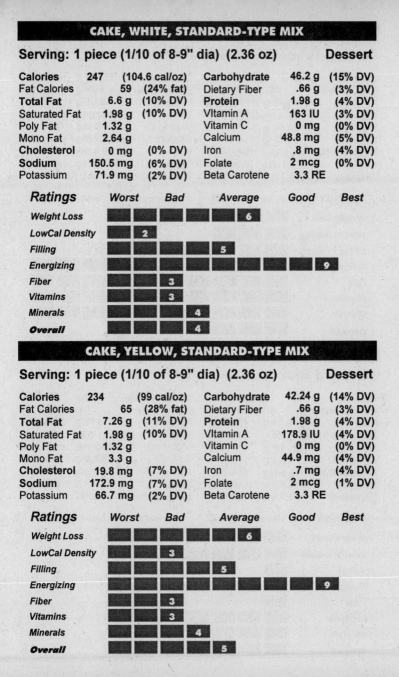

CALZONE, WITH MEAT & CHEESE

Serving: 1 calzone or stromboli (15.14 oz)   **Entree**

Calories	1476	(97.5 cal/oz)	Carbohydrate	131.02 g	(44% DV)
Fat Calories	687	(47% fat)	Dietary Fiber	8.48 g	(34% DV)
Total Fat	76.32 g	(117% DV)	Protein	63.6 g	(127% DV)
Saturated Fat	25.44 g	(127% DV)	Vitamin A	1992.8 IU	(40% DV)
Poly Fat	16.96 g		Vitamin C	0 mg	(0% DV)
Mono Fat	29.68 g		Calcium	771.7 mg	(77% DV)
Cholesterol	190.8 mg	(64% DV)	Iron	10.6 mg	(59% DV)
Sodium	1077 mg	(45% DV)	Folate	63.6 mcg	(67% DV)
Potassium	678.4 mg	(19% DV)	Beta Carotene	38.2 RE	

Ratings	Worst	Bad	Average	Good	Best
Weight Loss	1				
LowCal Density		3			
Filling				8	
Energizing					10
Fiber					10
Vitamins					10
Minerals					10
Overall			5		

CANADIAN BACON, COOKED

Serving: 1 slice (1 oz)   **Meat**

Calories	52	(51.8 cal/oz)	Carbohydrate	.39 g	(0% DV)
Fat Calories	20	(39% fat)	Dietary Fiber	0 g	(0% DV)
Total Fat	2.24 g	(3% DV)	Protein	6.72 g	(13% DV)
Saturated Fat	.84 g	(4% DV)	Vitamin A	0 IU	(0% DV)
Poly Fat	.28 g		Vitamin C	6.2 mg	(10% DV)
Mono Fat	1.12 g		Calcium	2.8 mg	(0% DV)
Cholesterol	16.2 mg	(5% DV)	Iron	.2 mg	(1% DV)
Sodium	432.9 mg	(18% DV)	Folate	6.7 mcg	(0% DV)
Potassium	109.2 mg	(3% DV)	Beta Carotene	0 RE	

Ratings	Worst	Bad	Average	Good	Best
Weight Loss				7	
LowCal Density				6	
Filling	1				
Energizing		2			
Fiber	1				
Vitamins			4		
Minerals		3			
Overall			5		

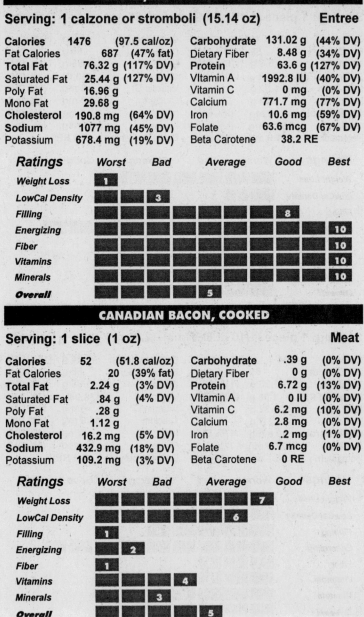

CANNELLONI, CHEESE & SPINACH-FILLED, NO SAUCE

Serving: 3 cannelloni (7.93 oz)   Entree

Calories	349	(44 cal/oz)	Carbohydrate	38.18 g	(13% DV)
Fat Calories	140	(40% fat)	Dietary Fiber	2.22 g	(9% DV)
Total Fat	15.54 g	(24% DV)	Protein	15.54 g	(31% DV)
Saturated Fat	6.66 g	(33% DV)	Vitamin A	4067 IU	(81% DV)
Poly Fat	0 g		Vitamin C	6.7 mg	(11% DV)
Mono Fat	6.66 g		Calcium	242 mg	(24% DV)
Cholesterol	99.9 mg	(33% DV)	Iron	4.1 mg	(23% DV)
Sodium	1216.6 mg	(51% DV)	Folate	15.5 mcg	(22% DV)
Potassium	381.8 mg	(11% DV)	Beta Carotene	373 RE	

Ratings	Worst	Bad	Average	Good	Best
Weight Loss		4			
LowCal Density			6		
Filling			6		
Energizing					9
Fiber			6		
Vitamins					9
Minerals				8	
Overall			6		

CANNELLONI,CHEESE-FILLED

Serving: 1 diet meal (9.25 oz)   Entree

Calories	298	(32.2 cal/oz)	Carbohydrate	24.35 g	(8% DV)
Fat Calories	117	(39% fat)	Dietary Fiber	2.59 g	(10% DV)
Total Fat	12.95 g	(20% DV)	Protein	20.72 g	(41% DV)
Saturated Fat	7.77 g	(39% DV)	Vitamin A	1209.5 IU	(24% DV)
Poly Fat	0 g		Vitamin C	10.4 mg	(17% DV)
Mono Fat	2.59 g		Calcium	269.4 mg	(27% DV)
Cholesterol	41.4 mg	(14% DV)	Iron	1.5 mg	(8% DV)
Sodium	1219.9 mg	(51% DV)	Folate	20.7 mcg	(5% DV)
Potassium	225.3 mg	(6% DV)	Beta Carotene	90.7 RE	

Ratings	Worst	Bad	Average	Good	Best
Weight Loss			5		
LowCal Density				7	
Filling			6		
Energizing			6		
Fiber				7	
Vitamins			6		
Minerals				7	
Overall			6		

CANTALOUPE (MUSKMELON), RAW

Serving: 1 wedge (1/8 melon) (2.46 oz)   Fruit

Calories	24	(9.8 cal/oz)	Carbohydrate	5.8 g	(2% DV)
Fat Calories	0	(0% fat)	Dietary Fiber	.69 g	(3% DV)
Total Fat	0 g	(0% DV)	Protein	.69 g	(1% DV)
Saturated Fat	0 g	(0% DV)	Vitamin A	2224.6 IU	(44% DV)
Poly Fat	0 g		Vitamin C	29 mg	(48% DV)
Mono Fat	0 g		Calcium	7.6 mg	(1% DV)
Cholesterol	0 mg	(0% DV)	Iron	.1 mg	(1% DV)
Sodium	6.2 mg	(0% DV)	Folate	.7 mcg	(3% DV)
Potassium	213.2 mg	(6% DV)	Beta Carotene	222.2 RE	

Ratings	Worst	Bad	Average	Good	Best
Weight Loss					10
LowCal Density					9
Filling			6		
Energizing		3			
Fiber		3			
Vitamins				7	
Minerals	2				
Overall				7	

CAP'N CRUNCH

Serving: 1 cup (1.32 oz)   Cereal

Calories	149	(113.2 cal/oz)	Carbohydrate	31.04 g	(10% DV)
Fat Calories	20	(13% fat)	Dietary Fiber	.74 g	(3% DV)
Total Fat	2.22 g	(3% DV)	Protein	1.85 g	(4% DV)
Saturated Fat	1.48 g	(7% DV)	Vitamin A	52.9 IU	(1% DV)
Poly Fat	.37 g		Vitamin C	0 mg	(0% DV)
Mono Fat	.37 g		Calcium	6.3 mg	(1% DV)
Cholesterol	0 mg	(0% DV)	Iron	6.3 mg	(35% DV)
Sodium	277.9 mg	(12% DV)	Folate	1.9 mcg	(59% DV)
Potassium	47.7 mg	(1% DV)	Beta Carotene	5.2 RE	

Ratings	Worst	Bad	Average	Good	Best
Weight Loss				7	
LowCal Density	2				
Filling		4			
Energizing				8	
Fiber		3			
Vitamins					9
Minerals				7	
Overall			5		

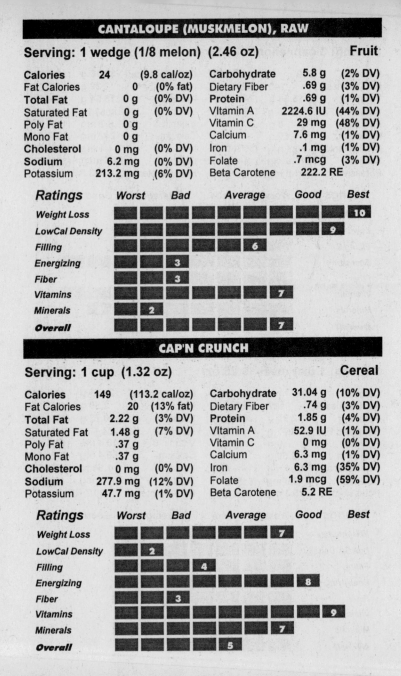

CAPPUCCINO

Serving: 1 mug (9.32 oz)   **Beverage**

Calories	86	(9.2 cal/oz)	Carbohydrate	7.05 g	(2% DV)
Fat Calories	47	(55% fat)	Dietary Fiber	0 g	(0% DV)
Total Fat	5.22 g	(8% DV)	Protein	5.22 g	(10% DV)
Saturated Fat	2.61 g	(13% DV)	Vitamin A	167 IU	(3% DV)
Poly Fat	0 g		Vitamin C	0 mg	(0% DV)
Mono Fat	0 g		Calcium	167 mg	(17% DV)
Cholesterol	18.3 mg	(6% DV)	Iron	.3 mg	(2% DV)
Sodium	67.9 mg	(3% DV)	Folate	5.2 mcg	(1% DV)
Potassium	271.4 mg	(8% DV)	Beta Carotene	5.2 RE	

Ratings

Rating	Worst — Bad — Average — Good — Best	Score
Weight Loss		4
LowCal Density		9
Filling		6
Energizing		4
Fiber		1
Vitamins		3
Minerals		5
Overall		6

CARAMBOLA (STAR FRUIT), RAW

Serving: 1 medium (3-5/8" long) (3.36 oz)   **Fruit**

Calories	31	(9.2 cal/oz)	Carbohydrate	7.33 g	(2% DV)
Fat Calories	0	(0% fat)	Dietary Fiber	2.82 g	(11% DV)
Total Fat	0 g	(0% DV)	Protein	.94 g	(2% DV)
Saturated Fat	0 g	(0% DV)	Vitamin A	463.4 IU	(9% DV)
Poly Fat	0 g		Vitamin C	19.7 mg	(33% DV)
Mono Fat	0 g		Calcium	3.8 mg	(0% DV)
Cholesterol	0 mg	(0% DV)	Iron	.2 mg	(1% DV)
Sodium	1.9 mg	(0% DV)	Folate	.9 mcg	(3% DV)
Potassium	153.2 mg	(4% DV)	Beta Carotene	46.1 RE	

Ratings

Rating	Worst — Bad — Average — Good — Best	Score
Weight Loss		10
LowCal Density		9
Filling		7
Energizing		4
Fiber		8
Vitamins		5
Minerals		2
Overall		8

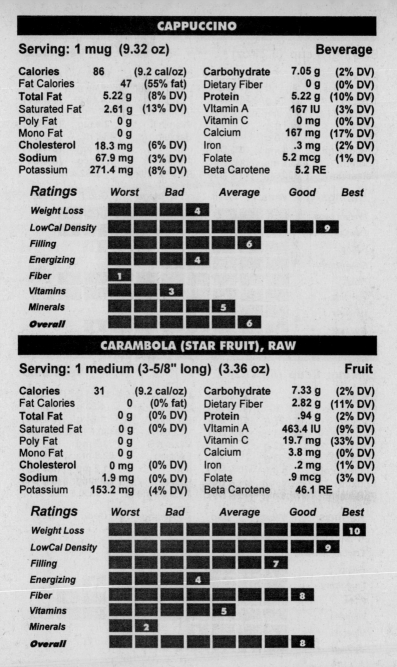

CARROTS, COOKED WITHOUT ADDED FAT

Serving: 1 cup (5.21 oz)   **Vegetable**

Calories	66	(12.6 cal/oz)	Carbohydrate	15.18 g	(5% DV)
Fat Calories	0	(0% fat)	Dietary Fiber	4.38 g	(18% DV)
Total Fat	0 g	(0% DV)	Protein	1.46 g	(3% DV)
Saturated Fat	0 g	(0% DV)	VItamin A	35635.7 IU	(713% DV)
Poly Fat	0 g		Vitamin C	2.9 mg	(5% DV)
Mono Fat	0 g		Calcium	45.3 mg	(5% DV)
Cholesterol	0 mg	(0% DV)	Iron	.9 mg	(5% DV)
Sodium	433.6 mg	(18% DV)	Folate	1.5 mcg	(5% DV)
Potassium	330 mg	(9% DV)	Beta Carotene	3562.4 RE	

Ratings	Worst	Bad	Average	Good	Best
Weight Loss					9
LowCal Density					9
Filling				8	
Energizing			5		
Fiber					9
Vitamins					10
Minerals		4			
Overall				8	

CARROTS, COOKED, GLAZED

Serving: 1 cup (5.75 oz)   **Vegetable**

Calories	233	(40.6 cal/oz)	Carbohydrate	33.65 g	(11% DV)
Fat Calories	101	(43% fat)	Dietary Fiber	4.83 g	(19% DV)
Total Fat	11.27 g	(17% DV)	Protein	1.61 g	(3% DV)
Saturated Fat	1.61 g	(8% DV)	VItamin A	33460.6 IU	(669% DV)
Poly Fat	3.22 g		Vitamin C	3.2 mg	(5% DV)
Mono Fat	4.83 g		Calcium	62.8 mg	(6% DV)
Cholesterol	0 mg	(0% DV)	Iron	1.2 mg	(7% DV)
Sodium	262.4 mg	(11% DV)	Folate	1.6 mcg	(5% DV)
Potassium	378.4 mg	(11% DV)	Beta Carotene	3300.5 RE	

Ratings	Worst	Bad	Average	Good	Best
Weight Loss	2				
LowCal Density			6		
Filling			6		
Energizing				8	
Fiber					9
Vitamins					10
Minerals		4			
Overall			5		

CARROTS, RAW, SALAD

Serving: 1 cup (6.25 oz)   **Salad**

Calories	418	(66.9 cal/oz)	Carbohydrate	40.77 g	(14% DV)
Fat Calories	268	(64% fat)	Dietary Fiber	5.25 g	(21% DV)
Total Fat	29.75 g	(46% DV)	Protein	1.75 g	(4% DV)
Saturated Fat	5.25 g	(26% DV)	VItamin A	26481 IU	(530% DV)
Poly Fat	15.75 g		Vitamin C	14 mg	(23% DV)
Mono Fat	8.75 g		Calcium	50.8 mg	(5% DV)
Cholesterol	21 mg	(7% DV)	Iron	1.4 mg	(8% DV)
Sodium	246.8 mg	(10% DV)	Folate	1.8 mcg	(4% DV)
Potassium	605.5 mg	(17% DV)	Beta Carotene	2637.3 RE	

Ratings	Worst	Bad	Average	Good	Best
Weight Loss	2				
LowCal Density			5		
Filling			6		
Energizing					9
Fiber					9
Vitamins					10
Minerals			5		
Overall			5		

CASHEW NUTS, DRY ROASTED

Serving: 18 kernels (1 oz)   **Snack**

Calories	161	(160.7 cal/oz)	Carbohydrate	9.16 g	(3% DV)
Fat Calories	116	(72% fat)	Dietary Fiber	.84 g	(3% DV)
Total Fat	12.88 g	(20% DV)	Protein	4.2 g	(8% DV)
Saturated Fat	2.52 g	(13% DV)	VItamin A	0 IU	(0% DV)
Poly Fat	2.24 g		Vitamin C	0 mg	(0% DV)
Mono Fat	7.56 g		Calcium	12.6 mg	(1% DV)
Cholesterol	0 mg	(0% DV)	Iron	1.7 mg	(9% DV)
Sodium	179.2 mg	(7% DV)	Folate	4.2 mcg	(5% DV)
Potassium	158.2 mg	(5% DV)	Beta Carotene	0 RE	

Ratings	Worst	Bad	Average	Good	Best
Weight Loss		3			
LowCal Density	1				
Filling	2				
Energizing			4		
Fiber			4		
Vitamins		3			
Minerals				6	
Overall		3			

CASHEW NUTS, ROASTED (ASSUME SALTED)

Serving: 18 kernels (1 oz)   **Snack**

Calories	161	(161.3 cal/oz)	Carbohydrate	7.98 g	(3% DV)
Fat Calories	121	(75% fat)	Dietary Fiber	1.68 g	(7% DV)
Total Fat	**13.44 g**	**(21% DV)**	**Protein**	**4.48 g**	**(9% DV)**
Saturated Fat	2.8 g	(14% DV)	VItamin A	0 IU	(0% DV)
Poly Fat	2.24 g		Vitamin C	0 mg	(0% DV)
Mono Fat	7.84 g		Calcium	11.5 mg	(1% DV)
Cholesterol	0 mg	(0% DV)	Iron	1.2 mg	(6% DV)
Sodium	175.3 mg	(7% DV)	Folate	4.5 mcg	(5% DV)
Potassium	148.4 mg	(4% DV)	Beta Carotene	0 RE	

Ratings	Worst	Bad	Average	Good	Best
Weight Loss		3			
LowCal Density	1				
Filling	2				
Energizing			4		
Fiber				5	
Vitamins		3			
Minerals				5	
Overall		3			

CATFISH, BAKED OR BROILED

Serving: 1 piece (3.04 oz)   **Fish**

Calories	184	(60.4 cal/oz)	Carbohydrate	.51 g	(0% DV)
Fat Calories	107	(58% fat)	Dietary Fiber	0 g	(0% DV)
Total Fat	**11.9 g**	**(18% DV)**	**Protein**	**17 g**	**(34% DV)**
Saturated Fat	2.55 g	(13% DV)	VItamin A	261.8 IU	(5% DV)
Poly Fat	3.4 g		Vitamin C	3.4 mg	(6% DV)
Mono Fat	5.95 g		Calcium	11.9 mg	(1% DV)
Cholesterol	51 mg	(17% DV)	Iron	.6 mg	(3% DV)
Sodium	484.5 mg	(20% DV)	Folate	17 mcg	(3% DV)
Potassium	332.4 mg	(9% DV)	Beta Carotene	4.3 RE	

Ratings	Worst	Bad	Average	Good	Best
Weight Loss			4		
LowCal Density				5	
Filling	1				
Energizing	2				
Fiber	1				
Vitamins				5	
Minerals				5	
Overall			4		

CATFISH, FLOURED OR BREADED, FRIED

Serving: 1 fillet (2.68 oz)   **Fish**

Calories	215	(80.3 cal/oz)	Carbohydrate	9.08 g	(3% DV)
Fat Calories	122	(56% fat)	Dietary Fiber	.75 g	(3% DV)
Total Fat	13.5 g	(21% DV)	Protein	13.5 g	(27% DV)
Saturated Fat	3 g	(15% DV)	Vitamin A	72 IU	(1% DV)
Poly Fat	3 g		Vitamin C	0 mg	(0% DV)
Mono Fat	6 g		Calcium	27 mg	(3% DV)
Cholesterol	60.8 mg	(20% DV)	Iron	1 mg	(5% DV)
Sodium	396.8 mg	(17% DV)	Folate	13.5 mcg	(3% DV)
Potassium	249.8 mg	(7% DV)	Beta Carotene	0 RE	

Ratings	Worst	Bad	Average	Good	Best
Weight Loss		3			
LowCal Density		3			
Filling	2				
Energizing			4		
Fiber		3			
Vitamins				5	
Minerals				5	
Overall		3			

CAULIFLOWER SOUP, CREAM OF, PREPARED WITH MILK

Serving: 1 cup (8.86 oz)   **Soup**

Calories	253	(28.6 cal/oz)	Carbohydrate	16.62 g	(6% DV)
Fat Calories	156	(62% fat)	Dietary Fiber	2.48 g	(10% DV)
Total Fat	17.36 g	(27% DV)	Protein	7.44 g	(15% DV)
Saturated Fat	7.44 g	(37% DV)	Vitamin A	642.3 IU	(13% DV)
Poly Fat	2.48 g		Vitamin C	29.8 mg	(50% DV)
Mono Fat	7.44 g		Calcium	255.4 mg	(26% DV)
Cholesterol	24.8 mg	(8% DV)	Iron	.4 mg	(2% DV)
Sodium	823.4 mg	(34% DV)	Folate	7.4 mcg	(9% DV)
Potassium	448.9 mg	(13% DV)	Beta Carotene	14.9 RE	

Ratings	Worst	Bad	Average	Good	Best
Weight Loss	2				
LowCal Density					8
Filling				6	
Energizing			5		
Fiber				7	
Vitamins				7	
Minerals				6	
Overall				6	

CAULIFLOWER, BATTER-DIPPED, FRIED

Serving: 1 cup (about 3 flowerets) (3.04 oz)   Vegetable

Calories	164	(54 cal/oz)	Carbohydrate	8.41 g	(3% DV)
Fat Calories	115	(70% fat)	Dietary Fiber	1.7 g	(7% DV)
Total Fat	**12.75 g**	**(20% DV)**	**Protein**	**4.25 g**	**(8% DV)**
Saturated Fat	3.4 g	(17% DV)	VItamin A	108 IU	(2% DV)
Poly Fat	5.95 g		Vitamin C	30.6 mg	(51% DV)
Mono Fat	3.4 g		Calcium	108.8 mg	(11% DV)
Cholesterol	19.6 mg	(7% DV)	Iron	.6 mg	(3% DV)
Sodium	156.4 mg	(7% DV)	Folate	4.3 mcg	(7% DV)
Potassium	217.6 mg	(6% DV)	Beta Carotene	2.6 RE	

Ratings	Worst	Bad	Average	Good	Best
Weight Loss	2				
LowCal Density				6	
Filling	3				
Energizing		4			
Fiber				6	
Vitamins				6	
Minerals			5		
Overall		4			

CAULIFLOWER, COOKED WITHOUT ADDED FAT

Serving: 1 cup (5.14 oz)   Vegetable

Calories	33	(6.4 cal/oz)	Carbohydrate	6.34 g	(2% DV)
Fat Calories	0	(0% fat)	Dietary Fiber	2.88 g	(12% DV)
Total Fat	**0 g**	**(0% DV)**	**Protein**	**2.88 g**	**(6% DV)**
Saturated Fat	0 g	(0% DV)	VItamin A	23 IU	(0% DV)
Poly Fat	0 g		Vitamin C	70.6 mg	(118% DV)
Mono Fat	0 g		Calcium	36 mg	(4% DV)
Cholesterol	0 mg	(0% DV)	Iron	.6 mg	(3% DV)
Sodium	345.6 mg	(14% DV)	Folate	2.9 mcg	(17% DV)
Potassium	396 mg	(11% DV)	Beta Carotene	1.4 RE	

Ratings	Worst	Bad	Average	Good	Best
Weight Loss					10
LowCal Density					10
Filling				8	
Energizing		4			
Fiber				8	
Vitamins				8	
Minerals		4			
Overall					9

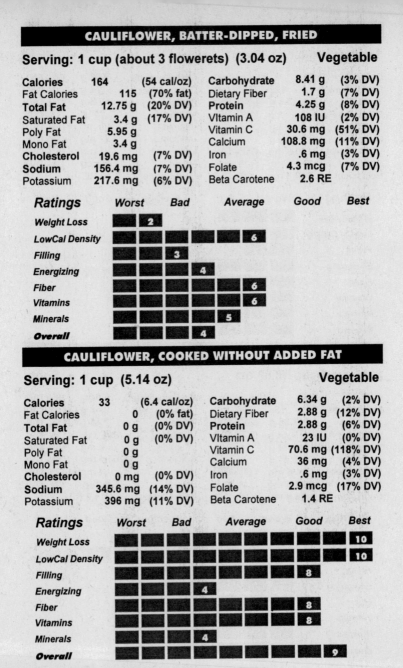

CELERY SOUP, CREAM OF, PREPARED WITH MILK

Serving: 1 cup (8.86 oz)   **Soup**

Calories	164	(18.5 cal/oz)	Carbohydrate	14.63 g	(5% DV)
Fat Calories	89	(55% fat)	Dietary Fiber	0 g	(0% DV)
Total Fat	9.92 g	(15% DV)	Protein	4.96 g	(10% DV)
Saturated Fat	4.96 g	(25% DV)	Vitamin A	461.3 IU	(9% DV)
Poly Fat	2.48 g		Vitamin C	2.5 mg	(4% DV)
Mono Fat	2.48 g		Calcium	186 mg	(19% DV)
Cholesterol	32.2 mg	(11% DV)	Iron	.7 mg	(4% DV)
Sodium	1009.4 mg	(42% DV)	Folate	5 mcg	(2% DV)
Potassium	310 mg	(9% DV)	Beta Carotene	29.8 RE	

Ratings	Worst	Bad	Average	Good	Best
Weight Loss		3			
LowCal Density				8	
Filling			6		
Energizing			5		
Fiber	1				
Vitamins		4			
Minerals			5		
Overall			5		

CELERY, RAW

Serving: 1 small stalk (5" long) (.61 oz)   **Vegetable**

Calories	3	(4.5 cal/oz)	Carbohydrate	.63 g	(0% DV)
Fat Calories	0	(0% fat)	Dietary Fiber	.34 g	(1% DV)
Total Fat	0 g	(0% DV)	Protein	.17 g	(0% DV)
Saturated Fat	0 g	(0% DV)	Vitamin A	22.8 IU	(0% DV)
Poly Fat	0 g		Vitamin C	1.2 mg	(2% DV)
Mono Fat	0 g		Calcium	6.8 mg	(1% DV)
Cholesterol	0 mg	(0% DV)	Iron	.1 mg	(0% DV)
Sodium	14.8 mg	(1% DV)	Folate	.2 mcg	(1% DV)
Potassium	48.8 mg	(1% DV)	Beta Carotene	2.2 RE	

Ratings	Worst	Bad	Average	Good	Best
Weight Loss					10
LowCal Density					10
Filling		3			
Energizing	2				
Fiber	2				
Vitamins	2				
Minerals	2				
Overall				7	

CELERY, STUFFED WITH CHEESE

Serving: 1 small stalk (5" long) (1.14 oz)   **Vegetable**

Calories	44	(38.7 cal/oz)	Carbohydrate	.99 g	(0% DV)
Fat Calories	35	(78% fat)	Dietary Fiber	.32 g	(1% DV)
Total Fat	3.84 g	(6% DV)	Protein	1.92 g	(4% DV)
Saturated Fat	2.24 g	(11% DV)	VItamin A	181.1 IU	(4% DV)
Poly Fat	0 g		Vitamin C	1.6 mg	(3% DV)
Mono Fat	.96 g		Calcium	44.8 mg	(4% DV)
Cholesterol	11.5 mg	(4% DV)	Iron	.2 mg	(1% DV)
Sodium	110.1 mg	(5% DV)	Folate	1.9 mcg	(2% DV)
Potassium	74.9 mg	(2% DV)	Beta Carotene	6.7 RE	

Ratings	Worst	Bad	Average	Good	Best
Weight Loss		4			
LowCal Density				7	
Filling	1				
Energizing	2				
Fiber	2				
Vitamins		3			
Minerals		3			
Overall		4			

CHALUPA WITH BEANS, CHICKEN, CHEESE, VEGETABLE

Serving: 1 chalupa (5.36 oz)   **Entree**

Calories	329	(61.3 cal/oz)	Carbohydrate	21.45 g	(7% DV)
Fat Calories	162	(49% fat)	Dietary Fiber	3 g	(12% DV)
Total Fat	18 g	(28% DV)	Protein	19.5 g	(39% DV)
Saturated Fat	9 g	(45% DV)	VItamin A	661.5 IU	(13% DV)
Poly Fat	1.5 g		Vitamin C	9 mg	(15% DV)
Mono Fat	7.5 g		Calcium	274.5 mg	(27% DV)
Cholesterol	58.5 mg	(20% DV)	Iron	2.1 mg	(12% DV)
Sodium	348 mg	(14% DV)	Folate	19.5 mcg	(20% DV)
Potassium	399 mg	(11% DV)	Beta Carotene	39 RE	

Ratings	Worst	Bad	Average	Good	Best
Weight Loss		4			
LowCal Density			5		
Filling			5		
Energizing			6		
Fiber				8	
Vitamins			6		
Minerals				8	
Overall			5		

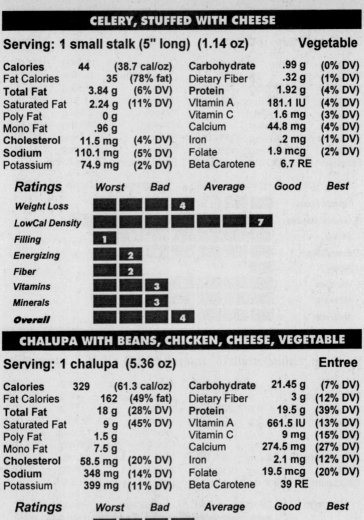

CHEDDAR CHEESE SOUP

Serving: 1 cup (8.96 oz)   **Soup**

Calories	231	(25.8 cal/oz)	Carbohydrate	16.31 g	(5% DV)
Fat Calories	136	(59% fat)	Dietary Fiber	0 g	(0% DV)
Total Fat	15.06 g	(23% DV)	Protein	10.04 g	(20% DV)
Saturated Fat	10.04 g	(50% DV)	VItamin A	1242.5 IU	(25% DV)
Poly Fat	0 g		Vitamin C	2.5 mg	(4% DV)
Mono Fat	5.02 g		Calcium	288.7 mg	(29% DV)
Cholesterol	47.7 mg	(16% DV)	Iron	.8 mg	(4% DV)
Sodium	1019.1 mg	(42% DV)	Folate	10 mcg	(3% DV)
Potassium	341.4 mg	(10% DV)	Beta Carotene	105.4 RE	

Ratings

	Worst	Bad	Average	Good	Best
Weight Loss	2				
LowCal Density				8	
Filling			5		
Energizing			5		
Fiber	1				
Vitamins			5		
Minerals				7	
Overall			5		

CHEERIOS

Serving: 1 cup (1 oz)   **Cereal**

Calories	109	(109.5 cal/oz)	Carbohydrate	19.35 g	(6% DV)
Fat Calories	15	(14% fat)	Dietary Fiber	3.08 g	(12% DV)
Total Fat	1.68 g	(3% DV)	Protein	4.2 g	(8% DV)
Saturated Fat	.28 g	(1% DV)	VItamin A	1234.5 IU	(25% DV)
Poly Fat	.84 g		Vitamin C	14.8 mg	(25% DV)
Mono Fat	.56 g		Calcium	47.9 mg	(5% DV)
Cholesterol	0 mg	(0% DV)	Iron	8 mg	(44% DV)
Sodium	303.2 mg	(13% DV)	Folate	4.2 mcg	(25% DV)
Potassium	100 mg	(3% DV)	Beta Carotene	0 RE	

Ratings

	Worst	Bad	Average	Good	Best
Weight Loss				8	
LowCal Density	2				
Filling		3			
Energizing			6		
Fiber				8	
Vitamins				9	
Minerals			7		
Overall			5		

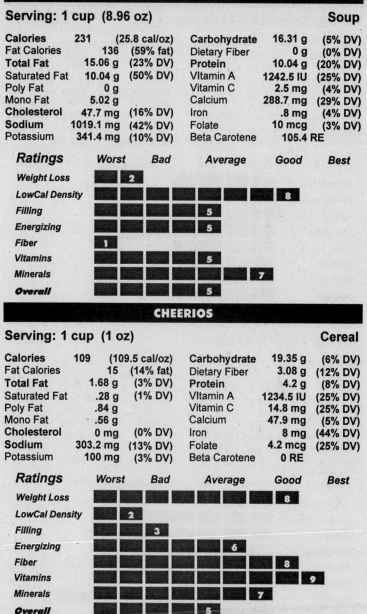

CHEESE SANDWICH, GRILLED

Serving: 1 sandwich (2.96 oz)   **Sandwich**

Calories	304	(102.6 cal/oz)	Carbohydrate	25.4 g	(8% DV)
Fat Calories	157	(52% fat)	Dietary Fiber	.83 g	(3% DV)
Total Fat	17.43 g	(27% DV)	Protein	9.96 g	(20% DV)
Saturated Fat	7.47 g	(37% DV)	Vitamin A	716.3 IU	(14% DV)
Poly Fat	3.32 g		Vitamin C	0 mg	(0% DV)
Mono Fat	6.64 g		Calcium	234.1 mg	(23% DV)
Cholesterol	27.4 mg	(9% DV)	Iron	1.6 mg	(9% DV)
Sodium	764.4 mg	(32% DV)	Folate	10 mcg	(3% DV)
Potassium	107.9 mg	(3% DV)	Beta Carotene	18.3 RE	

Ratings	Worst	Bad	Average	Good	Best
Weight Loss		4			
LowCal Density	2				
Filling		4			
Energizing			6		
Fiber		4			
Vitamins			5		
Minerals				7	
Overall		4			

CHEESE SAUCE

Serving: 1 cup (8.68 oz)   **Sauce**

Calories	267	(30.8 cal/oz)	Carbohydrate	20.17 g	(7% DV)
Fat Calories	131	(49% fat)	Dietary Fiber	0 g	(0% DV)
Total Fat	14.58 g	(22% DV)	Protein	14.58 g	(29% DV)
Saturated Fat	7.29 g	(36% DV)	Vitamin A	340.2 IU	(7% DV)
Poly Fat	2.43 g		Vitamin C	2.4 mg	(4% DV)
Mono Fat	4.86 g		Calcium	495.7 mg	(50% DV)
Cholesterol	46.2 mg	(15% DV)	Iron	.2 mg	(1% DV)
Sodium	1363.2 mg	(57% DV)	Folate	14.6 mcg	(3% DV)
Potassium	481.1 mg	(14% DV)	Beta Carotene	0 RE	

Ratings	Worst	Bad	Average	Good	Best
Weight Loss	2				
LowCal Density					7
Filling			6		
Energizing			6		
Fiber	1				
Vitamins		4			
Minerals					9
Overall			5		

CHEESE SAUCE MADE WITH LOWFAT CHEESE

Serving: 1 cup (8.68 oz)   **Sauce**

Calories	338	(38.9 cal/oz)	Carbohydrate	15.79 g	(5% DV)
Fat Calories	175	(52% fat)	Dietary Fiber	0 g	(0% DV)
Total Fat	19.44 g	(30% DV)	Protein	21.87 g	(44% DV)
Saturated Fat	7.29 g	(36% DV)	Vitamin A	921 IU	(18% DV)
Poly Fat	4.86 g		Vitamin C	2.4 mg	(4% DV)
Mono Fat	7.29 g		Calcium	661 mg	(66% DV)
Cholesterol	43.7 mg	(15% DV)	Iron	1 mg	(5% DV)
Sodium	1550.3 mg	(65% DV)	Folate	21.9 mcg	(4% DV)
Potassium	396.1 mg	(11% DV)	Beta Carotene	21.9 RE	

Ratings	Worst	Bad	Average	Good	Best
Weight Loss	1				
LowCal Density					7
Filling			5		
Energizing			5		
Fiber	1				
Vitamins			5		
Minerals					9
Overall		4			

CHEESE SPREAD, CHEDDAR OR AMERICAN CHEESE

Serving: 2 tbsp (1 oz)   **Cheese**

Calories	81	(81.2 cal/oz)	Carbohydrate	2.44 g	(1% DV)
Fat Calories	53	(65% fat)	Dietary Fiber	0 g	(0% DV)
Total Fat	5.88 g	(9% DV)	Protein	4.48 g	(9% DV)
Saturated Fat	3.64 g	(18% DV)	Vitamin A	220.6 IU	(4% DV)
Poly Fat	.28 g		Vitamin C	0 mg	(0% DV)
Mono Fat	1.68 g		Calcium	157.4 mg	(16% DV)
Cholesterol	15.4 mg	(5% DV)	Iron	.1 mg	(0% DV)
Sodium	376.6 mg	(16% DV)	Folate	4.5 mcg	(0% DV)
Potassium	67.8 mg	(2% DV)	Beta Carotene	6.4 RE	

Ratings	Worst	Bad	Average	Good	Best
Weight Loss			4		
LowCal Density		3			
Filling	1				
Energizing		3			
Fiber	1				
Vitamins	2				
Minerals			5		
Overall		3			

CHEESE, CHEDDAR OR COLBY, LOWFAT

Serving: 1 slice (1 oz)   Cheese

Calories	48	(48.4 cal/oz)	Carbohydrate	.53 g	(0% DV)
Fat Calories	18	(36% fat)	Dietary Fiber	0 g	(0% DV)
Total Fat	1.96 g	(3% DV)	Protein	6.72 g	(13% DV)
Saturated Fat	1.12 g	(6% DV)	Vitamin A	65.2 IU	(1% DV)
Poly Fat	0 g		Vitamin C	0 mg	(0% DV)
Mono Fat	.56 g		Calcium	196.8 mg	(20% DV)
Cholesterol	5.9 mg	(2% DV)	Iron	.2 mg	(1% DV)
Sodium	171.4 mg	(7% DV)	Folate	6.7 mcg	(1% DV)
Potassium	31.4 mg	(1% DV)	Beta Carotene	1.1 RE	

Ratings	Worst	Bad	Average	Good	Best
Weight Loss				7	
LowCal Density				6	
Filling	1				
Energizing	2				
Fiber	1				
Vitamins	2				
Minerals			5		
Overall			5		

CHEESE, COLBY

Serving: 1 slice (1 oz)   Cheese

Calories	110	(110.3 cal/oz)	Carbohydrate	.73 g	(0% DV)
Fat Calories	81	(73% fat)	Dietary Fiber	0 g	(0% DV)
Total Fat	8.96 g	(14% DV)	Protein	6.72 g	(13% DV)
Saturated Fat	5.6 g	(28% DV)	Vitamin A	289.5 IU	(6% DV)
Poly Fat	.28 g		Vitamin C	0 mg	(0% DV)
Mono Fat	2.52 g		Calcium	191.8 mg	(19% DV)
Cholesterol	26.6 mg	(9% DV)	Iron	.2 mg	(1% DV)
Sodium	169.1 mg	(7% DV)	Folate	6.7 mcg	(1% DV)
Potassium	35.6 mg	(1% DV)	Beta Carotene	5 RE	

Ratings	Worst	Bad	Average	Good	Best
Weight Loss		3			
LowCal Density	2				
Filling	1				
Energizing	2				
Fiber	1				
Vitamins	2				
Minerals			5		
Overall	2				

CHEESE, COTTAGE, CREAMED, LARGE OR SMALL CURD

Serving: 1 cup (7.5 oz)   **Cheese**

Calories	216	(28.8 cal/oz)	Carbohydrate	5.67 g	(2% DV)
Fat Calories	95	(44% fat)	Dietary Fiber	0 g	(0% DV)
Total Fat	10.5 g	(16% DV)	Protein	25.2 g	(50% DV)
Saturated Fat	6.3 g	(31% DV)	Vitamin A	342.3 IU	(7% DV)
Poly Fat	0 g		Vitamin C	0 mg	(0% DV)
Mono Fat	2.1 g		Calcium	126 mg	(13% DV)
Cholesterol	31.5 mg	(10% DV)	Iron	.3 mg	(2% DV)
Sodium	850.5 mg	(35% DV)	Folate	25.2 mcg	(6% DV)
Potassium	176.4 mg	(5% DV)	Beta Carotene	4.2 RE	

Ratings	Worst	Bad	Average	Good	Best
Weight Loss	2				
LowCal Density					8
Filling		3			
Energizing		3			
Fiber	1				
Vitamins		3			
Minerals				6	
Overall			4		

CHEESE, COTTAGE, LOWFAT (1-2% FAT)

Serving: 1 cup (8.07 oz)   **Cheese**

Calories	163	(20.2 cal/oz)	Carbohydrate	6.1 g	(2% DV)
Fat Calories	20	(12% fat)	Dietary Fiber	0 g	(0% DV)
Total Fat	2.26 g	(3% DV)	Protein	27.12 g	(54% DV)
Saturated Fat	2.26 g	(11% DV)	Vitamin A	83.6 IU	(2% DV)
Poly Fat	0 g		Vitamin C	0 mg	(0% DV)
Mono Fat	0 g		Calcium	137.9 mg	(14% DV)
Cholesterol	9 mg	(3% DV)	Iron	.3 mg	(2% DV)
Sodium	917.6 mg	(38% DV)	Folate	27.1 mcg	(7% DV)
Potassium	194.4 mg	(6% DV)	Beta Carotene	0 RE	

Ratings	Worst	Bad	Average	Good	Best
Weight Loss		4			
LowCal Density					8
Filling		4			
Energizing		4			
Fiber	1				
Vitamins		3			
Minerals				6	
Overall			5		

Serving: 1 tbsp (.52 oz)   **Cheese**

Calories	51	(97.3 cal/oz)	**Carbohydrate**	.39 g	(0% DV)
Fat Calories	46	(90% fat)	Dietary Fiber	0 g	(0% DV)
Total Fat	5.07 g	(8% DV)	**Protein**	1.16 g	(2% DV)
Saturated Fat	3.19 g	(16% DV)	VItamin A	206.9 IU	(4% DV)
Poly Fat	.15 g		Vitamin C	0 mg	(0% DV)
Mono Fat	1.45 g		Calcium	11.6 mg	(1% DV)
Cholesterol	16 mg	(5% DV)	Iron	.2 mg	(1% DV)
Sodium	42.9 mg	(2% DV)	Folate	1.2 mcg	(0% DV)
Potassium	17.3 mg	(0% DV)	Beta Carotene	3.3 RE	

Ratings	*Worst*	*Bad*	*Average*	*Good*	*Best*
Weight Loss		3			
LowCal Density		3			
Filling	1				
Energizing	2				
Fiber	1				
Vitamins	2				
Minerals	2				
Overall	2				

Serving: 1 tbsp (.54 oz)   **Cheese**

Calories	35	(64.2 cal/oz)	**Carbohydrate**	1.05 g	(0% DV)
Fat Calories	24	(70% fat)	Dietary Fiber	0 g	(0% DV)
Total Fat	2.7 g	(4% DV)	**Protein**	1.65 g	(3% DV)
Saturated Fat	1.65 g	(8% DV)	VItamin A	108 IU	(2% DV)
Poly Fat	.15 g		Vitamin C	0 mg	(0% DV)
Mono Fat	.75 g		Calcium	16.8 mg	(2% DV)
Cholesterol	8.4 mg	(3% DV)	Iron	.3 mg	(1% DV)
Sodium	44.4 mg	(2% DV)	Folate	1.7 mcg	(1% DV)
Potassium	25.1 mg	(1% DV)	Beta Carotene	1.8 RE	

Ratings	*Worst*	*Bad*	*Average*	*Good*	*Best*
Weight Loss			5		
LowCal Density			5		
Filling	1				
Energizing	2				
Fiber	1				
Vitamins	2				
Minerals	2				
Overall		4			

CHEESE, MOZZARELLA, PART SKIM

Serving: 1 slice (1 oz)   **Cheese**

Calories	78	(78.4 cal/oz)	Carbohydrate	.87 g	(0% DV)
Fat Calories	43	(55% fat)	Dietary Fiber	0 g	(0% DV)
Total Fat	4.76 g	(7% DV)	Protein	7.56 g	(15% DV)
Saturated Fat	3.08 g	(15% DV)	Vitamin A	175.8 IU	(4% DV)
Poly Fat	.28 g		Vitamin C	0 mg	(0% DV)
Mono Fat	1.4 g		Calcium	204.7 mg	(20% DV)
Cholesterol	15.1 mg	(5% DV)	Iron	.1 mg	(0% DV)
Sodium	147.8 mg	(6% DV)	Folate	7.6 mcg	(1% DV)
Potassium	26.6 mg	(1% DV)	Beta Carotene	2.8 RE	

Ratings	Worst	Bad	Average	Good	Best
Weight Loss			4		
LowCal Density			4		
Filling	1				
Energizing	2				
Fiber	1				
Vitamins	2				
Minerals				5	
Overall	3				

CHEESE, PARMESAN, DRY GRATED

Serving: 1 tbsp (.18 oz)   **Cheese**

Calories	23	(126.7 cal/oz)	Carbohydrate	.19 g	(0% DV)
Fat Calories	14	(59% fat)	Dietary Fiber	0 g	(0% DV)
Total Fat	1.5 g	(2% DV)	Protein	2.1 g	(4% DV)
Saturated Fat	.95 g	(5% DV)	Vitamin A	35.1 IU	(1% DV)
Poly Fat	.05 g		Vitamin C	0 mg	(0% DV)
Mono Fat	.45 g		Calcium	68.8 mg	(7% DV)
Cholesterol	4 mg	(1% DV)	Iron	.1 mg	(0% DV)
Sodium	93.1 mg	(4% DV)	Folate	2.1 mcg	(0% DV)
Potassium	5.4 mg	(0% DV)	Beta Carotene	1.6 RE	

Ratings	Worst	Bad	Average	Good	Best
Weight Loss					6
LowCal Density	2				
Filling	1				
Energizing	2				
Fiber	1				
Vitamins	2				
Minerals	3				
Overall	3				

CHEESE, PROCESSED CHEESE FOOD

Serving: 1 slice (.75 oz)   **Cheese**

Calories	69	(91.8 cal/oz)	Carbohydrate	1.53 g	(1% DV)
Fat Calories	47	(69% fat)	Dietary Fiber	0 g	(0% DV)
Total Fat	5.25 g	(8% DV)	Protein	4.2 g	(8% DV)
Saturated Fat	3.15 g	(16% DV)	Vitamin A	191.7 IU	(4% DV)
Poly Fat	.21 g		Vitamin C	0 mg	(0% DV)
Mono Fat	1.47 g		Calcium	120.5 mg	(12% DV)
Cholesterol	13.4 mg	(4% DV)	Iron	.2 mg	(1% DV)
Sodium	249.7 mg	(10% DV)	Folate	4.2 mcg	(0% DV)
Potassium	58.6 mg	(2% DV)	Beta Carotene	5.7 RE	

Ratings	Worst	Bad	Average	Good	Best
Weight Loss			4		
LowCal Density		3			
Filling	1				
Energizing		3			
Fiber	1				
Vitamins	2				
Minerals			4		
Overall		3			

CHEESE, PROCESSED, AMERICAN, LOWFAT

Serving: 1 slice (.75 oz)   **Cheese**

Calories	38	(50.4 cal/oz)	Carbohydrate	.74 g	(0% DV)
Fat Calories	13	(35% fat)	Dietary Fiber	0 g	(0% DV)
Total Fat	1.47 g	(2% DV)	Protein	5.25 g	(10% DV)
Saturated Fat	.84 g	(4% DV)	Vitamin A	56.9 IU	(1% DV)
Poly Fat	0 g		Vitamin C	0 mg	(0% DV)
Mono Fat	.42 g		Calcium	143.6 mg	(14% DV)
Cholesterol	7.4 mg	(2% DV)	Iron	.1 mg	(0% DV)
Sodium	300.3 mg	(13% DV)	Folate	5.3 mcg	(0% DV)
Potassium	37.8 mg	(1% DV)	Beta Carotene	1.7 RE	

Ratings	Worst	Bad	Average	Good	Best
Weight Loss				7	
LowCal Density				6	
Filling	1				
Energizing	2				
Fiber	1				
Vitamins	2				
Minerals			5		
Overall			5		

CHEESE, PROCESSED, CHEDDAR OR AMERICAN TYPE

Serving: 1 slice (.75 oz)   **Cheese**

Calories	79	(105 cal/oz)	**Carbohydrate**	.34 g	(0% DV)
Fat Calories	59	(74% fat)	Dietary Fiber	0 g	(0% DV)
Total Fat	6.51 g	(10% DV)	**Protein**	4.62 g	(9% DV)
Saturated Fat	4.2 g	(21% DV)	Vitamin A	254.1 IU	(5% DV)
Poly Fat	.21 g		Vitamin C	0 mg	(0% DV)
Mono Fat	1.89 g		Calcium	129.4 mg	(13% DV)
Cholesterol	19.7 mg	(7% DV)	Iron	.1 mg	(0% DV)
Sodium	300.3 mg	(13% DV)	Folate	4.6 mcg	(0% DV)
Potassium	34 mg	(1% DV)	Beta Carotene	7.6 RE	

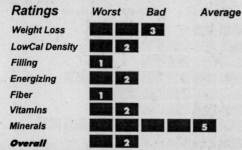

Ratings	Worst	Bad	Average	Good	Best
Weight Loss		3			
LowCal Density	2				
Filling	1				
Energizing	2				
Fiber	1				
Vitamins	2				
Minerals				5	
Overall	2				

CHEESE, SWISS

Serving: 1 slice (1 oz)   **Cheese**

Calories	105	(105.3 cal/oz)	**Carbohydrate**	.95 g	(0% DV)
Fat Calories	68	(65% fat)	Dietary Fiber	0 g	(0% DV)
Total Fat	7.56 g	(12% DV)	**Protein**	7.84 g	(16% DV)
Saturated Fat	5.04 g	(25% DV)	Vitamin A	236.6 IU	(5% DV)
Poly Fat	.28 g		Vitamin C	0 mg	(0% DV)
Mono Fat	1.96 g		Calcium	269.1 mg	(27% DV)
Cholesterol	25.8 mg	(9% DV)	Iron	.1 mg	(0% DV)
Sodium	72.8 mg	(3% DV)	Folate	7.8 mcg	(0% DV)
Potassium	31.1 mg	(1% DV)	Beta Carotene	2.2 RE	

Ratings	Worst	Bad	Average	Good	Best
Weight Loss		3			
LowCal Density	2				
Filling	1				
Energizing	2				
Fiber	1				
Vitamins	2				
Minerals				6	
Overall	2				

CHEESEBURGER, ¼ LB MEAT

Serving: 1 McDonald's (6.93 oz)   Sandwich

Calories	464	(66.9 cal/oz)	Carbohydrate	36.28 g	(12% DV)
Fat Calories	210	(45% fat)	Dietary Fiber	1.94 g	(8% DV)
Total Fat	23.28 g	(36% DV)	Protein	25.22 g	(50% DV)
Saturated Fat	9.7 g	(48% DV)	Vitamin A	504.4 IU	(10% DV)
Poly Fat	1.94 g		Vitamin C	3.9 mg	(6% DV)
Mono Fat	9.7 g		Calcium	221.2 mg	(22% DV)
Cholesterol	77.6 mg	(26% DV)	Iron	3.6 mg	(20% DV)
Sodium	1226.1 mg	(51% DV)	Folate	25.2 mcg	(11% DV)
Potassium	386.1 mg	(11% DV)	Beta Carotene	31 RE	

Ratings	Worst	Bad	Average	Good	Best
Weight Loss	3				
LowCal Density		5			
Filling		5			
Energizing				8	
Fiber			6		
Vitamins			6		
Minerals					9
Overall		5			

CHEESEBURGER, BACON, ¼ LB MEAT

Serving: 1 Wendy's (9.64 oz)   Sandwich

Calories	729	(75.6 cal/oz)	Carbohydrate	45.9 g	(15% DV)
Fat Calories	389	(53% fat)	Dietary Fiber	2.7 g	(11% DV)
Total Fat	43.2 g	(66% DV)	Protein	40.5 g	(81% DV)
Saturated Fat	18.9 g	(94% DV)	Vitamin A	637.2 IU	(13% DV)
Poly Fat	2.7 g		Vitamin C	10.8 mg	(18% DV)
Mono Fat	18.9 g		Calcium	283.5 mg	(28% DV)
Cholesterol	118.8 mg	(40% DV)	Iron	5 mg	(28% DV)
Sodium	1949.4 mg	(81% DV)	Folate	40.5 mcg	(14% DV)
Potassium	610.2 mg	(17% DV)	Beta Carotene	37.8 RE	

Ratings	Worst	Bad	Average	Good	Best
Weight Loss	2				
LowCal Density		4			
Filling		5			
Energizing					9
Fiber			7		
Vitamins				8	
Minerals					9
Overall		5			

CHEESEBURGER, BACON, DOUBLE (TWO ¼ LB PATTIES)

Serving: 1 Burger King (7.21 oz)   **Sandwich**

Calories	568	(78.7 cal/oz)	Carbohydrate	25.86 g	(9% DV)
Fat Calories	309	(54% fat)	Dietary Fiber	2.02 g	(8% DV)
Total Fat	34.34 g	(53% DV)	Protein	36.36 g	(73% DV)
Saturated Fat	14.14 g	(71% DV)	Vitamin A	299 IU	(6% DV)
Poly Fat	2.02 g		Vitamin C	6.1 mg	(10% DV)
Mono Fat	14.14 g		Calcium	177.8 mg	(18% DV)
Cholesterol	115.1 mg	(38% DV)	Iron	4.1 mg	(23% DV)
Sodium	1030.2 mg	(43% DV)	Folate	36.4 mcg	(9% DV)
Potassium	458.5 mg	(13% DV)	Beta Carotene	14.1 RE	

Ratings	Worst	Bad	Average	Good	Best	
Weight Loss		2				
LowCal Density			4			
Filling			4			
Energizing				6		
Fiber				6		
Vitamins				6		
Minerals						9
Overall			4			

CHEESEBURGER, DOUBLE (2 PATTIES), PLAIN, ON BUN

Serving: 1 double cheeseburger (5.64 oz)   **Sandwich**

Calories	483	(85.7 cal/oz)	Carbohydrate	34.44 g	(11% DV)
Fat Calories	228	(47% fat)	Dietary Fiber	1.58 g	(6% DV)
Total Fat	25.28 g	(39% DV)	Protein	26.86 g	(54% DV)
Saturated Fat	11.06 g	(55% DV)	Vitamin A	311.3 IU	(6% DV)
Poly Fat	1.58 g		Vitamin C	0 mg	(0% DV)
Mono Fat	11.06 g		Calcium	229.1 mg	(23% DV)
Cholesterol	85.3 mg	(28% DV)	Iron	3.6 mg	(20% DV)
Sodium	925.9 mg	(39% DV)	Folate	26.9 mcg	(8% DV)
Potassium	300.2 mg	(9% DV)	Beta Carotene	9.5 RE	

Ratings	Worst	Bad	Average	Good	Best	
Weight Loss		3				
LowCal Density		3				
Filling			5			
Energizing				8		
Fiber			5			
Vitamins			5			
Minerals						9
Overall		4				

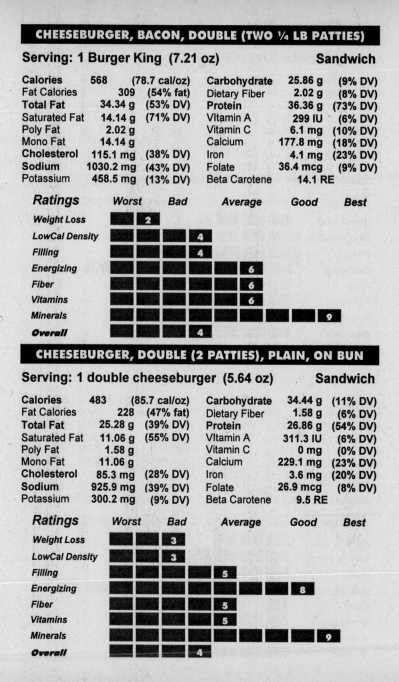

CHEESECAKE

Serving: 1 piece (1/12 of 9" dia) (4.57 oz)   **Dessert**

Calories	406	(88.8 cal/oz)	Carbohydrate	36.61 g	(12% DV)
Fat Calories	219	(54% fat)	Dietary Fiber	0 g	(0% DV)
Total Fat	24.32 g	(37% DV)	Protein	11.52 g	(23% DV)
Saturated Fat	10.24 g	(51% DV)	Vitamin A	1088 IU	(22% DV)
Poly Fat	3.84 g		Vitamin C	1.3 mg	(2% DV)
Mono Fat	8.96 g		Calcium	69.1 mg	(7% DV)
Cholesterol	85.8 mg	(29% DV)	Iron	1.1 mg	(6% DV)
Sodium	529.9 mg	(22% DV)	Folate	11.5 mcg	(4% DV)
Potassium	154.9 mg	(4% DV)	Beta Carotene	19.2 RE	

Ratings	Worst	Bad	Average	Good	Best
Weight Loss		3			
LowCal Density		3			
Filling			5		
Energizing					8
Fiber	1				
Vitamins			5		
Minerals			5		
Overall			4		

CHEESECAKE WITH FRUIT

Serving: 1 piece (1/12 of 9" dia) (5.07 oz)   **Dessert**

Calories	385	(75.9 cal/oz)	Carbohydrate	46.15 g	(15% DV)
Fat Calories	179	(46% fat)	Dietary Fiber	0 g	(0% DV)
Total Fat	19.88 g	(31% DV)	Protein	8.52 g	(17% DV)
Saturated Fat	8.52 g	(43% DV)	Vitamin A	1080.6 IU	(22% DV)
Poly Fat	2.84 g		Vitamin C	1.4 mg	(2% DV)
Mono Fat	7.1 g		Calcium	56.8 mg	(6% DV)
Cholesterol	66.7 mg	(22% DV)	Iron	1.3 mg	(7% DV)
Sodium	413.2 mg	(17% DV)	Folate	8.5 mcg	(3% DV)
Potassium	153.4 mg	(4% DV)	Beta Carotene	38.3 RE	

Ratings	Worst	Bad	Average	Good	Best
Weight Loss		3			
LowCal Density			4		
Filling			5		
Energizing					9
Fiber	1				
Vitamins			4		
Minerals			5		
Overall			4		

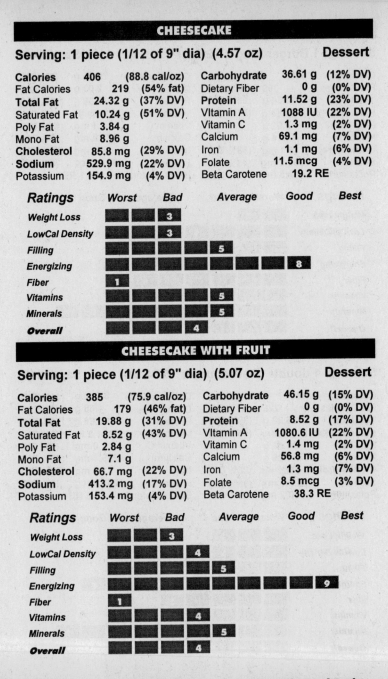

CHEESECAKE, DIET

Serving: 1 individual cake (4.04 oz)   **Dessert**

Calories	241	(59.6 cal/oz)	Carbohydrate	33 g	(11% DV)
Fat Calories	92	(38% fat)	Dietary Fiber	1.13 g	(5% DV)
Total Fat	10.17 g	(16% DV)	Protein	6.78 g	(14% DV)
Saturated Fat	5.65 g	(28% DV)	VItamin A	293.8 IU	(6% DV)
Poly Fat	1.13 g		Vitamin C	0 mg	(0% DV)
Mono Fat	3.39 g		Calcium	59.9 mg	(6% DV)
Cholesterol	22.6 mg	(8% DV)	Iron	1.8 mg	(10% DV)
Sodium	366.1 mg	(15% DV)	Folate	6.8 mcg	(3% DV)
Potassium	192.1 mg	(5% DV)	Beta Carotene	4.5 RE	

Ratings	Worst	Bad	Average	Good	Best
Weight Loss			5		
LowCal Density			5		
Filling			5		
Energizing				8	
Fiber		4			
Vitamins		4			
Minerals			5		
Overall			5		

CHERRIES, SWEET, RAW (QUEEN ANNE, BING)

Serving: 17 cherries (4.14 oz)   **Fruit**

Calories	84	(20.2 cal/oz)	Carbohydrate	19.26 g	(6% DV)
Fat Calories	10	(12% fat)	Dietary Fiber	1.16 g	(5% DV)
Total Fat	1.16 g	(2% DV)	Protein	1.16 g	(2% DV)
Saturated Fat	0 g	(0% DV)	VItamin A	248.2 IU	(5% DV)
Poly Fat	0 g		Vitamin C	8.1 mg	(14% DV)
Mono Fat	0 g		Calcium	17.4 mg	(2% DV)
Cholesterol	0 mg	(0% DV)	Iron	.5 mg	(3% DV)
Sodium	0 mg	(0% DV)	Folate	1.2 mcg	(1% DV)
Potassium	259.8 mg	(7% DV)	Beta Carotene	24.4 RE	

Ratings	Worst	Bad	Average	Good	Best
Weight Loss				8	
LowCal Density				8	
Filling				7	
Energizing			6		
Fiber		4			
Vitamins		4			
Minerals	3				
Overall				7	

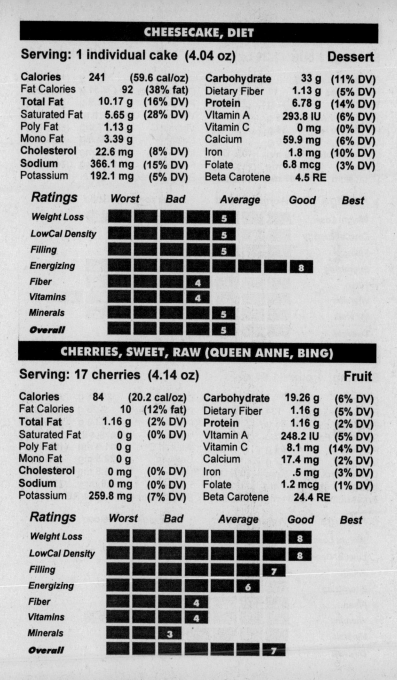

CHEX CEREAL

Serving: 1 cup (1.39 oz)   **Cereal**

Calories	143	(103 cal/oz)	Carbohydrate	32.06 g	(11% DV)
Fat Calories	11	(7% fat)	Dietary Fiber	3.51 g	(14% DV)
Total Fat	1.17 g	(2% DV)	Protein	3.9 g	(8% DV)
Saturated Fat	.39 g	(2% DV)	Vitamin A	0 IU	(0% DV)
Poly Fat	.39 g		Vitamin C	20.7 mg	(34% DV)
Mono Fat	0 g		Calcium	15.2 mg	(2% DV)
Cholesterol	0 mg	(0% DV)	Iron	11.1 mg	(62% DV)
Sodium	261.3 mg	(11% DV)	Folate	3.9 mcg	(34% DV)
Potassium	147 mg	(4% DV)	Beta Carotene	0 RE	

Ratings	Worst	Bad	Average	Good	Best
Weight Loss				8	
LowCal Density	2				
Filling		4			
Energizing				8	
Fiber				8	
Vitamins					9
Minerals				8	
Overall			6		

CHEX MIX, PRETZELS, CHEX CEREAL, NUTS

Serving: 1 cup (1.61 oz)   **Snack**

Calories	226	(140.3 cal/oz)	Carbohydrate	20.74 g	(7% DV)
Fat Calories	134	(59% fat)	Dietary Fiber	2.25 g	(9% DV)
Total Fat	14.85 g	(23% DV)	Protein	3.6 g	(7% DV)
Saturated Fat	2.7 g	(14% DV)	Vitamin A	478.4 IU	(10% DV)
Poly Fat	4.05 g		Vitamin C	11.3 mg	(19% DV)
Mono Fat	7.2 g		Calcium	22.5 mg	(2% DV)
Cholesterol	0 mg	(0% DV)	Iron	6.5 mg	(36% DV)
Sodium	506.3 mg	(21% DV)	Folate	3.6 mcg	(21% DV)
Potassium	131 mg	(4% DV)	Beta Carotene	13.1 RE	

Ratings	Worst	Bad	Average	Good	Best
Weight Loss		3			
LowCal Density	1				
Filling		3			
Energizing			6		
Fiber			6		
Vitamins				8	
Minerals			6		
Overall		3			

CHICKEN & VEGETABLE ENTREE WITH RICE, ORIENTAL

Serving: 1 diet meal (9.11 oz)   **Entree**

Calories	482	(52.9 cal/oz)	Carbohydrate	58.65 g	(20% DV)
Fat Calories	138	(29% fat)	Dietary Fiber	5.1 g	(20% DV)
Total Fat	15.3 g	(24% DV)	Protein	33.15 g	(66% DV)
Saturated Fat	2.55 g	(13% DV)	Vitamin A	4809.3 IU	(96% DV)
Poly Fat	5.1 g		Vitamin C	12.8 mg	(21% DV)
Mono Fat	5.1 g		Calcium	114.8 mg	(11% DV)
Cholesterol	71.4 mg	(24% DV)	Iron	4.7 mg	(26% DV)
Sodium	632.4 mg	(26% DV)	Folate	33.2 mcg	(8% DV)
Potassium	696.2 mg	(20% DV)	Beta Carotene	479.4 RE	

Ratings	Worst	Bad	Average	Good	Best
Weight Loss		4			
LowCal Density			6		
Filling			7		
Energizing					10
Fiber				9	
Vitamins				9	
Minerals				8	
Overall			6		

CHICKEN A LA KING WITH RICE

Serving: 1 Stouffer frozen meal (9.61 oz)   **Entree**

Calories	441	(45.9 cal/oz)	Carbohydrate	40.89 g	(14% DV)
Fat Calories	194	(44% fat)	Dietary Fiber	2.69 g	(11% DV)
Total Fat	21.52 g	(33% DV)	Protein	18.83 g	(38% DV)
Saturated Fat	8.07 g	(40% DV)	Vitamin A	1151.3 IU	(23% DV)
Poly Fat	5.38 g		Vitamin C	10.8 mg	(18% DV)
Mono Fat	8.07 g		Calcium	104.9 mg	(10% DV)
Cholesterol	123.7 mg	(41% DV)	Iron	2.5 mg	(14% DV)
Sodium	1027.6 mg	(43% DV)	Folate	18.8 mcg	(5% DV)
Potassium	309.4 mg	(9% DV)	Beta Carotene	37.7 RE	

Ratings	Worst	Bad	Average	Good	Best
Weight Loss		3			
LowCal Density			6		
Filling			6		
Energizing					9
Fiber			7		
Vitamins			7		
Minerals			7		
Overall			6		

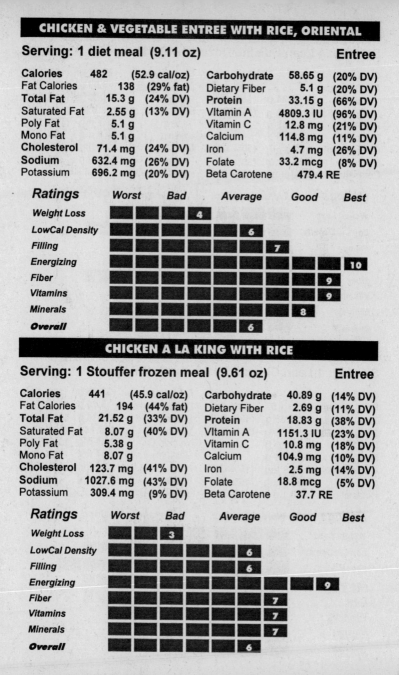

CHICKEN CACCIATORE, NOODLES

Serving: 1 Lean Cuisine frozen meal (11 oz)   Entree

Calories	290	(26.3 cal/oz)	Carbohydrate	29.57 g	(10% DV)
Fat Calories	83	(29% fat)	Dietary Fiber	3.08 g	(12% DV)
Total Fat	9.24 g	(14% DV)	Protein	21.56 g	(43% DV)
Saturated Fat	3.08 g	(15% DV)	Vitamin A	748.4 IU	(15% DV)
Poly Fat	3.08 g		Vitamin C	27.7 mg	(46% DV)
Mono Fat	3.08 g		Calcium	30.8 mg	(3% DV)
Cholesterol	58.5 mg	(20% DV)	Iron	2.5 mg	(14% DV)
Sodium	933.2 mg	(39% DV)	Folate	21.6 mcg	(8% DV)
Potassium	616 mg	(18% DV)	Beta Carotene	61.6 RE	

Ratings	Worst	Bad	Average	Good	Best
Weight Loss			6		
LowCal Density				8	
Filling			7		
Energizing			7		
Fiber				8	
Vitamins			7		
Minerals			7		
Overall			7		

CHICKEN CHOW MEIN WITH RICE

Serving: 1 Lean Cuisine frozen meal (11.39 oz)   Entree

Calories	290	(25.5 cal/oz)	Carbohydrate	37.96 g	(13% DV)
Fat Calories	57	(20% fat)	Dietary Fiber	3.19 g	(13% DV)
Total Fat	6.38 g	(10% DV)	Protein	19.14 g	(38% DV)
Saturated Fat	3.19 g	(16% DV)	Vitamin A	488.1 IU	(10% DV)
Poly Fat	0 g		Vitamin C	19.1 mg	(32% DV)
Mono Fat	3.19 g		Calcium	44.7 mg	(4% DV)
Cholesterol	47.9 mg	(16% DV)	Iron	2.5 mg	(14% DV)
Sodium	1068.7 mg	(45% DV)	Folate	19.1 mcg	(7% DV)
Potassium	338.1 mg	(10% DV)	Beta Carotene	44.7 RE	

Ratings	Worst	Bad	Average	Good	Best
Weight Loss			6		
LowCal Density				8	
Filling					9
Energizing				8	
Fiber				8	
Vitamins			7		
Minerals			6		
Overall			7		

CHICKEN CORDON BLEU, VEGETABLES

Serving: 1 diet meal (8.11 oz)   **Entree**

Calories	225	(27.7 cal/oz)	Carbohydrate	14.3 g	(5% DV)
Fat Calories	82	(36% fat)	Dietary Fiber	2.27 g	(9% DV)
Total Fat	9.08 g	(14% DV)	Protein	20.43 g	(41% DV)
Saturated Fat	4.54 g	(23% DV)	Vltamin A	6567.1 IU	(131% DV)
Poly Fat	2.27 g		Vitamin C	15.9 mg	(26% DV)
Mono Fat	2.27 g		Calcium	297.4 mg	(30% DV)
Cholesterol	54.5 mg	(18% DV)	Iron	1.4 mg	(8% DV)
Sodium	805.9 mg	(34% DV)	Folate	20.4 mcg	(7% DV)
Potassium	354.1 mg	(10% DV)	Beta Carotene	628.8 RE	

Ratings	Worst	Bad	Average	Good	Best
Weight Loss			6		
LowCal Density				8	
Filling			5		
Energizing			5		
Fiber			6		
Vitamins					9
Minerals				8	
Overall			7		

CHICKEN CURRY

Serving: ½ breast with sauce (4.61 oz)   **Entree**

Calories	160	(34.7 cal/oz)	Carbohydrate	5.68 g	(2% DV)
Fat Calories	81	(51% fat)	Dietary Fiber	1.29 g	(5% DV)
Total Fat	9.03 g	(14% DV)	Protein	15.48 g	(31% DV)
Saturated Fat	1.29 g	(6% DV)	Vltamin A	722.4 IU	(14% DV)
Poly Fat	2.58 g		Vitamin C	10.3 mg	(17% DV)
Mono Fat	3.87 g		Calcium	24.5 mg	(2% DV)
Cholesterol	46.4 mg	(15% DV)	Iron	1.1 mg	(6% DV)
Sodium	650.2 mg	(27% DV)	Folate	15.5 mcg	(3% DV)
Potassium	339.3 mg	(10% DV)	Beta Carotene	42.6 RE	

Ratings	Worst	Bad	Average	Good	Best
Weight Loss			6		
LowCal Density				7	
Filling		3			
Energizing		3			
Fiber			5		
Vitamins			6		
Minerals			5		
Overall			6		

CHICKEN DIVAN

Serving: 1 frozen meal (9.61 oz)　　　　　**Entree**

Calories	393	(40.9 cal/oz)	Carbohydrate	16.14 g	(5% DV)
Fat Calories	218	(55% fat)	Dietary Fiber	0 g	(0% DV)
Total Fat	24.21 g	(37% DV)	Protein	24.21 g	(48% DV)
Saturated Fat	10.76 g	(54% DV)	Vitamin A	1170.2 IU	(23% DV)
Poly Fat	2.69 g		Vitamin C	26.9 mg	(45% DV)
Mono Fat	8.07 g		Calcium	298.6 mg	(30% DV)
Cholesterol	96.8 mg	(32% DV)	Iron	1.8 mg	(10% DV)
Sodium	755.9 mg	(31% DV)	Folate	24.2 mcg	(10% DV)
Potassium	451.9 mg	(13% DV)	Beta Carotene	53.8 RE	

Ratings	Worst	Bad	Average	Good	Best
Weight Loss		3			
LowCal Density				6	
Filling			5		
Energizing			5		
Fiber	1				
Vitamins				7	
Minerals					8
Overall			5		

CHICKEN FAJITAS

Serving: 1 diet meal (6.82 oz)　　　　　**Entree**

Calories	235	(34.4 cal/oz)	Carbohydrate	30.37 g	(10% DV)
Fat Calories	52	(22% fat)	Dietary Fiber	1.91 g	(8% DV)
Total Fat	5.73 g	(9% DV)	Protein	17.19 g	(34% DV)
Saturated Fat	1.91 g	(10% DV)	Vitamin A	2446.7 IU	(49% DV)
Poly Fat	1.91 g		Vitamin C	70.7 mg	(118% DV)
Mono Fat	1.91 g		Calcium	32.5 mg	(3% DV)
Cholesterol	36.3 mg	(12% DV)	Iron	2.6 mg	(14% DV)
Sodium	590.2 mg	(25% DV)	Folate	17.2 mcg	(6% DV)
Potassium	317.1 mg	(9% DV)	Beta Carotene	242.6 RE	

Ratings	Worst	Bad	Average	Good	Best
Weight Loss				7	
LowCal Density				7	
Filling			6		
Energizing				7	
Fiber			6		
Vitamins					10
Minerals			6		
Overall				7	

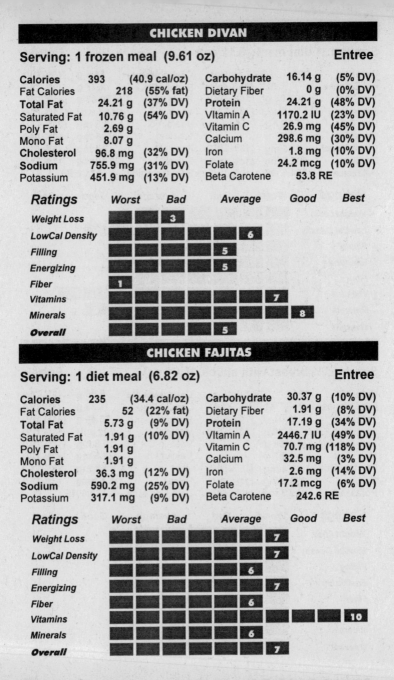

CHICKEN FILLET (BREADED, FRIED) SANDWICH

Serving: 1 sandwich (6.21 oz)   Sandwich

Calories	472	(75.9 cal/oz)	Carbohydrate	36.19 g	(12% DV)
Fat Calories	235	(50% fat)	Dietary Fiber	1.74 g	(7% DV)
Total Fat	26.1 g	(40% DV)	Protein	20.88 g	(42% DV)
Saturated Fat	5.22 g	(26% DV)	Vltamin A	264.5 IU	(5% DV)
Poly Fat	10.44 g		Vitamin C	3.5 mg	(6% DV)
Mono Fat	8.7 g		Calcium	74.8 mg	(7% DV)
Cholesterol	67.9 mg	(23% DV)	Iron	2.6 mg	(14% DV)
Sodium	563.8 mg	(23% DV)	Folate	20.9 mcg	(10% DV)
Potassium	257.5 mg	(7% DV)	Beta Carotene	17.4 RE	

Ratings	Worst	Bad	Average	Good	Best
Weight Loss		3			
LowCal Density		4			
Filling			5		
Energizing					8
Fiber			6		
Vitamins			7		
Minerals			6		
Overall			5		

CHICKEN FRANKFURTER, PLAIN, ON BUN

Serving: 1 frankfurter (3.04 oz)   Sandwich

Calories	235	(77.2 cal/oz)	Carbohydrate	24.23 g	(8% DV)
Fat Calories	99	(42% fat)	Dietary Fiber	.85 g	(3% DV)
Total Fat	11.05 g	(17% DV)	Protein	9.35 g	(19% DV)
Saturated Fat	3.4 g	(17% DV)	Vltamin A	58.7 IU	(1% DV)
Poly Fat	2.55 g		Vitamin C	0 mg	(0% DV)
Mono Fat	5.1 g		Calcium	82.5 mg	(8% DV)
Cholesterol	45.1 mg	(15% DV)	Iron	2 mg	(11% DV)
Sodium	818.6 mg	(34% DV)	Folate	9.4 mcg	(4% DV)
Potassium	75.7 mg	(2% DV)	Beta Carotene	0 RE	

Ratings	Worst	Bad	Average	Good	Best
Weight Loss			6		
LowCal Density		4			
Filling		4			
Energizing			6		
Fiber		4			
Vitamins		4			
Minerals			5		
Overall			5		

CHICKEN GUMBO SOUP

Serving: 1 cup (8.71 oz)   **Soup**

Calories	56	(6.4 cal/oz)	Carbohydrate	8.3 g	(3% DV)
Fat Calories	22	(39% fat)	Dietary Fiber	2.44 g	(10% DV)
Total Fat	2.44 g	(4% DV)	Protein	2.44 g	(5% DV)
Saturated Fat	0 g	(0% DV)	VItamin A	136.6 IU	(3% DV)
Poly Fat	0 g		Vitamin C	4.9 mg	(8% DV)
Mono Fat	0 g		Calcium	24.4 mg	(2% DV)
Cholesterol	4.9 mg	(2% DV)	Iron	.9 mg	(5% DV)
Sodium	954 mg	(40% DV)	Folate	2.4 mcg	(1% DV)
Potassium	75.6 mg	(2% DV)	Beta Carotene	14.6 RE	

Ratings	Worst	Bad	Average	Good	Best
Weight Loss				7	
LowCal Density					10
Filling				9	
Energizing		4			
Fiber				7	
Vitamins	3				
Minerals	3				
Overall				7	

CHICKEN KIEV, RICE-VEGETABLE MIX

Serving: 1 frozen meal (8.11 oz)   **Entree**

Calories	504	(62.1 cal/oz)	Carbohydrate	30.87 g	(10% DV)
Fat Calories	266	(53% fat)	Dietary Fiber	2.27 g	(9% DV)
Total Fat	29.51 g	(45% DV)	Protein	24.97 g	(50% DV)
Saturated Fat	11.35 g	(57% DV)	VItamin A	3332.4 IU	(67% DV)
Poly Fat	4.54 g		Vitamin C	6.8 mg	(11% DV)
Mono Fat	11.35 g		Calcium	56.8 mg	(6% DV)
Cholesterol	104.4 mg	(35% DV)	Iron	2.2 mg	(12% DV)
Sodium	696.9 mg	(29% DV)	Folate	25 mcg	(4% DV)
Potassium	299.6 mg	(9% DV)	Beta Carotene	299.6 RE	

Ratings	Worst	Bad	Average	Good	Best
Weight Loss	2				
LowCal Density			5		
Filling			5		
Energizing				7	
Fiber			6		
Vitamins				8	
Minerals			6		
Overall			5		

CHICKEN LIVER, COOKED

Serving: 1 liver (.71 oz)   **Meat**

Calories	45	(63.9 cal/oz)	Carbohydrate	2.12 g	(1% DV)
Fat Calories	16	(36% fat)	Dietary Fiber	0 g	(0% DV)
Total Fat	1.8 g	(3% DV)	Protein	4.8 g	(10% DV)
Saturated Fat	.6 g	(3% DV)	VItamin A	4009.4 IU	(80% DV)
Poly Fat	.4 g		Vitamin C	7 mg	(12% DV)
Mono Fat	.6 g		Calcium	5 mg	(0% DV)
Cholesterol	114.2 mg	(38% DV)	Iron	2.2 mg	(12% DV)
Sodium	95.8 mg	(4% DV)	Folate	4.8 mcg	(41% DV)
Potassium	53 mg	(2% DV)	Beta Carotene	0 RE	

Ratings	Worst	Bad	Average	Good	Best
Weight Loss					8
LowCal Density			5		
Filling	1				
Energizing		3			
Fiber	1				
Vitamins					9
Minerals		4			
Overall			5		

CHICKEN NOODLE SOUP

Serving: 1 cup (8.61 oz)   **Soup**

Calories	75	(8.7 cal/oz)	Carbohydrate	9.4 g	(3% DV)
Fat Calories	22	(29% fat)	Dietary Fiber	0 g	(0% DV)
Total Fat	2.41 g	(4% DV)	Protein	4.82 g	(10% DV)
Saturated Fat	0 g	(0% DV)	VItamin A	711 IU	(14% DV)
Poly Fat	0 g		Vitamin C	0 mg	(0% DV)
Mono Fat	0 g		Calcium	16.9 mg	(2% DV)
Cholesterol	7.2 mg	(2% DV)	Iron	.8 mg	(4% DV)
Sodium	1106.2 mg	(46% DV)	Folate	4.8 mcg	(1% DV)
Potassium	55.4 mg	(2% DV)	Beta Carotene	72.3 RE	

Ratings	Worst	Bad	Average	Good	Best
Weight Loss				7	
LowCal Density					9
Filling				7	
Energizing		4			
Fiber	1				
Vitamins		4			
Minerals	3				
Overall			6		

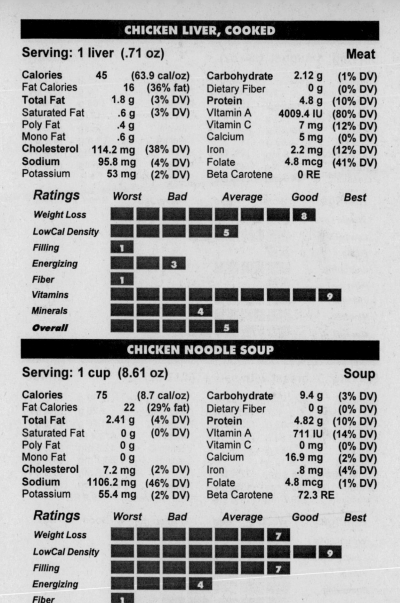

CHICKEN NUGGETS

Serving: 1 nugget (.64 oz)   **Poultry**

Calories	51	(79.9 cal/oz)	Carbohydrate	2.74 g	(1% DV)
Fat Calories	28	(54% fat)	Dietary Fiber	0 g	(0% DV)
Total Fat	3.06 g	(5% DV)	Protein	3.06 g	(6% DV)
Saturated Fat	.9 g	(5% DV)	VItamin A	18 IU	(0% DV)
Poly Fat	.36 g		Vitamin C	0 mg	(0% DV)
Mono Fat	1.62 g		Calcium	2.9 mg	(0% DV)
Cholesterol	10.8 mg	(4% DV)	Iron	.2 mg	(1% DV)
Sodium	95.8 mg	(4% DV)	Folate	3.1 mcg	(0% DV)
Potassium	44.3 mg	(1% DV)	Beta Carotene	7 RE	

Ratings	Worst	Bad	Average	Good	Best
Weight Loss				6	
LowCal Density			4		
Filling	1				
Energizing		3			
Fiber	1				
Vitamins		3			
Minerals		3			
Overall			4		

CHICKEN OR TURKEY CACCIATORE

Serving: ½ breast with sauce (4.57 oz)   **Entree**

Calories	241	(52.7 cal/oz)	Carbohydrate	6.66 g	(2% DV)
Fat Calories	127	(53% fat)	Dietary Fiber	1.28 g	(5% DV)
Total Fat	14.08 g	(22% DV)	Protein	21.76 g	(44% DV)
Saturated Fat	3.84 g	(19% DV)	VItamin A	573.4 IU	(11% DV)
Poly Fat	3.84 g		Vitamin C	12.8 mg	(21% DV)
Mono Fat	5.12 g		Calcium	30.7 mg	(3% DV)
Cholesterol	66.6 mg	(22% DV)	Iron	1.5 mg	(9% DV)
Sodium	309.8 mg	(13% DV)	Folate	21.8 mcg	(2% DV)
Potassium	359.7 mg	(10% DV)	Beta Carotene	49.9 RE	

Ratings	Worst	Bad	Average	Good	Best
Weight Loss			5		
LowCal Density			6		
Filling		3			
Energizing		4			
Fiber			5		
Vitamins			6		
Minerals			5		
Overall			5		

CHICKEN OR TURKEY CORDON BLEU

Serving: 1/2 breast with sauce (8.18 oz)　　　**Entree**

Calories	483	(59.1 cal/oz)	Carbohydrate	8.47 g	(3% DV)
Fat Calories	247	(51% fat)	Dietary Fiber	0 g	(0% DV)
Total Fat	27.48 g	(42% DV)	Protein	45.8 g	(92% DV)
Saturated Fat	13.74 g	(69% DV)	VItamin A	799.2 IU	(16% DV)
Poly Fat	2.29 g		Vitamin C	2.3 mg	(4% DV)
Mono Fat	9.16 g		Calcium	208.4 mg	(21% DV)
Cholesterol	190.1 mg	(63% DV)	Iron	2.2 mg	(12% DV)
Sodium	616 mg	(26% DV)	Folate	45.8 mcg	(4% DV)
Potassium	490.1 mg	(14% DV)	Beta Carotene	20.6 RE	

Ratings	Worst	Bad	Average	Good	Best
Weight Loss		3			
LowCal Density			5		
Filling		3			
Energizing		4			
Fiber	1				
Vitamins				8	
Minerals					9
Overall		4			

CHICKEN OR TURKEY DIVAN

Serving: 1 cup (8.43 oz)　　　**Entree**

Calories	316	(37.5 cal/oz)	Carbohydrate	8.26 g	(3% DV)
Fat Calories	127	(40% fat)	Dietary Fiber	2.36 g	(9% DV)
Total Fat	14.16 g	(22% DV)	Protein	40.12 g	(80% DV)
Saturated Fat	4.72 g	(24% DV)	VItamin A	2301 IU	(46% DV)
Poly Fat	2.36 g		Vitamin C	40.1 mg	(67% DV)
Mono Fat	4.72 g		Calcium	278.5 mg	(28% DV)
Cholesterol	134.5 mg	(45% DV)	Iron	1.9 mg	(10% DV)
Sodium	401.2 mg	(17% DV)	Folate	40.1 mcg	(9% DV)
Potassium	434.2 mg	(12% DV)	Beta Carotene	195.9 RE	

Ratings	Worst	Bad	Average	Good	Best
Weight Loss			5		
LowCal Density				7	
Filling		4			
Energizing		4			
Fiber			6		
Vitamins					9
Minerals				8	
Overall			6		

CHICKEN OR TURKEY PARMIGIANA

Serving: 1 piece with sauce & cheese (6.5 oz)   Entree

Calories	317	(48.7 cal/oz)	Carbohydrate	15.11 g	(5% DV)
Fat Calories	147	(47% fat)	Dietary Fiber	1.82 g	(7% DV)
Total Fat	16.38 g	(25% DV)	Protein	29.12 g	(58% DV)
Saturated Fat	5.46 g	(27% DV)	Vitamin A	831.7 IU	(17% DV)
Poly Fat	3.64 g		Vitamin C	9.1 mg	(15% DV)
Mono Fat	3.64 g		Calcium	189.3 mg	(19% DV)
Cholesterol	138.3 mg	(46% DV)	Iron	2.1 mg	(11% DV)
Sodium	768 mg	(32% DV)	Folate	29.1 mcg	(5% DV)
Potassium	464.1 mg	(13% DV)	Beta Carotene	54.6 RE	

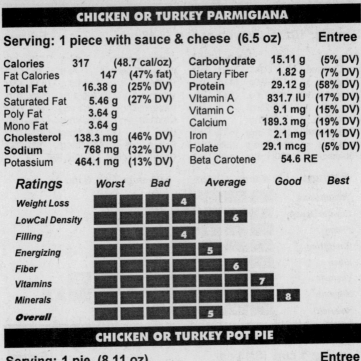

Ratings	Worst	Bad	Average	Good	Best
Weight Loss			4		
LowCal Density			6		
Filling			4		
Energizing			5		
Fiber			6		
Vitamins				7	
Minerals				8	
Overall			5		

CHICKEN OR TURKEY POT PIE

Serving: 1 pie (8.11 oz)   Entree

Calories	497	(61.3 cal/oz)	Carbohydrate	37 g	(12% DV)
Fat Calories	266	(53% fat)	Dietary Fiber	2.27 g	(9% DV)
Total Fat	29.51 g	(45% DV)	Protein	20.43 g	(41% DV)
Saturated Fat	9.08 g	(45% DV)	Vitamin A	5913.4 IU	(118% DV)
Poly Fat	6.81 g		Vitamin C	9.1 mg	(15% DV)
Mono Fat	11.35 g		Calcium	56.8 mg	(6% DV)
Cholesterol	61.3 mg	(20% DV)	Iron	3 mg	(17% DV)
Sodium	563 mg	(23% DV)	Folate	20.4 mcg	(7% DV)
Potassium	345 mg	(10% DV)	Beta Carotene	558.4 RE	

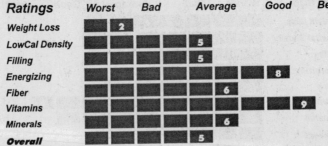

Ratings	Worst	Bad	Average	Good	Best
Weight Loss	2				
LowCal Density			5		
Filling			5		
Energizing				8	
Fiber			6		
Vitamins					9
Minerals			6		
Overall			5		

CHICKEN OR TURKEY SOUP, PREPARED WITH MILK

Serving: 1 cup (8.86 oz)   **Soup**

Calories	191	(21.6 cal/oz)	Carbohydrate	14.88 g	(5% DV)
Fat Calories	112	(58% fat)	Dietary Fiber	0 g	(0% DV)
Total Fat	12.4 g	(19% DV)	Protein	7.44 g	(15% DV)
Saturated Fat	4.96 g	(25% DV)	Vitamin A	714.2 IU	(14% DV)
Poly Fat	2.48 g		Vitamin C	2.5 mg	(4% DV)
Mono Fat	4.96 g		Calcium	181 mg	(18% DV)
Cholesterol	27.3 mg	(9% DV)	Iron	.7 mg	(4% DV)
Sodium	1046.6 mg	(44% DV)	Folate	7.4 mcg	(2% DV)
Potassium	272.8 mg	(8% DV)	Beta Carotene	54.6 RE	

Ratings	Worst	Bad	Average	Good	Best
Weight Loss		3			
LowCal Density				8	
Filling			6		
Energizing			5		
Fiber	1				
Vitamins		4			
Minerals			5		
Overall			5		

CHICKEN OR TURKEY STEW, POTATOES & VEGETABLES

Serving: 1 cup (9 oz)   **Entree**

Calories	287	(31.9 cal/oz)	Carbohydrate	15.12 g	(5% DV)
Fat Calories	136	(47% fat)	Dietary Fiber	2.52 g	(10% DV)
Total Fat	15.12 g	(23% DV)	Protein	25.2 g	(50% DV)
Saturated Fat	5.04 g	(25% DV)	Vitamin A	7673.4 IU	(153% DV)
Poly Fat	2.52 g		Vitamin C	12.6 mg	(21% DV)
Mono Fat	5.04 g		Calcium	32.8 mg	(3% DV)
Cholesterol	85.7 mg	(29% DV)	Iron	1.9 mg	(10% DV)
Sodium	458.6 mg	(19% DV)	Folate	25.2 mcg	(4% DV)
Potassium	632.5 mg	(18% DV)	Beta Carotene	753.5 RE	

Ratings	Worst	Bad	Average	Good	Best
Weight Loss			5		
LowCal Density				7	
Filling			5		
Energizing			5		
Fiber				7	
Vitamins					10
Minerals			6		
Overall			6		

CHICKEN OR TURKEY TETRAZZINI

Serving: 1 cup (8.79 oz)   **Entree**

Calories	371	(42.3 cal/oz)	Carbohydrate	28.29 g	(9% DV)
Fat Calories	177	(48% fat)	Dietary Fiber	2.46 g	(10% DV)
Total Fat	19.68 g	(30% DV)	Protein	19.68 g	(39% DV)
Saturated Fat	7.38 g	(37% DV)	Vitamin A	496.9 IU	(10% DV)
Poly Fat	4.92 g		Vitamin C	4.9 mg	(8% DV)
Mono Fat	4.92 g		Calcium	145.1 mg	(15% DV)
Cholesterol	49.2 mg	(16% DV)	Iron	2 mg	(11% DV)
Sodium	814.3 mg	(34% DV)	Folate	19.7 mcg	(3% DV)
Potassium	201.7 mg	(6% DV)	Beta Carotene	17.2 RE	

Ratings	Worst	Bad	Average	Good	Best
Weight Loss			4		
LowCal Density			6		
Filling			6		
Energizing			7		
Fiber			7		
Vitamins			6		
Minerals			7		
Overall			6		

CHICKEN OR TURKEY WITH DUMPLINGS

Serving: 1 cup (8.71 oz)   **Entree**

Calories	373	(42.9 cal/oz)	Carbohydrate	19.52 g	(7% DV)
Fat Calories	176	(47% fat)	Dietary Fiber	0 g	(0% DV)
Total Fat	19.52 g	(30% DV)	Protein	26.84 g	(54% DV)
Saturated Fat	4.88 g	(24% DV)	Vitamin A	170.8 IU	(3% DV)
Poly Fat	4.88 g		Vitamin C	2.4 mg	(4% DV)
Mono Fat	7.32 g		Calcium	109.8 mg	(11% DV)
Cholesterol	95.2 mg	(32% DV)	Iron	2.3 mg	(13% DV)
Sodium	1005.3 mg	(42% DV)	Folate	26.8 mcg	(2% DV)
Potassium	302.6 mg	(9% DV)	Beta Carotene	0 RE	

Ratings	Worst	Bad	Average	Good	Best
Weight Loss			4		
LowCal Density			6		
Filling			5		
Energizing			6		
Fiber	1				
Vitamins			6		
Minerals			7		
Overall			5		

CHICKEN OR TURKEY WITH STUFFING

Serving: 1 cup (7.14 oz)   **Entree**

Calories	270	(37.8 cal/oz)	Carbohydrate	18 g	(6% DV)
Fat Calories	54	(20% fat)	Dietary Fiber	0 g	(0% DV)
Total Fat	6 g	(9% DV)	Protein	36 g	(72% DV)
Saturated Fat	2 g	(10% DV)	Vitamin A	62 IU	(1% DV)
Poly Fat	2 g		Vitamin C	2 mg	(3% DV)
Mono Fat	2 g		Calcium	50 mg	(5% DV)
Cholesterol	104 mg	(35% DV)	Iron	2.1 mg	(12% DV)
Sodium	446 mg	(19% DV)	Folate	36 mcg	(5% DV)
Potassium	384 mg	(11% DV)	Beta Carotene	0 RE	

Ratings	Worst	Bad	Average	Good	Best
Weight Loss				7	
LowCal Density				7	
Filling			5		
Energizing			6		
Fiber	1				
Vitamins			6		
Minerals				7	
Overall			6		

CHICKEN OR TURKEY, RICE, & VEGETABLES

Serving: 1 cup (9 oz)   **Entree**

Calories	348	(38.6 cal/oz)	Carbohydrate	30.49 g	(10% DV)
Fat Calories	136	(39% fat)	Dietary Fiber	2.52 g	(10% DV)
Total Fat	15.12 g	(23% DV)	Protein	20.16 g	(40% DV)
Saturated Fat	5.04 g	(25% DV)	Vitamin A	1388.5 IU	(28% DV)
Poly Fat	2.52 g		Vitamin C	25.2 mg	(42% DV)
Mono Fat	7.56 g		Calcium	63 mg	(6% DV)
Cholesterol	68 mg	(23% DV)	Iron	2.6 mg	(15% DV)
Sodium	677.9 mg	(28% DV)	Folate	20.2 mcg	(11% DV)
Potassium	362.9 mg	(10% DV)	Beta Carotene	128.5 RE	

Ratings	Worst	Bad	Average	Good	Best
Weight Loss		4			
LowCal Density				7	
Filling			6		
Energizing				7	
Fiber				7	
Vitamins					8
Minerals			6		
Overall			6		

CHICKEN PATTY OR NUGGETS, BREADED, WITH PASTA

Serving: 1 meal (6.89 oz)   **Entree**

Calories	317	(45.9 cal/oz)	Carbohydrate	44.78 g	(15% DV)
Fat Calories	104	(33% fat)	Dietary Fiber	1.93 g	(8% DV)
Total Fat	11.58 g	(18% DV)	Protein	9.65 g	(19% DV)
Saturated Fat	3.86 g	(19% DV)	VItamin A	289.5 IU	(6% DV)
Poly Fat	1.93 g		Vitamin C	5.8 mg	(10% DV)
Mono Fat	5.79 g		Calcium	29 mg	(3% DV)
Cholesterol	36.7 mg	(12% DV)	Iron	2 mg	(11% DV)
Sodium	635 mg	(26% DV)	Folate	9.7 mcg	(3% DV)
Potassium	287.6 mg	(8% DV)	Beta Carotene	40.5 RE	

Ratings	Worst	Bad	Average	Good	Best
Weight Loss			5		
LowCal Density			6		
Filling				7	
Energizing					9
Fiber			6		
Vitamins			5		
Minerals			5		
Overall			6		

CHICKEN PATTY, BREADED, COOKED

Serving: 1 patty (2.68 oz)   **Poultry**

Calories	213	(79.5 cal/oz)	Carbohydrate	11.4 g	(4% DV)
Fat Calories	115	(54% fat)	Dietary Fiber	0 g	(0% DV)
Total Fat	12.75 g	(20% DV)	Protein	12.75 g	(26% DV)
Saturated Fat	3.75 g	(19% DV)	VItamin A	75 IU	(2% DV)
Poly Fat	1.5 g		Vitamin C	0 mg	(0% DV)
Mono Fat	6.75 g		Calcium	12 mg	(1% DV)
Cholesterol	45 mg	(15% DV)	Iron	.9 mg	(5% DV)
Sodium	399 mg	(17% DV)	Folate	12.8 mcg	(2% DV)
Potassium	184.5 mg	(5% DV)	Beta Carotene	29.3 RE	

Ratings	Worst	Bad	Average	Good	Best
Weight Loss		4			
LowCal Density		4			
Filling		3			
Energizing			5		
Fiber	1				
Vitamins			5		
Minerals			5		
Overall		4			

CHICKEN RICE SOUP

Serving: 1 cup (8.61 oz)　　　　　　　　　　**Soup**

Calories	60	(7 cal/oz)	Carbohydrate	7.23 g	(2% DV)
Fat Calories	22	(36% fat)	Dietary Fiber	0 g	(0% DV)
Total Fat	2.41 g	(4% DV)	Protein	2.41 g	(5% DV)
Saturated Fat	0 g	(0% DV)	Vitamin A	660.3 IU	(13% DV)
Poly Fat	0 g		Vitamin C	0 mg	(0% DV)
Mono Fat	0 g		Calcium	16.9 mg	(2% DV)
Cholesterol	7.2 mg	(2% DV)	Iron	.8 mg	(4% DV)
Sodium	814.6 mg	(34% DV)	Folate	2.4 mcg	(0% DV)
Potassium	101.2 mg	(3% DV)	Beta Carotene	65.1 RE	

Ratings	Worst	Bad	Average	Good	Best
Weight Loss				7	
LowCal Density					10
Filling				7	
Energizing			4		
Fiber	1				
Vitamins			4		
Minerals		3			
Overall				7	

CHICKEN SALAD OR CHICKEN SPREAD SANDWICH

Serving: 1 sandwich (4.04 oz)　　　　　　　**Sandwich**

Calories	277	(68.5 cal/oz)	Carbohydrate	25.65 g	(9% DV)
Fat Calories	112	(40% fat)	Dietary Fiber	1.13 g	(5% DV)
Total Fat	12.43 g	(19% DV)	Protein	14.69 g	(29% DV)
Saturated Fat	2.26 g	(11% DV)	Vitamin A	68.9 IU	(1% DV)
Poly Fat	5.65 g		Vitamin C	1.1 mg	(2% DV)
Mono Fat	3.39 g		Calcium	71.2 mg	(7% DV)
Cholesterol	37.3 mg	(12% DV)	Iron	2 mg	(11% DV)
Sodium	414.7 mg	(17% DV)	Folate	14.7 mcg	(6% DV)
Potassium	171.8 mg	(5% DV)	Beta Carotene	2.3 RE	

Ratings	Worst	Bad	Average	Good	Best
Weight Loss			5		
LowCal Density		4			
Filling		4			
Energizing			6		
Fiber		4			
Vitamins			5		
Minerals			5		
Overall			5		

CHICKEN TERIYAKI, RICE, VEGETABLE (FROZEN MEAL)

Serving: 1 meal (10.14 oz)   Entree

Calories	364	(35.9 cal/oz)	Carbohydrate	34.08 g	(11% DV)
Fat Calories	128	(35% fat)	Dietary Fiber	2.84 g	(11% DV)
Total Fat	14.2 g	(22% DV)	Protein	22.72 g	(45% DV)
Saturated Fat	5.68 g	(28% DV)	Vitamin A	17687.5 IU	(354% DV)
Poly Fat	2.84 g		Vitamin C	2.8 mg	(5% DV)
Mono Fat	5.68 g		Calcium	56.8 mg	(6% DV)
Cholesterol	68.2 mg	(23% DV)	Iron	2.8 mg	(15% DV)
Sodium	1976.6 mg	(82% DV)	Folate	22.7 mcg	(6% DV)
Potassium	420.3 mg	(12% DV)	Beta Carotene	1749.4 RE	

Ratings	Worst	Bad	Average	Good	Best
Weight Loss			5		
LowCal Density				7	
Filling				7	
Energizing				8	
Fiber				8	
Vitamins					10
Minerals				7	
Overall				7	

CHICKEN WING WITH HOT PEPPER SAUCE

Serving: 4 wings (1.71 oz)   Entree

Calories	147	(85.9 cal/oz)	Carbohydrate	.1 g	(0% DV)
Fat Calories	95	(65% fat)	Dietary Fiber	0 g	(0% DV)
Total Fat	10.56 g	(16% DV)	Protein	12.48 g	(25% DV)
Saturated Fat	2.88 g	(14% DV)	Vitamin A	111.4 IU	(2% DV)
Poly Fat	2.4 g		Vitamin C	0 mg	(0% DV)
Mono Fat	4.32 g		Calcium	7.2 mg	(1% DV)
Cholesterol	38.9 mg	(13% DV)	Iron	.6 mg	(3% DV)
Sodium	91.7 mg	(4% DV)	Folate	12.5 mcg	(0% DV)
Potassium	87.8 mg	(3% DV)	Beta Carotene	3.8 RE	

Ratings	Worst	Bad	Average	Good	Best
Weight Loss			5		
LowCal Density		3			
Filling	1				
Energizing		2			
Fiber	1				
Vitamins			4		
Minerals			4		
Overall		3			

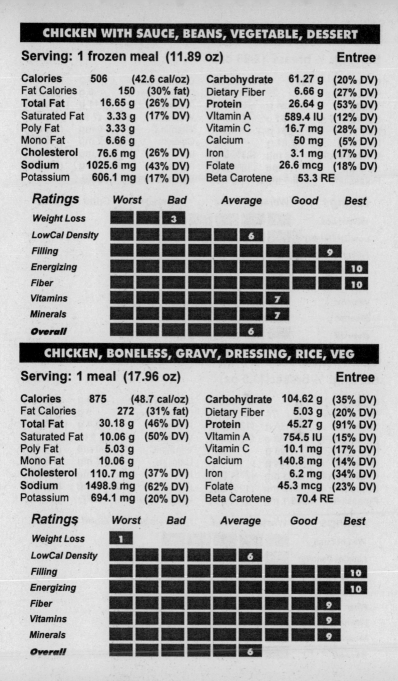

CHICKEN WITH SAUCE, BEANS, VEGETABLE, DESSERT

Serving: 1 frozen meal (11.89 oz)   **Entree**

Calories	506	(42.6 cal/oz)	Carbohydrate	61.27 g	(20% DV)
Fat Calories	150	(30% fat)	Dietary Fiber	6.66 g	(27% DV)
Total Fat	16.65 g	(26% DV)	Protein	26.64 g	(53% DV)
Saturated Fat	3.33 g	(17% DV)	VItamin A	589.4 IU	(12% DV)
Poly Fat	3.33 g		Vitamin C	16.7 mg	(28% DV)
Mono Fat	6.66 g		Calcium	50 mg	(5% DV)
Cholesterol	76.6 mg	(26% DV)	Iron	3.1 mg	(17% DV)
Sodium	1025.6 mg	(43% DV)	Folate	26.6 mcg	(18% DV)
Potassium	606.1 mg	(17% DV)	Beta Carotene	53.3 RE	

Ratings	Worst	Bad	Average	Good	Best
Weight Loss	3				
LowCal Density			6		
Filling				9	
Energizing					10
Fiber					10
Vitamins			7		
Minerals			7		
Overall			6		

CHICKEN, BONELESS, GRAVY, DRESSING, RICE, VEG

Serving: 1 meal (17.96 oz)   **Entree**

Calories	875	(48.7 cal/oz)	Carbohydrate	104.62 g	(35% DV)
Fat Calories	272	(31% fat)	Dietary Fiber	5.03 g	(20% DV)
Total Fat	30.18 g	(46% DV)	Protein	45.27 g	(91% DV)
Saturated Fat	10.06 g	(50% DV)	VItamin A	754.5 IU	(15% DV)
Poly Fat	5.03 g		Vitamin C	10.1 mg	(17% DV)
Mono Fat	10.06 g		Calcium	140.8 mg	(14% DV)
Cholesterol	110.7 mg	(37% DV)	Iron	6.2 mg	(34% DV)
Sodium	1498.9 mg	(62% DV)	Folate	45.3 mcg	(23% DV)
Potassium	694.1 mg	(20% DV)	Beta Carotene	70.4 RE	

Ratings	Worst	Bad	Average	Good	Best
Weight Loss	1				
LowCal Density			6		
Filling					10
Energizing					10
Fiber				9	
Vitamins				9	
Minerals				9	
Overall			6		

CHICKEN, BREAST, BROILED, SKIN NOT EATEN

Serving: ½ breast (2.89 oz)   **Poultry**

Calories	133	(46 cal/oz)	Carbohydrate	0 g	(0% DV)
Fat Calories	29	(22% fat)	Dietary Fiber	0 g	(0% DV)
Total Fat	3.24 g	(5% DV)	Protein	25.11 g	(50% DV)
Saturated Fat	.81 g	(4% DV)	VItamin A	17 IU	(0% DV)
Poly Fat	.81 g		Vitamin C	0 mg	(0% DV)
Mono Fat	.81 g		Calcium	12.2 mg	(1% DV)
Cholesterol	68 mg	(23% DV)	Iron	.8 mg	(5% DV)
Sodium	247.1 mg	(10% DV)	Folate	25.1 mcg	(1% DV)
Potassium	206.6 mg	(6% DV)	Beta Carotene	0 RE	

Ratings	Worst	Bad	Average	Good	Best
Weight Loss				7	
LowCal Density			6		
Filling	1				
Energizing	1				
Fiber	1				
Vitamins				7	
Minerals			5		
Overall			5		

CHICKEN, BREAST, WITH OR WITHOUT BONE

Serving: ½ breast (3.5 oz)   **Poultry**

Calories	192	(54.9 cal/oz)	Carbohydrate	0 g	(0% DV)
Fat Calories	71	(37% fat)	Dietary Fiber	0 g	(0% DV)
Total Fat	7.84 g	(12% DV)	Protein	29.4 g	(59% DV)
Saturated Fat	1.96 g	(10% DV)	VItamin A	90.2 IU	(2% DV)
Poly Fat	1.96 g		Vitamin C	0 mg	(0% DV)
Mono Fat	2.94 g		Calcium	13.7 mg	(1% DV)
Cholesterol	81.3 mg	(27% DV)	Iron	1 mg	(6% DV)
Sodium	296 mg	(12% DV)	Folate	29.4 mcg	(1% DV)
Potassium	239.1 mg	(7% DV)	Beta Carotene	0 RE	

Ratings	Worst	Bad	Average	Good	Best
Weight Loss			5		
LowCal Density			5		
Filling	1				
Energizing	1				
Fiber	1				
Vitamins				7	
Minerals			5		
Overall		4			

CHICKEN, BROTH, BOUILLON, OR CONSOMME

Serving: 1 cup (8.71 oz)   **Soup**

Calories	39	(4.5 cal/oz)	Carbohydrate	.98 g	(0% DV)
Fat Calories	22	(56% fat)	Dietary Fiber	0 g	(0% DV)
Total Fat	2.44 g	(4% DV)	Protein	4.88 g	(10% DV)
Saturated Fat	0 g	(0% DV)	Vitamin A	0 IU	(0% DV)
Poly Fat	0 g		Vitamin C	0 mg	(0% DV)
Mono Fat	0 g		Calcium	9.8 mg	(1% DV)
Cholesterol	0 mg	(0% DV)	Iron	.5 mg	(3% DV)
Sodium	775.9 mg	(32% DV)	Folate	4.9 mcg	(1% DV)
Potassium	209.8 mg	(6% DV)	Beta Carotene	0 RE	

Ratings	Worst	Bad	Average	Good	Best
Weight Loss			6		
LowCal Density					10
Filling	3				
Energizing	2				
Fiber	1				
Vitamins	3				
Minerals	3				
Overall			6		

CHICKEN, CANNED, LIGHT & DARK MEAT ONLY

Serving: 1 can (4.46 oz)   **Poultry**

Calories	206	(46.2 cal/oz)	Carbohydrate	0 g	(0% DV)
Fat Calories	90	(44% fat)	Dietary Fiber	0 g	(0% DV)
Total Fat	10 g	(15% DV)	Protein	27.5 g	(55% DV)
Saturated Fat	2.5 g	(12% DV)	Vitamin A	146.3 IU	(3% DV)
Poly Fat	2.5 g		Vitamin C	2.5 mg	(4% DV)
Mono Fat	3.75 g		Calcium	17.5 mg	(2% DV)
Cholesterol	77.5 mg	(26% DV)	Iron	2 mg	(11% DV)
Sodium	628.8 mg	(26% DV)	Folate	27.5 mcg	(1% DV)
Potassium	172.5 mg	(5% DV)	Beta Carotene	0 RE	

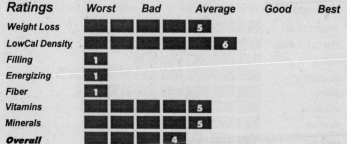

Ratings	Worst	Bad	Average	Good	Best
Weight Loss			5		
LowCal Density			6		
Filling	1				
Energizing	1				
Fiber	1				
Vitamins			5		
Minerals			5		
Overall		4			

CHICKEN, CHICKEN ROLL, ROASTED, LIGHT & DARK MEAT

Serving: 1 slice (1 oz)   **Poultry**

Calories	45	(44.5 cal/oz)	Carbohydrate	.7 g	(0% DV)
Fat Calories	18	(40% fat)	Dietary Fiber	0 g	(0% DV)
Total Fat	1.96 g	(3% DV)	Protein	5.6 g	(11% DV)
Saturated Fat	.56 g	(3% DV)	VItamin A	23 IU	(0% DV)
Poly Fat	.56 g		Vitamin C	0 mg	(0% DV)
Mono Fat	.84 g		Calcium	12 mg	(1% DV)
Cholesterol	14 mg	(5% DV)	Iron	.3 mg	(2% DV)
Sodium	163.5 mg	(7% DV)	Folate	5.6 mcg	(0% DV)
Potassium	63.8 mg	(2% DV)	Beta Carotene	0 RE	

Ratings	Worst	Bad	Average	Good	Best
Weight Loss				8	
LowCal Density			6		
Filling	1				
Energizing	2				
Fiber	1				
Vitamins	3				
Minerals	3				
Overall		5			

CHICKEN, FRIED, WITH POTATOES

Serving: 1 frozen meal (8.11 oz)   **Entree**

Calories	470	(57.9 cal/oz)	Carbohydrate	31.33 g	(10% DV)
Fat Calories	245	(52% fat)	Dietary Fiber	2.27 g	(9% DV)
Total Fat	27.24 g	(42% DV)	Protein	24.97 g	(50% DV)
Saturated Fat	6.81 g	(34% DV)	VItamin A	547.1 IU	(11% DV)
Poly Fat	9.08 g		Vitamin C	6.8 mg	(11% DV)
Mono Fat	9.08 g		Calcium	72.6 mg	(7% DV)
Cholesterol	68.1 mg	(23% DV)	Iron	2.3 mg	(13% DV)
Sodium	1246.2 mg	(52% DV)	Folate	25 mcg	(3% DV)
Potassium	388.2 mg	(11% DV)	Beta Carotene	9.1 RE	

Ratings	Worst	Bad	Average	Good	Best
Weight Loss	3				
LowCal Density			5		
Filling			5		
Energizing				8	
Fiber			6		
Vitamins			7		
Minerals			7		
Overall			5		

CHICKEN, LEG WITH SKIN, FRIED & BREADED

Serving: 1 leg (5.64 oz)   Poultry

Calories	416	(73.7 cal/oz)	Carbohydrate	8.22 g	(3% DV)
Fat Calories	213	(51% fat)	Dietary Fiber	0 g	(0% DV)
Total Fat	23.7 g	(36% DV)	Protein	41.08 g	(82% DV)
Saturated Fat	6.32 g	(32% DV)	VItamin A	135.9 IU	(3% DV)
Poly Fat	4.74 g		Vitamin C	0 mg	(0% DV)
Mono Fat	9.48 g		Calcium	26.9 mg	(3% DV)
Cholesterol	140.6 mg	(47% DV)	Iron	2.3 mg	(13% DV)
Sodium	598.8 mg	(25% DV)	Folate	41.1 mcg	(3% DV)
Potassium	371.3 mg	(11% DV)	Beta Carotene	0 RE	

Ratings	Worst	Bad	Average	Good	Best
Weight Loss	2				
LowCal Density			4		
Filling	2				
Energizing			4		
Fiber	1				
Vitamins				6	
Minerals					7
Overall		3			

CHICKEN, LEG WITHOUT SKIN, BROILED

Serving: 1 leg (3.46 oz)   Poultry

Calories	184	(53.3 cal/oz)	Carbohydrate	0 g	(0% DV)
Fat Calories	70	(38% fat)	Dietary Fiber	0 g	(0% DV)
Total Fat	7.76 g	(12% DV)	Protein	26.19 g	(52% DV)
Saturated Fat	1.94 g	(10% DV)	VItamin A	61.1 IU	(1% DV)
Poly Fat	1.94 g		Vitamin C	0 mg	(0% DV)
Mono Fat	2.91 g		Calcium	11.6 mg	(1% DV)
Cholesterol	90.2 mg	(30% DV)	Iron	1.3 mg	(7% DV)
Sodium	312.3 mg	(13% DV)	Folate	26.2 mcg	(2% DV)
Potassium	233.8 mg	(7% DV)	Beta Carotene	0 RE	

Ratings	Worst	Bad	Average	Good	Best
Weight Loss			5		
LowCal Density				6	
Filling	1				
Energizing	1				
Fiber	1				
Vitamins			5		
Minerals				6	
Overall			4		

CHICKEN, MEATLESS, VEGETARIAN

Serving: 1 cup (6 oz)   **Poultry**

Calories	370	(61.6 cal/oz)	Carbohydrate	11.76 g	(4% DV)
Fat Calories	212	(57% fat)	Dietary Fiber	8.4 g	(34% DV)
Total Fat	23.52 g	(36% DV)	Protein	28.56 g	(57% DV)
Saturated Fat	3.36 g	(17% DV)	VItamin A	0 IU	(0% DV)
Poly Fat	11.76 g		Vitamin C	0 mg	(0% DV)
Mono Fat	5.04 g		Calcium	58.8 mg	(6% DV)
Cholesterol	0 mg	(0% DV)	Iron	2.2 mg	(12% DV)
Sodium	1327.2 mg	(55% DV)	Folate	28.6 mcg	(32% DV)
Potassium	554.4 mg	(16% DV)	Beta Carotene	0 RE	

Ratings	Worst	Bad	Average	Good	Best
Weight Loss	2				
LowCal Density			5		
Filling		4			
Energizing			5		
Fiber					10
Vitamins					10
Minerals				8	
Overall			5		

CHICKEN, THIGH, FRIED & BREADED

Serving: 1 thigh (3.07 oz)   **Poultry**

Calories	231	(75.4 cal/oz)	Carbohydrate	4.47 g	(1% DV)
Fat Calories	116	(50% fat)	Dietary Fiber	0 g	(0% DV)
Total Fat	12.9 g	(20% DV)	Protein	22.36 g	(45% DV)
Saturated Fat	3.44 g	(17% DV)	VItamin A	80 IU	(2% DV)
Poly Fat	3.44 g		Vitamin C	0 mg	(0% DV)
Mono Fat	5.16 g		Calcium	14.6 mg	(1% DV)
Cholesterol	80 mg	(27% DV)	Iron	1.3 mg	(7% DV)
Sodium	325.9 mg	(14% DV)	Folate	22.4 mcg	(2% DV)
Potassium	205.5 mg	(6% DV)	Beta Carotene	0 RE	

Ratings	Worst	Bad	Average	Good	Best
Weight Loss		4			
LowCal Density		4			
Filling	2				
Energizing	3				
Fiber	1				
Vitamins			5		
Minerals			5		
Overall		4			

CHICKEN, THIGH, WITHOUT SKIN, COOKED

Serving: 1 thigh (1.86 oz)   **Poultry**

Calories	108	(58.2 cal/oz)	Carbohydrate	0 g	(0% DV)
Fat Calories	51	(48% fat)	Dietary Fiber	0 g	(0% DV)
Total Fat	5.72 g	(9% DV)	Protein	13.52 g	(27% DV)
Saturated Fat	1.56 g	(8% DV)	VItamin A	33.8 IU	(1% DV)
Poly Fat	1.04 g		Vitamin C	0 mg	(0% DV)
Mono Fat	2.08 g		Calcium	6.2 mg	(1% DV)
Cholesterol	48.9 mg	(16% DV)	Iron	.7 mg	(4% DV)
Sodium	165.9 mg	(7% DV)	Folate	13.5 mcg	(1% DV)
Potassium	123.2 mg	(4% DV)	Beta Carotene	0 RE	

Ratings	Worst	Bad	Average	Good	Best
Weight Loss				6	
LowCal Density			5		
Filling	1				
Energizing	1				
Fiber	1				
Vitamins			4		
Minerals			4		
Overall			4		

CHICKEN, WING, FRIED & BREADED

Serving: 1 wing (1.75 oz)   **Poultry**

Calories	159	(91 cal/oz)	Carbohydrate	2.55 g	(1% DV)
Fat Calories	97	(61% fat)	Dietary Fiber	0 g	(0% DV)
Total Fat	10.78 g	(17% DV)	Protein	12.25 g	(24% DV)
Saturated Fat	2.94 g	(15% DV)	VItamin A	57.8 IU	(1% DV)
Poly Fat	2.45 g		Vitamin C	0 mg	(0% DV)
Mono Fat	4.41 g		Calcium	9.3 mg	(1% DV)
Cholesterol	37.2 mg	(12% DV)	Iron	.6 mg	(3% DV)
Sodium	180.8 mg	(8% DV)	Folate	12.3 mcg	(0% DV)
Potassium	89.2 mg	(3% DV)	Beta Carotene	0 RE	

Ratings	Worst	Bad	Average	Good	Best
Weight Loss		4			
LowCal Density		3			
Filling	1				
Energizing		3			
Fiber	1				
Vitamins			4		
Minerals			4		
Overall		3			

CHICKEN, WING, WITHOUT SKIN, COOKED

Serving: 1 wing (.71 oz)   **Poultry**

Calories	40	(56.9 cal/oz)	Carbohydrate	0 g	(0% DV)
Fat Calories	14	(36% fat)	Dietary Fiber	0 g	(0% DV)
Total Fat	1.6 g	(2% DV)	**Protein**	6 g	(12% DV)
Saturated Fat	.4 g	(2% DV)	VItamin A	12.2 IU	(0% DV)
Poly Fat	.4 g		Vitamin C	0 mg	(0% DV)
Mono Fat	.6 g		Calcium	3.2 mg	(0% DV)
Cholesterol	16.8 mg	(6% DV)	Iron	.2 mg	(1% DV)
Sodium	64.6 mg	(3% DV)	Folate	6 mcg	(0% DV)
Potassium	41.8 mg	(1% DV)	Beta Carotene	0 RE	

Ratings	Worst	Bad	Average	Good	Best
Weight Loss				8	
LowCal Density			5		
Filling	1				
Energizing	1				
Fiber	1				
Vitamins		3			
Minerals		3			
Overall		4			

CHICKPEAS, DRY, COOKED WITHOUT ADDED FAT

Serving: 1 cup (5.86 oz)   **Vegetable**

Calories	295	(50.4 cal/oz)	Carbohydrate	49.2 g	(16% DV)
Fat Calories	44	(15% fat)	Dietary Fiber	13.12 g	(52% DV)
Total Fat	4.92 g	(8% DV)	**Protein**	16.4 g	(33% DV)
Saturated Fat	0 g	(0% DV)	VItamin A	49.2 IU	(1% DV)
Poly Fat	1.64 g		Vitamin C	1.6 mg	(3% DV)
Mono Fat	1.64 g		Calcium	78.7 mg	(8% DV)
Cholesterol	0 mg	(0% DV)	Iron	4.1 mg	(23% DV)
Sodium	398.5 mg	(17% DV)	Folate	16.4 mcg	(39% DV)
Potassium	496.9 mg	(14% DV)	Beta Carotene	4.9 RE	

Ratings	Worst	Bad	Average	Good	Best
Weight Loss	2				
LowCal Density			6		
Filling				7	
Energizing					9
Fiber					10
Vitamins			5		
Minerals				8	
Overall			6		

CHILI BEEF SOUP

Serving: 1 cup (8.93 oz)   **Soup**

Calories	170	(19 cal/oz)	Carbohydrate	21.5 g	(7% DV)
Fat Calories	68	(40% fat)	Dietary Fiber	10 g	(40% DV)
Total Fat	7.5 g	(12% DV)	Protein	7.5 g	(15% DV)
Saturated Fat	2.5 g	(12% DV)	Vitamin A	1510 IU	(30% DV)
Poly Fat	0 g		Vitamin C	5 mg	(8% DV)
Mono Fat	2.5 g		Calcium	42.5 mg	(4% DV)
Cholesterol	12.5 mg	(4% DV)	Iron	2.1 mg	(12% DV)
Sodium	1035 mg	(43% DV)	Folate	7.5 mcg	(4% DV)
Potassium	525 mg	(15% DV)	Beta Carotene	150 RE	

Ratings	Worst	Bad	Average	Good	Best
Weight Loss		4			
LowCal Density				8	
Filling				9	
Energizing			6		
Fiber					10
Vitamins			5		
Minerals			6		
Overall				7	

CHILI CON CARNE WITH BEANS

Serving: 1 cup (9.07 oz)   **Entree**

Calories	320	(35.3 cal/oz)	Carbohydrate	27.18 g	(9% DV)
Fat Calories	137	(43% fat)	Dietary Fiber	5.08 g	(20% DV)
Total Fat	15.24 g	(23% DV)	Protein	22.86 g	(46% DV)
Saturated Fat	5.08 g	(25% DV)	Vitamin A	1191.3 IU	(24% DV)
Poly Fat	2.54 g		Vitamin C	20.3 mg	(34% DV)
Mono Fat	5.08 g		Calcium	61 mg	(6% DV)
Cholesterol	58.4 mg	(19% DV)	Iron	3.8 mg	(21% DV)
Sodium	1277.6 mg	(53% DV)	Folate	22.9 mcg	(11% DV)
Potassium	762 mg	(22% DV)	Beta Carotene	119.4 RE	

Ratings	Worst	Bad	Average	Good	Best
Weight Loss			5		
LowCal Density				7	
Filling			6		
Energizing				7	
Fiber					9
Vitamins				7	
Minerals				8	
Overall				7	

CHILI CON QUESO (TOMATO, PEPPER & CHEESE DIP)

Serving: 1 tbsp (.54 oz)   **Sauce**

Calories	31	(58.1 cal/oz)	Carbohydrate	1.11 g	(0% DV)
Fat Calories	20	(65% fat)	Dietary Fiber	0 g	(0% DV)
Total Fat	2.25 g	(3% DV)	Protein	1.8 g	(4% DV)
Saturated Fat	1.35 g	(7% DV)	VItamin A	110 IU	(2% DV)
Poly Fat	0 g		Vitamin C	.9 mg	(2% DV)
Mono Fat	.6 g		Calcium	60 mg	(6% DV)
Cholesterol	5.9 mg	(2% DV)	Iron	.1 mg	(0% DV)
Sodium	147.8 mg	(6% DV)	Folate	1.8 mcg	(0% DV)
Potassium	36.6 mg	(1% DV)	Beta Carotene	5.1 RE	

Ratings	Worst	Bad	Average	Good	Best
Weight Loss				6	
LowCal Density			5		
Filling	1				
Energizing	2				
Fiber	1				
Vitamins	2				
Minerals			4		
Overall			4		

CHILI DOG (FRANKFURTER, CHILI CON CARNE, NO BUN)

Serving: 1 frankfurter (4.46 oz)   **Entree**

Calories	234	(52.4 cal/oz)	Carbohydrate	10.63 g	(4% DV)
Fat Calories	158	(67% fat)	Dietary Fiber	2.5 g	(10% DV)
Total Fat	17.5 g	(27% DV)	Protein	10 g	(20% DV)
Saturated Fat	6.25 g	(31% DV)	VItamin A	268.8 IU	(5% DV)
Poly Fat	1.25 g		Vitamin C	12.5 mg	(21% DV)
Mono Fat	7.5 g		Calcium	42.5 mg	(4% DV)
Cholesterol	36.3 mg	(12% DV)	Iron	3.3 mg	(18% DV)
Sodium	922.5 mg	(38% DV)	Folate	10 mcg	(5% DV)
Potassium	367.5 mg	(10% DV)	Beta Carotene	27.5 RE	

Ratings	Worst	Bad	Average	Good	Best
Weight Loss		4			
LowCal Density			6		
Filling		4			
Energizing		4			
Fiber				7	
Vitamins			5		
Minerals			6		
Overall			5		

CHILI, VEGETARIAN (MADE WITH MEAT SUBSTITUTE)

Serving: 1 cup (9.07 oz) **Entree**

Calories	335	(37 cal/oz)	Carbohydrate	35.81 g	(12% DV)
Fat Calories	46	(14% fat)	Dietary Fiber	10.16 g	(41% DV)
Total Fat	5.08 g	(8% DV)	Protein	45.72 g	(91% DV)
Saturated Fat	0 g	(0% DV)	Vitamin A	1846.6 IU	(37% DV)
Poly Fat	2.54 g		Vitamin C	38.1 mg	(64% DV)
Mono Fat	2.54 g		Calcium	127 mg	(13% DV)
Cholesterol	0 mg	(0% DV)	Iron	10.1 mg	(56% DV)
Sodium	1249.7 mg	(52% DV)	Folate	45.7 mcg	(49% DV)
Potassium	861.1 mg	(25% DV)	Beta Carotene	185.4 RE	

Ratings	Worst	Bad	Average	Good	Best
Weight Loss			6		
LowCal Density			7		
Filling			7		
Energizing				8	
Fiber					10
Vitamins				9	
Minerals				9	
Overall			7		

CHIMICHANGA WITH BEEF, BEANS, LETTUCE & TOMATO

Serving: 1 chimichanga (4.21 oz) **Entree**

Calories	249	(59.1 cal/oz)	Carbohydrate	25.61 g	(9% DV)
Fat Calories	106	(43% fat)	Dietary Fiber	3.54 g	(14% DV)
Total Fat	11.8 g	(18% DV)	Protein	10.62 g	(21% DV)
Saturated Fat	3.54 g	(18% DV)	Vitamin A	402.4 IU	(8% DV)
Poly Fat	2.36 g		Vitamin C	9.4 mg	(16% DV)
Mono Fat	4.72 g		Calcium	46 mg	(5% DV)
Cholesterol	23.6 mg	(8% DV)	Iron	2.6 mg	(15% DV)
Sodium	241.9 mg	(10% DV)	Folate	10.6 mcg	(14% DV)
Potassium	385.9 mg	(11% DV)	Beta Carotene	40.1 RE	

Ratings	Worst	Bad	Average	Good	Best
Weight Loss			5		
LowCal Density			5		
Filling			5		
Energizing			6		
Fiber				8	
Vitamins			6		
Minerals			6		
Overall			5		

CHIMICHANGA WITH CHICKEN, SOUR CREAM, LETTUCE

Serving: 1 chimichanga (4.21 oz)   **Entree**

Calories	230	(54.7 cal/oz)	Carbohydrate	22.07 g	(7% DV)
Fat Calories	96	(42% fat)	Dietary Fiber	1.18 g	(5% DV)
Total Fat	10.62 g	(16% DV)	Protein	10.62 g	(21% DV)
Saturated Fat	4.72 g	(24% DV)	VItamin A	408.3 IU	(8% DV)
Poly Fat	1.18 g		Vitamin C	4.7 mg	(8% DV)
Mono Fat	3.54 g		Calcium	72 mg	(7% DV)
Cholesterol	33 mg	(11% DV)	Iron	1.6 mg	(9% DV)
Sodium	205.3 mg	(9% DV)	Folate	10.6 mcg	(4% DV)
Potassium	190 mg	(5% DV)	Beta Carotene	21.2 RE	

Ratings	Worst	Bad	Average	Good	Best
Weight Loss				6	
LowCal Density				6	
Filling			5		
Energizing				6	
Fiber			4		
Vitamins			5		
Minerals			5		
Overall				6	

CHOP SUEY, MEATLESS

Serving: 1 cup (7.86 oz)   **Entree**

Calories	249	(31.6 cal/oz)	Carbohydrate	39.82 g	(13% DV)
Fat Calories	59	(24% fat)	Dietary Fiber	2.2 g	(9% DV)
Total Fat	6.6 g	(10% DV)	Protein	4.4 g	(9% DV)
Saturated Fat	2.2 g	(11% DV)	VItamin A	118.8 IU	(2% DV)
Poly Fat	4.4 g		Vitamin C	19.8 mg	(33% DV)
Mono Fat	2.2 g		Calcium	30.8 mg	(3% DV)
Cholesterol	0 mg	(0% DV)	Iron	2.1 mg	(12% DV)
Sodium	444.4 mg	(19% DV)	Folate	4.4 mcg	(9% DV)
Potassium	288.2 mg	(8% DV)	Beta Carotene	11 RE	

Ratings	Worst	Bad	Average	Good	Best
Weight Loss				6	
LowCal Density				7	
Filling				8	
Energizing					9
Fiber				6	
Vitamins				6	
Minerals			5		
Overall				7	

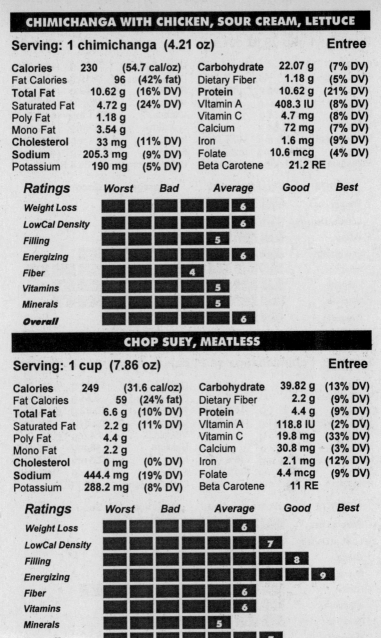

CINNAMON TOAST CRUNCH

Serving: 1 cup (1.36 oz)   **Cereal**

Calories	161	(118.2 cal/oz)	Carbohydrate	29.98 g	(10% DV)
Fat Calories	34	(21% fat)	Dietary Fiber	1.9 g	(8% DV)
Total Fat	3.8 g	(6% DV)	Protein	1.9 g	(4% DV)
Saturated Fat	3.42 g	(17% DV)	Vitamin A	1672 IU	(33% DV)
Poly Fat	0 g		Vitamin C	20.1 mg	(34% DV)
Mono Fat	.38 g		Calcium	60 mg	(6% DV)
Cholesterol	0 mg	(0% DV)	Iron	6 mg	(33% DV)
Sodium	297.5 mg	(12% DV)	Folate	1.9 mcg	(34% DV)
Potassium	55.5 mg	(2% DV)	Beta Carotene	0 RE	

Ratings	Worst	Bad	Average	Good	Best
Weight Loss				6	
LowCal Density	2				
Filling		4			
Energizing				7	
Fiber			6		
Vitamins					10
Minerals			5		
Overall			5		

CLAM CHOWDER, MANHATTAN

Serving: 1 cup (8.57 oz)   **Soup**

Calories	106	(12.3 cal/oz)	Carbohydrate	15.36 g	(5% DV)
Fat Calories	22	(20% fat)	Dietary Fiber	2.4 g	(10% DV)
Total Fat	2.4 g	(4% DV)	Protein	4.8 g	(10% DV)
Saturated Fat	2.4 g	(12% DV)	Vitamin A	2121.6 IU	(42% DV)
Poly Fat	0 g		Vitamin C	7.2 mg	(12% DV)
Mono Fat	0 g		Calcium	48 mg	(5% DV)
Cholesterol	9.6 mg	(3% DV)	Iron	2.1 mg	(12% DV)
Sodium	784.8 mg	(33% DV)	Folate	4.8 mcg	(2% DV)
Potassium	285.6 mg	(8% DV)	Beta Carotene	139.2 RE	

Ratings	Worst	Bad	Average	Good	Best
Weight Loss				7	
LowCal Density					9
Filling				8	
Energizing			5		
Fiber				7	
Vitamins			6		
Minerals			5		
Overall				7	

CLAM CHOWDER, NEW ENGLAND, WITH MILK

Serving: 1 cup (8.86 oz)   **Soup**

Calories	164	(18.5 cal/oz)	Carbohydrate	16.62 g	(6% DV)
Fat Calories	67	(41% fat)	Dietary Fiber	2.48 g	(10% DV)
Total Fat	7.44 g	(11% DV)	Protein	9.92 g	(20% DV)
Saturated Fat	2.48 g	(12% DV)	Vitamin A	163.7 IU	(3% DV)
Poly Fat	0 g		Vitamin C	2.5 mg	(4% DV)
Mono Fat	2.48 g		Calcium	186 mg	(19% DV)
Cholesterol	22.3 mg	(7% DV)	Iron	1.5 mg	(8% DV)
Sodium	992 mg	(41% DV)	Folate	9.9 mcg	(2% DV)
Potassium	300.1 mg	(9% DV)	Beta Carotene	0 RE	

Ratings	Worst	Bad	Average	Good	Best
Weight Loss			4		
LowCal Density					8
Filling				7	
Energizing			5		
Fiber				7	
Vitamins			4		
Minerals			6		
Overall			6		

CLAM SAUCE, WHITE

Serving: 1 cup (8.57 oz)   **Sauce**

Calories	598	(69.7 cal/oz)	Carbohydrate	9.6 g	(3% DV)
Fat Calories	389	(65% fat)	Dietary Fiber	0 g	(0% DV)
Total Fat	43.2 g	(66% DV)	Protein	43.2 g	(86% DV)
Saturated Fat	4.8 g	(24% DV)	Vitamin A	996 IU	(20% DV)
Poly Fat	4.8 g		Vitamin C	38.4 mg	(64% DV)
Mono Fat	28.8 g		Calcium	165.6 mg	(17% DV)
Cholesterol	110.4 mg	(37% DV)	Iron	46.7 mg	(260% DV)
Sodium	979.2 mg	(41% DV)	Folate	43.2 mcg	(12% DV)
Potassium	1060.8 mg	(30% DV)	Beta Carotene	4.8 RE	

Ratings	Worst	Bad	Average	Good	Best
Weight Loss	1				
LowCal Density			4		
Filling	2				
Energizing			4		
Fiber	1				
Vitamins					9
Minerals					10
Overall		3			

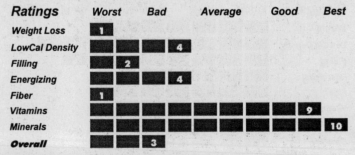

CLAMS, CANNED

Serving: 1 cup, solids only (5.71 oz) **Shellfish**

Calories	149	(26.1 cal/oz)	Carbohydrate	5.12 g	(2% DV)
Fat Calories	14	(10% fat)	Dietary Fiber	0 g	(0% DV)
Total Fat	1.6 g	(2% DV)	Protein	25.6 g	(51% DV)
Saturated Fat	0 g	(0% DV)	Vitamin A	539.2 IU	(11% DV)
Poly Fat	0 g		Vitamin C	20.8 mg	(35% DV)
Mono Fat	0 g		Calcium	92.8 mg	(9% DV)
Cholesterol	68.8 mg	(23% DV)	Iron	25.2 mg	(140% DV)
Sodium	112 mg	(5% DV)	Folate	25.6 mcg	(6% DV)
Potassium	564.8 mg	(16% DV)	Beta Carotene	0 RE	

Ratings	Worst	Bad	Average	Good	Best
Weight Loss				6	
LowCal Density					8
Filling		3			
Energizing		3			
Fiber	1				
Vitamins				7	
Minerals					10
Overall				6	

COBB SALAD WITH DRESSING

Serving: 1 cup (4.61 oz) **Salad**

Calories	182	(39.5 cal/oz)	Carbohydrate	5.03 g	(2% DV)
Fat Calories	128	(70% fat)	Dietary Fiber	1.29 g	(5% DV)
Total Fat	14.19 g	(22% DV)	Protein	9.03 g	(18% DV)
Saturated Fat	3.87 g	(19% DV)	Vitamin A	1052.6 IU	(21% DV)
Poly Fat	3.87 g		Vitamin C	12.9 mg	(22% DV)
Mono Fat	5.16 g		Calcium	72.2 mg	(7% DV)
Cholesterol	78.7 mg	(26% DV)	Iron	.9 mg	(5% DV)
Sodium	303.2 mg	(13% DV)	Folate	9 mcg	(15% DV)
Potassium	331.5 mg	(9% DV)	Beta Carotene	90.3 RE	

Ratings	Worst	Bad	Average	Good	Best
Weight Loss		3			
LowCal Density				6	
Filling		3			
Energizing		3			
Fiber			5		
Vitamins				6	
Minerals			5		
Overall		4			

COBBLER, APPLE

Serving: 1 cup (7.75 oz)   **Dessert**

Calories	469	(60.5 cal/oz)	Carbohydrate	86.8 g	(29% DV)
Fat Calories		117 (25% fat)	Dietary Fiber	2.17 g	(9% DV)
Total Fat	13.02 g	(20% DV)	Protein	4.34 g	(9% DV)
Saturated Fat	4.34 g	(22% DV)	Vitamin A	119.4 IU	(2% DV)
Poly Fat	4.34 g		Vitamin C	2.2 mg	(4% DV)
Mono Fat	4.34 g		Calcium	117.2 mg	(12% DV)
Cholesterol	4.3 mg	(1% DV)	Iron	1.6 mg	(9% DV)
Sodium	375.4 mg	(16% DV)	Folate	4.3 mcg	(2% DV)
Potassium	177.9 mg	(5% DV)	Beta Carotene	4.3 RE	

Ratings	Worst	Bad	Average	Good	Best
Weight Loss		3			
LowCal Density			5		
Filling				8	
Energizing					10
Fiber			6		
Vitamins			5		
Minerals			5		
Overall			5		

COCOA PUFFS

Serving: 1 cup (1.07 oz)   **Cereal**

Calories	117	(109.3 cal/oz)	Carbohydrate	26.1 g	(9% DV)
Fat Calories		5 (5% fat)	Dietary Fiber	.3 g	(1% DV)
Total Fat	.6 g	(1% DV)	Protein	1.8 g	(4% DV)
Saturated Fat	0 g	(0% DV)	Vitamin A	52.8 IU	(1% DV)
Poly Fat	.3 g		Vitamin C	15.9 mg	(27% DV)
Mono Fat	0 g		Calcium	.3 mg	(0% DV)
Cholesterol	0 mg	(0% DV)	Iron	4.8 mg	(26% DV)
Sodium	180 mg	(8% DV)	Folate	1.8 mcg	(26% DV)
Potassium	45 mg	(1% DV)	Beta Carotene	5.4 RE	

Ratings	Worst	Bad	Average	Good	Best
Weight Loss					9
LowCal Density	2				
Filling		4			
Energizing				7	
Fiber	2				
Vitamins					9
Minerals			5		
Overall			5		

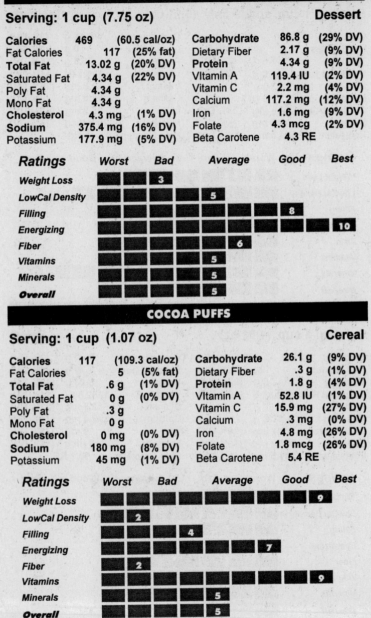

COCOA, SUGAR, & DRY MILK MIXTURE, WATER ADDED

Serving: 1 packet with 6 fl oz water (7.36 oz)   **Beverage**

Calories	103	(14 cal/oz)	Carbohydrate	22.45 g	(7% DV)
Fat Calories	19	(18% fat)	Dietary Fiber	0 g	(0% DV)
Total Fat	2.06 g	(3% DV)	Protein	2.06 g	(4% DV)
Saturated Fat	0 g	(0% DV)	Vitamin A	4.1 IU	(0% DV)
Poly Fat	0 g		Vitamin C	0 mg	(0% DV)
Mono Fat	0 g		Calcium	96.8 mg	(10% DV)
Cholesterol	2.1 mg	(1% DV)	Iron	.4 mg	(2% DV)
Sodium	148.3 mg	(6% DV)	Folate	2.1 mcg	(0% DV)
Potassium	201.9 mg	(6% DV)	Beta Carotene	0 RE	

Ratings	Worst	Bad	Average	Good	Best
Weight Loss			6		
LowCal Density					9
Filling					9
Energizing			6		
Fiber	1				
Vitamins	2				
Minerals		4			
Overall				7	

COCOA, WHEY, & LOW CALORIE SWEETENER, FORTIFIED

Serving: 1 cup (8.89 oz)   **Beverage**

Calories	50	(5.6 cal/oz)	Carbohydrate	8.72 g	(3% DV)
Fat Calories	0	(0% fat)	Dietary Fiber	0 g	(0% DV)
Total Fat	0 g	(0% DV)	Protein	4.98 g	(10% DV)
Saturated Fat	0 g	(0% DV)	Vitamin A	244 IU	(5% DV)
Poly Fat	0 g		Vitamin C	0 mg	(0% DV)
Mono Fat	0 g		Calcium	224.1 mg	(22% DV)
Cholesterol	0 mg	(0% DV)	Iron	.8 mg	(4% DV)
Sodium	107.1 mg	(4% DV)	Folate	5 mcg	(1% DV)
Potassium	413.3 mg	(12% DV)	Beta Carotene	0 RE	

Ratings	Worst	Bad	Average	Good	Best
Weight Loss				9	
LowCal Density					10
Filling				8	
Energizing		4			
Fiber	1				
Vitamins		3			
Minerals			6		
Overall				8	

COD, BAKED OR BROILED

Serving: 1 piece (3.04 oz)   **Fish**

Calories	105	(34.4 cal/oz)	Carbohydrate	.34 g	(0% DV)
Fat Calories	31	(29% fat)	Dietary Fiber	0 g	(0% DV)
Total Fat	3.4 g	(5% DV)	Protein	17.85 g	(36% DV)
Saturated Fat	.85 g	(4% DV)	Vitamin A	166.6 IU	(3% DV)
Poly Fat	.85 g		Vitamin C	2.6 mg	(4% DV)
Mono Fat	.85 g		Calcium	17 mg	(2% DV)
Cholesterol	42.5 mg	(14% DV)	Iron	.4 mg	(2% DV)
Sodium	316.2 mg	(13% DV)	Folate	17.9 mcg	(2% DV)
Potassium	415.7 mg	(12% DV)	Beta Carotene	2.6 RE	

Ratings	Worst	Bad	Average	Good	Best
Weight Loss				7	
LowCal Density				7	
Filling	1				
Energizing	2				
Fiber	1				
Vitamins			4		
Minerals			5		
Overall			5		

COD, FLOURED OR BREADED, FRIED

Serving: 1 fillet (3.93 oz)   **Fish**

Calories	230	(58.5 cal/oz)	Carbohydrate	8.69 g	(3% DV)
Fat Calories	109	(47% fat)	Dietary Fiber	0 g	(0% DV)
Total Fat	12.1 g	(19% DV)	Protein	20.9 g	(42% DV)
Saturated Fat	3.3 g	(16% DV)	Vitamin A	74.8 IU	(1% DV)
Poly Fat	3.3 g		Vitamin C	1.1 mg	(2% DV)
Mono Fat	5.5 g		Calcium	36.3 mg	(4% DV)
Cholesterol	70.4 mg	(23% DV)	Iron	1 mg	(5% DV)
Sodium	397.1 mg	(17% DV)	Folate	20.9 mcg	(3% DV)
Potassium	462 mg	(13% DV)	Beta Carotene	0 RE	

Ratings	Worst	Bad	Average	Good	Best
Weight Loss			4		
LowCal Density			5		
Filling		3			
Energizing			4		
Fiber	1				
Vitamins			4		
Minerals			5		
Overall			4		

COFFEE CAKE, CRUMB OR QUICK-BREAD TYPE

Serving: 1 piece (1/12 of 8" square) (1.5 oz)   **Bakery**

Calories	135	(90.2 cal/oz)	Carbohydrate	21.84 g	(7% DV)
Fat Calories	38	(28% fat)	Dietary Fiber	0 g	(0% DV)
Total Fat	4.2 g	(6% DV)	Protein	2.94 g	(6% DV)
Saturated Fat	1.26 g	(6% DV)	Vitamin A	60.1 IU	(1% DV)
Poly Fat	.42 g		Vitamin C	0 mg	(0% DV)
Mono Fat	2.1 g		Calcium	15.1 mg	(2% DV)
Cholesterol	40.3 mg	(13% DV)	Iron	.7 mg	(4% DV)
Sodium	185.2 mg	(8% DV)	Folate	2.9 mcg	(1% DV)
Potassium	36.1 mg	(1% DV)	Beta Carotene	0 RE	

Ratings	Worst	Bad	Average	Good	Best
Weight Loss				5	
LowCal Density		3			
Filling			4		
Energizing				6	
Fiber	1				
Vitamins		3			
Minerals		3			
Overall			4		

COFFEE CAKE, YEAST TYPE

Serving: 1 piece (1/12 of 9" square) (1.68 oz)   **Bakery**

Calories	149	(88.4 cal/oz)	Carbohydrate	23.17 g	(8% DV)
Fat Calories	38	(26% fat)	Dietary Fiber	.47 g	(2% DV)
Total Fat	4.23 g	(7% DV)	Protein	4.23 g	(8% DV)
Saturated Fat	.94 g	(5% DV)	Vitamin A	32.9 IU	(1% DV)
Poly Fat	.47 g		Vitamin C	0 mg	(0% DV)
Mono Fat	2.35 g		Calcium	49.4 mg	(5% DV)
Cholesterol	15.5 mg	(5% DV)	Iron	1 mg	(6% DV)
Sodium	182.8 mg	(8% DV)	Folate	4.2 mcg	(4% DV)
Potassium	58.3 mg	(2% DV)	Beta Carotene	0 RE	

Ratings	Worst	Bad	Average	Good	Best
Weight Loss				5	
LowCal Density		3			
Filling			4		
Energizing				6	
Fiber		3			
Vitamins			4		
Minerals			4		
Overall			4		

COFFEE CAKE, YEAST TYPE, LOW FAT, NO CHOLESTEROL

Serving: 1 piece (5"x 7/8"x 1-1/8") (1.18 oz)   **Bakery**

Calories	94	(79.4 cal/oz)	Carbohydrate	20.49 g	(7% DV)
Fat Calories	0	(0% fat)	Dietary Fiber	.66 g	(3% DV)
Total Fat	0 g	(0% DV)	Protein	2.97 g	(6% DV)
Saturated Fat	0 g	(0% DV)	Vitamin A	20.5 IU	(0% DV)
Poly Fat	0 g		Vitamin C	.7 mg	(1% DV)
Mono Fat	0 g		Calcium	15.5 mg	(2% DV)
Cholesterol	.3 mg	(0% DV)	Iron	.7 mg	(4% DV)
Sodium	53.5 mg	(2% DV)	Folate	3 mcg	(4% DV)
Potassium	59.1 mg	(2% DV)	Beta Carotene	.3 RE	

Ratings	Worst	Bad	Average	Good	Best
Weight Loss					9
LowCal Density		4			
Filling		4			
Energizing			6		
Fiber	3				
Vitamins	3				
Minerals	3				
Overall			5		

COFFEE, FROM MIX, WHITENER, LOW CAL SWEETENER

Serving: 1 mug (8.57 oz)   **Beverage**

Calories	38	(4.5 cal/oz)	Carbohydrate	3.84 g	(1% DV)
Fat Calories	22	(56% fat)	Dietary Fiber	0 g	(0% DV)
Total Fat	2.4 g	(4% DV)	Protein	0 g	(0% DV)
Saturated Fat	2.4 g	(12% DV)	Vitamin A	0 IU	(0% DV)
Poly Fat	0 g		Vitamin C	0 mg	(0% DV)
Mono Fat	0 g		Calcium	12 mg	(1% DV)
Cholesterol	0 mg	(0% DV)	Iron	.3 mg	(2% DV)
Sodium	33.6 mg	(1% DV)	Folate	0 mcg	(0% DV)
Potassium	156 mg	(4% DV)	Beta Carotene	0 RE	

Ratings	Worst	Bad	Average	Good	Best
Weight Loss			6		
LowCal Density					10
Filling			6		
Energizing		3			
Fiber	1				
Vitamins	2				
Minerals		3			
Overall			6		

COFFEE, FROM MIX, WITH WHITENER & SUGAR

Serving: 1 mug (8.57 oz)   **Beverage**

Calories	74	(8.7 cal/oz)	Carbohydrate	10.8 g	(4% DV)
Fat Calories	22	(29% fat)	Dietary Fiber	0 g	(0% DV)
Total Fat	2.4 g	(4% DV)	Protein	0 g	(0% DV)
Saturated Fat	2.4 g	(12% DV)	Vitamin A	0 IU	(0% DV)
Poly Fat	0 g		Vitamin C	0 mg	(0% DV)
Mono Fat	0 g		Calcium	9.6 mg	(1% DV)
Cholesterol	0 mg	(0% DV)	Iron	.2 mg	(1% DV)
Sodium	79.2 mg	(3% DV)	Folate	0 mcg	(0% DV)
Potassium	163.2 mg	(5% DV)	Beta Carotene	0 RE	

Ratings	Worst	Bad	Average	Good	Best
Weight Loss			6		
LowCal Density					9
Filling			7		
Energizing		4			
Fiber	1				
Vitamins	2				
Minerals	3				
Overall			6		

COFFEE, MADE FROM GROUND, REGULAR

Serving: 1 mug (8.57 oz)   **Beverage**

Calories	5	(.6 cal/oz)	Carbohydrate	.96 g	(0% DV)
Fat Calories	0	(0% fat)	Dietary Fiber	0 g	(0% DV)
Total Fat	0 g	(0% DV)	Protein	0 g	(0% DV)
Saturated Fat	0 g	(0% DV)	Vitamin A	0 IU	(0% DV)
Poly Fat	0 g		Vitamin C	0 mg	(0% DV)
Mono Fat	0 g		Calcium	4.8 mg	(0% DV)
Cholesterol	0 mg	(0% DV)	Iron	.1 mg	(1% DV)
Sodium	4.8 mg	(0% DV)	Folate	0 mcg	(0% DV)
Potassium	129.6 mg	(4% DV)	Beta Carotene	0 RE	

Ratings	Worst	Bad	Average	Good	Best
Weight Loss					10
LowCal Density					10
Filling					9
Energizing	2				
Fiber	1				
Vitamins	2				
Minerals	2				
Overall				8	

COOKIE, BROWNIE, WITH ICING

Serving: 1 brownie (2" x 2") (1.5 oz)   **Bakery**

Calories	176	(117.3 cal/oz)	Carbohydrate	25.49 g	(8% DV)
Fat Calories	79	(45% fat)	Dietary Fiber	.84 g	(3% DV)
Total Fat	8.82 g	(14% DV)	Protein	2.1 g	(4% DV)
Saturated Fat	2.1 g	(11% DV)	VItamin A	123.1 IU	(2% DV)
Poly Fat	1.26 g		Vitamin C	0 mg	(0% DV)
Mono Fat	4.62 g		Calcium	16.8 mg	(2% DV)
Cholesterol	7.1 mg	(2% DV)	Iron	1 mg	(6% DV)
Sodium	84 mg	(4% DV)	Folate	2.1 mcg	(1% DV)
Potassium	75.2 mg	(2% DV)	Beta Carotene	3.8 RE	

Ratings	Worst	Bad	Average	Good	Best
Weight Loss		3			
LowCal Density	2				
Filling		3			
Energizing				6	
Fiber			4		
Vitamins		3			
Minerals			4		
Overall		3			

COOKIE, BROWNIE, WITH ICING, DIETETIC

Serving: 1 brownie (2" x 2") (1.21 oz)   **Bakery**

Calories	104	(86 cal/oz)	Carbohydrate	22.1 g	(7% DV)
Fat Calories	31	(29% fat)	Dietary Fiber	5.1 g	(20% DV)
Total Fat	3.4 g	(5% DV)	Protein	2.38 g	(5% DV)
Saturated Fat	1.36 g	(7% DV)	VItamin A	29.9 IU	(1% DV)
Poly Fat	.68 g		Vitamin C	.3 mg	(1% DV)
Mono Fat	1.02 g		Calcium	10.5 mg	(1% DV)
Cholesterol	18 mg	(6% DV)	Iron	.8 mg	(5% DV)
Sodium	133.6 mg	(6% DV)	Folate	2.4 mcg	(1% DV)
Potassium	121.4 mg	(3% DV)	Beta Carotene	.3 RE	

Ratings	Worst	Bad	Average	Good	Best
Weight Loss			6		
LowCal Density		3			
Filling			4		
Energizing			6		
Fiber					9
Vitamins	2				
Minerals			4		
Overall			5		

Serving: 1 cookie (.57 oz)   **Bakery**

Calories	72	(126.3 cal/oz)	Carbohydrate	12.18 g	(4% DV)
Fat Calories	20	(28% fat)	Dietary Fiber	.16 g	(1% DV)
Total Fat	2.24 g	(3% DV)	Protein	.8 g	(2% DV)
Saturated Fat	.64 g	(3% DV)	Vitamin A	31.2 IU	(1% DV)
Poly Fat	.48 g		Vitamin C	0 mg	(0% DV)
Mono Fat	.96 g		Calcium	12.5 mg	(1% DV)
Cholesterol	7.2 mg	(2% DV)	Iron	.3 mg	(2% DV)
Sodium	44.5 mg	(2% DV)	Folate	.8 mcg	(0% DV)
Potassium	10.7 mg	(0% DV)	Beta Carotene	.5 RE	

Ratings	Worst	Bad	Average	Good	Best
Weight Loss				7	
LowCal Density	2				
Filling	2				
Energizing			5		
Fiber	2				
Vitamins	2				
Minerals	2				
Overall		4			

Serving: 1 cookie (.46 oz)   **Bakery**

Calories	51	(111.6 cal/oz)	Carbohydrate	8.52 g	(3% DV)
Fat Calories	20	(39% fat)	Dietary Fiber	.78 g	(3% DV)
Total Fat	2.21 g	(3% DV)	Protein	1.17 g	(2% DV)
Saturated Fat	.39 g	(2% DV)	Vitamin A	12.2 IU	(0% DV)
Poly Fat	.65 g		Vitamin C	0 mg	(0% DV)
Mono Fat	1.04 g		Calcium	35.1 mg	(4% DV)
Cholesterol	7.8 mg	(3% DV)	Iron	.3 mg	(2% DV)
Sodium	40.2 mg	(2% DV)	Folate	1.2 mcg	(1% DV)
Potassium	69.9 mg	(2% DV)	Beta Carotene	0 RE	

Ratings	Worst	Bad	Average	Good	Best
Weight Loss				7	
LowCal Density	2				
Filling	2				
Energizing			4		
Fiber		3			
Vitamins	2				
Minerals		3			
Overall		4			

COOKIE, CHOCOLATE CHIP

Serving: 1 cookie (approx 2" dia) (.36 oz)   **Bakery**

Calories	47	(130.8 cal/oz)	Carbohydrate	6.97 g	(2% DV)
Fat Calories	19	(40% fat)	Dietary Fiber	.3 g	(1% DV)
Total Fat	2.1 g	(3% DV)	Protein	.5 g	(1% DV)
Saturated Fat	.7 g	(3% DV)	Vitamin A	12 IU	(0% DV)
Poly Fat	.2 g		Vitamin C	0 mg	(0% DV)
Mono Fat	1.1 g		Calcium	3.9 mg	(0% DV)
Cholesterol	0 mg	(0% DV)	Iron	.3 mg	(2% DV)
Sodium	40.1 mg	(2% DV)	Folate	.5 mcg	(0% DV)
Potassium	13.4 mg	(0% DV)	Beta Carotene	0 RE	

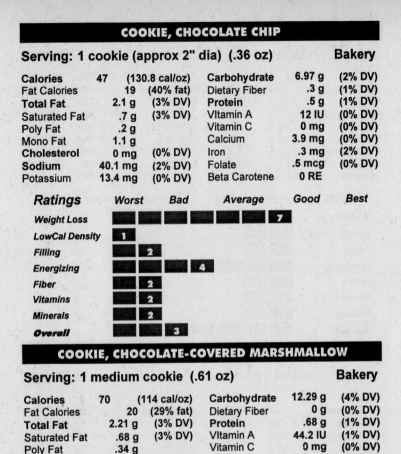

Ratings   Worst   Bad   Average   Good   Best

Weight Loss	7
LowCal Density	1
Filling	2
Energizing	4
Fiber	2
Vitamins	2
Minerals	2
Overall	3

COOKIE, CHOCOLATE-COVERED MARSHMALLOW

Serving: 1 medium cookie (.61 oz)   **Bakery**

Calories	70	(114 cal/oz)	Carbohydrate	12.29 g	(4% DV)
Fat Calories	20	(29% fat)	Dietary Fiber	0 g	(0% DV)
Total Fat	2.21 g	(3% DV)	Protein	.68 g	(1% DV)
Saturated Fat	.68 g	(3% DV)	Vitamin A	44.2 IU	(1% DV)
Poly Fat	.34 g		Vitamin C	0 mg	(0% DV)
Mono Fat	1.19 g		Calcium	3.6 mg	(0% DV)
Cholesterol	0 mg	(0% DV)	Iron	.3 mg	(2% DV)
Sodium	35.5 mg	(1% DV)	Folate	.7 mcg	(1% DV)
Potassium	15.5 mg	(0% DV)	Beta Carotene	.3 RE	

Ratings   Worst   Bad   Average   Good   Best

Weight Loss	7
LowCal Density	2
Filling	2
Energizing	5
Fiber	1
Vitamins	2
Minerals	2
Overall	4

COOKIE, DIETETIC, CHOCOLATE CHIP

Serving: 2 cookies (.5 oz)   **Bakery**

Calories	70	(139.4 cal/oz)	Carbohydrate	8.76 g	(3% DV)
Fat Calories	34	(49% fat)	Dietary Fiber	.7 g	(3% DV)
Total Fat	3.78 g	(6% DV)	Protein	.7 g	(1% DV)
Saturated Fat	1.26 g	(6% DV)	Vitamin A	4.3 IU	(0% DV)
Poly Fat	1.12 g		Vitamin C	0 mg	(0% DV)
Mono Fat	1.26 g		Calcium	4.3 mg	(0% DV)
Cholesterol	1.7 mg	(1% DV)	Iron	.2 mg	(1% DV)
Sodium	1.7 mg	(0% DV)	Folate	.7 mcg	(0% DV)
Potassium	11.6 mg	(0% DV)	Beta Carotene	0 RE	

Ratings	Worst	Bad	Average	Good	Best
Weight Loss				6	
LowCal Density	1				
Filling	2				
Energizing			4		
Fiber		3			
Vitamins	2				
Minerals	2				
Overall		3			

COOKIE, DIETETIC, OATMEAL WITH RAISINS

Serving: 2 cookies (.5 oz)   **Bakery**

Calories	61	(121.8 cal/oz)	Carbohydrate	8.93 g	(3% DV)
Fat Calories	23	(37% fat)	Dietary Fiber	.28 g	(1% DV)
Total Fat	2.52 g	(4% DV)	Protein	.84 g	(2% DV)
Saturated Fat	.7 g	(3% DV)	Vitamin A	.1 IU	(0% DV)
Poly Fat	.7 g		Vitamin C	0 mg	(0% DV)
Mono Fat	1.12 g		Calcium	3.1 mg	(0% DV)
Cholesterol	.6 mg	(0% DV)	Iron	.3 mg	(2% DV)
Sodium	.4 mg	(0% DV)	Folate	.8 mcg	(0% DV)
Potassium	23.5 mg	(1% DV)	Beta Carotene	0 RE	

Ratings	Worst	Bad	Average	Good	Best
Weight Loss				7	
LowCal Density	2				
Filling	2				
Energizing			4		
Fiber	2				
Vitamins	2				
Minerals	2				
Overall		4			

COOKIE, DIETETIC, SANDWICH TYPE

Serving: 1 cookie (.43 oz)   **Bakery**

Calories	55	(127.5 cal/oz)	Carbohydrate	6.68 g	(2% DV)
Fat Calories	27	(49% fat)	Dietary Fiber	.12 g	(0% DV)
Total Fat	3 g	(5% DV)	Protein	.6 g	(1% DV)
Saturated Fat	.72 g	(4% DV)	VItamin A	.1 IU	(0% DV)
Poly Fat	.84 g		Vitamin C	0 mg	(0% DV)
Mono Fat	1.32 g		Calcium	4.3 mg	(0% DV)
Cholesterol	0 mg	(0% DV)	Iron	.1 mg	(1% DV)
Sodium	1.4 mg	(0% DV)	Folate	.6 mcg	(0% DV)
Potassium	11.6 mg	(0% DV)	Beta Carotene	0 RE	

Ratings	Worst	Bad	Average	Good	Best
Weight Loss				6	
LowCal Density	2				
Filling	2				
Energizing			4		
Fiber	2				
Vitamins	2				
Minerals	2				
Overall	3				

COOKIE, DIETETIC, SUGAR OR PLAIN

Serving: 2 cookies (.5 oz)   **Bakery**

Calories	65	(129.9 cal/oz)	Carbohydrate	8.25 g	(3% DV)
Fat Calories	30	(47% fat)	Dietary Fiber	0 g	(0% DV)
Total Fat	3.36 g	(5% DV)	Protein	.7 g	(1% DV)
Saturated Fat	.7 g	(3% DV)	VItamin A	0 IU	(0% DV)
Poly Fat	.98 g		Vitamin C	0 mg	(0% DV)
Mono Fat	1.4 g		Calcium	1 mg	(0% DV)
Cholesterol	8.5 mg	(3% DV)	Iron	.2 mg	(1% DV)
Sodium	.1 mg	(0% DV)	Folate	.7 mcg	(0% DV)
Potassium	5.7 mg	(0% DV)	Beta Carotene	0 RE	

Ratings	Worst	Bad	Average	Good	Best
Weight Loss				6	
LowCal Density	2				
Filling	2				
Energizing			4		
Fiber	1				
Vitamins	2				
Minerals	2				
Overall	3				

COOKIE, FIG BAR

Serving: 1 cookie (.57 oz)   **Bakery**

Calories	57	(100.5 cal/oz)	Carbohydrate	12.06 g	(4% DV)
Fat Calories	9	(15% fat)	Dietary Fiber	.8 g	(3% DV)
Total Fat	.96 g	(1% DV)	Protein	.64 g	(1% DV)
Saturated Fat	.16 g	(1% DV)	Vitamin A	17.6 IU	(0% DV)
Poly Fat	.16 g		Vitamin C	0 mg	(0% DV)
Mono Fat	.48 g		Calcium	12.5 mg	(1% DV)
Cholesterol	0 mg	(0% DV)	Iron	.4 mg	(2% DV)
Sodium	40.3 mg	(2% DV)	Folate	.6 mcg	(0% DV)
Potassium	31.7 mg	(1% DV)	Beta Carotene	1.8 RE	

Ratings	Worst	Bad	Average	Good	Best
Weight Loss					9
LowCal Density	2				
Filling	2				
Energizing			5		
Fiber		4			
Vitamins	2				
Minerals	2				
Overall		4			

COOKIE, FORTUNE

Serving: 1 cookie (.29 oz)   **Bakery**

Calories	30	(104.3 cal/oz)	Carbohydrate	6.7 g	(2% DV)
Fat Calories	2	(7% fat)	Dietary Fiber	.16 g	(1% DV)
Total Fat	.24 g	(0% DV)	Protein	.4 g	(1% DV)
Saturated Fat	0 g	(0% DV)	Vitamin A	.8 IU	(0% DV)
Poly Fat	.08 g		Vitamin C	0 mg	(0% DV)
Mono Fat	0 g		Calcium	1 mg	(0% DV)
Cholesterol	.9 mg	(0% DV)	Iron	.1 mg	(1% DV)
Sodium	21.9 mg	(1% DV)	Folate	.4 mcg	(0% DV)
Potassium	3.3 mg	(0% DV)	Beta Carotene	0 RE	

Ratings	Worst	Bad	Average	Good	Best
Weight Loss					9
LowCal Density	2				
Filling	2				
Energizing		4			
Fiber	2				
Vitamins	2				
Minerals	2				
Overall		4			

COOKIE, GRANOLA

Serving: 1 cookie (.46 oz) **Bakery**

Calories	60	(129.7 cal/oz)	Carbohydrate	8.72 g	(3% DV)
Fat Calories	20	(33% fat)	Dietary Fiber	.52 g	(2% DV)
Total Fat	2.21 g	(3% DV)	Protein	1.17 g	(2% DV)
Saturated Fat	1.82 g	(9% DV)	VItamin A	1.3 IU	(0% DV)
Poly Fat	0 g		Vitamin C	.1 mg	(0% DV)
Mono Fat	.13 g		Calcium	8.8 mg	(1% DV)
Cholesterol	0 mg	(0% DV)	Iron	.4 mg	(2% DV)
Sodium	42.9 mg	(2% DV)	Folate	1.2 mcg	(3% DV)
Potassium	46.8 mg	(1% DV)	Beta Carotene	.1 RE	

Ratings	Worst	Bad	Average	Good	Best
Weight Loss					7
LowCal Density	2				
Filling	2				
Energizing		4			
Fiber		3			
Vitamins		3			
Minerals		3			
Overall		4			

COOKIE, MACAROON

Serving: 1 cookie (.86 oz) **Bakery**

Calories	96	(112.2 cal/oz)	Carbohydrate	17.28 g	(6% DV)
Fat Calories	28	(29% fat)	Dietary Fiber	.48 g	(2% DV)
Total Fat	3.12 g	(5% DV)	Protein	.96 g	(2% DV)
Saturated Fat	2.64 g	(13% DV)	VItamin A	0 IU	(0% DV)
Poly Fat	0 g		Vitamin C	0 mg	(0% DV)
Mono Fat	.24 g		Calcium	2.2 mg	(0% DV)
Cholesterol	0 mg	(0% DV)	Iron	.2 mg	(1% DV)
Sodium	58.6 mg	(2% DV)	Folate	1 mcg	(0% DV)
Potassium	37.4 mg	(1% DV)	Beta Carotene	0 RE	

Ratings	Worst	Bad	Average	Good	Best
Weight Loss			6		
LowCal Density	2				
Filling		3			
Energizing			6		
Fiber		3			
Vitamins	2				
Minerals	2				
Overall		4			

COOKIE, OATMEAL, WITH CHOCOLATE CHIPS

Serving: 1 cookie (.64 oz)   **Bakery**

Calories	92	(144.3 cal/oz)	Carbohydrate	10.17 g	(3% DV)
Fat Calories	52	(56% fat)	Dietary Fiber	.36 g	(1% DV)
Total Fat	5.76 g	(9% DV)	Protein	.9 g	(2% DV)
Saturated Fat	1.62 g	(8% DV)	VItamin A	103.7 IU	(2% DV)
Poly Fat	1.62 g		Vitamin C	0 mg	(0% DV)
Mono Fat	2.34 g		Calcium	6.8 mg	(1% DV)
Cholesterol	4.3 mg	(1% DV)	Iron	.4 mg	(2% DV)
Sodium	62.6 mg	(3% DV)	Folate	.9 mcg	(0% DV)
Potassium	36.4 mg	(1% DV)	Beta Carotene	2.2 RE	

Ratings	Worst	Bad	Average	Good	Best
Weight Loss			5		
LowCal Density	1				
Filling	2				
Energizing		4			
Fiber	2				
Vitamins	2				
Minerals	3				
Overall	3				

COOKIE, OATMEAL, WITH RAISINS

Serving: 1 cookie (.46 oz)   **Bakery**

Calories	59	(127.5 cal/oz)	Carbohydrate	9.56 g	(3% DV)
Fat Calories	18	(30% fat)	Dietary Fiber	.39 g	(2% DV)
Total Fat	1.95 g	(3% DV)	Protein	.78 g	(2% DV)
Saturated Fat	.39 g	(2% DV)	VItamin A	10.4 IU	(0% DV)
Poly Fat	.26 g		Vitamin C	0 mg	(0% DV)
Mono Fat	1.17 g		Calcium	2.7 mg	(0% DV)
Cholesterol	0 mg	(0% DV)	Iron	.4 mg	(2% DV)
Sodium	21.1 mg	(1% DV)	Folate	.8 mcg	(0% DV)
Potassium	48.1 mg	(1% DV)	Beta Carotene	0 RE	

Ratings	Worst	Bad	Average	Good	Best
Weight Loss				7	
LowCal Density	2				
Filling	2				
Energizing		4			
Fiber	2				
Vitamins	2				
Minerals	2				
Overall		4			

COOKIE, PEANUT BUTTER

Serving: 1 cookie (.57 oz)   **Bakery**

Calories	81	(142 cal/oz)	Carbohydrate	9.74 g	(3% DV)
Fat Calories	37	(46% fat)	Dietary Fiber	.32 g	(1% DV)
Total Fat	4.16 g	(6% DV)	Protein	1.44 g	(3% DV)
Saturated Fat	.96 g	(5% DV)	Vitamin A	8.2 IU	(0% DV)
Poly Fat	1.12 g		Vitamin C	0 mg	(0% DV)
Mono Fat	1.92 g		Calcium	5.3 mg	(1% DV)
Cholesterol	5.3 mg	(2% DV)	Iron	.4 mg	(2% DV)
Sodium	32.3 mg	(1% DV)	Folate	1.4 mcg	(1% DV)
Potassium	39.5 mg	(1% DV)	Beta Carotene	0 RE	

Ratings	Worst	Bad	Average	Good	Best
Weight Loss				6	
LowCal Density	1				
Filling	2				
Energizing			4		
Fiber	2				
Vitamins	3				
Minerals	3				
Overall	3				

COOKIE, PFEFFERNUSSE

Serving: 1 cookie (.46 oz)   **Bakery**

Calories	52	(113.6 cal/oz)	Carbohydrate	9.41 g	(3% DV)
Fat Calories	12	(22% fat)	Dietary Fiber	.13 g	(1% DV)
Total Fat	1.3 g	(2% DV)	Protein	.78 g	(2% DV)
Saturated Fat	.26 g	(1% DV)	Vitamin A	65.4 IU	(1% DV)
Poly Fat	.39 g		Vitamin C	0 mg	(0% DV)
Mono Fat	.52 g		Calcium	8.7 mg	(1% DV)
Cholesterol	5.2 mg	(2% DV)	Iron	.5 mg	(3% DV)
Sodium	38.9 mg	(2% DV)	Folate	.8 mcg	(0% DV)
Potassium	52.7 mg	(2% DV)	Beta Carotene	1.3 RE	

Ratings	Worst	Bad	Average	Good	Best
Weight Loss					8
LowCal Density	2				
Filling	2				
Energizing			4		
Fiber	2				
Vitamins	2				
Minerals	3				
Overall		4			

COOKIE, SANDWICH-TYPE, NOT CHOCOLATE OR VANILLA

Serving: 1 sandwich (.39 oz)   **Bakery**

Calories	54	(139.6 cal/oz)	Carbohydrate	7.62 g	(3% DV)
Fat Calories	23	(42% fat)	Dietary Fiber	.22 g	(1% DV)
Total Fat	2.53 g	(4% DV)	Protein	.55 g	(1% DV)
Saturated Fat	.44 g	(2% DV)	VItamin A	0 IU	(0% DV)
Poly Fat	.33 g		Vitamin C	0 mg	(0% DV)
Mono Fat	1.43 g		Calcium	2.9 mg	(0% DV)
Cholesterol	0 mg	(0% DV)	Iron	.2 mg	(1% DV)
Sodium	53.1 mg	(2% DV)	Folate	.6 mcg	(0% DV)
Potassium	4.2 mg	(0% DV)	Beta Carotene	0 RE	

Ratings	Worst	Bad	Average	Good	Best
Weight Loss				7	
LowCal Density	1				
Filling	2				
Energizing		4			
Fiber	2				
Vitamins	2				
Minerals	2				
Overall	3				

COOKIE, SHORT BREAD

Serving: 1 cookie (.54 oz)   **Bakery**

Calories	75	(138.3 cal/oz)	Carbohydrate	9.76 g	(3% DV)
Fat Calories	31	(42% fat)	Dietary Fiber	.3 g	(1% DV)
Total Fat	3.45 g	(5% DV)	Protein	1.05 g	(2% DV)
Saturated Fat	.9 g	(5% DV)	VItamin A	12 IU	(0% DV)
Poly Fat	.45 g		Vitamin C	0 mg	(0% DV)
Mono Fat	1.95 g		Calcium	10.5 mg	(1% DV)
Cholesterol	5 mg	(2% DV)	Iron	.5 mg	(3% DV)
Sodium	9 mg	(0% DV)	Folate	1.1 mcg	(0% DV)
Potassium	9.9 mg	(0% DV)	Beta Carotene	0 RE	

Ratings	Worst	Bad	Average	Good	Best
Weight Loss			6		
LowCal Density	1				
Filling	2				
Energizing		4			
Fiber	2				
Vitamins	3				
Minerals	2				
Overall	3				

COOKIE, SUGAR WAFER

Serving: 2 cookies (.5 oz)   **Bakery**

Calories	68	(135.8 cal/oz)	Carbohydrate	10.28 g	(3% DV)
Fat Calories	24	(35% fat)	Dietary Fiber	.14 g	(1% DV)
Total Fat	2.66 g	(4% DV)	Protein	.7 g	(1% DV)
Saturated Fat	.56 g	(3% DV)	VItamin A	19.6 IU	(0% DV)
Poly Fat	.42 g		Vitamin C	0 mg	(0% DV)
Mono Fat	1.54 g		Calcium	5 mg	(1% DV)
Cholesterol	0 mg	(0% DV)	Iron	.3 mg	(2% DV)
Sodium	26.5 mg	(1% DV)	Folate	.7 mcg	(0% DV)
Potassium	8.4 mg	(0% DV)	Beta Carotene	0 RE	

Ratings	Worst	Bad	Average	Good	Best
Weight Loss				7	
LowCal Density	1				
Filling	2				
Energizing			4		
Fiber	2				
Vitamins	2				
Minerals	2				
Overall		3			

COOKIE, TOFFEE BAR

Serving: 1 bar (.68 oz)   **Bakery**

Calories	89	(131.6 cal/oz)	Carbohydrate	13.24 g	(4% DV)
Fat Calories	36	(40% fat)	Dietary Fiber	.57 g	(2% DV)
Total Fat	3.99 g	(6% DV)	Protein	.95 g	(2% DV)
Saturated Fat	1.71 g	(9% DV)	VItamin A	22.8 IU	(0% DV)
Poly Fat	.38 g		Vitamin C	0 mg	(0% DV)
Mono Fat	1.71 g		Calcium	7.4 mg	(1% DV)
Cholesterol	4.4 mg	(1% DV)	Iron	.5 mg	(3% DV)
Sodium	76.2 mg	(3% DV)	Folate	1 mcg	(0% DV)
Potassium	25.5 mg	(1% DV)	Beta Carotene	0 RE	

Ratings	Worst	Bad	Average	Good	Best
Weight Loss			6		
LowCal Density	1				
Filling	2				
Energizing			5		
Fiber	3				
Vitamins	2				
Minerals	3				
Overall	3				

COOKIE, VANILLA WAFER

Serving: 3 cookies (.43 oz)　　　　　　　　**Bakery**

Calories	55	(128.9 cal/oz)	Carbohydrate	8.93 g	(3% DV)
Fat Calories	17	(31% fat)	Dietary Fiber	0 g	(0% DV)
Total Fat	1.92 g	(3% DV)	Protein	.6 g	(1% DV)
Saturated Fat	.48 g	(2% DV)	Vitamin A	15.6 IU	(0% DV)
Poly Fat	.48 g		Vitamin C	0 mg	(0% DV)
Mono Fat	.84 g		Calcium	4.9 mg	(0% DV)
Cholesterol	7.4 mg	(2% DV)	Iron	.3 mg	(2% DV)
Sodium	30.2 mg	(1% DV)	Folate	.6 mcg	(0% DV)
Potassium	8.6 mg	(0% DV)	Beta Carotene	.2 RE	

Ratings	Worst	Bad	Average	Good	Best
Weight Loss				7	
LowCal Density	2				
Filling	2				
Energizing			4		
Fiber	1				
Vitamins	2				
Minerals	2				
Overall		4			

CORN CHIPS SALTY SNACKS, CORN BASE, CORN-CHEESE

Serving: 10 chips (.64 oz)　　　　　　　　**Snack**

Calories	97	(151.6 cal/oz)	Carbohydrate	10.24 g	(3% DV)
Fat Calories	53	(55% fat)	Dietary Fiber	.72 g	(3% DV)
Total Fat	5.94 g	(9% DV)	Protein	1.26 g	(3% DV)
Saturated Fat	.9 g	(5% DV)	Vitamin A	16.9 IU	(0% DV)
Poly Fat	2.88 g		Vitamin C	0 mg	(0% DV)
Mono Fat	1.8 g		Calcium	22.9 mg	(2% DV)
Cholesterol	0 mg	(0% DV)	Iron	.2 mg	(1% DV)
Sodium	113.4 mg	(5% DV)	Folate	1.3 mcg	(1% DV)
Potassium	25.6 mg	(1% DV)	Beta Carotene	1.6 RE	

Ratings	Worst	Bad	Average	Good	Best
Weight Loss			5		
LowCal Density	1				
Filling	2				
Energizing			4		
Fiber		3			
Vitamins	2				
Minerals		3			
Overall		3			

CORN DOG (FRANKFURTER WITH CORNBREAD COATING)

Serving: 1 corn dog (3.14 oz)   **Sandwich**

Calories	275	(87.4 cal/oz)	Carbohydrate	20.5 g	(7% DV)
Fat Calories	158	(58% fat)	Dietary Fiber	.88 g	(4% DV)
Total Fat	17.6 g	(27% DV)	**Protein**	8.8 g	(18% DV)
Saturated Fat	7.04 g	(35% DV)	Vitamin A	104.7 IU	(2% DV)
Poly Fat	1.76 g		Vitamin C	11.4 mg	(19% DV)
Mono Fat	7.92 g		Calcium	93.3 mg	(9% DV)
Cholesterol	47.5 mg	(16% DV)	Iron	1.6 mg	(9% DV)
Sodium	646.8 mg	(27% DV)	Folate	8.8 mcg	(3% DV)
Potassium	141.7 mg	(4% DV)	Beta Carotene	6.2 RE	

Ratings	Worst	Bad	Average	Good	Best
Weight Loss		4			
LowCal Density	3				
Filling		4			
Energizing			6		
Fiber		4			
Vitamins			5		
Minerals			5		
Overall		4			

CORN FLAKES

Serving: 1 cup (.89 oz)   **Cereal**

Calories	97	(109.3 cal/oz)	Carbohydrate	21.53 g	(7% DV)
Fat Calories	0	(0% fat)	Dietary Fiber	.5 g	(2% DV)
Total Fat	0 g	(0% DV)	**Protein**	2 g	(4% DV)
Saturated Fat	0 g	(0% DV)	Vitamin A	648.8 IU	(13% DV)
Poly Fat	0 g		Vitamin C	10.5 mg	(18% DV)
Mono Fat	0 g		Calcium	1 mg	(0% DV)
Cholesterol	0 mg	(0% DV)	Iron	1.4 mg	(8% DV)
Sodium	254.8 mg	(11% DV)	Folate	2 mcg	(20% DV)
Potassium	23.5 mg	(1% DV)	Beta Carotene	1 RE	

Ratings	Worst	Bad	Average	Good	Best
Weight Loss					9
LowCal Density	2				
Filling		3			
Energizing			6		
Fiber		3			
Vitamins				8	
Minerals		3			
Overall			5		

CORN FRITTER

Serving: 1 fritter (1.25 oz)   **Vegetable**

Calories	131	(104.7 cal/oz)	Carbohydrate	13.65 g	(5% DV)
Fat Calories	66	(51% fat)	Dietary Fiber	.7 g	(3% DV)
Total Fat	7.35 g	(11% DV)	Protein	2.8 g	(6% DV)
Saturated Fat	2.1 g	(11% DV)	VItamin A	82.3 IU	(2% DV)
Poly Fat	1.75 g		Vitamin C	1.4 mg	(2% DV)
Mono Fat	3.15 g		Calcium	35 mg	(4% DV)
Cholesterol	24.5 mg	(8% DV)	Iron	.8 mg	(5% DV)
Sodium	164.2 mg	(7% DV)	Folate	2.8 mcg	(3% DV)
Potassium	67.2 mg	(2% DV)	Beta Carotene	3.2 RE	

Ratings	Worst	Bad	Average	Good	Best
Weight Loss			4		
LowCal Density	2				
Filling	2				
Energizing			5		
Fiber		3			
Vitamins		3			
Minerals		4			
Overall		3			

CORN OIL

Serving: 1 tbsp (.49 oz)   **Fat & Oil**

Calories	120	(245.3 cal/oz)	Carbohydrate	0 g	(0% DV)
Fat Calories	122	(102% fat)	Dietary Fiber	0 g	(0% DV)
Total Fat	13.6 g	(21% DV)	Protein	0 g	(0% DV)
Saturated Fat	1.77 g	(9% DV)	VItamin A	0 IU	(0% DV)
Poly Fat	8.02 g		Vitamin C	0 mg	(0% DV)
Mono Fat	3.26 g		Calcium	0 mg	(0% DV)
Cholesterol	0 mg	(0% DV)	Iron	0 mg	(0% DV)
Sodium	0 mg	(0% DV)	Folate	0 mcg	(0% DV)
Potassium	0 mg	(0% DV)	Beta Carotene	0 RE	

Ratings	Worst	Bad	Average	Good	Best
Weight Loss	1				
LowCal Density	1				
Filling	1				
Energizing	1				
Fiber	1				
Vitamins		3			
Minerals	1				
Overall	1				

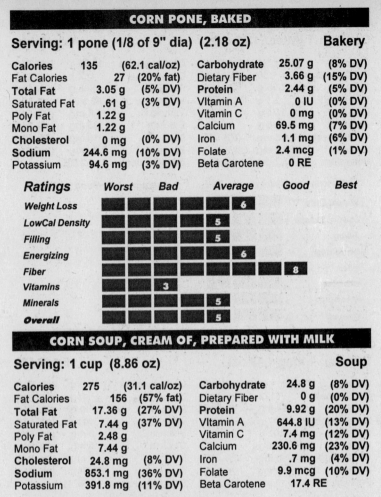

CORN PONE, BAKED

Serving: 1 pone (1/8 of 9" dia) (2.18 oz)　　　　**Bakery**

Calories	135	(62.1 cal/oz)	Carbohydrate	25.07 g	(8% DV)
Fat Calories	27	(20% fat)	Dietary Fiber	3.66 g	(15% DV)
Total Fat	3.05 g	(5% DV)	Protein	2.44 g	(5% DV)
Saturated Fat	.61 g	(3% DV)	Vitamin A	0 IU	(0% DV)
Poly Fat	1.22 g		Vitamin C	0 mg	(0% DV)
Mono Fat	1.22 g		Calcium	69.5 mg	(7% DV)
Cholesterol	0 mg	(0% DV)	Iron	1.1 mg	(6% DV)
Sodium	244.6 mg	(10% DV)	Folate	2.4 mcg	(1% DV)
Potassium	94.6 mg	(3% DV)	Beta Carotene	0 RE	

Ratings	Worst	Bad	Average	Good	Best
Weight Loss				6	
LowCal Density			5		
Filling			5		
Energizing			6		
Fiber					8
Vitamins		3			
Minerals			5		
Overall			5		

CORN SOUP, CREAM OF, PREPARED WITH MILK

Serving: 1 cup (8.86 oz)　　　　**Soup**

Calories	275	(31.1 cal/oz)	Carbohydrate	24.8 g	(8% DV)
Fat Calories	156	(57% fat)	Dietary Fiber	0 g	(0% DV)
Total Fat	17.36 g	(27% DV)	Protein	9.92 g	(20% DV)
Saturated Fat	7.44 g	(37% DV)	Vitamin A	644.8 IU	(13% DV)
Poly Fat	2.48 g		Vitamin C	7.4 mg	(12% DV)
Mono Fat	7.44 g		Calcium	230.6 mg	(23% DV)
Cholesterol	24.8 mg	(8% DV)	Iron	.7 mg	(4% DV)
Sodium	853.1 mg	(36% DV)	Folate	9.9 mcg	(10% DV)
Potassium	391.8 mg	(11% DV)	Beta Carotene	17.4 RE	

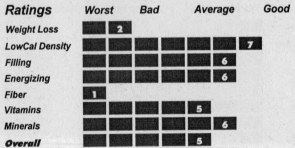

Ratings	Worst	Bad	Average	Good	Best
Weight Loss	2				
LowCal Density					7
Filling			6		
Energizing			6		
Fiber	1				
Vitamins			5		
Minerals			6		
Overall			5		

CORN, CREAM STYLE

Serving: 1 cup (9.14 oz)   **Vegetable**

Calories	184	(20.2 cal/oz)	Carbohydrate	46.34 g	(15% DV)
Fat Calories	0	(0% fat)	Dietary Fiber	2.56 g	(10% DV)
Total Fat	0 g	(0% DV)	Protein	5.12 g	(10% DV)
Saturated Fat	0 g	(0% DV)	Vitamin A	248.3 IU	(5% DV)
Poly Fat	0 g		Vitamin C	12.8 mg	(21% DV)
Mono Fat	0 g		Calcium	7.7 mg	(1% DV)
Cholesterol	0 mg	(0% DV)	Iron	1 mg	(5% DV)
Sodium	729.6 mg	(30% DV)	Folate	5.1 mcg	(29% DV)
Potassium	343 mg	(10% DV)	Beta Carotene	25.6 RE	

Ratings	Worst	Bad	Average	Good	Best
Weight Loss			5		
LowCal Density				8	
Filling					10
Energizing				9	
Fiber				7	
Vitamins			6		
Minerals			5		
Overall				7	

CORN, YELLOW, COOKED WITHOUT ADDED FAT

Serving: 1 cup (5.86 oz)   **Vegetable**

Calories	175	(29.9 cal/oz)	Carbohydrate	41 g	(14% DV)
Fat Calories	15	(8% fat)	Dietary Fiber	6.56 g	(26% DV)
Total Fat	1.64 g	(3% DV)	Protein	4.92 g	(10% DV)
Saturated Fat	0 g	(0% DV)	Vitamin A	354.2 IU	(7% DV)
Poly Fat	1.64 g		Vitamin C	9.8 mg	(16% DV)
Mono Fat	0 g		Calcium	3.3 mg	(0% DV)
Cholesterol	0 mg	(0% DV)	Iron	1 mg	(6% DV)
Sodium	406.7 mg	(17% DV)	Folate	4.9 mcg	(19% DV)
Potassium	406.7 mg	(12% DV)	Beta Carotene	36.1 RE	

Ratings	Worst	Bad	Average	Good	Best
Weight Loss			5		
LowCal Density				7	
Filling				9	
Energizing				9	
Fiber					10
Vitamins			6		
Minerals			5		
Overall				7	

CORNBREAD MUFFIN, STICK, ROUND

Serving: 1 muffin (1.86 oz)   **Bakery**

Calories	165	(88.6 cal/oz)	Carbohydrate	26.1 g	(9% DV)
Fat Calories	47	(28% fat)	Dietary Fiber	.52 g	(2% DV)
Total Fat	5.2 g	(8% DV)	Protein	3.12 g	(6% DV)
Saturated Fat	1.56 g	(8% DV)	Vitamin A	101.4 IU	(2% DV)
Poly Fat	.52 g		Vitamin C	0 mg	(0% DV)
Mono Fat	2.6 g		Calcium	48.9 mg	(5% DV)
Cholesterol	24.4 mg	(8% DV)	Iron	.9 mg	(5% DV)
Sodium	247 mg	(10% DV)	Folate	3.1 mcg	(1% DV)
Potassium	58.2 mg	(2% DV)	Beta Carotene	5.2 RE	

Ratings	Worst	Bad	Average	Good	Best
Weight Loss			5		
LowCal Density		3			
Filling		4			
Energizing				7	
Fiber		3			
Vitamins		3			
Minerals			5		
Overall		4			

CORNED BEEF HASH

Serving: 1 cup, canned (7.86 oz)   **Entree**

Calories	398	(50.7 cal/oz)	Carbohydrate	23.54 g	(8% DV)
Fat Calories	218	(55% fat)	Dietary Fiber	2.2 g	(9% DV)
Total Fat	24.2 g	(37% DV)	Protein	19.8 g	(40% DV)
Saturated Fat	11 g	(55% DV)	Vitamin A	0 IU	(0% DV)
Poly Fat	0 g		Vitamin C	0 mg	(0% DV)
Mono Fat	11 g		Calcium	28.6 mg	(3% DV)
Cholesterol	72.6 mg	(24% DV)	Iron	4.4 mg	(24% DV)
Sodium	1188 mg	(50% DV)	Folate	19.8 mcg	(4% DV)
Potassium	440 mg	(13% DV)	Beta Carotene	0 RE	

Ratings	Worst	Bad	Average	Good	Best
Weight Loss		3			
LowCal Density			6		
Filling			5		
Energizing			6		
Fiber			6		
Vitamins		4			
Minerals				7	
Overall			5		

CORNED BEEF SANDWICH

Serving: 1 sandwich (4.64 oz)   Sandwich

Calories	268	(57.7 cal/oz)	Carbohydrate	23.53 g	(8% DV)
Fat Calories	94	(35% fat)	Dietary Fiber	1.3 g	(5% DV)
Total Fat	10.4 g	(16% DV)	Protein	19.5 g	(39% DV)
Saturated Fat	3.9 g	(19% DV)	Vitamin A	28.6 IU	(1% DV)
Poly Fat	1.3 g		Vitamin C	2.6 mg	(4% DV)
Mono Fat	3.9 g		Calcium	67.6 mg	(7% DV)
Cholesterol	48.1 mg	(16% DV)	Iron	2.6 mg	(14% DV)
Sodium	1196 mg	(50% DV)	Folate	19.5 mcg	(5% DV)
Potassium	185.9 mg	(5% DV)	Beta Carotene	2.6 RE	

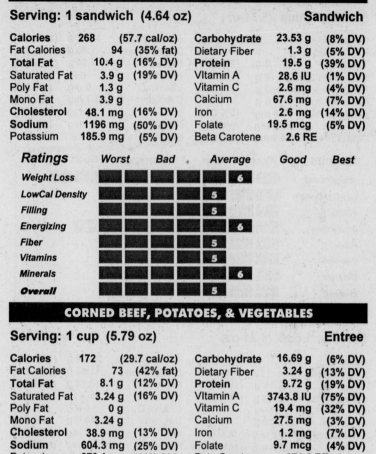

Ratings	Worst	Bad	Average	Good	Best
Weight Loss				6	
LowCal Density			5		
Filling			5		
Energizing				6	
Fiber			5		
Vitamins			5		
Minerals				6	
Overall			5		

CORNED BEEF, POTATOES, & VEGETABLES

Serving: 1 cup (5.79 oz)   Entree

Calories	172	(29.7 cal/oz)	Carbohydrate	16.69 g	(6% DV)
Fat Calories	73	(42% fat)	Dietary Fiber	3.24 g	(13% DV)
Total Fat	8.1 g	(12% DV)	Protein	9.72 g	(19% DV)
Saturated Fat	3.24 g	(16% DV)	Vitamin A	3743.8 IU	(75% DV)
Poly Fat	0 g		Vitamin C	19.4 mg	(32% DV)
Mono Fat	3.24 g		Calcium	27.5 mg	(3% DV)
Cholesterol	38.9 mg	(13% DV)	Iron	1.2 mg	(7% DV)
Sodium	604.3 mg	(25% DV)	Folate	9.7 mcg	(4% DV)
Potassium	379.1 mg	(11% DV)	Beta Carotene	374.2 RE	

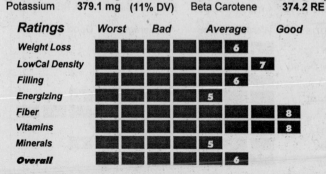

Ratings	Worst	Bad	Average	Good	Best
Weight Loss				6	
LowCal Density				7	
Filling				6	
Energizing			5		
Fiber					8
Vitamins					8
Minerals			5		
Overall				6	

COUSCOUS, PLAIN, COOKED WITHOUT ADDED FAT

Serving: 1 cup (5.21 oz)   **Entree**

Calories	164	(31.4 cal/oz)	Carbohydrate	33.87 g	(11% DV)
Fat Calories	0	(0% fat)	Dietary Fiber	1.46 g	(6% DV)
Total Fat	0 g	(0% DV)	Protein	5.84 g	(12% DV)
Saturated Fat	0 g	(0% DV)	Vitamin A	0 IU	(0% DV)
Poly Fat	0 g		Vitamin C	0 mg	(0% DV)
Mono Fat	0 g		Calcium	11.7 mg	(1% DV)
Cholesterol	0 mg	(0% DV)	Iron	.6 mg	(3% DV)
Sodium	7.3 mg	(0% DV)	Folate	5.8 mcg	(5% DV)
Potassium	84.7 mg	(2% DV)	Beta Carotene	0 RE	

Ratings	Worst	Bad	Average	Good	Best	
Weight Loss						9
LowCal Density				7		
Filling				7		
Energizing				8		
Fiber			5			
Vitamins		3				
Minerals		3				
Overall				7		

COWPEAS, DRY, COOKED WITH ADDED FAT

Serving: 1 cup (6.21 oz)   **Vegetable**

Calories	289	(46.5 cal/oz)	Carbohydrate	33.06 g	(11% DV)
Fat Calories	110	(38% fat)	Dietary Fiber	15.66 g	(63% DV)
Total Fat	12.18 g	(19% DV)	Protein	12.18 g	(24% DV)
Saturated Fat	3.48 g	(17% DV)	Vitamin A	24.4 IU	(0% DV)
Poly Fat	1.74 g		Vitamin C	0 mg	(0% DV)
Mono Fat	5.22 g		Calcium	40 mg	(4% DV)
Cholesterol	12.2 mg	(4% DV)	Iron	4.1 mg	(23% DV)
Sodium	605.5 mg	(25% DV)	Folate	12.2 mcg	(83% DV)
Potassium	452.4 mg	(13% DV)	Beta Carotene	3.5 RE	

Ratings	Worst	Bad	Average	Good	Best	
Weight Loss	2					
LowCal Density			6			
Filling			7			
Energizing				8		
Fiber						10
Vitamins			7			
Minerals				8		
Overall			6			

CRAB, BAKED OR BROILED

Serving: 1 king crab leg, 19" (4.25 oz)　　　Shellfish

Calories	164	(38.6 cal/oz)	Carbohydrate	.12 g	(0% DV)
Fat Calories	64	(39% fat)	Dietary Fiber	0 g	(0% DV)
Total Fat	7.14 g	(11% DV)	Protein	22.61 g	(45% DV)
Saturated Fat	1.19 g	(6% DV)	Vitamin A	298.7 IU	(6% DV)
Poly Fat	2.38 g		Vitamin C	3.6 mg	(6% DV)
Mono Fat	2.38 g		Calcium	117.8 mg	(12% DV)
Cholesterol	111.9 mg	(37% DV)	Iron	1 mg	(6% DV)
Sodium	642.6 mg	(27% DV)	Folate	22.6 mcg	(14% DV)
Potassium	364.1 mg	(10% DV)	Beta Carotene	6 RE	

Ratings	Worst	Bad	Average	Good	Best
Weight Loss			4		
LowCal Density				7	
Filling	1				
Energizing	2				
Fiber	1				
Vitamins			5		
Minerals				7	
Overall			4		

CRACKERS, GRAHAM

Serving: 1 large piece (.5 oz)　　　Snack

Calories	54	(107.5 cal/oz)	Carbohydrate	10.26 g	(3% DV)
Fat Calories	11	(21% fat)	Dietary Fiber	.42 g	(2% DV)
Total Fat	1.26 g	(2% DV)	Protein	1.12 g	(2% DV)
Saturated Fat	.28 g	(1% DV)	Vitamin A	0 IU	(0% DV)
Poly Fat	.14 g		Vitamin C	0 mg	(0% DV)
Mono Fat	.7 g		Calcium	5.6 mg	(1% DV)
Cholesterol	0 mg	(0% DV)	Iron	.5 mg	(3% DV)
Sodium	93.8 mg	(4% DV)	Folate	1.1 mcg	(1% DV)
Potassium	53.8 mg	(2% DV)	Beta Carotene	0 RE	

Ratings	Worst	Bad	Average	Good	Best
Weight Loss					9
LowCal Density	2				
Filling	2				
Energizing			4		
Fiber		3			
Vitamins		3			
Minerals		3			
Overall			4		

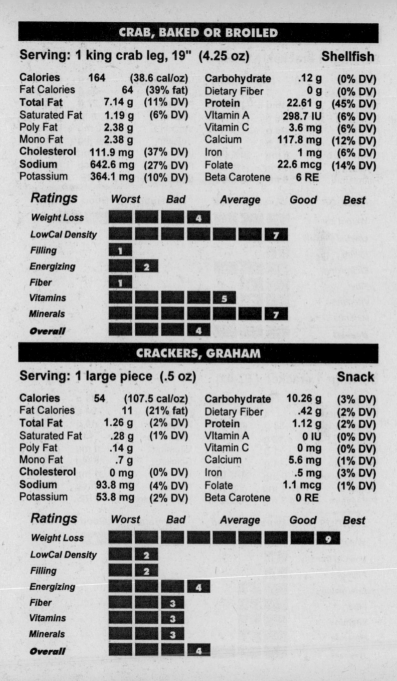

CRACKERS, SALTINE

Serving: 1 cracker (.11 oz)   **Snack**

Calories	13	(118.1 cal/oz)	Carbohydrate	2.15 g	(1% DV)
Fat Calories	3	(25% fat)	Dietary Fiber	.09 g	(0% DV)
Total Fat	.36 g	(1% DV)	Protein	.27 g	(1% DV)
Saturated Fat	.06 g	(0% DV)	VItamin A	0 IU	(0% DV)
Poly Fat	.06 g		Vitamin C	0 mg	(0% DV)
Mono Fat	.21 g		Calcium	.6 mg	(0% DV)
Cholesterol	0 mg	(0% DV)	Iron	.1 mg	(1% DV)
Sodium	33 mg	(1% DV)	Folate	.3 mcg	(0% DV)
Potassium	3.6 mg	(0% DV)	Beta Carotene	0 RE	

Ratings	Worst	Bad	Average	Good	Best
Weight Loss					9
LowCal Density	2				
Filling	1				
Energizing	3				
Fiber	2				
Vitamins	2				
Minerals	2				
Overall	4				

CRACKERS, TOAST THINS (RYE, PUMPERNICKEL, WHITE)

Serving: 1 cracker (.07 oz)   **Snack**

Calories	9	(131.1 cal/oz)	Carbohydrate	1.35 g	(0% DV)
Fat Calories	3	(37% fat)	Dietary Fiber	.04 g	(0% DV)
Total Fat	.38 g	(1% DV)	Protein	.16 g	(0% DV)
Saturated Fat	.12 g	(1% DV)	VItamin A	1 IU	(0% DV)
Poly Fat	.1 g		Vitamin C	0 mg	(0% DV)
Mono Fat	.14 g		Calcium	.6 mg	(0% DV)
Cholesterol	0 mg	(0% DV)	Iron	.1 mg	(0% DV)
Sodium	17.1 mg	(1% DV)	Folate	.2 mcg	(0% DV)
Potassium	4.3 mg	(0% DV)	Beta Carotene	0 RE	

Ratings	Worst	Bad	Average	Good	Best
Weight Loss					8
LowCal Density	1				
Filling	1				
Energizing	2				
Fiber	2				
Vitamins	2				
Minerals	2				
Overall	3				

CRANBERRIES, COOKED OR CANNED

Serving: 1 slice (½" thick) (2.04 oz)   **Fruit**

Calories	86	(42.2 cal/oz)	Carbohydrate	22.17 g	(7% DV)
Fat Calories	0	(0% fat)	Dietary Fiber	.57 g	(2% DV)
Total Fat	0 g	(0% DV)	Protein	0 g	(0% DV)
Saturated Fat	0 g	(0% DV)	Vitamin A	11.4 IU	(0% DV)
Poly Fat	0 g		Vitamin C	1.1 mg	(2% DV)
Mono Fat	0 g		Calcium	2.3 mg	(0% DV)
Cholesterol	0 mg	(0% DV)	Iron	.1 mg	(1% DV)
Sodium	16.5 mg	(1% DV)	Folate	0 mcg	(0% DV)
Potassium	14.8 mg	(0% DV)	Beta Carotene	1.1 RE	

Ratings	Worst	Bad	Average	Good	Best
Weight Loss					9
LowCal Density			6		
Filling			5		
Energizing			6		
Fiber		3			
Vitamins	2				
Minerals	2				
Overall			6		

CRANBERRY JUICE DRINK WITH VITAMIN C ADDED

Serving: 1 cup (9.04 oz)   **Beverage**

Calories	144	(16 cal/oz)	Carbohydrate	36.43 g	(12% DV)
Fat Calories	0	(0% fat)	Dietary Fiber	0 g	(0% DV)
Total Fat	0 g	(0% DV)	Protein	0 g	(0% DV)
Saturated Fat	0 g	(0% DV)	Vitamin A	10.1 IU	(0% DV)
Poly Fat	0 g		Vitamin C	88.6 mg	(148% DV)
Mono Fat	0 g		Calcium	7.6 mg	(1% DV)
Cholesterol	0 mg	(0% DV)	Iron	.4 mg	(2% DV)
Sodium	5.1 mg	(0% DV)	Folate	0 mcg	(0% DV)
Potassium	45.5 mg	(1% DV)	Beta Carotene	0 RE	

Ratings	Worst	Bad	Average	Good	Best
Weight Loss			6		
LowCal Density				9	
Filling					10
Energizing				8	
Fiber	1				
Vitamins				8	
Minerals	2				
Overall				7	

CRANBERRY JUICE DRINK, LOW CALORIE, WITH VITAMIN C

Serving: 1 cup (8.57 oz)   Beverage

Calories	46	(5.3 cal/oz)	Carbohydrate	11.28 g	(4% DV)
Fat Calories	0	(0% fat)	Dietary Fiber	0 g	(0% DV)
Total Fat	0 g	(0% DV)	Protein	0 g	(0% DV)
Saturated Fat	0 g	(0% DV)	Vitamin A	9.6 IU	(0% DV)
Poly Fat	0 g		Vitamin C	76.8 mg	(128% DV)
Mono Fat	0 g		Calcium	21.6 mg	(2% DV)
Cholesterol	0 mg	(0% DV)	Iron	.1 mg	(1% DV)
Sodium	7.2 mg	(0% DV)	Folate	0 mcg	(0% DV)
Potassium	52.8 mg	(2% DV)	Beta Carotene	0 RE	

Ratings	Worst	Bad	Average	Good	Best
Weight Loss				9	
LowCal Density					10
Filling					10
Energizing			5		
Fiber	1				
Vitamins				8	
Minerals	2				
Overall				8	

CRAYFISH, BOILED OR STEAMED

Serving: about 6 (3.04 oz)   Shellfish

Calories	97	(31.9 cal/oz)	Carbohydrate	0 g	(0% DV)
Fat Calories	8	(8% fat)	Dietary Fiber	0 g	(0% DV)
Total Fat	.85 g	(1% DV)	Protein	20.4 g	(41% DV)
Saturated Fat	0 g	(0% DV)	Vitamin A	62.1 IU	(1% DV)
Poly Fat	0 g		Vitamin C	2.6 mg	(4% DV)
Mono Fat	0 g		Calcium	25.5 mg	(3% DV)
Cholesterol	151.3 mg	(50% DV)	Iron	2.7 mg	(15% DV)
Sodium	57.8 mg	(2% DV)	Folate	20.4 mcg	(1% DV)
Potassium	298.4 mg	(9% DV)	Beta Carotene	0 RE	

Ratings	Worst	Bad	Average	Good	Best
Weight Loss				8	
LowCal Density				7	
Filling	1				
Energizing	1				
Fiber	1				
Vitamins			4		
Minerals			6		
Overall			5		

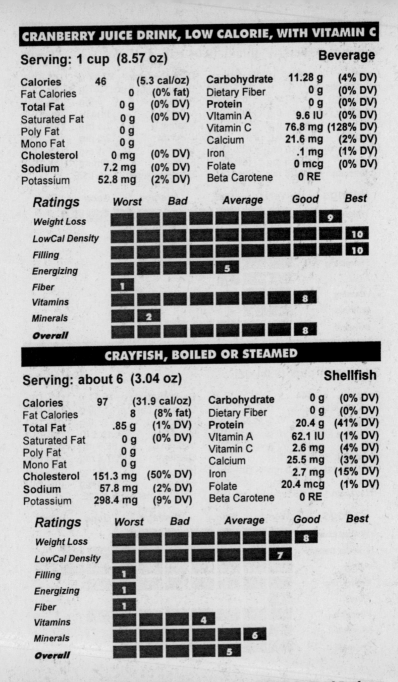

CREAM OF RICE, MADE WITH MILK

Serving: 1 cup, cooked (8.75 oz)   **Cereal**

Calories	296	(33.9 cal/oz)	Carbohydrate	46.06 g	(15% DV)
Fat Calories	66	(22% fat)	Dietary Fiber	0 g	(0% DV)
Total Fat	7.35 g	(11% DV)	Protein	9.8 g	(20% DV)
Saturated Fat	4.9 g	(25% DV)	Vitamin A	264.6 IU	(5% DV)
Poly Fat	0 g		Vitamin C	2.5 mg	(4% DV)
Mono Fat	2.45 g		Calcium	294 mg	(29% DV)
Cholesterol	31.9 mg	(11% DV)	Iron	1.2 mg	(7% DV)
Sodium	355.3 mg	(15% DV)	Folate	9.8 mcg	(2% DV)
Potassium	357.7 mg	(10% DV)	Beta Carotene	2.5 RE	

Ratings	Worst	Bad	Average	Good	Best
Weight Loss			4		
LowCal Density				7	
Filling				8	
Energizing					9
Fiber	1				
Vitamins			4		
Minerals				7	
Overall			6		

CREAM OF WHEAT, COOKED, WITH MILK & SUGAR

Serving: 1 cup, cooked (8.75 oz)   **Cereal**

Calories	309	(35.3 cal/oz)	Carbohydrate	47.04 g	(16% DV)
Fat Calories	88	(29% fat)	Dietary Fiber	0 g	(0% DV)
Total Fat	9.8 g	(15% DV)	Protein	9.8 g	(20% DV)
Saturated Fat	4.9 g	(25% DV)	Vitamin A	269.5 IU	(5% DV)
Poly Fat	0 g		Vitamin C	2.5 mg	(4% DV)
Mono Fat	2.45 g		Calcium	328.3 mg	(33% DV)
Cholesterol	31.9 mg	(11% DV)	Iron	7.4 mg	(41% DV)
Sodium	360.2 mg	(15% DV)	Folate	9.8 mcg	(4% DV)
Potassium	367.5 mg	(10% DV)	Beta Carotene	2.5 RE	

Ratings	Worst	Bad	Average	Good	Best
Weight Loss		3			
LowCal Density				7	
Filling				8	
Energizing					9
Fiber	1				
Vitamins			4		
Minerals					9
Overall			6		

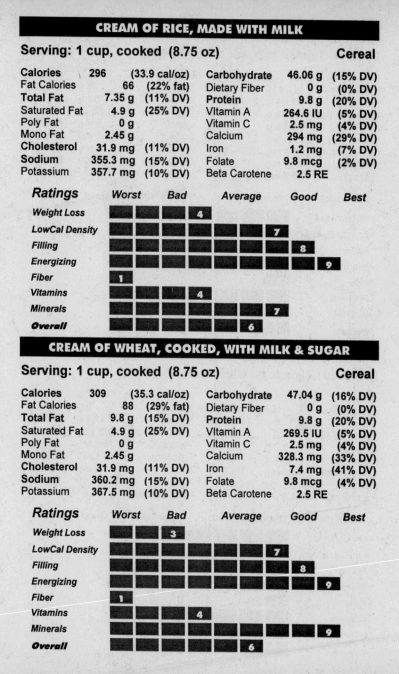

CREAM PUFF, ECLAIR, CUSTARD OR CREAM FILLED, ICED

Serving: 1 eclair (5"x 2"x 1¾") (3.64 oz)   **Dessert**

Calories	219	(60.2 cal/oz)	Carbohydrate	22.24 g	(7% DV)
Fat Calories	110	(50% fat)	Dietary Fiber	0 g	(0% DV)
Total Fat	12.24 g	(19% DV)	Protein	6.12 g	(12% DV)
Saturated Fat	3.06 g	(15% DV)	VItamin A	603.8 IU	(12% DV)
Poly Fat	3.06 g		Vitamin C	0 mg	(0% DV)
Mono Fat	5.1 g		Calcium	87.7 mg	(9% DV)
Cholesterol	105.1 mg	(35% DV)	Iron	.9 mg	(5% DV)
Sodium	163.2 mg	(7% DV)	Folate	6.1 mcg	(3% DV)
Potassium	136.7 mg	(4% DV)	Beta Carotene	10.2 RE	

Ratings	Worst	Bad	Average	Good	Best
Weight Loss			5		
LowCal Density			5		
Filling		4			
Energizing			6		
Fiber	1				
Vitamins		4			
Minerals			5		
Overall			5		

CREAMED DRIED BEEF ON TOAST

Serving: 1 slice toast with sauce (5.18 oz)   **Entree**

Calories	241	(46.5 cal/oz)	Carbohydrate	21.17 g	(7% DV)
Fat Calories	104	(43% fat)	Dietary Fiber	0 g	(0% DV)
Total Fat	11.6 g	(18% DV)	Protein	11.6 g	(23% DV)
Saturated Fat	4.35 g	(22% DV)	VItamin A	503.2 IU	(10% DV)
Poly Fat	2.9 g		Vitamin C	2.9 mg	(5% DV)
Mono Fat	4.35 g		Calcium	158.1 mg	(16% DV)
Cholesterol	21.8 mg	(7% DV)	Iron	1.8 mg	(10% DV)
Sodium	867.1 mg	(36% DV)	Folate	11.6 mcg	(4% DV)
Potassium	272.6 mg	(8% DV)	Beta Carotene	11.6 RE	

Ratings	Worst	Bad	Average	Good	Best
Weight Loss			5		
LowCal Density			6		
Filling			5		
Energizing			6		
Fiber	1				
Vitamins			5		
Minerals			6		
Overall			5		

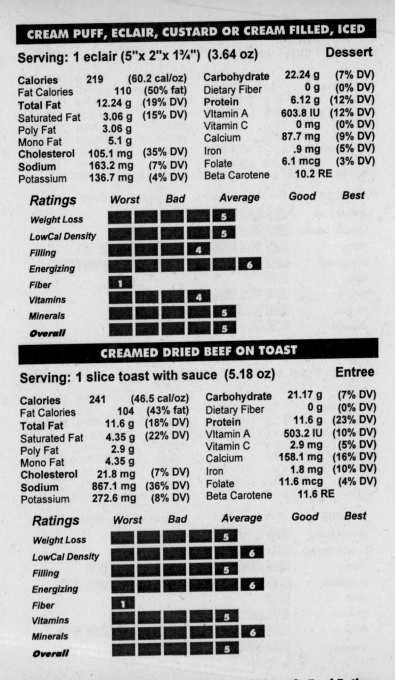

CREPE, DESSERT TYPE, FRUIT-FILLED

Serving: 1 crepe with filling (2.79 oz)   **Dessert**

Calories	131	(47 cal/oz)	Carbohydrate	20.75 g	(7% DV)
Fat Calories	35	(27% fat)	Dietary Fiber	.78 g	(3% DV)
Total Fat	3.9 g	(6% DV)	Protein	3.9 g	(8% DV)
Saturated Fat	1.56 g	(8% DV)	Vitamin A	234 IU	(5% DV)
Poly Fat	.78 g		Vitamin C	3.9 mg	(6% DV)
Mono Fat	1.56 g		Calcium	38.2 mg	(4% DV)
Cholesterol	63.2 mg	(21% DV)	Iron	.7 mg	(4% DV)
Sodium	124 mg	(5% DV)	Folate	3.9 mcg	(2% DV)
Potassium	89.7 mg	(3% DV)	Beta Carotene	5.5 RE	

Ratings	Worst	Bad	Average	Good	Best
Weight Loss				8	
LowCal Density			6		
Filling			5		
Energizing			6		
Fiber		3			
Vitamins		4			
Minerals		4			
Overall			6		

CREPES, FILLED WITH MEAT, FISH, OR POULTRY

Serving: 1 crepe, with sauce (5.5 oz)   **Entree**

Calories	291	(52.9 cal/oz)	Carbohydrate	12.17 g	(4% DV)
Fat Calories	152	(52% fat)	Dietary Fiber	0 g	(0% DV)
Total Fat	16.94 g	(26% DV)	Protein	21.56 g	(43% DV)
Saturated Fat	6.16 g	(31% DV)	Vitamin A	589.8 IU	(12% DV)
Poly Fat	1.54 g		Vitamin C	1.5 mg	(3% DV)
Mono Fat	6.16 g		Calcium	172.5 mg	(17% DV)
Cholesterol	110.9 mg	(37% DV)	Iron	2 mg	(11% DV)
Sodium	588.3 mg	(25% DV)	Folate	21.6 mcg	(3% DV)
Potassium	274.1 mg	(8% DV)	Beta Carotene	23.1 RE	

Ratings	Worst	Bad	Average	Good	Best
Weight Loss		4			
LowCal Density			6		
Filling		4			
Energizing			5		
Fiber	1				
Vitamins			5		
Minerals			7		
Overall			5		

Serving: 1 croissant (2 oz) · Bakery

Calories	227	(113.4 cal/oz)	Carbohydrate	24.25 g	(8% DV)
Fat Calories	111	(49% fat)	Dietary Fiber	1.12 g	(4% DV)
Total Fat	12.32 g	(19% DV)	Protein	5.04 g	(10% DV)
Saturated Fat	7.28 g	(36% DV)	Vitamin A	459.2 IU	(9% DV)
Poly Fat	.56 g		Vitamin C	0 mg	(0% DV)
Mono Fat	3.36 g		Calcium	29.1 mg	(3% DV)
Cholesterol	62.2 mg	(21% DV)	Iron	1.5 mg	(8% DV)
Sodium	285 mg	(12% DV)	Folate	5 mcg	(5% DV)
Potassium	73.9 mg	(2% DV)	Beta Carotene	11.2 RE	

Ratings	Worst	Bad	Average	Good	Best
Weight Loss	2				
LowCal Density	2				
Filling	3				
Energizing				6	
Fiber		4			
Vitamins			5		
Minerals		4			
Overall	3				

Serving: 1 croissant (4.04 oz) · Entree

Calories	338	(83.6 cal/oz)	Carbohydrate	25.42 g	(8% DV)
Fat Calories	173	(51% fat)	Dietary Fiber	1.13 g	(5% DV)
Total Fat	19.21 g	(30% DV)	Protein	14.69 g	(29% DV)
Saturated Fat	11.3 g	(57% DV)	Vitamin A	643 IU	(13% DV)
Poly Fat	1.13 g		Vitamin C	6.8 mg	(11% DV)
Mono Fat	5.65 g		Calcium	163.9 mg	(16% DV)
Cholesterol	64.4 mg	(21% DV)	Iron	1.9 mg	(10% DV)
Sodium	876.9 mg	(37% DV)	Folate	14.7 mcg	(3% DV)
Potassium	233.9 mg	(7% DV)	Beta Carotene	14.7 RE	

Ratings	Worst	Bad	Average	Good	Best
Weight Loss		4			
LowCal Density		3			
Filling		4			
Energizing				6	
Fiber		4			
Vitamins				6	
Minerals				7	
Overall		4			

CROUTONS

Serving: 1 fast food package (.36 oz)   **Bread**

Calories	46	(128.6 cal/oz)	Carbohydrate	6.36 g	(2% DV)
Fat Calories	16	(35% fat)	Dietary Fiber	.5 g	(2% DV)
Total Fat	1.8 g	(3% DV)	Protein	1.1 g	(2% DV)
Saturated Fat	.4 g	(2% DV)	Vitamin A	.5 IU	(0% DV)
Poly Fat	.5 g		Vitamin C	0 mg	(0% DV)
Mono Fat	.7 g		Calcium	9.6 mg	(1% DV)
Cholesterol	0 mg	(0% DV)	Iron	.3 mg	(2% DV)
Sodium	93.6 mg	(4% DV)	Folate	1.1 mcg	(1% DV)
Potassium	18.1 mg	(1% DV)	Beta Carotene	0 RE	

Ratings	Worst	Bad	Average	Good	Best
Weight Loss					7
LowCal Density	2				
Filling	2				
Energizing		4			
Fiber	3				
Vitamins	2				
Minerals	2				
Overall		4			

CUCUMBER SALAD WITH CREAMY DRESSING

Serving: 1 cup (4.75 oz)   **Salad**

Calories	67	(14 cal/oz)	Carbohydrate	4.92 g	(2% DV)
Fat Calories	48	(72% fat)	Dietary Fiber	0 g	(0% DV)
Total Fat	5.32 g	(8% DV)	Protein	1.33 g	(3% DV)
Saturated Fat	2.66 g	(13% DV)	Vitamin A	179.6 IU	(4% DV)
Poly Fat	0 g		Vitamin C	6.7 mg	(11% DV)
Mono Fat	1.33 g		Calcium	45.2 mg	(5% DV)
Cholesterol	10.6 mg	(4% DV)	Iron	.4 mg	(2% DV)
Sodium	14.6 mg	(1% DV)	Folate	1.3 mcg	(5% DV)
Potassium	236.7 mg	(7% DV)	Beta Carotene	5.3 RE	

Ratings	Worst	Bad	Average	Good	Best
Weight Loss		5			
LowCal Density					9
Filling		4			
Energizing	3				
Fiber	1				
Vitamins		4			
Minerals		4			
Overall			5		

CUCUMBER, RAW

Serving: 1 stick, 4" long (.32 oz)   **Vegetable**

Calories	1	(4.5 cal/oz)	Carbohydrate	.32 g	(0% DV)
Fat Calories	0	(0% fat)	Dietary Fiber	.09 g	(0% DV)
Total Fat	0 g	(0% DV)	Protein	.09 g	(0% DV)
Saturated Fat	0 g	(0% DV)	Vitamin A	0 IU	
Poly Fat	0 g		Vitamin C	.5 mg	(1% DV)
Mono Fat	0 g		Calcium	1.5 mg	(0% DV)
Cholesterol	0 mg	(0% DV)	Iron	0 mg	(0% DV)
Sodium	.2 mg	(0% DV)	Folate	.1 mcg	(0% DV)
Potassium	16.7 mg	(0% DV)	Beta Carotene	0 RE	

Ratings	Worst	Bad	Average	Good	Best
Weight Loss					10
LowCal Density					10
Filling	2				
Energizing	2				
Fiber	2				
Vitamins	2				
Minerals	2				
Overall			7		

DANISH PASTRY

Serving: 1 small (approx 3" dia) (1.25 oz)   **Bakery**

Calories	148	(118.2 cal/oz)	Carbohydrate	15.96 g	(5% DV)
Fat Calories	76	(51% fat)	Dietary Fiber	.35 g	(1% DV)
Total Fat	8.4 g	(13% DV)	Protein	2.45 g	(5% DV)
Saturated Fat	2.45 g	(12% DV)	Vitamin A	37.5 IU	(1% DV)
Poly Fat	1.05 g		Vitamin C	0 mg	(0% DV)
Mono Fat	4.2 g		Calcium	17.5 mg	(2% DV)
Cholesterol	30.1 mg	(10% DV)	Iron	.8 mg	(4% DV)
Sodium	128.1 mg	(5% DV)	Folate	2.5 mcg	(2% DV)
Potassium	39.2 mg	(1% DV)	Beta Carotene	.7 RE	

Ratings	Worst	Bad	Average	Good	Best
Weight Loss			4		
LowCal Density	2				
Filling	2				
Energizing			5		
Fiber	2				
Vitamins		3			
Minerals		3			
Overall		3			

DANISH PASTRY, CHEESE, LOW FAT, NO CHOLESTEROL

Serving: 1 slice (3¾x 1¼x ¾") (1.14 oz)   **Bakery**

Calories	94	(82.8 cal/oz)	Carbohydrate	20.54 g	(7% DV)
Fat Calories	3	(3% fat)	Dietary Fiber	.32 g	(1% DV)
Total Fat	.32 g	(0% DV)	Protein	2.56 g	(5% DV)
Saturated Fat	0 g	(0% DV)	Vitamin A	15 IU	(0% DV)
Poly Fat	0 g		Vitamin C	0 mg	(0% DV)
Mono Fat	0 g		Calcium	13.4 mg	(1% DV)
Cholesterol	.3 mg	(0% DV)	Iron	.6 mg	(3% DV)
Sodium	88.3 mg	(4% DV)	Folate	2.6 mcg	(2% DV)
Potassium	38.4 mg	(1% DV)	Beta Carotene	0 RE	

Ratings	Worst	Bad	Average	Good	Best
Weight Loss				8	
LowCal Density	3				
Filling		4			
Energizing			6		
Fiber	2				
Vitamins	3				
Minerals	3				
Overall			5		

DANISH PASTRY, WITH CHEESE

Serving: 1 small (approx 3" dia) (1.96 oz)   **Bakery**

Calories	211	(107.8 cal/oz)	Carbohydrate	21.01 g	(7% DV)
Fat Calories	109	(52% fat)	Dietary Fiber	.55 g	(2% DV)
Total Fat	12.1 g	(19% DV)	Protein	4.4 g	(9% DV)
Saturated Fat	3.3 g	(16% DV)	Vitamin A	74.8 IU	(1% DV)
Poly Fat	2.75 g		Vitamin C	0 mg	(0% DV)
Mono Fat	5.5 g		Calcium	27 mg	(3% DV)
Cholesterol	35.2 mg	(12% DV)	Iron	1.1 mg	(6% DV)
Sodium	128.2 mg	(5% DV)	Folate	4.4 mcg	(4% DV)
Potassium	64.4 mg	(2% DV)	Beta Carotene	.6 RE	

Ratings	Worst	Bad	Average	Good	Best
Weight Loss	2				
LowCal Density	2				
Filling	3				
Energizing			6		
Fiber	3				
Vitamins	4				
Minerals	4				
Overall	3				

DIM SUM, MEAT FILLED (EGG ROLL-TYPE)

Serving: 1 piece (1 oz)   **Entree**

Calories	49	(49.3 cal/oz)	Carbohydrate	3.75 g	(1% DV)
Fat Calories	20	(41% fat)	Dietary Fiber	.28 g	(1% DV)
Total Fat	2.24 g	(3% DV)	Protein	3.36 g	(7% DV)
Saturated Fat	.56 g	(3% DV)	VItamin A	35.6 IU	(1% DV)
Poly Fat	.56 g		Vitamin C	.6 mg	(1% DV)
Mono Fat	.84 g		Calcium	6.7 mg	(1% DV)
Cholesterol	17.4 mg	(6% DV)	Iron	.4 mg	(2% DV)
Sodium	32.2 mg	(1% DV)	Folate	3.4 mcg	(1% DV)
Potassium	44 mg	(1% DV)	Beta Carotene	2.5 RE	

Ratings	Worst	Bad	Average	Good	Best
Weight Loss					8
LowCal Density				6	
Filling	2				
Energizing	3				
Fiber	2				
Vitamins	3				
Minerals	3				
Overall			5		

DIP, CREAM CHEESE BASE

Serving: 1 tbsp (.54 oz)   **Snack**

Calories	49	(90 cal/oz)	Carbohydrate	.81 g	(0% DV)
Fat Calories	42	(86% fat)	Dietary Fiber	0 g	(0% DV)
Total Fat	4.65 g	(7% DV)	Protein	.9 g	(2% DV)
Saturated Fat	2.7 g	(14% DV)	VItamin A	175.7 IU	(4% DV)
Poly Fat	.45 g		Vitamin C	0 mg	(0% DV)
Mono Fat	1.35 g		Calcium	11.3 mg	(1% DV)
Cholesterol	13.7 mg	(5% DV)	Iron	.2 mg	(1% DV)
Sodium	87.2 mg	(4% DV)	Folate	.9 mcg	(0% DV)
Potassium	19.1 mg	(1% DV)	Beta Carotene	2.9 RE	

Ratings	Worst	Bad	Average	Good	Best
Weight Loss		4			
LowCal Density	3				
Filling	1				
Energizing	2				
Fiber	1				
Vitamins	2				
Minerals	2				
Overall	3				

DIRTY RICE

Serving: 1 cup (7.07 oz)   **Entree**

Calories	285	(40.3 cal/oz)	Carbohydrate	37.03 g	(12% DV)
Fat Calories	89	(31% fat)	Dietary Fiber	0 g	(0% DV)
Total Fat	9.9 g	(15% DV)	Protein	11.88 g	(24% DV)
Saturated Fat	5.94 g	(30% DV)	Vitamin A	2530.4 IU	(51% DV)
Poly Fat	0 g		Vitamin C	4 mg	(7% DV)
Mono Fat	1.98 g		Calcium	21.8 mg	(2% DV)
Cholesterol	103 mg	(34% DV)	Iron	4 mg	(22% DV)
Sodium	455.4 mg	(19% DV)	Folate	11.9 mcg	(20% DV)
Potassium	221.8 mg	(6% DV)	Beta Carotene	7.9 RE	

Ratings	Worst	Bad	Average	Good	Best
Weight Loss			6		
LowCal Density			6		
Filling			6		
Energizing				8	
Fiber	1				
Vitamins				7	
Minerals			6		
Overall			6		

DONUTZ CEREAL

Serving: 1 cup (1.18 oz)   **Cereal**

Calories	140	(118.3 cal/oz)	Carbohydrate	25.61 g	(9% DV)
Fat Calories	33	(23% fat)	Dietary Fiber	.66 g	(3% DV)
Total Fat	3.63 g	(6% DV)	Protein	2.31 g	(5% DV)
Saturated Fat	2.97 g	(15% DV)	Vitamin A	1455.3 IU	(29% DV)
Poly Fat	0 g		Vitamin C	17.5 mg	(29% DV)
Mono Fat	.33 g		Calcium	23.1 mg	(2% DV)
Cholesterol	0 mg	(0% DV)	Iron	5.2 mg	(29% DV)
Sodium	212.9 mg	(9% DV)	Folate	2.3 mcg	(0% DV)
Potassium	0 mg	(0% DV)	Beta Carotene	0 RE	

Ratings	Worst	Bad	Average	Good	Best
Weight Loss				7	
LowCal Density	2				
Filling		3			
Energizing			6		
Fiber		3			
Vitamins					9
Minerals			5		
Overall			5		

DOUGHNUT, CAKE TYPE

Serving: 1 medium (1.5 oz)   **Bakery**

Calories	164	(109.5 cal/oz)	Carbohydrate	21.59 g	(7% DV)
Fat Calories	72	(44% fat)	Dietary Fiber	.84 g	(3% DV)
Total Fat	7.98 g	(12% DV)	Protein	2.1 g	(4% DV)
Saturated Fat	2.1 g	(11% DV)	Vitamin A	14.3 IU	(0% DV)
Poly Fat	.84 g		Vitamin C	0 mg	(0% DV)
Mono Fat	4.2 g		Calcium	16.8 mg	(2% DV)
Cholesterol	10.9 mg	(4% DV)	Iron	.8 mg	(5% DV)
Sodium	210.4 mg	(9% DV)	Folate	2.1 mcg	(1% DV)
Potassium	37.8 mg	(1% DV)	Beta Carotene	0 RE	

Ratings	Worst	Bad	Average	Good	Best
Weight Loss			4		
LowCal Density	2				
Filling		3			
Energizing				6	
Fiber			4		
Vitamins		3			
Minerals			4		
Overall		3			

DOUGHNUT, JELLY

Serving: 1 doughnut (2.32 oz)   **Bakery**

Calories	253	(109 cal/oz)	Carbohydrate	28.27 g	(9% DV)
Fat Calories	129	(51% fat)	Dietary Fiber	1.3 g	(5% DV)
Total Fat	14.3 g	(22% DV)	Protein	3.25 g	(6% DV)
Saturated Fat	6.5 g	(32% DV)	Vitamin A	6.5 IU	(0% DV)
Poly Fat	1.3 g		Vitamin C	0 mg	(0% DV)
Mono Fat	5.85 g		Calcium	21.5 mg	(2% DV)
Cholesterol	22.1 mg	(7% DV)	Iron	1.2 mg	(6% DV)
Sodium	129.4 mg	(5% DV)	Folate	3.3 mcg	(4% DV)
Potassium	50.1 mg	(1% DV)	Beta Carotene	0 RE	

Ratings	Worst	Bad	Average	Good	Best
Weight Loss	2				
LowCal Density	2				
Filling			4		
Energizing				7	
Fiber			5		
Vitamins			4		
Minerals			4		
Overall		3			

DOUGHNUT, RAISED OR YEAST

Serving: 1 medium (2.14 oz)   Bakery

Calories	243	(113.6 cal/oz)	Carbohydrate	26.7 g	(9% DV)
Fat Calories	124	(51% fat)	Dietary Fiber	1.2 g	(5% DV)
Total Fat	13.8 g	(21% DV)	Protein	3 g	(6% DV)
Saturated Fat	5.4 g	(27% DV)	VItamin A	4.8 IU	(0% DV)
Poly Fat	1.2 g		Vitamin C	0 mg	(0% DV)
Mono Fat	5.4 g		Calcium	19.2 mg	(2% DV)
Cholesterol	21 mg	(7% DV)	Iron	1.1 mg	(6% DV)
Sodium	120 mg	(5% DV)	Folate	3 mcg	(3% DV)
Potassium	41.4 mg	(1% DV)	Beta Carotene	0 RE	

Ratings	Worst	Bad	Average	Good	Best
Weight Loss	2				
LowCal Density	2				
Filling		4			
Energizing				7	
Fiber			5		
Vitamins		4			
Minerals		4			
Overall		3			

DUMPLING, POTATO-FILLED OR CHEESE-FILLED

Serving: 1 piece (1.36 oz)   Entree

Calories	70	(51.1 cal/oz)	Carbohydrate	11.1 g	(4% DV)
Fat Calories	14	(20% fat)	Dietary Fiber	.38 g	(2% DV)
Total Fat	1.52 g	(2% DV)	Protein	2.66 g	(5% DV)
Saturated Fat	.76 g	(4% DV)	VItamin A	70.3 IU	(1% DV)
Poly Fat	.38 g		Vitamin C	.8 mg	(1% DV)
Mono Fat	.38 g		Calcium	22.4 mg	(2% DV)
Cholesterol	21.7 mg	(7% DV)	Iron	.7 mg	(4% DV)
Sodium	88.2 mg	(4% DV)	Folate	2.7 mcg	(1% DV)
Potassium	58.9 mg	(2% DV)	Beta Carotene	.8 RE	

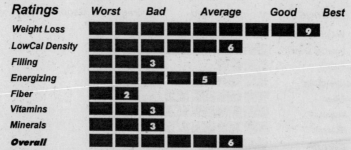

Ratings	Worst	Bad	Average	Good	Best
Weight Loss					9
LowCal Density			6		
Filling	3				
Energizing			5		
Fiber	2				
Vitamins	3				
Minerals	3				
Overall			6		

EGG DROP SOUP

Serving: 1 cup (8.71 oz)   Soup

Calories	73	(8.4 cal/oz)	Carbohydrate	1.22 g	(0% DV)
Fat Calories	44	(60% fat)	Dietary Fiber	0 g	(0% DV)
Total Fat	4.88 g	(8% DV)	Protein	7.32 g	(15% DV)
Saturated Fat	0 g	(0% DV)	Vitamin A	136.6 IU	(3% DV)
Poly Fat	0 g		Vitamin C	0 mg	(0% DV)
Mono Fat	2.44 g		Calcium	22 mg	(2% DV)
Cholesterol	102.5 mg	(34% DV)	Iron	.8 mg	(4% DV)
Sodium	729.6 mg	(30% DV)	Folate	7.3 mcg	(4% DV)
Potassium	219.6 mg	(6% DV)	Beta Carotene	0 RE	

Ratings	Worst	Bad	Average	Good	Best
Weight Loss			5		
LowCal Density					9
Filling		3			
Energizing	2				
Fiber	1				
Vitamins			4		
Minerals			4		
Overall			5		

EGG FOO YUNG

Serving: 1 patty (3.07 oz)   Entree

Calories	113	(36.7 cal/oz)	Carbohydrate	3.35 g	(1% DV)
Fat Calories	77	(69% fat)	Dietary Fiber	.86 g	(3% DV)
Total Fat	8.6 g	(13% DV)	Protein	6.02 g	(12% DV)
Saturated Fat	1.72 g	(9% DV)	Vitamin A	305.3 IU	(6% DV)
Poly Fat	1.72 g		Vitamin C	5.2 mg	(9% DV)
Mono Fat	3.44 g		Calcium	31.8 mg	(3% DV)
Cholesterol	184 mg	(61% DV)	Iron	1 mg	(6% DV)
Sodium	309.6 mg	(13% DV)	Folate	6 mcg	(7% DV)
Potassium	117.8 mg	(3% DV)	Beta Carotene	2.6 RE	

Ratings	Worst	Bad	Average	Good	Best
Weight Loss			5		
LowCal Density				7	
Filling		2			
Energizing		3			
Fiber			4		
Vitamins			4		
Minerals			4		
Overall			5		

EGG OMELET OR SCRAMBLED EGG, WITH POTATOES

Serving: 1 large egg (4.21 oz)   **Breakfast**

Calories	136	(32.2 cal/oz)	Carbohydrate	10.27 g	(3% DV)
Fat Calories	64	(47% fat)	Dietary Fiber	1.18 g	(5% DV)
Total Fat	7.08 g	(11% DV)	Protein	7.08 g	(14% DV)
Saturated Fat	2.36 g	(12% DV)	Vitamin A	405.9 IU	(8% DV)
Poly Fat	1.18 g		Vitamin C	3.5 mg	(6% DV)
Mono Fat	2.36 g		Calcium	33 mg	(3% DV)
Cholesterol	217.1 mg	(72% DV)	Iron	.9 mg	(5% DV)
Sodium	302.1 mg	(13% DV)	Folate	7.1 mcg	(6% DV)
Potassium	221.8 mg	(6% DV)	Beta Carotene	2.4 RE	

Ratings	Worst	Bad	Average	Good	Best
Weight Loss			5		
LowCal Density				7	
Filling		4			
Energizing		4			
Fiber		4			
Vitamins		4			
Minerals		4			
Overall			5		

EGG OMELET OR SCRAMBLED, FAT ADDED IN COOKING

Serving: 1 large egg (2.21 oz)   **Breakfast**

Calories	100	(45.4 cal/oz)	Carbohydrate	1.55 g	(1% DV)
Fat Calories	67	(67% fat)	Dietary Fiber	0 g	(0% DV)
Total Fat	7.44 g	(11% DV)	Protein	6.82 g	(14% DV)
Saturated Fat	2.48 g	(12% DV)	Vitamin A	429 IU	(9% DV)
Poly Fat	1.24 g		Vitamin C	0 mg	(0% DV)
Mono Fat	3.1 g		Calcium	47.7 mg	(5% DV)
Cholesterol	208.3 mg	(69% DV)	Iron	.7 mg	(4% DV)
Sodium	167.4 mg	(7% DV)	Folate	6.8 mcg	(4% DV)
Potassium	89.3 mg	(3% DV)	Beta Carotene	2.5 RE	

Ratings	Worst	Bad	Average	Good	Best
Weight Loss			5		
LowCal Density				6	
Filling	1				
Energizing		3			
Fiber	1				
Vitamins		3			
Minerals		4			
Overall		4			

EGG OMELET OR SCRAMBLED, PEPPER, ONION, HAM

Serving: 1 large egg (2.82 oz)   **Breakfast**

Calories	116	(41.2 cal/oz)	Carbohydrate	1.34 g	(0% DV)
Fat Calories	78	(67% fat)	Dietary Fiber	0 g	(0% DV)
Total Fat	8.69 g	(13% DV)	Protein	7.9 g	(16% DV)
Saturated Fat	2.37 g	(12% DV)	Vitamin A	429.8 IU	(9% DV)
Poly Fat	1.58 g		Vitamin C	4.7 mg	(8% DV)
Mono Fat	3.16 g		Calcium	27.7 mg	(3% DV)
Cholesterol	219.6 mg	(73% DV)	Iron	.8 mg	(5% DV)
Sodium	261.5 mg	(11% DV)	Folate	7.9 mcg	(5% DV)
Potassium	101.1 mg	(3% DV)	Beta Carotene	5.5 RE	

Ratings	Worst	Bad	Average	Good	Best
Weight Loss		4			
LowCal Density			6		
Filling	1				
Energizing	2				
Fiber	1				
Vitamins		4			
Minerals		4			
Overall		4			

EGG OMELET OR SCRAMBLED, WITH HAM OR BACON

Serving: 1 large egg (2.68 oz)   **Breakfast**

Calories	126	(47 cal/oz)	Carbohydrate	.68 g	(0% DV)
Fat Calories	81	(64% fat)	Dietary Fiber	0 g	(0% DV)
Total Fat	9 g	(14% DV)	Protein	9 g	(18% DV)
Saturated Fat	3 g	(15% DV)	Vitamin A	402.8 IU	(8% DV)
Poly Fat	1.5 g		Vitamin C	0 mg	(0% DV)
Mono Fat	3.75 g		Calcium	27 mg	(3% DV)
Cholesterol	223.5 mg	(74% DV)	Iron	.9 mg	(5% DV)
Sodium	326.3 mg	(14% DV)	Folate	9 mcg	(4% DV)
Potassium	100.5 mg	(3% DV)	Beta Carotene	2.3 RE	

Ratings	Worst	Bad	Average	Good	Best
Weight Loss		4			
LowCal Density			6		
Filling	1				
Energizing	2				
Fiber	1				
Vitamins		4			
Minerals		4			
Overall		4			

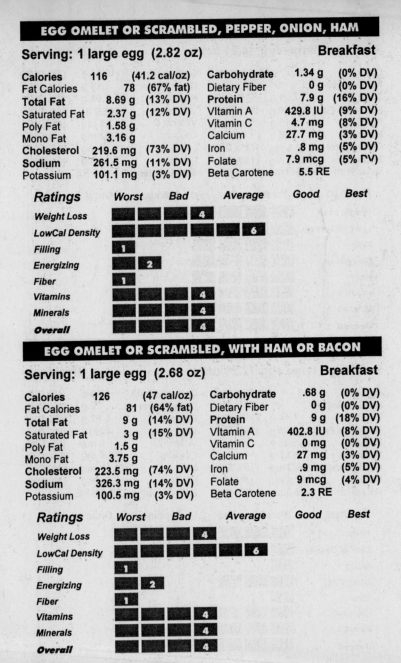

EGG ROLL, MEATLESS

Serving: 1 egg roll (2.29 oz)   Entree

Calories	102	(44.4 cal/oz)	Carbohydrate	9.98 g	(3% DV)
Fat Calories	52	(51% fat)	Dietary Fiber	.64 g	(3% DV)
Total Fat	5.76 g	(9% DV)	Protein	2.56 g	(5% DV)
Saturated Fat	1.28 g	(6% DV)	Vitamin A	57 IU	(1% DV)
Poly Fat	1.92 g		Vitamin C	3.2 mg	(5% DV)
Mono Fat	2.56 g		Calcium	12.2 mg	(1% DV)
Cholesterol	30.1 mg	(10% DV)	Iron	.8 mg	(4% DV)
Sodium	306.6 mg	(13% DV)	Folate	2.6 mcg	(3% DV)
Potassium	97.9 mg	(3% DV)	Beta Carotene	1.3 RE	

Ratings	Worst	Bad	Average	Good	Best
Weight Loss				6	
LowCal Density				6	
Filling		4			
Energizing		4			
Fiber		3			
Vitamins		4			
Minerals		3			
Overall			5		

EGG ROLL, WITH BEEF AND/OR PORK

Serving: 1 egg roll (2.29 oz)   Entree

Calories	115	(50 cal/oz)	Carbohydrate	9.41 g	(3% DV)
Fat Calories	58	(50% fat)	Dietary Fiber	.64 g	(3% DV)
Total Fat	6.4 g	(10% DV)	Protein	5.12 g	(10% DV)
Saturated Fat	1.28 g	(6% DV)	Vitamin A	55 IU	(1% DV)
Poly Fat	1.28 g		Vitamin C	1.9 mg	(3% DV)
Mono Fat	2.56 g		Calcium	12.8 mg	(1% DV)
Cholesterol	37.1 mg	(12% DV)	Iron	.8 mg	(4% DV)
Sodium	303.4 mg	(13% DV)	Folate	5.1 mcg	(2% DV)
Potassium	124.2 mg	(4% DV)	Beta Carotene	1.3 RE	

Ratings	Worst	Bad	Average	Good	Best
Weight Loss				6	
LowCal Density				6	
Filling		3			
Energizing		4			
Fiber		3			
Vitamins		4			
Minerals		4			
Overall			5		

EGG SALAD SANDWICH

Serving: 1 sandwich (4.43 oz)   Sandwich

Calories	362	(81.7 cal/oz)	Carbohydrate	32.49 g	(11% DV)
Fat Calories	190	(52% fat)	Dietary Fiber	1.24 g	(5% DV)
Total Fat	21.08 g	(32% DV)	Protein	11.16 g	(22% DV)
Saturated Fat	3.72 g	(19% DV)	Vitamin A	284 IU	(6% DV)
Poly Fat	8.68 g		Vitamin C	0 mg	(0% DV)
Mono Fat	6.2 g		Calcium	98 mg	(10% DV)
Cholesterol	189.7 mg	(63% DV)	Iron	2.5 mg	(14% DV)
Sodium	554.3 mg	(23% DV)	Folate	11.2 mcg	(11% DV)
Potassium	133.9 mg	(4% DV)	Beta Carotene	0 RE	

Ratings	Worst	Bad	Average	Good	Best
Weight Loss			4		
LowCal Density		3			
Filling			5		
Energizing				8	
Fiber			5		
Vitamins			5		
Minerals			6		
Overall			4		

EGG, CHEESE, & BACON ON BISCUIT

Serving: 1 Great Starts sandwich (4.25 oz)   Breakfast

Calories	339	(79.8 cal/oz)	Carbohydrate	33.92 g	(11% DV)
Fat Calories	150	(44% fat)	Dietary Fiber	1.19 g	(5% DV)
Total Fat	16.66 g	(26% DV)	Protein	14.28 g	(29% DV)
Saturated Fat	5.95 g	(30% DV)	Vitamin A	426 IU	(9% DV)
Poly Fat	1.19 g		Vitamin C	2.4 mg	(4% DV)
Mono Fat	7.14 g		Calcium	242.8 mg	(24% DV)
Cholesterol	130.9 mg	(44% DV)	Iron	2.1 mg	(12% DV)
Sodium	1238.8 mg	(52% DV)	Folate	14.3 mcg	(3% DV)
Potassium	180.9 mg	(5% DV)	Beta Carotene	7.1 RE	

Ratings	Worst	Bad	Average	Good	Best
Weight Loss	2				
LowCal Density		4			
Filling			5		
Energizing				8	
Fiber		4			
Vitamins			5		
Minerals				8	
Overall		4			

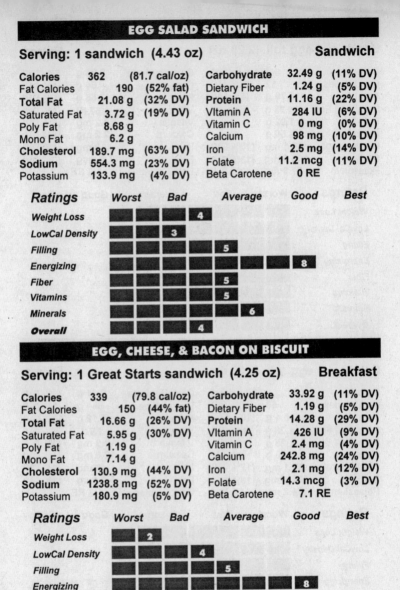

EGG, CHEESE, & HAM ON ENGLISH MUFFIN

Serving: 1 egg muffin (4.93 oz)   Breakfast

Calories	311	(63 cal/oz)	Carbohydrate	22.91 g	(8% DV)
Fat Calories	137	(44% fat)	Dietary Fiber	1.38 g	(6% DV)
Total Fat	15.18 g	(23% DV)	Protein	20.7 g	(41% DV)
Saturated Fat	5.52 g	(28% DV)	VItamin A	581 IU	(12% DV)
Poly Fat	1.38 g		Vitamin C	0 mg	(0% DV)
Mono Fat	5.52 g		Calcium	220.8 mg	(22% DV)
Cholesterol	224.9 mg	(75% DV)	Iron	2.6 mg	(14% DV)
Sodium	892.9 mg	(37% DV)	Folate	20.7 mcg	(17% DV)
Potassium	233.2 mg	(7% DV)	Beta Carotene	8.3 RE	

Ratings	Worst	Bad	Average	Good	Best
Weight Loss		3			
LowCal Density			5		
Filling		4			
Energizing			6		
Fiber			5		
Vitamins			6		
Minerals				8	
Overall			5		

EGG, CHEESE, & SAUSAGE ON BISCUIT

Serving: 1 Great Starts sandwich (6.29 oz)   Breakfast

Calories	600	(95.4 cal/oz)	Carbohydrate	40.83 g	(14% DV)
Fat Calories	348	(58% fat)	Dietary Fiber	0 g	(0% DV)
Total Fat	38.72 g	(60% DV)	Protein	22.88 g	(46% DV)
Saturated Fat	14.08 g	(70% DV)	VItamin A	797.3 IU	(16% DV)
Poly Fat	5.28 g		Vitamin C	1.8 mg	(3% DV)
Mono Fat	15.84 g		Calcium	318.6 mg	(32% DV)
Cholesterol	167.2 mg	(56% DV)	Iron	2.9 mg	(16% DV)
Sodium	1760 mg	(73% DV)	Folate	22.9 mcg	(4% DV)
Potassium	327.4 mg	(9% DV)	Beta Carotene	15.8 RE	

Ratings	Worst	Bad	Average	Good	Best
Weight Loss	1				
LowCal Density		3			
Filling			5		
Energizing					9
Fiber	1				
Vitamins				7	
Minerals					9
Overall		4			

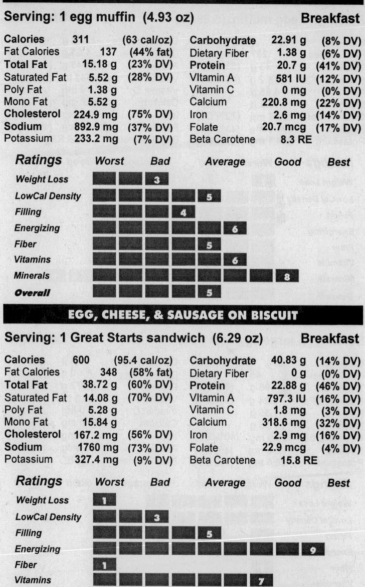

EGG, CHEESE, & SAUSAGE ON ENGLISH MUFFIN

Serving: 1 egg muffin (5.89 oz)   **Breakfast**

Calories	492	(83.5 cal/oz)	Carbohydrate	27.22 g	(9% DV)
Fat Calories	297	(60% fat)	Dietary Fiber	1.65 g	(7% DV)
Total Fat	**33 g**	**(51% DV)**	Protein	21.45 g	(43% DV)
Saturated Fat	13.2 g	(66% DV)	Vitamin A	863 IU	(17% DV)
Poly Fat	4.95 g		Vitamin C	0 mg	(0% DV)
Mono Fat	13.2 g		Calcium	308.6 mg	(31% DV)
Cholesterol	214.5 mg	(72% DV)	Iron	2.9 mg	(16% DV)
Sodium	1026.3 mg	(43% DV)	Folate	21.5 mcg	(18% DV)
Potassium	254.1 mg	(7% DV)	Beta Carotene	16.5 RE	

Ratings	Worst	Bad	Average	Good	Best
Weight Loss	1				
LowCal Density		3			
Filling			4		
Energizing				7	
Fiber			5		
Vitamins			6		
Minerals					9
Overall			4		

EGG, DEVILED

Serving: ½ large egg (1.11 oz)   **Breakfast**

Calories	63	(56.4 cal/oz)	Carbohydrate	.4 g	(0% DV)
Fat Calories	45	(71% fat)	Dietary Fiber	0 g	(0% DV)
Total Fat	**4.96 g**	**(8% DV)**	Protein	3.72 g	(7% DV)
Saturated Fat	1.24 g	(6% DV)	Vitamin A	164.3 IU	(3% DV)
Poly Fat	1.55 g		Vitamin C	0 mg	(0% DV)
Mono Fat	1.86 g		Calcium	14.6 mg	(1% DV)
Cholesterol	120.9 mg	(40% DV)	Iron	.4 mg	(2% DV)
Sodium	93.6 mg	(4% DV)	Folate	3.7 mcg	(3% DV)
Potassium	36.6 mg	(1% DV)	Beta Carotene	0 RE	

Ratings	Worst	Bad	Average	Good	Best
Weight Loss			5		
LowCal Density			5		
Filling	1				
Energizing	2				
Fiber	1				
Vitamins		3			
Minerals		3			
Overall		4			

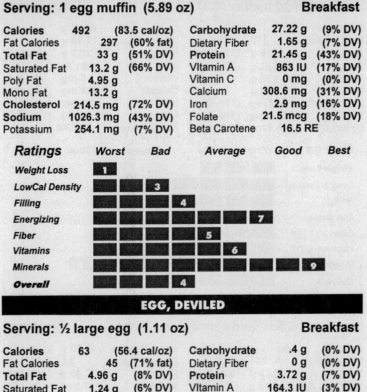

EGG, FRIED, SANDWICH

Serving: 1 sandwich (3.43 oz)

Sandwich

Calories	225	(65.5 cal/oz)	Carbohydrate	25.34 g	(8% DV)
Fat Calories	78	(35% fat)	Dietary Fiber	.96 g	(4% DV)
Total Fat	8.64 g	(13% DV)	Protein	10.56 g	(21% DV)
Saturated Fat	1.92 g	(10% DV)	Vitamin A	394.6 IU	(8% DV)
Poly Fat	1.92 g		Vitamin C	0 mg	(0% DV)
Mono Fat	3.84 g		Calcium	83.5 mg	(8% DV)
Cholesterol	211.2 mg	(70% DV)	Iron	2.2 mg	(12% DV)
Sodium	437.8 mg	(18% DV)	Folate	10.6 mcg	(9% DV)
Potassium	119 mg	(3% DV)	Beta Carotene	1.9 RE	

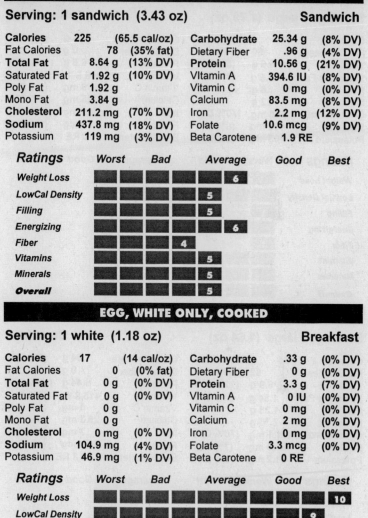

Ratings	Worst	Bad	Average	Good	Best
Weight Loss				6	
LowCal Density			5		
Filling			5		
Energizing				6	
Fiber		4			
Vitamins			5		
Minerals			5		
Overall			5		

EGG, WHITE ONLY, COOKED

Serving: 1 white (1.18 oz)

Breakfast

Calories	17	(14 cal/oz)	Carbohydrate	.33 g	(0% DV)
Fat Calories	0	(0% fat)	Dietary Fiber	0 g	(0% DV)
Total Fat	0 g	(0% DV)	Protein	3.3 g	(7% DV)
Saturated Fat	0 g	(0% DV)	Vitamin A	0 IU	(0% DV)
Poly Fat	0 g		Vitamin C	0 mg	(0% DV)
Mono Fat	0 g		Calcium	2 mg	(0% DV)
Cholesterol	0 mg	(0% DV)	Iron	0 mg	(0% DV)
Sodium	104.9 mg	(4% DV)	Folate	3.3 mcg	(0% DV)
Potassium	46.9 mg	(1% DV)	Beta Carotene	0 RE	

Ratings	Worst	Bad	Average	Good	Best
Weight Loss					10
LowCal Density				9	
Filling	1				
Energizing	2				
Fiber	1				
Vitamins	2				
Minerals	2				
Overall			6		

EGG, WHOLE, BOILED

Serving: 1 large (1.79 oz)   **Breakfast**

Calories	77	(43 cal/oz)	Carbohydrate	.55 g	(0% DV)
Fat Calories	50	(64% fat)	Dietary Fiber	0 g	(0% DV)
Total Fat	5.5 g	(8% DV)	Protein	6.5 g	(13% DV)
Saturated Fat	1.5 g	(8% DV)	Vitamin A	276.5 IU	(6% DV)
Poly Fat	.5 g		Vitamin C	0 mg	(0% DV)
Mono Fat	2 g		Calcium	25 mg	(2% DV)
Cholesterol	210 mg	(70% DV)	Iron	.6 mg	(3% DV)
Sodium	139 mg	(6% DV)	Folate	6.5 mcg	(6% DV)
Potassium	63 mg	(2% DV)	Beta Carotene	0 RE	

Ratings	Worst	Bad	Average	Good	Best
Weight Loss			5		
LowCal Density			6		
Filling	1				
Energizing	2				
Fiber	1				
Vitamins			5		
Minerals		4			
Overall		4			

EGG, WHOLE, FRIED

Serving: 1 large (1.64 oz)   **Breakfast**

Calories	91	(55.5 cal/oz)	Carbohydrate	.64 g	(0% DV)
Fat Calories	62	(68% fat)	Dietary Fiber	0 g	(0% DV)
Total Fat	6.9 g	(11% DV)	Protein	6.44 g	(13% DV)
Saturated Fat	1.84 g	(9% DV)	Vitamin A	415.8 IU	(8% DV)
Poly Fat	1.38 g		Vitamin C	0 mg	(0% DV)
Mono Fat	2.76 g		Calcium	25.3 mg	(3% DV)
Cholesterol	211.1 mg	(70% DV)	Iron	.7 mg	(4% DV)
Sodium	161.9 mg	(7% DV)	Folate	6.4 mcg	(4% DV)
Potassium	61.2 mg	(2% DV)	Beta Carotene	2.3 RE	

Ratings	Worst	Bad	Average	Good	Best
Weight Loss			5		
LowCal Density			5		
Filling	1				
Energizing	2				
Fiber	1				
Vitamins			5		
Minerals		4			
Overall		4			

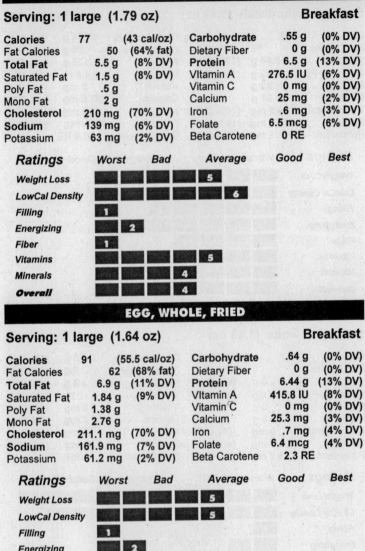

EGGNOG, MADE WITH 2% LOWFAT MILK

Serving: 1 cup (9.07 oz)   **Beverage**

Calories	188	(20.7 cal/oz)	Carbohydrate	16.51 g	(6% DV)
Fat Calories	69	(36% fat)	Dietary Fiber	0 g	(0% DV)
Total Fat	7.62 g	(12% DV)	Protein	12.7 g	(25% DV)
Saturated Fat	2.54 g	(13% DV)	VItamin A	685.8 IU	(14% DV)
Poly Fat	0 g		Vitamin C	2.5 mg	(4% DV)
Mono Fat	2.54 g		Calcium	269.2 mg	(27% DV)
Cholesterol	193 mg	(64% DV)	Iron	.7 mg	(4% DV)
Sodium	154.9 mg	(6% DV)	Folate	12.7 mcg	(8% DV)
Potassium	365.8 mg	(10% DV)	Beta Carotene	5.1 RE	

Ratings

	Worst	Bad	Average	Good	Best
Weight Loss	2				
LowCal Density					8
Filling			6		
Energizing			5		
Fiber	1				
Vitamins		4			
Minerals				7	
Overall			5		

EGGPLANT & MEAT CASSEROLE

Serving: 1 piece (3"x 2"x 1") (3.07 oz)   **Entree**

Calories	120	(39.2 cal/oz)	Carbohydrate	5.5 g	(2% DV)
Fat Calories	77	(64% fat)	Dietary Fiber	1.72 g	(7% DV)
Total Fat	8.6 g	(13% DV)	Protein	6.88 g	(14% DV)
Saturated Fat	1.72 g	(9% DV)	VItamin A	295 IU	(6% DV)
Poly Fat	2.58 g		Vitamin C	5.2 mg	(9% DV)
Mono Fat	2.58 g		Calcium	45.6 mg	(5% DV)
Cholesterol	19.8 mg	(7% DV)	Iron	.9 mg	(5% DV)
Sodium	104.1 mg	(4% DV)	Folate	6.9 mcg	(3% DV)
Potassium	217.6 mg	(6% DV)	Beta Carotene	20.6 RE	

Ratings

	Worst	Bad	Average	Good	Best
Weight Loss			5		
LowCal Density			6		
Filling		3			
Energizing		3			
Fiber			6		
Vitamins		4			
Minerals		4			
Overall			5		

EGGPLANT IN TOMATO SAUCE, WITHOUT ADDED FAT

Serving: 1 cup (8.25 oz)　　　　　　　**Vegetable**

Calories	67	(8.1 cal/oz)	Carbohydrate	15.71 g	(5% DV)
Fat Calories	0	(0% fat)	Dietary Fiber	4.62 g	(18% DV)
Total Fat	**0 g**	**(0% DV)**	Protein	2.31 g	(5% DV)
Saturated Fat	0 g	(0% DV)	Vitamin A	926.3 IU	(19% DV)
Poly Fat	0 g		Vitamin C	13.9 mg	(23% DV)
Mono Fat	0 g		Calcium	20.8 mg	(2% DV)
Cholesterol	**0 mg**	**(0% DV)**	Iron	1.2 mg	(6% DV)
Sodium	**857 mg**	**(36% DV)**	Folate	2.3 mcg	(8% DV)
Potassium	674.5 mg	(19% DV)	Beta Carotene	92.4 RE	

Ratings	Worst	Bad	Average	Good	Best
Weight Loss					9
LowCal Density					9
Filling					10
Energizing			5		
Fiber					9
Vitamins			6		
Minerals		4			
Overall				8	

EGGPLANT, BATTER-DIPPED, FRIED

Serving: 1 slice (3" dia, ½" thick) (1.79 oz)　　**Vegetable**

Calories	75	(41.9 cal/oz)	Carbohydrate	6.05 g	(2% DV)
Fat Calories	50	(66% fat)	Dietary Fiber	1 g	(4% DV)
Total Fat	**5.5 g**	**(8% DV)**	Protein	1 g	(2% DV)
Saturated Fat	1.5 g	(8% DV)	Vitamin A	34.5 IU	(1% DV)
Poly Fat	1.5 g		Vitamin C	.5 mg	(1% DV)
Mono Fat	2.5 g		Calcium	27 mg	(3% DV)
Cholesterol	**9 mg**	**(3% DV)**	Iron	.5 mg	(3% DV)
Sodium	**31.5 mg**	**(1% DV)**	Folate	1 mcg	(2% DV)
Potassium	106.5 mg	(3% DV)	Beta Carotene	2.5 RE	

Ratings	Worst	Bad	Average	Good	Best
Weight Loss		4			
LowCal Density			6		
Filling	3				
Energizing		4			
Fiber		4			
Vitamins	3				
Minerals	3				
Overall		4			

EGGS BENEDICT

Serving: 1 large egg (5.54 oz)   **Breakfast**

Calories	287	(51.8 cal/oz)	Carbohydrate	13.95 g	(5% DV)
Fat Calories	153	(54% fat)	Dietary Fiber	1.55 g	(6% DV)
Total Fat	17.05 g	(26% DV)	Protein	17.05 g	(34% DV)
Saturated Fat	6.2 g	(31% DV)	VItamin A	556.5 IU	(11% DV)
Poly Fat	3.1 g		Vitamin C	0 mg	(0% DV)
Mono Fat	7.75 g		Calcium	88.4 mg	(9% DV)
Cholesterol	226.3 mg	(75% DV)	Iron	1.9 mg	(11% DV)
Sodium	962.6 mg	(40% DV)	Folate	17.1 mcg	(10% DV)
Potassium	223.2 mg	(6% DV)	Beta Carotene	3.1 RE	

Ratings	Worst	Bad	Average	Good	Best
Weight Loss		3			
LowCal Density				6	
Filling		4			
Energizing			5		
Fiber			5		
Vitamins				6	
Minerals				6	
Overall			5		

EMPANADA, FRUIT-FILLED

Serving: 1 empanada (3.07 oz)   **Dessert**

Calories	358	(116.5 cal/oz)	Carbohydrate	38.44 g	(13% DV)
Fat Calories	194	(54% fat)	Dietary Fiber	1.72 g	(7% DV)
Total Fat	21.5 g	(33% DV)	Protein	3.44 g	(7% DV)
Saturated Fat	4.3 g	(21% DV)	VItamin A	12 IU	(0% DV)
Poly Fat	6.88 g		Vitamin C	0 mg	(0% DV)
Mono Fat	9.46 g		Calcium	36.1 mg	(4% DV)
Cholesterol	0 mg	(0% DV)	Iron	1.6 mg	(9% DV)
Sodium	183.2 mg	(8% DV)	Folate	3.4 mcg	(1% DV)
Potassium	55 mg	(2% DV)	Beta Carotene	1.7 RE	

Ratings	Worst	Bad	Average	Good	Best
Weight Loss		3			
LowCal Density	2				
Filling		4			
Energizing					9
Fiber			6		
Vitamins		4			
Minerals		4			
Overall		4			

ENCHILADA WITH BEEF, BEANS, & CHEESE

Serving: 1 enchilada or enchirito (4.61 oz) **Entree**

Calories	250	(54.3 cal/oz)	Carbohydrate	26.7 g	(9% DV)
Fat Calories	104	(42% fat)	Dietary Fiber	3.87 g	(15% DV)
Total Fat	11.61 g	(18% DV)	Protein	10.32 g	(21% DV)
Saturated Fat	5.16 g	(26% DV)	Vitamin A	1741.5 IU	(35% DV)
Poly Fat	1.29 g		Vitamin C	14.2 mg	(24% DV)
Mono Fat	3.87 g		Calcium	161.3 mg	(16% DV)
Cholesterol	25.8 mg	(9% DV)	Iron	1.8 mg	(10% DV)
Sodium	318.6 mg	(13% DV)	Folate	10.3 mcg	(11% DV)
Potassium	437.3 mg	(12% DV)	Beta Carotene	165.1 RE	

Ratings	Worst	Bad	Average	Good	Best
Weight Loss			5		
LowCal Density			6		
Filling			5		
Energizing			7		
Fiber					9
Vitamins			6		
Minerals			7		
Overall			6		

ENCHILADA WITH CHICKEN, BEANS, & CHEESE

Serving: 1 enchilada (4.5 oz) **Entree**

Calories	232	(51.5 cal/oz)	Carbohydrate	26.59 g	(9% DV)
Fat Calories	91	(39% fat)	Dietary Fiber	3.78 g	(15% DV)
Total Fat	10.08 g	(16% DV)	Protein	10.08 g	(20% DV)
Saturated Fat	3.78 g	(19% DV)	Vitamin A	1741.3 IU	(35% DV)
Poly Fat	2.52 g		Vitamin C	13.9 mg	(23% DV)
Mono Fat	3.78 g		Calcium	161.3 mg	(16% DV)
Cholesterol	23.9 mg	(8% DV)	Iron	1.6 mg	(9% DV)
Sodium	308.7 mg	(13% DV)	Folate	10.1 mcg	(10% DV)
Potassium	409.5 mg	(12% DV)	Beta Carotene	163.8 RE	

Ratings	Worst	Bad	Average	Good	Best
Weight Loss			6		
LowCal Density			6		
Filling			5		
Energizing			7		
Fiber					9
Vitamins			6		
Minerals			7		
Overall			6		

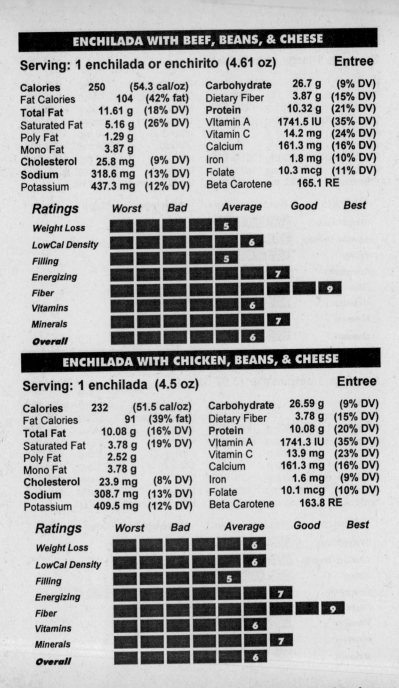

ENGLISH MUFFIN, 100% WHOLE WHEAT

Serving: 1 muffin (2.07 oz)   **Bread**

Calories	132	(63.9 cal/oz)	Carbohydrate	26.39 g	(9% DV)
Fat Calories	16	(12% fat)	Dietary Fiber	5.22 g	(21% DV)
Total Fat	1.74 g	(3% DV)	Protein	5.8 g	(12% DV)
Saturated Fat	.58 g	(3% DV)	VItamin A	0 IU	(0% DV)
Poly Fat	.58 g		Vitamin C	0 mg	(0% DV)
Mono Fat	.58 g		Calcium	60.9 mg	(6% DV)
Cholesterol	0 mg	(0% DV)	Iron	1.7 mg	(9% DV)
Sodium	171.7 mg	(7% DV)	Folate	5.8 mcg	(15% DV)
Potassium	185.6 mg	(5% DV)	Beta Carotene	0 RE	

Ratings	Worst	Bad	Average	Good	Best
Weight Loss			5		
LowCal Density			5		
Filling			5		
Energizing				7	
Fiber					9
Vitamins			5		
Minerals			6		
Overall			6		

ENGLISH MUFFIN, MULTIGRAIN

Serving: 1 muffin (2.07 oz)   **Bread**

Calories	143	(68.9 cal/oz)	Carbohydrate	27.49 g	(9% DV)
Fat Calories	16	(11% fat)	Dietary Fiber	4.06 g	(16% DV)
Total Fat	1.74 g	(3% DV)	Protein	5.22 g	(10% DV)
Saturated Fat	.58 g	(3% DV)	VItamin A	3.5 IU	(0% DV)
Poly Fat	.58 g		Vitamin C	1.2 mg	(2% DV)
Mono Fat	.58 g		Calcium	58.6 mg	(6% DV)
Cholesterol	0 mg	(0% DV)	Iron	1.9 mg	(11% DV)
Sodium	189.7 mg	(8% DV)	Folate	5.2 mcg	(15% DV)
Potassium	141.5 mg	(4% DV)	Beta Carotene	0 RE	

Ratings	Worst	Bad	Average	Good	Best
Weight Loss			5		
LowCal Density		4			
Filling			5		
Energizing				7	
Fiber					9
Vitamins			5		
Minerals			5		
Overall			5		

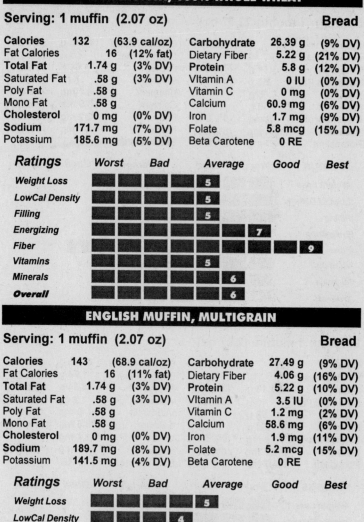

ENGLISH MUFFIN, WHEAT BRAN

Serving: 1 muffin (2.07 oz)   **Bread**

Calories	126	(60.8 cal/oz)	Carbohydrate	24.65 g	(8% DV)
Fat Calories	16	(12% fat)	Dietary Fiber	2.9 g	(12% DV)
Total Fat	1.74 g	(3% DV)	Protein	4.64 g	(9% DV)
Saturated Fat	.58 g	(3% DV)	Vitamin A	0 IU	(0% DV)
Poly Fat	.58 g		Vitamin C	4.1 mg	(7% DV)
Mono Fat	.58 g		Calcium	53.9 mg	(5% DV)
Cholesterol	0 mg	(0% DV)	Iron	2.2 mg	(12% DV)
Sodium	198.4 mg	(8% DV)	Folate	4.6 mcg	(14% DV)
Potassium	124.7 mg	(4% DV)	Beta Carotene	0 RE	

Ratings	Worst	Bad	Average	Good	Best
Weight Loss			6		
LowCal Density			5		
Filling			5		
Energizing			6		
Fiber				8	
Vitamins				7	
Minerals			5		
Overall			6		

ENGLISH MUFFIN, WITH RAISINS

Serving: 1 muffin (2.07 oz)   **Bread**

Calories	137	(66.4 cal/oz)	Carbohydrate	27.43 g	(9% DV)
Fat Calories	10	(8% fat)	Dietary Fiber	1.74 g	(7% DV)
Total Fat	1.16 g	(2% DV)	Protein	4.64 g	(9% DV)
Saturated Fat	0 g	(0% DV)	Vitamin A	.6 IU	(0% DV)
Poly Fat	.58 g		Vitamin C	0 mg	(0% DV)
Mono Fat	.58 g		Calcium	108.5 mg	(11% DV)
Cholesterol	0 mg	(0% DV)	Iron	1.7 mg	(10% DV)
Sodium	142.7 mg	(6% DV)	Folate	4.6 mcg	(12% DV)
Potassium	113.7 mg	(3% DV)	Beta Carotene	0 RE	

Ratings	Worst	Bad	Average	Good	Best
Weight Loss			5		
LowCal Density			5		
Filling			5		
Energizing			7		
Fiber			6		
Vitamins			5		
Minerals			5		
Overall			5		

FAJITA WITH BEEF & VEGETABLES

Serving: 1 tortilla (7.96 oz)   **Entree**

Calories	410	(51.5 cal/oz)	Carbohydrate	46.16 g	(15% DV)
Fat Calories	161	(39% fat)	Dietary Fiber	4.46 g	(18% DV)
Total Fat	17.84 g	(27% DV)	Protein	17.84 g	(36% DV)
Saturated Fat	4.46 g	(22% DV)	Vltamin A	521.8 IU	(10% DV)
Poly Fat	4.46 g		Vitamin C	29 mg	(48% DV)
Mono Fat	6.69 g		Calcium	75.8 mg	(8% DV)
Cholesterol	26.8 mg	(9% DV)	Iron	3.7 mg	(20% DV)
Sodium	849.6 mg	(35% DV)	Folate	17.8 mcg	(6% DV)
Potassium	425.9 mg	(12% DV)	Beta Carotene	51.3 RE	

Ratings	Worst	Bad	Average	Good	Best
Weight Loss			4		
LowCal Density			6		
Filling			6		
Energizing					9
Fiber					9
Vitamins				8	
Minerals				7	
Overall			6		

FAJITA WITH CHICKEN & VEGETABLES

Serving: 1 tortilla (7.96 oz)   **Entree**

Calories	406	(51 cal/oz)	Carbohydrate	50.4 g	(17% DV)
Fat Calories	120	(30% fat)	Dietary Fiber	4.46 g	(18% DV)
Total Fat	13.38 g	(21% DV)	Protein	22.3 g	(45% DV)
Saturated Fat	2.23 g	(11% DV)	Vltamin A	508.4 IU	(10% DV)
Poly Fat	4.46 g		Vitamin C	22.3 mg	(37% DV)
Mono Fat	6.69 g		Calcium	82.5 mg	(8% DV)
Cholesterol	40.1 mg	(13% DV)	Iron	3.7 mg	(21% DV)
Sodium	439.3 mg	(18% DV)	Folate	22.3 mcg	(10% DV)
Potassium	530.7 mg	(15% DV)	Beta Carotene	49.1 RE	

Ratings	Worst	Bad	Average	Good	Best
Weight Loss			5		
LowCal Density			6		
Filling			7		
Energizing					10
Fiber				9	
Vitamins				8	
Minerals			7		
Overall			7		

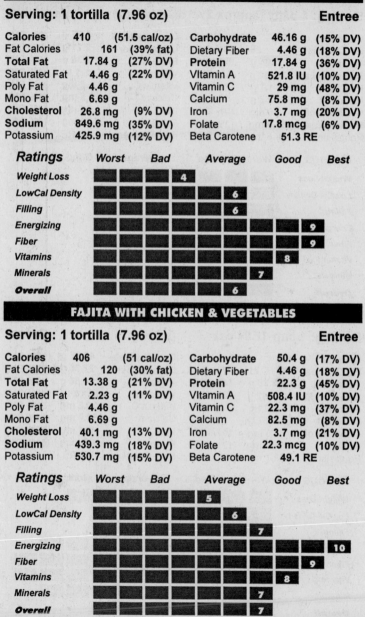

FALAFEL

Serving: 1 patty (approx 2¼" dia) (.61 oz) Vegetable

Calories	57	(92.8 cal/oz)	Carbohydrate	5.37 g	(2% DV)
Fat Calories	28	(49% fat)	Dietary Fiber	2.21 g	(9% DV)
Total Fat	3.06 g	(5% DV)	Protein	2.38 g	(5% DV)
Saturated Fat	.51 g	(3% DV)	Vitamin A	5.1 IU	(0% DV)
Poly Fat	1.7 g		Vitamin C	.2 mg	(0% DV)
Mono Fat	.68 g		Calcium	9.2 mg	(1% DV)
Cholesterol	0 mg	(0% DV)	Iron	.5 mg	(3% DV)
Sodium	64.8 mg	(3% DV)	Folate	2.4 mcg	(3% DV)
Potassium	68.5 mg	(2% DV)	Beta Carotene	.5 RE	

Ratings	Worst	Bad	Average	Good	Best
Weight Loss				6	
LowCal Density	3				
Filling	2				
Energizing	3				
Fiber				6	
Vitamins	2				
Minerals	3				
Overall		4			

FIBER ONE

Serving: 1 cup (2.04 oz) Cereal

Calories	121	(59.2 cal/oz)	Carbohydrate	45.88 g	(15% DV)
Fat Calories	21	(17% fat)	Dietary Fiber	27.36 g	(109% DV)
Total Fat	2.28 g	(4% DV)	Protein	4.56 g	(9% DV)
Saturated Fat	.57 g	(3% DV)	Vitamin A	2513.7 IU	(50% DV)
Poly Fat	1.71 g		Vitamin C	30.2 mg	(50% DV)
Mono Fat	.57 g		Calcium	131.7 mg	(13% DV)
Cholesterol	0 mg	(0% DV)	Iron	9.1 mg	(50% DV)
Sodium	281.6 mg	(12% DV)	Folate	4.6 mcg	(51% DV)
Potassium	502.7 mg	(14% DV)	Beta Carotene	0 RE	

Ratings	Worst	Bad	Average	Good	Best
Weight Loss				8	
LowCal Density			5		
Filling			7		
Energizing				9	
Fiber					10
Vitamins					10
Minerals				9	
Overall			7		

FILBERTS, HAZEL NUTS

Serving: about 20 nuts (1 oz)   **Snack**

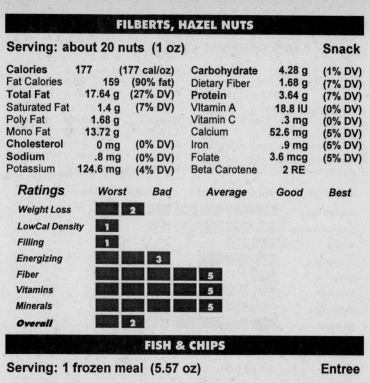

Calories	177	(177 cal/oz)	Carbohydrate	4.28 g	(1% DV)
Fat Calories	159	(90% fat)	Dietary Fiber	1.68 g	(7% DV)
Total Fat	17.64 g	(27% DV)	Protein	3.64 g	(7% DV)
Saturated Fat	1.4 g	(7% DV)	Vitamin A	18.8 IU	(0% DV)
Poly Fat	1.68 g		Vitamin C	.3 mg	(0% DV)
Mono Fat	13.72 g		Calcium	52.6 mg	(5% DV)
Cholesterol	0 mg	(0% DV)	Iron	.9 mg	(5% DV)
Sodium	.8 mg	(0% DV)	Folate	3.6 mcg	(5% DV)
Potassium	124.6 mg	(4% DV)	Beta Carotene	2 RE	

Ratings	Worst	Bad	Average	Good	Best
Weight Loss	2				
LowCal Density	1				
Filling	1				
Energizing		3			
Fiber				5	
Vitamins				5	
Minerals				5	
Overall	2				

FISH & CHIPS

Serving: 1 frozen meal (5.57 oz)   **Entree**

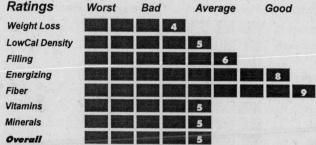

Calories	324	(58.3 cal/oz)	Carbohydrate	34.79 g	(12% DV)
Fat Calories	140	(43% fat)	Dietary Fiber	4.68 g	(19% DV)
Total Fat	15.6 g	(24% DV)	Protein	14.04 g	(28% DV)
Saturated Fat	4.68 g	(23% DV)	Vitamin A	64 IU	(1% DV)
Poly Fat	4.68 g		Vitamin C	7.8 mg	(13% DV)
Mono Fat	4.68 g		Calcium	25 mg	(2% DV)
Cholesterol	23.4 mg	(8% DV)	Iron	1.6 mg	(9% DV)
Sodium	620.9 mg	(26% DV)	Folate	14 mcg	(4% DV)
Potassium	553.8 mg	(16% DV)	Beta Carotene	3.1 RE	

Ratings	Worst	Bad	Average	Good	Best
Weight Loss			4		
LowCal Density			5		
Filling			6		
Energizing				8	
Fiber					9
Vitamins			5		
Minerals			5		
Overall			5		

FISH STICK, BREADED OR BATTERED, BAKED

Serving: 1 stick (4"x 1"x ½") (1 oz)   **Fish**

Calories	58	(58 cal/oz)	Carbohydrate	2.27 g	(1% DV)
Fat Calories	23	(39% fat)	Dietary Fiber	0 g	(0% DV)
Total Fat	2.52 g	(4% DV)	Protein	5.88 g	(12% DV)
Saturated Fat	.56 g	(3% DV)	Vitamin A	126.3 IU	(3% DV)
Poly Fat	.84 g		Vitamin C	0 mg	(0% DV)
Mono Fat	1.12 g		Calcium	22.1 mg	(2% DV)
Cholesterol	25.8 mg	(9% DV)	Iron	.3 mg	(2% DV)
Sodium	136.1 mg	(6% DV)	Folate	5.9 mcg	(1% DV)
Potassium	105.3 mg	(3% DV)	Beta Carotene	2.2 RE	

Ratings	Worst	Bad	Average	Good	Best
Weight Loss					7
LowCal Density			5		
Filling	2				
Energizing		3			
Fiber	1				
Vitamins		3			
Minerals		4			
Overall			5		

FLAUTA

Serving: 1 flauta (4.04 oz)   **Entree**

Calories	351	(87 cal/oz)	Carbohydrate	12.77 g	(4% DV)
Fat Calories	244	(69% fat)	Dietary Fiber	1.13 g	(5% DV)
Total Fat	27.12 g	(42% DV)	Protein	14.69 g	(29% DV)
Saturated Fat	4.52 g	(23% DV)	Vitamin A	159.3 IU	(3% DV)
Poly Fat	9.04 g		Vitamin C	13.6 mg	(23% DV)
Mono Fat	11.3 g		Calcium	50.9 mg	(5% DV)
Cholesterol	41.8 mg	(14% DV)	Iron	1.6 mg	(9% DV)
Sodium	188.7 mg	(8% DV)	Folate	14.7 mcg	(2% DV)
Potassium	267.8 mg	(8% DV)	Beta Carotene	14.7 RE	

Ratings	Worst	Bad	Average	Good	Best
Weight Loss		3			
LowCal Density		3			
Filling		3			
Energizing			5		
Fiber		4			
Vitamins			5		
Minerals			6		
Overall		4			

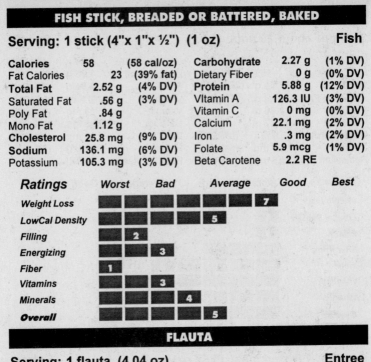

FLOUNDER WITH CHOPPED BROCCOLI

Serving: 1 diet meal (12.54 oz)

Entree

Calories	270	(21.6 cal/oz)	Carbohydrate	22.82 g	(8% DV)
Fat Calories	63	(23% fat)	Dietary Fiber	3.51 g	(14% DV)
Total Fat	7.02 g	(11% DV)	Protein	31.59 g	(63% DV)
Saturated Fat	3.51 g	(18% DV)	VItamin A	1519.8 IU	(30% DV)
Poly Fat	0 g		Vitamin C	63.2 mg	(105% DV)
Mono Fat	0 g		Calcium	273.8 mg	(27% DV)
Cholesterol	66.7 mg	(22% DV)	Iron	1.8 mg	(10% DV)
Sodium	649.4 mg	(27% DV)	Folate	31.6 mcg	(16% DV)
Potassium	905.6 mg	(26% DV)	Beta Carotene	115.8 RE	

Ratings	Worst	Bad	Average	Good	Best
Weight Loss			6		
LowCal Density				8	
Filling			7		
Energizing			6		
Fiber				8	
Vitamins					9
Minerals					9
Overall			7		

FLOUNDER, BAKED OR BROILED

Serving: 1 fillet (4.64 oz)

Fish

Calories	173	(37.3 cal/oz)	Carbohydrate	.52 g	(0% DV)
Fat Calories	47	(27% fat)	Dietary Fiber	0 g	(0% DV)
Total Fat	5.2 g	(8% DV)	Protein	28.6 g	(57% DV)
Saturated Fat	1.3 g	(7% DV)	VItamin A	245.7 IU	(5% DV)
Poly Fat	1.3 g		Vitamin C	3.9 mg	(6% DV)
Mono Fat	2.6 g		Calcium	29.9 mg	(3% DV)
Cholesterol	72.8 mg	(24% DV)	Iron	.6 mg	(3% DV)
Sodium	523.9 mg	(22% DV)	Folate	28.6 mcg	(3% DV)
Potassium	556.4 mg	(16% DV)	Beta Carotene	3.9 RE	

Ratings	Worst	Bad	Average	Good	Best
Weight Loss			6		
LowCal Density				7	
Filling	1				
Energizing		2			
Fiber	1				
Vitamins			5		
Minerals			6		
Overall			5		

FLOUNDER, FLOURED OR BREADED, FRIED

Serving: 1 fillet (5.54 oz)   **Fish**

Calories	338	(61 cal/oz)	Carbohydrate	12.25 g	(4% DV)
Fat Calories	153	(45% fat)	Dietary Fiber	0 g	(0% DV)
Total Fat	17.05 g	(26% DV)	Protein	31 g	(62% DV)
Saturated Fat	4.65 g	(23% DV)	VItamin A	96.1 IU	(2% DV)
Poly Fat	4.65 g		Vitamin C	1.6 mg	(3% DV)
Mono Fat	7.75 g		Calcium	54.3 mg	(5% DV)
Cholesterol	107 mg	(36% DV)	Iron	1.3 mg	(7% DV)
Sodium	599.9 mg	(25% DV)	Folate	31 mcg	(5% DV)
Potassium	573.5 mg	(16% DV)	Beta Carotene	0 RE	

Ratings	Worst	Bad	Average	Good	Best
Weight Loss	2				
LowCal Density			5		
Filling		3			
Energizing			5		
Fiber	1				
Vitamins			5		
Minerals				6	
Overall			4		

FRANKFURTER, MEATLESS, VEGETARIAN

Serving: 1 frankfurter (2.5 oz)   **Entree**

Calories	140	(56 cal/oz)	Carbohydrate	5.6 g	(2% DV)
Fat Calories	63	(45% fat)	Dietary Fiber	3.5 g	(14% DV)
Total Fat	7 g	(11% DV)	Protein	14 g	(28% DV)
Saturated Fat	1.4 g	(7% DV)	VItamin A	0 IU	(0% DV)
Poly Fat	3.5 g		Vitamin C	0 mg	(0% DV)
Mono Fat	1.4 g		Calcium	23.1 mg	(2% DV)
Cholesterol	0 mg	(0% DV)	Iron	1.3 mg	(7% DV)
Sodium	301 mg	(13% DV)	Folate	14 mcg	(14% DV)
Potassium	105 mg	(3% DV)	Beta Carotene	0 RE	

Ratings	Worst	Bad	Average	Good	Best
Weight Loss			6		
LowCal Density			5		
Filling		3			
Energizing		3			
Fiber				8	
Vitamins					9
Minerals			5		
Overall			5		

FRANKFURTER, PLAIN, ON BUN

Serving: 1 frankfurter (3.04 oz)   **Sandwich**

Calories	264	(86.7 cal/oz)	Carbohydrate	22.36 g	(7% DV)
Fat Calories	138	(52% fat)	Dietary Fiber	.85 g	(3% DV)
Total Fat	15.3 g	(24% DV)	Protein	8.5 g	(17% DV)
Saturated Fat	5.1 g	(25% DV)	Vitamin A	0 IU	(0% DV)
Poly Fat	1.7 g		Vitamin C	11.9 mg	(20% DV)
Mono Fat	7.65 g		Calcium	45.1 mg	(5% DV)
Cholesterol	22.1 mg	(7% DV)	Iron	1.6 mg	(9% DV)
Sodium	706.4 mg	(29% DV)	Folate	8.5 mcg	(4% DV)
Potassium	113.1 mg	(3% DV)	Beta Carotene	0 RE	

Ratings

	Worst	Bad	Average	Good	Best
Weight Loss			5		
LowCal Density		3			
Filling			4		
Energizing			6		
Fiber			4		
Vitamins			5		
Minerals			5		
Overall			4		

FRANKFURTER, TURKEY

Serving: 1 frankfurter (1.61 oz)   **Meat**

Calories	104	(64.6 cal/oz)	Carbohydrate	.72 g	(0% DV)
Fat Calories	73	(70% fat)	Dietary Fiber	0 g	(0% DV)
Total Fat	8.1 g	(12% DV)	Protein	6.75 g	(14% DV)
Saturated Fat	2.7 g	(14% DV)	Vitamin A	0 IU	(0% DV)
Poly Fat	2.25 g		Vitamin C	0 mg	(0% DV)
Mono Fat	2.25 g		Calcium	50.9 mg	(5% DV)
Cholesterol	50.9 mg	(17% DV)	Iron	.9 mg	(5% DV)
Sodium	648.5 mg	(27% DV)	Folate	6.8 mcg	(1% DV)
Potassium	81.5 mg	(2% DV)	Beta Carotene	0 RE	

Ratings

	Worst	Bad	Average	Good	Best
Weight Loss		4			
LowCal Density			5		
Filling	1				
Energizing	2				
Fiber	1				
Vitamins		3			
Minerals		4			
Overall		3			

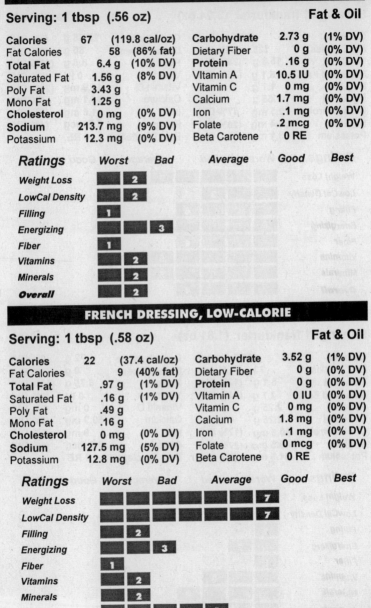

FRENCH DRESSING

Serving: 1 tbsp (.56 oz) — Fat & Oil

Calories	67	(119.8 cal/oz)	Carbohydrate	2.73 g	(1% DV)
Fat Calories	58	(86% fat)	Dietary Fiber	0 g	(0% DV)
Total Fat	6.4 g	(10% DV)	Protein	.16 g	(0% DV)
Saturated Fat	1.56 g	(8% DV)	VItamin A	10.5 IU	(0% DV)
Poly Fat	3.43 g		Vitamin C	0 mg	(0% DV)
Mono Fat	1.25 g		Calcium	1.7 mg	(0% DV)
Cholesterol	0 mg	(0% DV)	Iron	.1 mg	(0% DV)
Sodium	213.7 mg	(9% DV)	Folate	.2 mcg	(0% DV)
Potassium	12.3 mg	(0% DV)	Beta Carotene	0 RE	

Ratings	Worst	Bad	Average	Good	Best
Weight Loss	2				
LowCal Density	2				
Filling	1				
Energizing		3			
Fiber	1				
Vitamins	2				
Minerals	2				
Overall	2				

FRENCH DRESSING, LOW-CALORIE

Serving: 1 tbsp (.58 oz) — Fat & Oil

Calories	22	(37.4 cal/oz)	Carbohydrate	3.52 g	(1% DV)
Fat Calories	9	(40% fat)	Dietary Fiber	0 g	(0% DV)
Total Fat	.97 g	(1% DV)	Protein	0 g	(0% DV)
Saturated Fat	.16 g	(1% DV)	VItamin A	0 IU	(0% DV)
Poly Fat	.49 g		Vitamin C	0 mg	(0% DV)
Mono Fat	.16 g		Calcium	1.8 mg	(0% DV)
Cholesterol	0 mg	(0% DV)	Iron	.1 mg	(0% DV)
Sodium	127.5 mg	(5% DV)	Folate	0 mcg	(0% DV)
Potassium	12.8 mg	(0% DV)	Beta Carotene	0 RE	

Ratings	Worst	Bad	Average	Good	Best
Weight Loss					7
LowCal Density					7
Filling	2				
Energizing		3			
Fiber	1				
Vitamins	2				
Minerals	2				
Overall			5		

FRENCH TOAST, PLAIN

Serving: 1 slice (2.32 oz)   **Breakfast**

Calories	161	(69.5 cal/oz)	Carbohydrate	19.24 g	(6% DV)
Fat Calories	59	(36% fat)	Dietary Fiber	.65 g	(3% DV)
Total Fat	6.5 g	(10% DV)	Protein	5.85 g	(12% DV)
Saturated Fat	1.95 g	(10% DV)	VItamin A	150.8 IU	(3% DV)
Poly Fat	1.3 g		Vitamin C	0 mg	(0% DV)
Mono Fat	2.6 g		Calcium	63.1 mg	(6% DV)
Cholesterol	92.3 mg	(31% DV)	Iron	1.3 mg	(7% DV)
Sodium	430.3 mg	(18% DV)	Folate	5.9 mcg	(4% DV)
Potassium	82.6 mg	(2% DV)	Beta Carotene	.7 RE	

Ratings	Worst	Bad	Average	Good	Best
Weight Loss					6
LowCal Density			4		
Filling			4		
Energizing				6	
Fiber		3			
Vitamins			4		
Minerals			4		
Overall			5		

FRITTER, APPLE

Serving: 1 Mrs Paul's apple fritter (2 oz)   **Dessert**

Calories	204	(101.9 cal/oz)	Carbohydrate	18.2 g	(6% DV)
Fat Calories	121	(59% fat)	Dietary Fiber	.56 g	(2% DV)
Total Fat	13.44 g	(21% DV)	Protein	3.36 g	(7% DV)
Saturated Fat	3.36 g	(17% DV)	VItamin A	99.7 IU	(2% DV)
Poly Fat	3.36 g		Vitamin C	.6 mg	(1% DV)
Mono Fat	5.6 g		Calcium	29.1 mg	(3% DV)
Cholesterol	48.7 mg	(16% DV)	Iron	.8 mg	(4% DV)
Sodium	23 mg	(1% DV)	Folate	3.4 mcg	(2% DV)
Potassium	77.8 mg	(2% DV)	Beta Carotene	1.1 RE	

Ratings	Worst	Bad	Average	Good	Best
Weight Loss		4			
LowCal Density	2				
Filling		3			
Energizing				6	
Fiber		3			
Vitamins		3			
Minerals		3			
Overall		3			

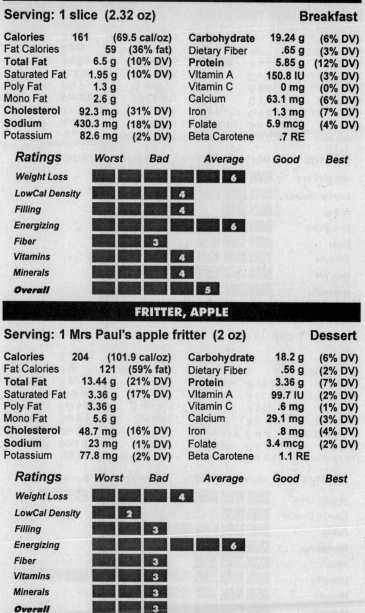

FROG LEGS

Serving: 2 legs (1.71 oz)   **Fish**

Calories	120	(70.5 cal/oz)	Carbohydrate	8.64 g	(3% DV)
Fat Calories	52	(43% fat)	Dietary Fiber	.48 g	(2% DV)
Total Fat	5.76 g	(9% DV)	Protein	8.16 g	(16% DV)
Saturated Fat	1.44 g	(7% DV)	Vitamin A	86.9 IU	(2% DV)
Poly Fat	1.44 g		Vitamin C	1.4 mg	(2% DV)
Mono Fat	2.4 g		Calcium	25.4 mg	(3% DV)
Cholesterol	64.3 mg	(21% DV)	Iron	1.1 mg	(6% DV)
Sodium	237.6 mg	(10% DV)	Folate	8.2 mcg	(3% DV)
Potassium	130.6 mg	(4% DV)	Beta Carotene	0 RE	

Ratings	Worst	Bad	Average	Good	Best
Weight Loss			6		
LowCal Density		4			
Filling	2				
Energizing		4			
Fiber	3				
Vitamins		4			
Minerals		4			
Overall		4			

FROOT LOOPS

Serving: 1 cup (1 oz)   **Cereal**

Calories	110	(109.8 cal/oz)	Carbohydrate	24.72 g	(8% DV)
Fat Calories	5	(5% fat)	Dietary Fiber	.56 g	(2% DV)
Total Fat	.56 g	(1% DV)	Protein	1.68 g	(3% DV)
Saturated Fat	.28 g	(1% DV)	Vitamin A	740.6 IU	(15% DV)
Poly Fat	.28 g		Vitamin C	59.4 mg	(99% DV)
Mono Fat	0 g		Calcium	2.8 mg	(0% DV)
Cholesterol	0 mg	(0% DV)	Iron	4.5 mg	(25% DV)
Sodium	142.8 mg	(6% DV)	Folate	1.7 mcg	(25% DV)
Potassium	25.8 mg	(1% DV)	Beta Carotene	0 RE	

Ratings	Worst	Bad	Average	Good	Best
Weight Loss				9	
LowCal Density	2				
Filling		4			
Energizing			6		
Fiber	3				
Vitamins					10
Minerals			6		
Overall			6		

FROSTED FLAKES, KELLOGG

Serving: 1 cup (1.25 oz)   **Cereal**

Calories	133	(106.7 cal/oz)	Carbohydrate	31.71 g	(11% DV)
Fat Calories	0	(0% fat)	Dietary Fiber	.7 g	(3% DV)
Total Fat	0 g	(0% DV)	Protein	1.75 g	(4% DV)
Saturated Fat	0 g	(0% DV)	Vitamin A	925.8 IU	(19% DV)
Poly Fat	0 g		Vitamin C	18.6 mg	(31% DV)
Mono Fat	0 g		Calcium	1.4 mg	(0% DV)
Cholesterol	0 mg	(0% DV)	Iron	2.2 mg	(12% DV)
Sodium	283.5 mg	(12% DV)	Folate	1.8 mcg	(31% DV)
Potassium	22.4 mg	(1% DV)	Beta Carotene	0 RE	

Ratings	Worst	Bad	Average	Good	Best
Weight Loss					9
LowCal Density	2				
Filling		4			
Energizing				8	
Fiber		3			
Vitamins					9
Minerals		4			
Overall			5		

FRUIT COCKTAIL, COOKED OR CANNED

Serving: 1 cup (8.86 oz)   **Fruit**

Calories	186	(21 cal/oz)	Carbohydrate	48.36 g	(16% DV)
Fat Calories	0	(0% fat)	Dietary Fiber	2.48 g	(10% DV)
Total Fat	0 g	(0% DV)	Protein	0 g	(0% DV)
Saturated Fat	0 g	(0% DV)	Vitamin A	691.9 IU	(14% DV)
Poly Fat	0 g		Vitamin C	9.9 mg	(17% DV)
Mono Fat	0 g		Calcium	17.4 mg	(2% DV)
Cholesterol	0 mg	(0% DV)	Iron	.8 mg	(4% DV)
Sodium	12.4 mg	(1% DV)	Folate	0 mcg	(2% DV)
Potassium	228.2 mg	(7% DV)	Beta Carotene	69.4 RE	

Ratings	Worst	Bad	Average	Good	Best
Weight Loss			7		
LowCal Density				8	
Filling					10
Energizing				9	
Fiber			7		
Vitamins		5			
Minerals		3			
Overall			7		

FRUIT JUICE BAR, 90% FRUIT JUICE, FROZEN

Serving: 1 bar (1.86 oz)   **Dessert**

Calories	18	(9.8 cal/oz)	Carbohydrate	4.68 g	(2% DV)
Fat Calories	0	(0% fat)	Dietary Fiber	0 g	(0% DV)
Total Fat	0 g	(0% DV)	**Protein**	0 g	(0% DV)
Saturated Fat	0 g	(0% DV)	Vitamin A	17.2 IU	(0% DV)
Poly Fat	0 g		Vitamin C	6.8 mg	(11% DV)
Mono Fat	0 g		Calcium	2.6 mg	(0% DV)
Cholesterol	0 mg	(0% DV)	Iron	.1 mg	(1% DV)
Sodium	7.3 mg	(0% DV)	Folate	0 mcg	(1% DV)
Potassium	40.6 mg	(1% DV)	Beta Carotene	1.6 RE	

Ratings	Worst	Bad	Average	Good	Best
Weight Loss					10
LowCal Density					9
Filling			5		
Energizing		3			
Fiber	1				
Vitamins		3			
Minerals	2				
Overall				7	

FRUIT LEATHER

Serving: 1 roll-up (.5 oz)   **Sweets**

Calories	49	(98 cal/oz)	Carbohydrate	11.8 g	(4% DV)
Fat Calories	4	(8% fat)	Dietary Fiber	.56 g	(2% DV)
Total Fat	.42 g	(1% DV)	**Protein**	.14 g	(0% DV)
Saturated Fat	.14 g	(1% DV)	Vitamin A	16.2 IU	(0% DV)
Poly Fat	.14 g		Vitamin C	.8 mg	(1% DV)
Mono Fat	.14 g		Calcium	4.5 mg	(0% DV)
Cholesterol	0 mg	(0% DV)	Iron	.1 mg	(1% DV)
Sodium	8.5 mg	(0% DV)	Folate	.1 mcg	(0% DV)
Potassium	41.2 mg	(1% DV)	Beta Carotene	1.7 RE	

Ratings	Worst	Bad	Average	Good	Best
Weight Loss				7	
LowCal Density		3			
Filling	2				
Energizing			5		
Fiber		3			
Vitamins	2				
Minerals	2				
Overall		4			

FRUIT PUNCH, FRUIT DRINK, OR FRUITADE, VITAMIN C

Serving: 1 cup (8.82 oz)   **Beverage**

Calories	116	(13.2 cal/oz)	Carbohydrate	29.39 g	(10% DV)
Fat Calories	0	(0% fat)	Dietary Fiber	0 g	(0% DV)
Total Fat	0 g	(0% DV)	Protein	0 g	(0% DV)
Saturated Fat	0 g	(0% DV)	VItamin A	34.6 IU	(1% DV)
Poly Fat	0 g		Vitamin C	74.1 mg	(123% DV)
Mono Fat	0 g		Calcium	19.8 mg	(2% DV)
Cholesterol	0 mg	(0% DV)	Iron	.5 mg	(3% DV)
Sodium	54.3 mg	(2% DV)	Folate	0 mcg	(1% DV)
Potassium	61.8 mg	(2% DV)	Beta Carotene	2.5 RE	

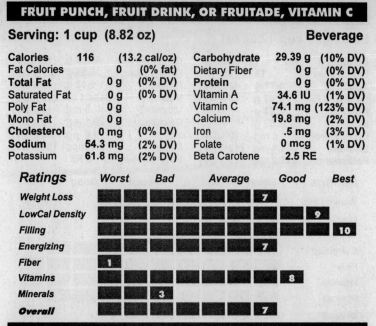

Ratings	Worst	Bad	Average	Good	Best
Weight Loss				7	
LowCal Density					9
Filling					10
Energizing				7	
Fiber	1				
Vitamins				8	
Minerals		3			
Overall				7	

FRUIT SALAD (EXCLUDING CITRUS FRUITS) WITH CREAM

Serving: 1 cup (6.5 oz)   **Salad**

Calories	166	(25.5 cal/oz)	Carbohydrate	28.39 g	(9% DV)
Fat Calories	66	(40% fat)	Dietary Fiber	3.64 g	(15% DV)
Total Fat	7.28 g	(11% DV)	Protein	1.82 g	(4% DV)
Saturated Fat	3.64 g	(18% DV)	VItamin A	283.9 IU	(6% DV)
Poly Fat	0 g		Vitamin C	14.6 mg	(24% DV)
Mono Fat	1.82 g		Calcium	18.2 mg	(2% DV)
Cholesterol	18.2 mg	(6% DV)	Iron	.5 mg	(3% DV)
Sodium	7.3 mg	(0% DV)	Folate	1.8 mcg	(5% DV)
Potassium	358.5 mg	(10% DV)	Beta Carotene	10.9 RE	

Ratings	Worst	Bad	Average	Good	Best
Weight Loss			6		
LowCal Density				8	
Filling			7		
Energizing			7		
Fiber				8	
Vitamins		5			
Minerals		4			
Overall			7		

FRUIT'N FIBER

Serving: 1 cup (2.04 oz)   Cereal

Calories	187	(91.6 cal/oz)	Carbohydrate	44.23 g	(15% DV)
Fat Calories	15	(8% fat)	Dietary Fiber	6.84 g	(27% DV)
Total Fat	1.71 g	(3% DV)	Protein	5.13 g	(10% DV)
Saturated Fat	.57 g	(3% DV)	VItamin A	2464.1 IU	(49% DV)
Poly Fat	.57 g		Vitamin C	0 mg	(0% DV)
Mono Fat	.57 g		Calcium	29.1 mg	(3% DV)
Cholesterol	0 mg	(0% DV)	Iron	9.6 mg	(53% DV)
Sodium	296.4 mg	(12% DV)	Folate	5.1 mcg	(50% DV)
Potassium	315.2 mg	(9% DV)	Beta Carotene	0 RE	

Ratings	Worst	Bad	Average	Good	Best
Weight Loss				7	
LowCal Density		3			
Filling			5		
Energizing					9
Fiber					10
Vitamins					10
Minerals					9
Overall			6		

GARLIC, RAW

Serving: 1 clove (.11 oz)   Vegetable

Calories	4	(40.6 cal/oz)	Carbohydrate	.99 g	(0% DV)
Fat Calories	0	(6% fat)	Dietary Fiber	.06 g	(0% DV)
Total Fat	.03 g	(0% DV)	Protein	.18 g	(0% DV)
Saturated Fat	0 g	(0% DV)	VItamin A	0 IU	(0% DV)
Poly Fat	0 g		Vitamin C	.9 mg	(2% DV)
Mono Fat	0 g		Calcium	5.4 mg	(1% DV)
Cholesterol	0 mg	(0% DV)	Iron	.1 mg	(0% DV)
Sodium	.5 mg	(0% DV)	Folate	.2 mcg	(0% DV)
Potassium	12 mg	(0% DV)	Beta Carotene	0 RE	

Ratings	Worst	Bad	Average	Good	Best
Weight Loss					10
LowCal Density			6		
Filling	1				
Energizing		2			
Fiber		2			
Vitamins		2			
Minerals		2			
Overall			5		

GAZPACHO

Serving: 1 cup (8.71 oz)   **Soup**

Calories	56	(6.4 cal/oz)	Carbohydrate	.73 g	(0% DV)
Fat Calories	0	(0% fat)	Dietary Fiber	4.88 g	(20% DV)
Total Fat	0 g	(0% DV)	Protein	7.32 g	(15% DV)
Saturated Fat	0 g	(0% DV)	Vitamin A	2603.5 IU	(52% DV)
Poly Fat	2.44 g		Vitamin C	7.3 mg	(12% DV)
Mono Fat	0 g		Calcium	24.4 mg	(2% DV)
Cholesterol	0 mg	(0% DV)	Iron	1 mg	(5% DV)
Sodium	739.3 mg	(31% DV)	Folate	7.3 mcg	(2% DV)
Potassium	224.5 mg	(6% DV)	Beta Carotene	261.1 RE	

Ratings	Worst	Bad	Average	Good	Best
Weight Loss				9	
LowCal Density					10
Filling			6		
Energizing	2				
Fiber				9	
Vitamins			6		
Minerals		3			
Overall				8	

GELATIN DESSERT

Serving: 1 cup (8.57 oz)   **Dessert**

Calories	142	(16.5 cal/oz)	Carbohydrate	33.6 g	(11% DV)
Fat Calories	0	(0% fat)	Dietary Fiber	0 g	(0% DV)
Total Fat	0 g	(0% DV)	Protein	2.4 g	(5% DV)
Saturated Fat	0 g	(0% DV)	Vitamin A	0 IU	(0% DV)
Poly Fat	0 g		Vitamin C	0 mg	(0% DV)
Mono Fat	0 g		Calcium	4.8 mg	(0% DV)
Cholesterol	0 mg	(0% DV)	Iron	.1 mg	(0% DV)
Sodium	100.8 mg	(4% DV)	Folate	2.4 mcg	(0% DV)
Potassium	2.4 mg	(0% DV)	Beta Carotene	0 RE	

Ratings	Worst	Bad	Average	Good	Best
Weight Loss				9	
LowCal Density				9	
Filling					10
Energizing				8	
Fiber	1				
Vitamins	1				
Minerals		3			
Overall				8	

GELATIN DESSERT WITH FRUIT

Serving: 1 cup (8.57 oz)   **Dessert**

Calories	158	(18.5 cal/oz)	Carbohydrate	38.88 g	(13% DV)
Fat Calories	0	(0% fat)	Dietary Fiber	0 g	(0% DV)
Total Fat	0 g	(0% DV)	Protein	2.4 g	(5% DV)
Saturated Fat	0 g	(0% DV)	Vitamin A	67.2 IU	(1% DV)
Poly Fat	0 g		Vitamin C	9.6 mg	(16% DV)
Mono Fat	0 g		Calcium	12 mg	(1% DV)
Cholesterol	0 mg	(0% DV)	Iron	.3 mg	(2% DV)
Sodium	64.8 mg	(3% DV)	Folate	2.4 mcg	(2% DV)
Potassium	247.2 mg	(7% DV)	Beta Carotene	7.2 RE	

Ratings	Worst	Bad	Average	Good	Best
Weight Loss					9
LowCal Density				8	
Filling					10
Energizing					9
Fiber	1				
Vitamins		4			
Minerals		3			
Overall				8	

GELATIN DESSERT, DIETETIC, LOW CALORIE SWEETENER

Serving: 1 cup (8.57 oz)   **Dessert**

Calories	17	(2 cal/oz)	Carbohydrate	1.68 g	(1% DV)
Fat Calories	0	(0% fat)	Dietary Fiber	0 g	(0% DV)
Total Fat	0 g	(0% DV)	Protein	2.4 g	(5% DV)
Saturated Fat	0 g	(0% DV)	Vitamin A	0 IU	(0% DV)
Poly Fat	0 g		Vitamin C	0 mg	(0% DV)
Mono Fat	0 g		Calcium	4.8 mg	(0% DV)
Cholesterol	0 mg	(0% DV)	Iron	0 mg	(0% DV)
Sodium	117.6 mg	(5% DV)	Folate	2.4 mcg	(0% DV)
Potassium	0 mg	(0% DV)	Beta Carotene	0 RE	

Ratings	Worst	Bad	Average	Good	Best
Weight Loss					10
LowCal Density					10
Filling			6		
Energizing		3			
Fiber	1				
Vitamins	1				
Minerals		3			
Overall				7	

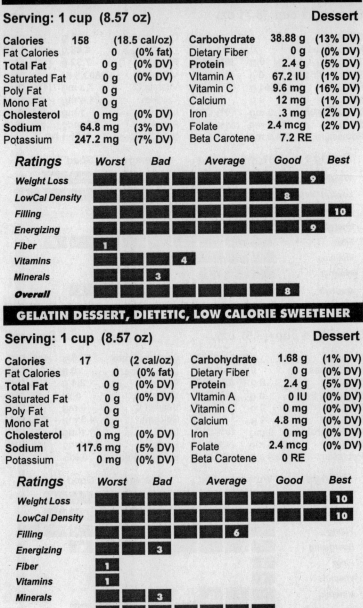

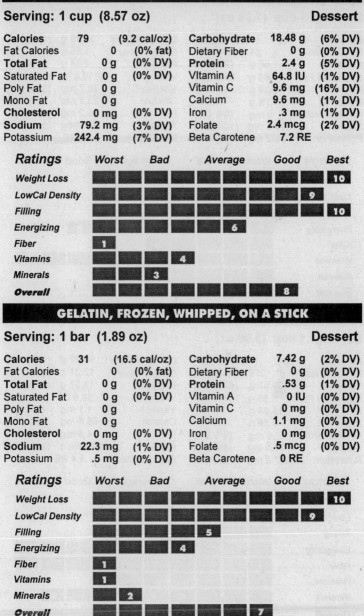

GELATIN DESSERT, DIETETIC, WITH FRUIT

Serving: 1 cup (8.57 oz)   **Dessert**

Calories	79	(9.2 cal/oz)	Carbohydrate	18.48 g	(6% DV)
Fat Calories	0	(0% fat)	Dietary Fiber	0 g	(0% DV)
Total Fat	0 g	(0% DV)	Protein	2.4 g	(5% DV)
Saturated Fat	0 g	(0% DV)	VItamin A	64.8 IU	(1% DV)
Poly Fat	0 g		Vitamin C	9.6 mg	(16% DV)
Mono Fat	0 g		Calcium	9.6 mg	(1% DV)
Cholesterol	0 mg	(0% DV)	Iron	.3 mg	(1% DV)
Sodium	79.2 mg	(3% DV)	Folate	2.4 mcg	(2% DV)
Potassium	242.4 mg	(7% DV)	Beta Carotene	7.2 RE	

Ratings	Worst	Bad	Average	Good	Best
Weight Loss					10
LowCal Density				9	
Filling					10
Energizing			6		
Fiber	1				
Vitamins		4			
Minerals		3			
Overall				8	

GELATIN, FROZEN, WHIPPED, ON A STICK

Serving: 1 bar (1.89 oz)   **Dessert**

Calories	31	(16.5 cal/oz)	Carbohydrate	7.42 g	(2% DV)
Fat Calories	0	(0% fat)	Dietary Fiber	0 g	(0% DV)
Total Fat	0 g	(0% DV)	Protein	.53 g	(1% DV)
Saturated Fat	0 g	(0% DV)	VItamin A	0 IU	(0% DV)
Poly Fat	0 g		Vitamin C	0 mg	(0% DV)
Mono Fat	0 g		Calcium	1.1 mg	(0% DV)
Cholesterol	0 mg	(0% DV)	Iron	0 mg	(0% DV)
Sodium	22.3 mg	(1% DV)	Folate	.5 mcg	(0% DV)
Potassium	.5 mg	(0% DV)	Beta Carotene	0 RE	

Ratings	Worst	Bad	Average	Good	Best
Weight Loss					10
LowCal Density				9	
Filling			5		
Energizing			4		
Fiber	1				
Vitamins	1				
Minerals		2			
Overall				7	

GOLDEN GRAHAMS

Serving: 1 cup (1.39 oz)   **Cereal**

Calories	150	(108 cal/oz)	**Carbohydrate**	33.19 g	(11% DV)
Fat Calories	14	(9% fat)	Dietary Fiber	1.56 g	(6% DV)
Total Fat	1.56 g	(2% DV)	**Protein**	2.34 g	(5% DV)
Saturated Fat	.39 g	(2% DV)	VItamin A	1719.5 IU	(34% DV)
Poly Fat	.39 g		Vitamin C	20.7 mg	(34% DV)
Mono Fat	.78 g		Calcium	23.8 mg	(2% DV)
Cholesterol	0 mg	(0% DV)	Iron	6.2 mg	(34% DV)
Sodium	385.3 mg	(16% DV)	Folate	2.3 mcg	(34% DV)
Potassium	86.2 mg	(2% DV)	Beta Carotene	0 RE	

Ratings	Worst	Bad	Average	Good	Best
Weight Loss				7	
LowCal Density	2				
Filling		4			
Energizing				8	
Fiber			5		
Vitamins					10
Minerals			6		
Overall			5		

GRANOLA

Serving: 1 cup (3.96 oz)   **Cereal**

Calories	541	(136.5 cal/oz)	**Carbohydrate**	61.27 g	(20% DV)
Fat Calories	270	(50% fat)	Dietary Fiber	12.21 g	(49% DV)
Total Fat	29.97 g	(46% DV)	**Protein**	13.32 g	(27% DV)
Saturated Fat	5.55 g	(28% DV)	VItamin A	38.9 IU	(1% DV)
Poly Fat	15.54 g		Vitamin C	1.1 mg	(2% DV)
Mono Fat	8.88 g		Calcium	68.8 mg	(7% DV)
Cholesterol	0 mg	(0% DV)	Iron	4.4 mg	(25% DV)
Sodium	11.1 mg	(0% DV)	Folate	13.3 mcg	(22% DV)
Potassium	557.2 mg	(16% DV)	Beta Carotene	4.4 RE	

Ratings	Worst	Bad	Average	Good	Best
Weight Loss	1				
LowCal Density	1				
Filling			5		
Energizing					10
Fiber					10
Vitamins			7		
Minerals				9	
Overall		4			

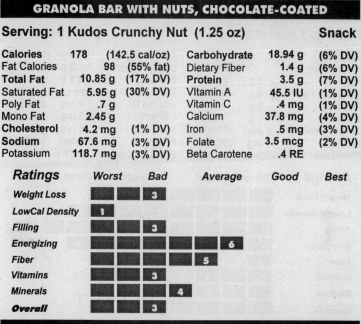

GRANOLA BAR WITH NUTS, CHOCOLATE-COATED

Serving: 1 Kudos Crunchy Nut (1.25 oz)   **Snack**

Calories	178	(142.5 cal/oz)	Carbohydrate	18.94 g	(6% DV)
Fat Calories	98	(55% fat)	Dietary Fiber	1.4 g	(6% DV)
Total Fat	10.85 g	(17% DV)	Protein	3.5 g	(7% DV)
Saturated Fat	5.95 g	(30% DV)	VItamin A	45.5 IU	(1% DV)
Poly Fat	.7 g		Vitamin C	.4 mg	(1% DV)
Mono Fat	2.45 g		Calcium	37.8 mg	(4% DV)
Cholesterol	4.2 mg	(1% DV)	Iron	.5 mg	(3% DV)
Sodium	67.6 mg	(3% DV)	Folate	3.5 mcg	(2% DV)
Potassium	118.7 mg	(3% DV)	Beta Carotene	.4 RE	

Ratings	Worst	Bad	Average	Good	Best
Weight Loss		3			
LowCal Density	1				
Filling		3			
Energizing				6	
Fiber			5		
Vitamins		3			
Minerals			4		
Overall		3			

GRANOLA BAR, OATS, SUGAR, RAISINS, COCONUT

Serving: 1 Quaker Oats bar (1 oz)   **Snack**

Calories	127	(127.1 cal/oz)	Carbohydrate	18.68 g	(6% DV)
Fat Calories	45	(36% fat)	Dietary Fiber	.84 g	(3% DV)
Total Fat	5.04 g	(8% DV)	Protein	2.8 g	(6% DV)
Saturated Fat	3.36 g	(17% DV)	VItamin A	2.8 IU	(0% DV)
Poly Fat	.56 g		Vitamin C	.3 mg	(0% DV)
Mono Fat	.84 g		Calcium	16.8 mg	(2% DV)
Cholesterol	0 mg	(0% DV)	Iron	.9 mg	(5% DV)
Sodium	77.8 mg	(3% DV)	Folate	2.8 mcg	(6% DV)
Potassium	91.3 mg	(3% DV)	Beta Carotene	.3 RE	

Ratings	Worst	Bad	Average	Good	Best
Weight Loss				6	
LowCal Density	2				
Filling		3			
Energizing				6	
Fiber			4		
Vitamins		3			
Minerals			4		
Overall			4		

GRAPE JUICE, UNSWEETENED

Serving: 1 cup (8.93 oz)   **Beverage**

Calories	153	(17.1 cal/oz)	Carbohydrate	37.5 g	(12% DV)
Fat Calories	0	(0% fat)	Dietary Fiber	0 g	(0% DV)
Total Fat	0 g	(0% DV)	Protein	2.5 g	(5% DV)
Saturated Fat	0 g	(0% DV)	Vitamin A	20 IU	(0% DV)
Poly Fat	0 g		Vitamin C	0 mg	(0% DV)
Mono Fat	0 g		Calcium	22.5 mg	(2% DV)
Cholesterol	0 mg	(0% DV)	Iron	.6 mg	(3% DV)
Sodium	7.5 mg	(0% DV)	Folate	2.5 mcg	(2% DV)
Potassium	330 mg	(9% DV)	Beta Carotene	2.5 RE	

Ratings	Worst	Bad	Average	Good	Best
Weight Loss			6		
LowCal Density				8	
Filling					10
Energizing				8	
Fiber	1				
Vitamins		3			
Minerals		3			
Overall				7	

GRAPE-NUTS

Serving: 1 cup (3.89 oz)   **Cereal**

Calories	389	(100 cal/oz)	Carbohydrate	89.38 g	(30% DV)
Fat Calories	0	(0% fat)	Dietary Fiber	7.63 g	(31% DV)
Total Fat	0 g	(0% DV)	Protein	13.08 g	(26% DV)
Saturated Fat	0 g	(0% DV)	Vitamin A	4805.8 IU	(96% DV)
Poly Fat	0 g		Vitamin C	0 mg	(0% DV)
Mono Fat	0 g		Calcium	10.9 mg	(1% DV)
Cholesterol	0 mg	(0% DV)	Iron	31.2 mg	(173% DV)
Sodium	757.6 mg	(32% DV)	Folate	13.1 mcg	(96% DV)
Potassium	364.1 mg	(10% DV)	Beta Carotene	0 RE	

Ratings	Worst	Bad	Average	Good	Best
Weight Loss		3			
LowCal Density	2				
Filling			6		
Energizing					10
Fiber					10
Vitamins					10
Minerals					10
Overall			5		

GRAPEFRUIT, RAW

Serving: ½ medium (approx 4" dia) (4.57 oz)   **Fruit**

Calories	41	(9 cal/oz)	Carbohydrate	10.37 g	(3% DV)
Fat Calories	0	(0% fat)	Dietary Fiber	1.28 g	(5% DV)
Total Fat	0 g	(0% DV)	Protein	1.28 g	(3% DV)
Saturated Fat	0 g	(0% DV)	Vitamin A	158.7 IU	(3% DV)
Poly Fat	0 g		Vitamin C	43.5 mg	(73% DV)
Mono Fat	0 g		Calcium	15.4 mg	(2% DV)
Cholesterol	0 mg	(0% DV)	Iron	.1 mg	(1% DV)
Sodium	0 mg	(0% DV)	Folate	1.3 mcg	(3% DV)
Potassium	177.9 mg	(5% DV)	Beta Carotene	15.4 RE	

Ratings	Worst	Bad	Average	Good	Best
Weight Loss					10
LowCal Density				9	
Filling				8	
Energizing		4			
Fiber			5		
Vitamins			6		
Minerals	2				
Overall				8	

GRAPES, RAW

Serving: 32 grape, seedless (5.71 oz)   **Fruit**

Calories	114	(19.9 cal/oz)	Carbohydrate	28.48 g	(9% DV)
Fat Calories	14	(13% fat)	Dietary Fiber	1.6 g	(6% DV)
Total Fat	1.6 g	(2% DV)	Protein	1.6 g	(3% DV)
Saturated Fat	0 g	(0% DV)	Vitamin A	116.8 IU	(2% DV)
Poly Fat	0 g		Vitamin C	17.6 mg	(29% DV)
Mono Fat	0 g		Calcium	17.6 mg	(2% DV)
Cholesterol	0 mg	(0% DV)	Iron	.4 mg	(2% DV)
Sodium	3.2 mg	(0% DV)	Folate	1.6 mcg	(2% DV)
Potassium	296 mg	(8% DV)	Beta Carotene	11.2 RE	

Ratings	Worst	Bad	Average	Good	Best
Weight Loss				8	
LowCal Density				8	
Filling				8	
Energizing			7		
Fiber			5		
Vitamins			5		
Minerals		3			
Overall			7		

Serving: 1 cup (8.43 oz)   **Sauce**

Calories	156	(18.5 cal/oz)	Carbohydrate	12.04 g	(4% DV)
Fat Calories	85	(55% fat)	Dietary Fiber	0 g	(0% DV)
Total Fat	9.44 g	(15% DV)	Protein	7.08 g	(14% DV)
Saturated Fat	2.36 g	(12% DV)	Vitamin A	436.6 IU	(9% DV)
Poly Fat	2.36 g		Vitamin C	0 mg	(0% DV)
Mono Fat	4.72 g		Calcium	30.7 mg	(3% DV)
Cholesterol	7.1 mg	(2% DV)	Iron	1.4 mg	(8% DV)
Sodium	1342.8 mg	(56% DV)	Folate	7.1 mcg	(1% DV)
Potassium	224.2 mg	(6% DV)	Beta Carotene	0 RE	

Ratings	Worst	Bad	Average	Good	Best
Weight Loss		3			
LowCal Density					8
Filling			6		
Energizing			5		
Fiber	1				
Vitamins			4		
Minerals			5		
Overall			5		

Serving: 1 cup (3.75 oz)   **Salad**

Calories	107	(28.6 cal/oz)	Carbohydrate	3.15 g	(1% DV)
Fat Calories	66	(62% fat)	Dietary Fiber	1.05 g	(4% DV)
Total Fat	7.35 g	(11% DV)	Protein	7.35 g	(15% DV)
Saturated Fat	3.15 g	(16% DV)	Vitamin A	846.3 IU	(17% DV)
Poly Fat	1.05 g		Vitamin C	6.3 mg	(10% DV)
Mono Fat	2.1 g		Calcium	121.8 mg	(12% DV)
Cholesterol	118.7 mg	(40% DV)	Iron	1.1 mg	(6% DV)
Sodium	405.3 mg	(17% DV)	Folate	7.4 mcg	(12% DV)
Potassium	186.9 mg	(5% DV)	Beta Carotene	64.1 RE	

Ratings	Worst	Bad	Average	Good	Best
Weight Loss			5		
LowCal Density					8
Filling		3			
Energizing		3			
Fiber		4			
Vitamins			5		
Minerals			5		
Overall			5		

GREEN BEANS, STRING, COOKED WITHOUT ADDED FAT

Serving: 1 cup (4.82 oz)   Vegetable

Calories	47	(9.8 cal/oz)	Carbohydrate	10.53 g	(4% DV)
Fat Calories	0	(0% fat)	Dietary Fiber	1.35 g	(5% DV)
Total Fat	0 g	(0% DV)	Protein	2.7 g	(5% DV)
Saturated Fat	0 g	(0% DV)	Vitamin A	893.7 IU	(18% DV)
Poly Fat	0 g		Vitamin C	13.5 mg	(22% DV)
Mono Fat	0 g		Calcium	62.1 mg	(6% DV)
Cholesterol	0 mg	(0% DV)	Iron	1.7 mg	(10% DV)
Sodium	315.9 mg	(13% DV)	Folate	2.7 mcg	(11% DV)
Potassium	401 mg	(11% DV)	Beta Carotene	90.5 RE	

Ratings	Worst	Bad	Average	Good	Best
Weight Loss					9
LowCal Density					9
Filling			7		
Energizing		4			
Fiber		5			
Vitamins		5			
Minerals		5			
Overall				8	

GREEN BEANS, STRING, WITH MUSHROOM SAUCE

Serving: 1 cup (8.14 oz)   Vegetable

Calories	137	(16.8 cal/oz)	Carbohydrate	14.82 g	(5% DV)
Fat Calories	62	(45% fat)	Dietary Fiber	2.28 g	(9% DV)
Total Fat	6.84 g	(11% DV)	Protein	4.56 g	(9% DV)
Saturated Fat	2.28 g	(11% DV)	Vitamin A	631.6 IU	(13% DV)
Poly Fat	2.28 g		Vitamin C	11.4 mg	(19% DV)
Mono Fat	2.28 g		Calcium	100.3 mg	(10% DV)
Cholesterol	4.6 mg	(2% DV)	Iron	1.3 mg	(7% DV)
Sodium	1051.1 mg	(44% DV)	Folate	4.6 mcg	(3% DV)
Potassium	221.2 mg	(6% DV)	Beta Carotene	61.6 RE	

Ratings	Worst	Bad	Average	Good	Best
Weight Loss		4			
LowCal Density				8	
Filling			7		
Energizing			5		
Fiber			6		
Vitamins			5		
Minerals			5		
Overall			6		

GREEN BEANS, WITH ALMONDS, WITHOUT ADDED FAT

Serving: 1 cup (4.36 oz)   **Vegetable**

Calories	193	(44.2 cal/oz)	Carbohydrate	12.44 g	(4% DV)
Fat Calories	132	(68% fat)	Dietary Fiber	3.66 g	(15% DV)
Total Fat	14.64 g	(23% DV)	Protein	7.32 g	(15% DV)
Saturated Fat	1.22 g	(6% DV)	Vitamin A	627.1 IU	(13% DV)
Poly Fat	3.66 g		Vitamin C	9.8 mg	(16% DV)
Mono Fat	9.76 g		Calcium	111 mg	(11% DV)
Cholesterol	0 mg	(0% DV)	Iron	2.2 mg	(12% DV)
Sodium	239.1 mg	(10% DV)	Folate	7.3 mcg	(10% DV)
Potassium	485.6 mg	(14% DV)	Beta Carotene	63.4 RE	

Ratings	Worst	Bad	Average	Good	Best
Weight Loss	2				
LowCal Density				6	
Filling		4			
Energizing			5		
Fiber					8
Vitamins			6		
Minerals				7	
Overall			5		

GREEN GODDESS DRESSING

Serving: 1 tbsp (.55 oz)   **Fat & Oil**

Calories	78	(141.3 cal/oz)	Carbohydrate	2.36 g	(1% DV)
Fat Calories	69	(89% fat)	Dietary Fiber	0 g	(0% DV)
Total Fat	7.65 g	(12% DV)	Protein	.31 g	(1% DV)
Saturated Fat	1.07 g	(5% DV)	Vitamin A	15.6 IU	(0% DV)
Poly Fat	2.75 g		Vitamin C	0 mg	(0% DV)
Mono Fat	3.21 g		Calcium	5.2 mg	(1% DV)
Cholesterol	6.1 mg	(2% DV)	Iron	.1 mg	(0% DV)
Sodium	165.7 mg	(7% DV)	Folate	.3 mcg	(0% DV)
Potassium	8.9 mg	(0% DV)	Beta Carotene	1.5 RE	

Ratings	Worst	Bad	Average	Good	Best
Weight Loss	2				
LowCal Density	1				
Filling	1				
Energizing		3			
Fiber	1				
Vitamins	2				
Minerals	2				
Overall	2				

GRITS, CORN OR HOMINY, REGULAR, WITHOUT ADDED FAT

Serving: 1 cup, cooked (8.64 oz)

Cereal

Calories	145	(16.8 cal/oz)	Carbohydrate	31.22 g	(10% DV)
Fat Calories	0	(0% fat)	Dietary Fiber	0 g	(0% DV)
Total Fat	0 g	(0% DV)	Protein	2.42 g	(5% DV)
Saturated Fat	0 g	(0% DV)	Vitamin A	0 IU	(0% DV)
Poly Fat	0 g		Vitamin C	0 mg	(0% DV)
Mono Fat	0 g		Calcium	0 mg	(0% DV)
Cholesterol	0 mg	(0% DV)	Iron	1.5 mg	(9% DV)
Sodium	559 mg	(23% DV)	Folate	2.4 mcg	(1% DV)
Potassium	53.2 mg	(2% DV)	Beta Carotene	0 RE	

Ratings

	Worst	Bad	Average	Good	Best
Weight Loss				8	
LowCal Density				8	
Filling					9
Energizing				8	
Fiber	1				
Vitamins			4		
Minerals		3			
Overall				7	

GUACAMOLE

Serving: 1 cup (8.32 oz)

Fruit

Calories	363	(43.7 cal/oz)	Carbohydrate	17.24 g	(6% DV)
Fat Calories	315	(87% fat)	Dietary Fiber	4.66 g	(19% DV)
Total Fat	34.95 g	(54% DV)	Protein	4.66 g	(9% DV)
Saturated Fat	4.66 g	(23% DV)	Vitamin A	1372.4 IU	(27% DV)
Poly Fat	4.66 g		Vitamin C	18.6 mg	(31% DV)
Mono Fat	20.97 g		Calcium	25.6 mg	(3% DV)
Cholesterol	0 mg	(0% DV)	Iron	2.3 mg	(13% DV)
Sodium	305.2 mg	(13% DV)	Folate	4.7 mcg	(35% DV)
Potassium	1356.1 mg	(39% DV)	Beta Carotene	137.5 RE	

Ratings

	Worst	Bad	Average	Good	Best
Weight Loss	1				
LowCal Density			6		
Filling			5		
Energizing			6		
Fiber					9
Vitamins				8	
Minerals			6		
Overall			5		

GUMBO WITH RICE (NEW ORLEANS TYPE)

Serving: 1 cup (8.71 oz)　　　　　　　　　**Entree**

Calories	193	(22.1 cal/oz)	Carbohydrate	17.08 g	(6% DV)
Fat Calories	66	(34% fat)	Dietary Fiber	2.44 g	(10% DV)
Total Fat	7.32 g	(11% DV)	Protein	14.64 g	(29% DV)
Saturated Fat	2.44 g	(12% DV)	VItamin A	561.2 IU	(11% DV)
Poly Fat	2.44 g		Vitamin C	14.6 mg	(24% DV)
Mono Fat	2.44 g		Calcium	70.8 mg	(7% DV)
Cholesterol	41.5 mg	(14% DV)	Iron	2.6 mg	(14% DV)
Sodium	888.2 mg	(37% DV)	Folate	14.6 mcg	(12% DV)
Potassium	453.8 mg	(13% DV)	Beta Carotene	48.8 RE	

Ratings	Worst	Bad	Average	Good	Best
Weight Loss			6		
LowCal Density				8	
Filling			6		
Energizing			6		
Fiber			7		
Vitamins			6		
Minerals				9	
Overall			7		

GYRO SANDWICH (PITA, BEEF, LAMB, CONDIMENTS)

Serving: 1 gyro (3.75 oz)　　　　　　　　　**Sandwich**

Calories	169	(45.1 cal/oz)	Carbohydrate	20.47 g	(7% DV)
Fat Calories	38	(22% fat)	Dietary Fiber	1.05 g	(4% DV)
Total Fat	4.2 g	(6% DV)	Protein	12.6 g	(25% DV)
Saturated Fat	1.05 g	(5% DV)	VItamin A	104 IU	(2% DV)
Poly Fat	0 g		Vitamin C	4.2 mg	(7% DV)
Mono Fat	1.05 g		Calcium	44.1 mg	(4% DV)
Cholesterol	34.7 mg	(12% DV)	Iron	2.2 mg	(12% DV)
Sodium	212.1 mg	(9% DV)	Folate	12.6 mcg	(8% DV)
Potassium	209 mg	(6% DV)	Beta Carotene	10.5 RE	

Ratings	Worst	Bad	Average	Good	Best
Weight Loss				8	
LowCal Density			6		
Filling			5		
Energizing			6		
Fiber		4			
Vitamins			5		
Minerals			6		
Overall			6		

HADDOCK WITH CHOPPED SPINACH

Serving: 1 diet meal (9.11 oz)   **Entree**

Calories	196	(21.6 cal/oz)	Carbohydrate	13.52 g	(5% DV)
Fat Calories	46	(23% fat)	Dietary Fiber	0 g	(0% DV)
Total Fat	5.1 g	(8% DV)	Protein	25.5 g	(51% DV)
Saturated Fat	2.55 g	(13% DV)	Vitamin A	2088.5 IU	(42% DV)
Poly Fat	0 g		Vitamin C	2.6 mg	(4% DV)
Mono Fat	0 g		Calcium	229.5 mg	(23% DV)
Cholesterol	68.9 mg	(23% DV)	Iron	2.3 mg	(13% DV)
Sodium	482 mg	(20% DV)	Folate	25.5 mcg	(13% DV)
Potassium	632.4 mg	(18% DV)	Beta Carotene	173.4 RE	

Ratings	Worst	Bad	Average	Good	Best
Weight Loss				7	
LowCal Density				8	
Filling			5		
Energizing			5		
Fiber	1				
Vitamins			6		
Minerals				8	
Overall			6		

HADDOCK, BAKED OR BROILED

Serving: 1 fillet (5.5 oz)   **Fish**

Calories	199	(36.1 cal/oz)	Carbohydrate	.62 g	(0% DV)
Fat Calories	55	(28% fat)	Dietary Fiber	0 g	(0% DV)
Total Fat	6.16 g	(9% DV)	Protein	33.88 g	(68% DV)
Saturated Fat	1.54 g	(8% DV)	Vitamin A	446.6 IU	(9% DV)
Poly Fat	1.54 g		Vitamin C	3.1 mg	(5% DV)
Mono Fat	1.54 g		Calcium	61.6 mg	(6% DV)
Cholesterol	101.6 mg	(34% DV)	Iron	1.9 mg	(11% DV)
Sodium	597.5 mg	(25% DV)	Folate	33.9 mcg	(5% DV)
Potassium	572.9 mg	(16% DV)	Beta Carotene	16.9 RE	

Ratings	Worst	Bad	Average	Good	Best
Weight Loss			5		
LowCal Density				7	
Filling	1				
Energizing	2				
Fiber	1				
Vitamins			5		
Minerals				7	
Overall			5		

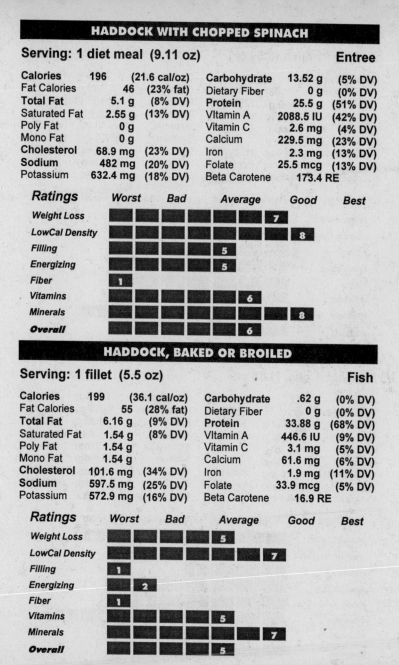

HADDOCK, FLOURED OR BREADED, FRIED

Serving: 1 fillet (6.54 oz)   Fish

Calories	428	(65.5 cal/oz)	Carbohydrate	22.69 g	(8% DV)
Fat Calories	181	(42% fat)	Dietary Fiber	1.83 g	(7% DV)
Total Fat	20.13 g	(31% DV)	Protein	34.77 g	(70% DV)
Saturated Fat	5.49 g	(27% DV)	Vitamin A	175.7 IU	(4% DV)
Poly Fat	5.49 g		Vitamin C	0 mg	(0% DV)
Mono Fat	9.15 g		Calcium	102.5 mg	(10% DV)
Cholesterol	155.6 mg	(52% DV)	Iron	3.1 mg	(17% DV)
Sodium	845.5 mg	(35% DV)	Folate	34.8 mcg	(8% DV)
Potassium	*558.2 mg	(16% DV)	Beta Carotene	0 RE	

Ratings	Worst	Bad	Average	Good	Best
Weight Loss	2				
LowCal Density			5		
Filling		4			
Energizing			6		
Fiber			6		
Vitamins			5		
Minerals				8	
Overall		4			

HALFSIES

Serving: 1 cup (1.18 oz)   Cereal

Calories	132	(111.9 cal/oz)	Carbohydrate	28.02 g	(9% DV)
Fat Calories	12	(9% fat)	Dietary Fiber	2.31 g	(9% DV)
Total Fat	1.32 g	(2% DV)	Protein	1.98 g	(4% DV)
Saturated Fat	.33 g	(2% DV)	Vitamin A	0 IU	(0% DV)
Poly Fat	.66 g		Vitamin C	0 mg	(0% DV)
Mono Fat	.33 g		Calcium	13.9 mg	(1% DV)
Cholesterol	0 mg	(0% DV)	Iron	6.9 mg	(38% DV)
Sodium	271.6 mg	(11% DV)	Folate	2 mcg	(40% DV)
Potassium	45.5 mg	(1% DV)	Beta Carotene	0 RE	

Ratings	Worst	Bad	Average	Good	Best
Weight Loss				8	
LowCal Density	2				
Filling		4			
Energizing				7	
Fiber			6		
Vitamins					9
Minerals				7	
Overall			6		

HAM & CHEESE HOT SANDWICH, ON BUN

Serving: 1 Burger King (7.43 oz)   **Sandwich**

Calories	487	(65.5 cal/oz)	Carbohydrate	30.78 g	(10% DV)
Fat Calories	243	(50% fat)	Dietary Fiber	2.08 g	(8% DV)
Total Fat	27.04 g	(42% DV)	Protein	27.04 g	(54% DV)
Saturated Fat	10.4 g	(52% DV)	VItamin A	528.3 IU	(11% DV)
Poly Fat	6.24 g		Vitamin C	22.9 mg	(38% DV)
Mono Fat	10.4 g		Calcium	216.3 mg	(22% DV)
Cholesterol	74.9 mg	(25% DV)	Iron	2.9 mg	(16% DV)
Sodium	1845 mg	(77% DV)	Folate	27 mcg	(10% DV)
Potassium	486.7 mg	(14% DV)	Beta Carotene	29.1 RE	

Ratings	Worst	Bad	Average	Good	Best
Weight Loss	3				
LowCal Density		5			
Filling		5			
Energizing			7		
Fiber		6			
Vitamins				8	
Minerals					9
Overall		5			

HAM & CHEESE SANDWICH, ON BUN, LETTUCE, SPREAD

Serving: 1 sandwich (5.5 oz)   **Sandwich**

Calories	367	(66.6 cal/oz)	Carbohydrate	24.02 g	(8% DV)
Fat Calories	194	(53% fat)	Dietary Fiber	1.54 g	(6% DV)
Total Fat	21.56 g	(33% DV)	Protein	20.02 g	(40% DV)
Saturated Fat	9.24 g	(46% DV)	VItamin A	628.3 IU	(13% DV)
Poly Fat	3.08 g		Vitamin C	16.9 mg	(28% DV)
Mono Fat	7.7 g		Calcium	221.8 mg	(22% DV)
Cholesterol	58.5 mg	(20% DV)	Iron	1.9 mg	(11% DV)
Sodium	1402.9 mg	(58% DV)	Folate	20 mcg	(8% DV)
Potassium	312.6 mg	(9% DV)	Beta Carotene	23.1 RE	

Ratings	Worst	Bad	Average	Good	Best
Weight Loss	4				
LowCal Density		5			
Filling	4				
Energizing			6		
Fiber		5			
Vitamins				8	
Minerals				8	
Overall		5			

HAM SALAD SANDWICH

Serving: 1 sandwich (3.82 oz)   **Sandwich**

Calories	256	(66.9 cal/oz)	Carbohydrate	30.82 g	(10% DV)
Fat Calories	96	(38% fat)	Dietary Fiber	1.07 g	(4% DV)
Total Fat	10.7 g	(16% DV)	Protein	8.56 g	(17% DV)
Saturated Fat	3.21 g	(16% DV)	Vitamin A	0 IU	(0% DV)
Poly Fat	2.14 g		Vitamin C	3.2 mg	(5% DV)
Mono Fat	4.28 g		Calcium	62.1 mg	(6% DV)
Cholesterol	21.4 mg	(7% DV)	Iron	1.8 mg	(10% DV)
Sodium	795 mg	(33% DV)	Folate	8.6 mcg	(4% DV)
Potassium	143.4 mg	(4% DV)	Beta Carotene	0 RE	

Ratings	Worst	Bad	Average	Good	Best
Weight Loss				6	
LowCal Density			5		
Filling			5		
Energizing				7	
Fiber		4			
Vitamins			5		
Minerals			5		
Overall			5		

HAM, GLAZED, SWEET POTATO, VEGETABLE

Serving: 1 frozen meal (10.14 oz)   **Entree**

Calories	318	(31.4 cal/oz)	Carbohydrate	43.74 g	(15% DV)
Fat Calories	77	(24% fat)	Dietary Fiber	2.84 g	(11% DV)
Total Fat	8.52 g	(13% DV)	Protein	17.04 g	(34% DV)
Saturated Fat	2.84 g	(14% DV)	Vitamin A	11570.2 IU	(231% DV)
Poly Fat	2.84 g		Vitamin C	62.5 mg	(104% DV)
Mono Fat	2.84 g		Calcium	51.1 mg	(5% DV)
Cholesterol	36.9 mg	(12% DV)	Iron	1.9 mg	(11% DV)
Sodium	1587.6 mg	(66% DV)	Folate	17 mcg	(6% DV)
Potassium	514 mg	(15% DV)	Beta Carotene	1147.4 RE	

Ratings	Worst	Bad	Average	Good	Best
Weight Loss			6		
LowCal Density				7	
Filling				8	
Energizing				9	
Fiber				8	
Vitamins					10
Minerals			6		
Overall				7	

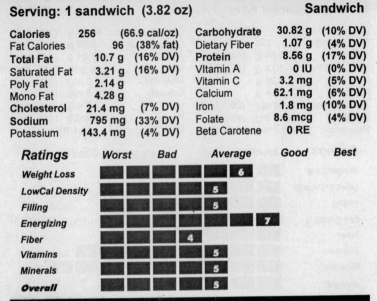

HAM, PROSCIUTTO

Serving: 1 piece (1 oz)   **Meat**

Calories	55	(54.6 cal/oz)	Carbohydrate	.08 g	(0% DV)
Fat Calories	20	(37% fat)	Dietary Fiber	0 g	(0% DV)
Total Fat	2.24 g	(3% DV)	Protein	7.84 g	(16% DV)
Saturated Fat	.84 g	(4% DV)	VItamin A	0 IU	(0% DV)
Poly Fat	.28 g		Vitamin C	0 mg	(0% DV)
Mono Fat	1.12 g		Calcium	2.8 mg	(0% DV)
Cholesterol	19.6 mg	(7% DV)	Iron	.3 mg	(2% DV)
Sodium	754.6 mg	(31% DV)	Folate	7.8 mcg	(0% DV)
Potassium	142.8 mg	(4% DV)	Beta Carotene	0 RE	

Ratings	Worst	Bad	Average	Good	Best
Weight Loss				7	
LowCal Density				6	
Filling	1				
Energizing		2			
Fiber	1				
Vitamins			3		
Minerals			4		
Overall			5		

HAM, SMOKED OR CURED, COOKED, LEAN ONLY

Serving: 1 piece (3.04 oz)   **Meat**

Calories	123	(40.5 cal/oz)	Carbohydrate	1.28 g	(0% DV)
Fat Calories	46	(37% fat)	Dietary Fiber	0 g	(0% DV)
Total Fat	5.1 g	(8% DV)	Protein	17.85 g	(36% DV)
Saturated Fat	1.7 g	(8% DV)	VItamin A	0 IU	(0% DV)
Poly Fat	.85 g		Vitamin C	17.9 mg	(30% DV)
Mono Fat	2.55 g		Calcium	6.8 mg	(1% DV)
Cholesterol	45.1 mg	(15% DV)	Iron	1.3 mg	(7% DV)
Sodium	1022.6 mg	(43% DV)	Folate	17.9 mcg	(1% DV)
Potassium	244 mg	(7% DV)	Beta Carotene	0 RE	

Ratings	Worst	Bad	Average	Good	Best
Weight Loss			6		
LowCal Density			6		
Filling	1				
Energizing		2			
Fiber	1				
Vitamins				7	
Minerals			5		
Overall			5		

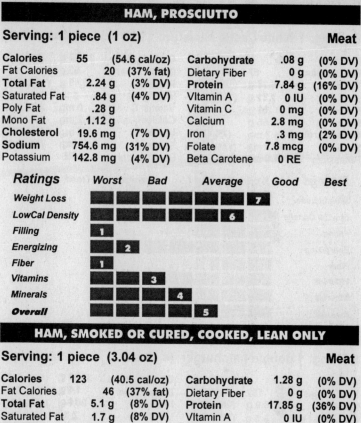

HAMBURGER, 1 OZ MEAT, PLAIN, ON MINIATURE BUN

Serving: 1 White Castle Miniature (1.89 oz)   Sandwich

Calories	150	(79.4 cal/oz)	Carbohydrate	14.47 g	(5% DV)
Fat Calories	57	(38% fat)	Dietary Fiber	.53 g	(2% DV)
Total Fat	6.36 g	(10% DV)	Protein	8.48 g	(17% DV)
Saturated Fat	2.12 g	(11% DV)	VItamin A	0 IU	(0% DV)
Poly Fat	.53 g		Vitamin C	0 mg	(0% DV)
Mono Fat	2.65 g		Calcium	30.2 mg	(3% DV)
Cholesterol	21.7 mg	(7% DV)	Iron	1.3 mg	(7% DV)
Sodium	345.6 mg	(14% DV)	Folate	8.5 mcg	(3% DV)
Potassium	101.8 mg	(3% DV)	Beta Carotene	0 RE	

Ratings	Worst	Bad	Average	Good	Best
Weight Loss				7	
LowCal Density		4			
Filling	3				
Energizing			5		
Fiber	3				
Vitamins		4			
Minerals		4			
Overall			5		

HAMBURGER, DOUBLE (2 PATTIES), PLAIN, ON BUN

Serving: 1 double hamburger (4.64 oz)   Sandwich

Calories	380	(81.8 cal/oz)	Carbohydrate	33.41 g	(11% DV)
Fat Calories	152	(40% fat)	Dietary Fiber	1.3 g	(5% DV)
Total Fat	16.9 g	(26% DV)	Protein	20.8 g	(42% DV)
Saturated Fat	6.5 g	(32% DV)	VItamin A	0 IU	(0% DV)
Poly Fat	1.3 g		Vitamin C	0 mg	(0% DV)
Mono Fat	7.8 g		Calcium	70.2 mg	(7% DV)
Cholesterol	59.8 mg	(20% DV)	Iron	3.4 mg	(19% DV)
Sodium	548.6 mg	(23% DV)	Folate	20.8 mcg	(7% DV)
Potassium	253.5 mg	(7% DV)	Beta Carotene	0 RE	

Ratings	Worst	Bad	Average	Good	Best
Weight Loss		4			
LowCal Density	3				
Filling			5		
Energizing				8	
Fiber			5		
Vitamins			5		
Minerals				7	
Overall			5		

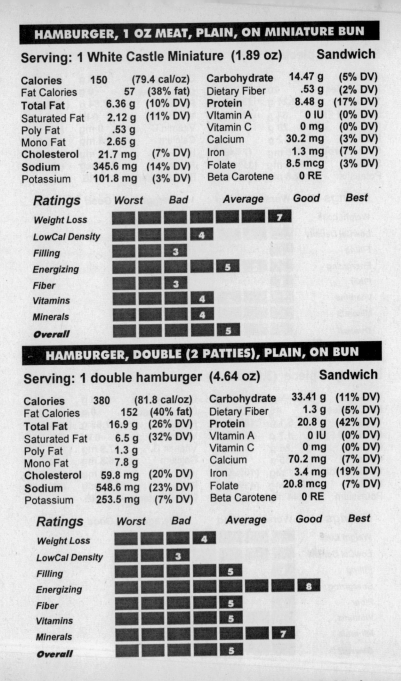

HAMBURGER, PLAIN, ON BUN

Serving: 1 Wendy's Kid's Meal (3.54 oz)   Sandwich

Calories	291	(82.2 cal/oz)	Carbohydrate	31.58 g	(11% DV)
Fat Calories	107	(37% fat)	Dietary Fiber	.99 g	(4% DV)
Total Fat	11.88 g	(18% DV)	Protein	13.86 g	(28% DV)
Saturated Fat	3.96 g	(20% DV)	Vitamin A	0 IU	(0% DV)
Poly Fat	.99 g		Vitamin C	0 mg	(0% DV)
Mono Fat	4.95 g		Calcium	64.4 mg	(6% DV)
Cholesterol	35.6 mg	(12% DV)	Iron	2.6 mg	(15% DV)
Sodium	416.8 mg	(17% DV)	Folate	13.9 mcg	(6% DV)
Potassium	171.3 mg	(5% DV)	Beta Carotene	0 RE	

Ratings	Worst	Bad	Average	Good	Best
Weight Loss				6	
LowCal Density		3			
Filling			5		
Energizing					8
Fiber		4			
Vitamins			5		
Minerals			6		
Overall			5		

HEARTLAND NATURAL CEREAL, PLAIN

Serving: 1 cup (4.11 oz)   Cereal

Calories	499	(121.4 cal/oz)	Carbohydrate	78.55 g	(26% DV)
Fat Calories	155	(31% fat)	Dietary Fiber	6.9 g	(28% DV)
Total Fat	17.25 g	(27% DV)	Protein	11.5 g	(23% DV)
Saturated Fat	9.2 g	(46% DV)	Vitamin A	64.4 IU	(1% DV)
Poly Fat	3.45 g		Vitamin C	1.2 mg	(2% DV)
Mono Fat	3.45 g		Calcium	74.8 mg	(7% DV)
Cholesterol	0 mg	(0% DV)	Iron	4.3 mg	(24% DV)
Sodium	293.3 mg	(12% DV)	Folate	11.5 mcg	(16% DV)
Potassium	385.3 mg	(11% DV)	Beta Carotene	6.9 RE	

Ratings	Worst	Bad	Average	Good	Best
Weight Loss	1				
LowCal Density	2				
Filling			6		
Energizing					10
Fiber					10
Vitamins			5		
Minerals				9	
Overall		4			

HOMINY, COOKED WITHOUT ADDED FAT

Serving: 1 cup (5.89 oz)   **Vegetable**

Calories	145	(24.7 cal/oz)	**Carbohydrate**	33.66 g	(11% DV)
Fat Calories	15	(10% fat)	**Dietary Fiber**	9.9 g	(40% DV)
Total Fat	1.65 g	(3% DV)	**Protein**	3.3 g	(7% DV)
Saturated Fat	0 g	(0% DV)	**Vitamin A**	0 IU	(0% DV)
Poly Fat	1.65 g		**Vitamin C**	0 mg	(0% DV)
Mono Fat	0 g		**Calcium**	16.5 mg	(2% DV)
Cholesterol	0 mg	(0% DV)	**Iron**	1.5 mg	(8% DV)
Sodium	292.1 mg	(12% DV)	**Folate**	3.3 mcg	(0% DV)
Potassium	16.5 mg	(0% DV)	**Beta Carotene**	0 RE	

Ratings	Worst	Bad	Average	Good	Best
Weight Loss			6		
LowCal Density				8	
Filling					9
Energizing				8	
Fiber					10
Vitamins	2				
Minerals			5		
Overall				7	

HONEY & NUT TOASTY O'S

Serving: 1 cup (1.36 oz)   **Cereal**

Calories	144	(105.6 cal/oz)	**Carbohydrate**	30.51 g	(10% DV)
Fat Calories	7	(5% fat)	**Dietary Fiber**	1.52 g	(6% DV)
Total Fat	.76 g	(1% DV)	**Protein**	4.18 g	(8% DV)
Saturated Fat	0 g	(0% DV)	**Vitamin A**	1675.4 IU	(34% DV)
Poly Fat	.38 g		**Vitamin C**	20.1 mg	(34% DV)
Mono Fat	.38 g		**Calcium**	26.6 mg	(3% DV)
Cholesterol	0 mg	(0% DV)	**Iron**	6 mg	(34% DV)
Sodium	343.9 mg	(14% DV)	**Folate**	4.2 mcg	(34% DV)
Potassium	132.6 mg	(4% DV)	**Beta Carotene**	0 RE	

Ratings	Worst	Bad	Average	Good	Best
Weight Loss				8	
LowCal Density	2				
Filling		4			
Energizing				7	
Fiber			5		
Vitamins					10
Minerals				7	
Overall			6		

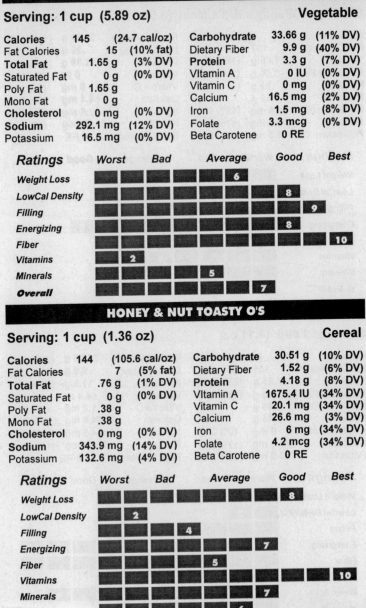

HONEY MUSTARD DRESSING

Serving: 1 tbsp (.56 oz)   **Fat & Oil**

Calories	50	(90 cal/oz)	Carbohydrate	6.88 g	(2% DV)
Fat Calories	25	(50% fat)	Dietary Fiber	.16 g	(1% DV)
Total Fat	2.81 g	(4% DV)	Protein	.16 g	(0% DV)
Saturated Fat	.47 g	(2% DV)	Vitamin A	0 IU	(0% DV)
Poly Fat	1.56 g		Vitamin C	0 mg	(0% DV)
Mono Fat	.78 g		Calcium	3.1 mg	(0% DV)
Cholesterol	0 mg	(0% DV)	Iron	.1 mg	(1% DV)
Sodium	90.6 mg	(4% DV)	Folate	.2 mcg	(0% DV)
Potassium	10.1 mg	(0% DV)	Beta Carotene	0 RE	

Ratings	Worst	Bad	Average	Good	Best
Weight Loss				5	
LowCal Density		3			
Filling	2				
Energizing			4		
Fiber	2				
Vitamins	2				
Minerals	2				
Overall		3			

HONEYCOMB, PLAIN

Serving: 1 cup (.79 oz)   **Cereal**

Calories	86	(108.9 cal/oz)	Carbohydrate	19.6 g	(7% DV)
Fat Calories	4	(5% fat)	Dietary Fiber	.44 g	(2% DV)
Total Fat	.44 g	(1% DV)	Protein	1.32 g	(3% DV)
Saturated Fat	0 g	(0% DV)	Vitamin A	970 IU	(19% DV)
Poly Fat	.22 g		Vitamin C	0 mg	(0% DV)
Mono Fat	.22 g		Calcium	3.7 mg	(0% DV)
Cholesterol	0 mg	(0% DV)	Iron	2.1 mg	(12% DV)
Sodium	123.9 mg	(5% DV)	Folate	1.3 mcg	(19% DV)
Potassium	25.3 mg	(1% DV)	Beta Carotene	0 RE	

Ratings	Worst	Bad	Average	Good	Best
Weight Loss					9
LowCal Density	2				
Filling		3			
Energizing				6	
Fiber		3			
Vitamins					8
Minerals		4			
Overall			5		

HONEYDEW MELON, RAW

Serving: 1 wedge (5.71 oz)   Fruit

Calories	56	(9.8 cal/oz)	Carbohydrate	14.72 g	(5% DV)
Fat Calories	0	(0% fat)	Dietary Fiber	1.6 g	(6% DV)
Total Fat	0 g	(0% DV)	Protein	0 g	(0% DV)
Saturated Fat	0 g	(0% DV)	Vitamin A	64 IU	(1% DV)
Poly Fat	0 g		Vitamin C	40 mg	(67% DV)
Mono Fat	0 g		Calcium	9.6 mg	(1% DV)
Cholesterol	0 mg	(0% DV)	Iron	.1 mg	(1% DV)
Sodium	16 mg	(1% DV)	Folate	0 mcg	(2% DV)
Potassium	433.6 mg	(12% DV)	Beta Carotene	6.4 RE	

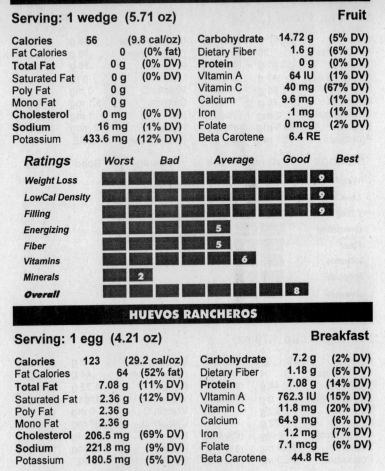

Ratings	Worst	Bad	Average	Good	Best
Weight Loss				9	
LowCal Density				9	
Filling				9	
Energizing			5		
Fiber			5		
Vitamins			6		
Minerals	2				
Overall				8	

HUEVOS RANCHEROS

Serving: 1 egg (4.21 oz)   Breakfast

Calories	123	(29.2 cal/oz)	Carbohydrate	7.2 g	(2% DV)
Fat Calories	64	(52% fat)	Dietary Fiber	1.18 g	(5% DV)
Total Fat	7.08 g	(11% DV)	Protein	7.08 g	(14% DV)
Saturated Fat	2.36 g	(12% DV)	Vitamin A	762.3 IU	(15% DV)
Poly Fat	2.36 g		Vitamin C	11.8 mg	(20% DV)
Mono Fat	2.36 g		Calcium	64.9 mg	(6% DV)
Cholesterol	206.5 mg	(69% DV)	Iron	1.2 mg	(7% DV)
Sodium	221.8 mg	(9% DV)	Folate	7.1 mcg	(6% DV)
Potassium	180.5 mg	(5% DV)	Beta Carotene	44.8 RE	

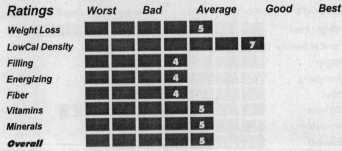

Ratings	Worst	Bad	Average	Good	Best
Weight Loss			5		
LowCal Density				7	
Filling		4			
Energizing		4			
Fiber		4			
Vitamins			5		
Minerals			5		
Overall			5		

HUMMUS

Serving: 1 cup (8.39 oz)   **Vegetable**

Calories	402	(47.9 cal/oz)	Carbohydrate	47.47 g	(16% DV)
Fat Calories	169	(42% fat)	Dietary Fiber	11.75 g	(47% DV)
Total Fat	18.8 g	(29% DV)	Protein	11.75 g	(24% DV)
Saturated Fat	2.35 g	(12% DV)	VItamin A	58.8 IU	(1% DV)
Poly Fat	7.05 g		Vitamin C	18.8 mg	(31% DV)
Mono Fat	9.4 g		Calcium	117.5 mg	(12% DV)
Cholesterol	0 mg	(0% DV)	Iron	3.7 mg	(20% DV)
Sodium	573.4 mg	(24% DV)	Folate	11.8 mcg	(35% DV)
Potassium	408.9 mg	(12% DV)	Beta Carotene	4.7 RE	

Ratings	Worst	Bad	Average	Good	Best
Weight Loss	1				
LowCal Density			6		
Filling			7		
Energizing				9	
Fiber					10
Vitamins			7		
Minerals				8	
Overall			5		

HUSH PUPPY

Serving: 1 hush puppy (.79 oz)   **Bakery**

Calories	73	(92.7 cal/oz)	Carbohydrate	8.32 g	(3% DV)
Fat Calories	34	(46% fat)	Dietary Fiber	.44 g	(2% DV)
Total Fat	3.74 g	(6% DV)	Protein	1.54 g	(3% DV)
Saturated Fat	1.1 g	(6% DV)	VItamin A	30.6 IU	(1% DV)
Poly Fat	.88 g		Vitamin C	.2 mg	(0% DV)
Mono Fat	1.54 g		Calcium	22.7 mg	(2% DV)
Cholesterol	16.3 mg	(5% DV)	Iron	.5 mg	(3% DV)
Sodium	104.5 mg	(4% DV)	Folate	1.5 mcg	(1% DV)
Potassium	32.3 mg	(1% DV)	Beta Carotene	.2 RE	

Ratings	Worst	Bad	Average	Good	Best
Weight Loss			6		
LowCal Density		3			
Filling	2				
Energizing		4			
Fiber		3			
Vitamins		3			
Minerals		3			
Overall		4			

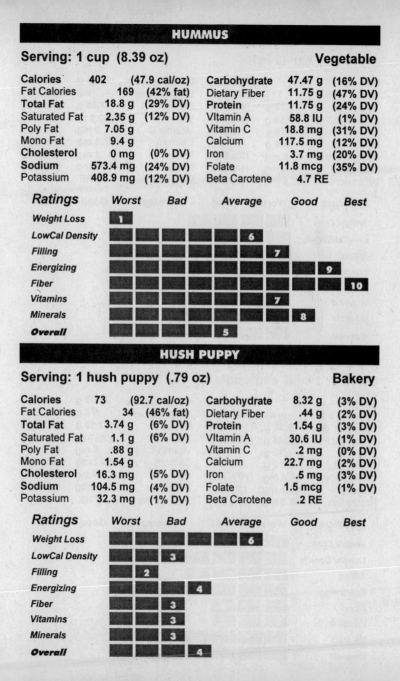

ICE CREAM BAR OR STICK, CHOCOLATE COVERED

Serving: 1 bar (2 oz)　　　　　　　　　　　　　**Dessert**

Calories	169	(84.6 cal/oz)	Carbohydrate	14.34 g	(5% DV)
Fat Calories	111	(66% fat)	Dietary Fiber	0 g	(0% DV)
Total Fat	12.32 g	(19% DV)	Protein	1.68 g	(3% DV)
Saturated Fat	9.52 g	(48% DV)	VItamin A	180.9 IU	(4% DV)
Poly Fat	.56 g		Vitamin C	0 mg	(0% DV)
Mono Fat	1.68 g		Calcium	57.1 mg	(6% DV)
Cholesterol	19.6 mg	(7% DV)	Iron	.1 mg	(1% DV)
Sodium	35.3 mg	(1% DV)	Folate	1.7 mcg	(1% DV)
Potassium	103.6 mg	(3% DV)	Beta Carotene	5 RE	

Ratings	Worst	Bad	Average	Good	Best
Weight Loss			4		
LowCal Density		3			
Filling		3			
Energizing			5		
Fiber	1				
Vitamins	2				
Minerals			4		
Overall		3			

ICE CREAM CONE, CHOCOLATE COVERED OR DIPPED

Serving: 1 cone and single dip (2.79 oz)　　　　**Dessert**

Calories	185	(66.3 cal/oz)	Carbohydrate	24.02 g	(8% DV)
Fat Calories	84	(46% fat)	Dietary Fiber	.78 g	(3% DV)
Total Fat	9.36 g	(14% DV)	Protein	3.12 g	(6% DV)
Saturated Fat	5.46 g	(27% DV)	VItamin A	270.7 IU	(5% DV)
Poly Fat	.78 g		Vitamin C	.8 mg	(1% DV)
Mono Fat	3.12 g		Calcium	95.2 mg	(10% DV)
Cholesterol	28.9 mg	(10% DV)	Iron	.4 mg	(2% DV)
Sodium	66.3 mg	(3% DV)	Folate	3.1 mcg	(1% DV)
Potassium	168.5 mg	(5% DV)	Beta Carotene	7 RE	

Ratings	Worst	Bad	Average	Good	Best
Weight Loss			5		
LowCal Density			5		
Filling			4		
Energizing				6	
Fiber		3			
Vitamins		3			
Minerals			4		
Overall			5		

ICE CREAM SANDWICH

Serving: 1 sandwich (2.11 oz)   Dessert

Calories	143	(67.9 cal/oz)	Carbohydrate	21.77 g	(7% DV)
Fat Calories	53	(37% fat)	Dietary Fiber	.59 g	(2% DV)
Total Fat	5.9 g	(9% DV)	Protein	2.36 g	(5% DV)
Saturated Fat	3.54 g	(18% DV)	Vitamin A	184.1 IU	(4% DV)
Poly Fat	.59 g		Vitamin C	0 mg	(0% DV)
Mono Fat	1.77 g		Calcium	60.2 mg	(6% DV)
Cholesterol	20.1 mg	(7% DV)	Iron	.3 mg	(2% DV)
Sodium	36.6 mg	(2% DV)	Folate	2.4 mcg	(1% DV)
Potassium	122.1 mg	(3% DV)	Beta Carotene	4.7 RE	

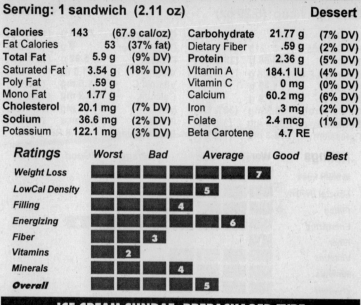

Ratings	Worst	Bad	Average	Good	Best
Weight Loss				7	
LowCal Density			5		
Filling			4		
Energizing			6		
Fiber		3			
Vitamins	2				
Minerals			4		
Overall			5		

ICE CREAM SUNDAE, PREPACKAGED TYPE

Serving: 1 sundae (2.32 oz)   Dessert

Calories	120	(51.8 cal/oz)	Carbohydrate	19.11 g	(6% DV)
Fat Calories	35	(29% fat)	Dietary Fiber	0 g	(0% DV)
Total Fat	3.9 g	(6% DV)	Protein	2.6 g	(5% DV)
Saturated Fat	2.6 g	(13% DV)	Vitamin A	97.5 IU	(2% DV)
Poly Fat	0 g		Vitamin C	1.3 mg	(2% DV)
Mono Fat	1.3 g		Calcium	78 mg	(8% DV)
Cholesterol	8.5 mg	(3% DV)	Iron	.2 mg	(1% DV)
Sodium	61.8 mg	(3% DV)	Folate	2.6 mcg	(1% DV)
Potassium	137.2 mg	(4% DV)	Beta Carotene	2.6 RE	

Ratings	Worst	Bad	Average	Good	Best
Weight Loss				8	
LowCal Density			6		
Filling			4		
Energizing			6		
Fiber	1				
Vitamins		3			
Minerals			4		
Overall			6		

ICE CREAM, RICH, FLAVORS OTHER THAN CHOCOLATE

Serving: 1 cup (5.29 oz)   **Dessert**

Calories	357	(67.4 cal/oz)	Carbohydrate	33.15 g	(11% DV)
Fat Calories	213	(60% fat)	Dietary Fiber	0 g	(0% DV)
Total Fat	23.68 g	(36% DV)	Protein	5.92 g	(12% DV)
Saturated Fat	14.8 g	(74% DV)	Vitamin A	951.6 IU	(19% DV)
Poly Fat	1.48 g		Vitamin C	1.5 mg	(2% DV)
Mono Fat	7.4 g		Calcium	173.2 mg	(17% DV)
Cholesterol	90.3 mg	(30% DV)	Iron	.1 mg	(0% DV)
Sodium	82.9 mg	(3% DV)	Folate	5.9 mcg	(2% DV)
Potassium	235.3 mg	(7% DV)	Beta Carotene	14.8 RE	

Ratings	Worst	Bad	Average	Good	Best
Weight Loss		3			
LowCal Density			5		
Filling			5		
Energizing					8
Fiber	1				
Vitamins		4			
Minerals			5		
Overall		4			

ICE CREAM, SOFT SERVE, OTHER THAN CHOCOLATE

Serving: 1 cup (6.18 oz)   **Dessert**

Calories	348	(56.3 cal/oz)	Carbohydrate	40.83 g	(14% DV)
Fat Calories	171	(49% fat)	Dietary Fiber	0 g	(0% DV)
Total Fat	19.03 g	(29% DV)	Protein	6.92 g	(14% DV)
Saturated Fat	12.11 g	(61% DV)	Vitamin A	707.6 IU	(14% DV)
Poly Fat	0 g		Vitamin C	1.7 mg	(3% DV)
Mono Fat	5.19 g		Calcium	221.4 mg	(22% DV)
Cholesterol	76.1 mg	(25% DV)	Iron	.2 mg	(1% DV)
Sodium	138.4 mg	(6% DV)	Folate	6.9 mcg	(2% DV)
Potassium	344.3 mg	(10% DV)	Beta Carotene	19 RE	

Ratings	Worst	Bad	Average	Good	Best
Weight Loss		3			
LowCal Density			5		
Filling			6		
Energizing					9
Fiber	1				
Vitamins		4			
Minerals			6		
Overall			5		

ICE MILK, REGULAR, FLAVORS OTHER THAN CHOCOLATE

Serving: 1 cup (4.68 oz)   **Dessert**

Calories	182	(38.9 cal/oz)	Carbohydrate	29.74 g	(10% DV)
Fat Calories	47	(26% fat)	Dietary Fiber	0 g	(0% DV)
Total Fat	5.24 g	(8% DV)	Protein	5.24 g	(10% DV)
Saturated Fat	3.93 g	(20% DV)	Vitamin A	216.2 IU	(4% DV)
Poly Fat	0 g		Vitamin C	1.3 mg	(2% DV)
Mono Fat	1.31 g		Calcium	182.1 mg	(18% DV)
Cholesterol	18.3 mg	(6% DV)	Iron	.1 mg	(1% DV)
Sodium	111.4 mg	(5% DV)	Folate	5.2 mcg	(2% DV)
Potassium	276.4 mg	(8% DV)	Beta Carotene	5.2 RE	

Ratings	Worst	Bad	Average	Good	Best
Weight Loss				7	
LowCal Density				7	
Filling			6		
Energizing				7	
Fiber	1				
Vitamins		3			
Minerals			5		
Overall			6		

ICE, FRUIT

Serving: 1 cup (6.89 oz)   **Dessert**

Calories	151	(21.9 cal/oz)	Carbohydrate	62.92 g	(21% DV)
Fat Calories	0	(0% fat)	Dietary Fiber	0 g	(0% DV)
Total Fat	0 g	(0% DV)	Protein	0 g	(0% DV)
Saturated Fat	0 g	(0% DV)	Vitamin A	0 IU	(0% DV)
Poly Fat	0 g		Vitamin C	1.9 mg	(3% DV)
Mono Fat	0 g		Calcium	3.9 mg	(0% DV)
Cholesterol	0 mg	(0% DV)	Iron	.3 mg	(2% DV)
Sodium	42.5 mg	(2% DV)	Folate	0 mcg	(0% DV)
Potassium	5.8 mg	(0% DV)	Beta Carotene	0 RE	

Ratings	Worst	Bad	Average	Good	Best
Weight Loss				9	
LowCal Density				8	
Filling					10
Energizing					10
Fiber	1				
Vitamins	2				
Minerals	2				
Overall				7	

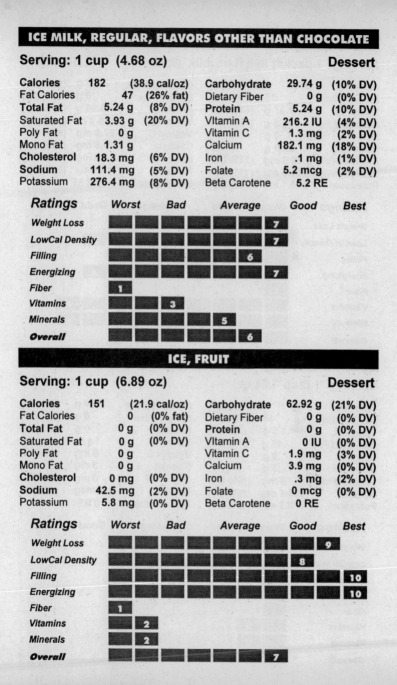

INSTANT BREAKFAST, POWDER, MILK ADDED

Serving: 1 packet in 8 fl oz milk (9.96 oz) Breakfast

Calories	273	(27.5 cal/oz)	Carbohydrate	34.6 g	(12% DV)
Fat Calories	75	(28% fat)	Dietary Fiber	0 g	(0% DV)
Total Fat	8.37 g	(13% DV)	Protein	13.95 g	(28% DV)
Saturated Fat	5.58 g	(28% DV)	VItamin A	2056.2 IU	(41% DV)
Poly Fat	0 g		Vitamin C	27.9 mg	(46% DV)
Mono Fat	2.79 g		Calcium	390.6 mg	(39% DV)
Cholesterol	36.3 mg	(12% DV)	Iron	4.6 mg	(26% DV)
Sodium	253.9 mg	(11% DV)	Folate	14 mcg	(28% DV)
Potassium	703.1 mg	(20% DV)	Beta Carotene	8.4 RE	

Ratings	Worst	Bad	Average	Good	Best
Weight Loss			4		
LowCal Density				8	
Filling				7	
Energizing				8	
Fiber	1				
Vitamins					9
Minerals					9
Overall				6	

ITALIAN DRESSING, LOW CALORIE

Serving: 1 tbsp (.54 oz) Fat & Oil

Calories	16	(29.2 cal/oz)	Carbohydrate	.74 g	(0% DV)
Fat Calories	14	(86% fat)	Dietary Fiber	0 g	(0% DV)
Total Fat	1.5 g	(2% DV)	Protein	0 g	(0% DV)
Saturated Fat	.15 g	(1% DV)	VItamin A	0 IU	(0% DV)
Poly Fat	.9 g		Vitamin C	0 mg	(0% DV)
Mono Fat	.3 g		Calcium	.3 mg	(0% DV)
Cholesterol	.9 mg	(0% DV)	Iron	0 mg	(0% DV)
Sodium	118.1 mg	(5% DV)	Folate	0 mcg	(0% DV)
Potassium	2.3 mg	(0% DV)	Beta Carotene	0 RE	

Ratings	Worst	Bad	Average	Good	Best
Weight Loss			4		
LowCal Density				7	
Filling	1				
Energizing		2			
Fiber	1				
Vitamins		2			
Minerals		2			
Overall			4		

ITALIAN DRESSING, MADE WITH VINEGAR & OIL

Serving: 1 tbsp (.53 oz)   **Fat & Oil**

Calories	69	(129.5 cal/oz)	Carbohydrate	1.5 g	(0% DV)
Fat Calories	64	(93% fat)	Dietary Fiber	0 g	(0% DV)
Total Fat	7.06 g	(11% DV)	Protein	.15 g	(0% DV)
Saturated Fat	1.03 g	(5% DV)	VItamin A	11.5 IU	(0% DV)
Poly Fat	4.12 g		Vitamin C	0 mg	(0% DV)
Mono Fat	1.62 g		Calcium	1.5 mg	(0% DV)
Cholesterol	0 mg	(0% DV)	Iron	0 mg	(0% DV)
Sodium	115.7 mg	(5% DV)	Folate	.2 mcg	(0% DV)
Potassium	2.2 mg	(0% DV)	Beta Carotene	0 RE	

Ratings	Worst	Bad	Average	Good	Best
Weight Loss	2				
LowCal Density	2				
Filling	1				
Energizing	3				
Fiber	1				
Vitamins	2				
Minerals	2				
Overall	2				

ITALIAN SAUSAGE

Serving: 1 link (5" long) (2.43 oz)   **Meat**

Calories	220	(90.4 cal/oz)	Carbohydrate	1.02 g	(0% DV)
Fat Calories	159	(72% fat)	Dietary Fiber	0 g	(0% DV)
Total Fat	17.68 g	(27% DV)	Protein	13.6 g	(27% DV)
Saturated Fat	6.12 g	(31% DV)	VItamin A	0 IU	(0% DV)
Poly Fat	2.04 g		Vitamin C	1.4 mg	(2% DV)
Mono Fat	8.16 g		Calcium	16.3 mg	(2% DV)
Cholesterol	53 mg	(18% DV)	Iron	1 mg	(6% DV)
Sodium	627 mg	(26% DV)	Folate	13.6 mcg	(1% DV)
Potassium	206.7 mg	(6% DV)	Beta Carotene	0 RE	

Ratings	Worst	Bad	Average	Good	Best
Weight Loss	2				
LowCal Density	3				
Filling	1				
Energizing	2				
Fiber	1				
Vitamins					5
Minerals					5
Overall	3				

Serving: 1 tbsp (.71 oz)   **Sweets**

Calories	48	(68.2 cal/oz)	Carbohydrate	12.88 g	(4% DV)
Fat Calories	0	(0% fat)	Dietary Fiber	.2 g	(1% DV)
Total Fat	0 g	(0% DV)	Protein	.2 g	(0% DV)
Saturated Fat	0 g	(0% DV)	Vitamin A	21.8 IU	(0% DV)
Poly Fat	0 g		Vitamin C	1.8 mg	(3% DV)
Mono Fat	0 g		Calcium	4 mg	(0% DV)
Cholesterol	0 mg	(0% DV)	Iron	.1 mg	(1% DV)
Sodium	8 mg	(0% DV)	Folate	.2 mcg	(2% DV)
Potassium	15.4 mg	(0% DV)	Beta Carotene	2.2 RE	

Ratings	Worst	Bad	Average	Good	Best
Weight Loss				8	
LowCal Density		4			
Filling		3			
Energizing			5		
Fiber	2				
Vitamins	2				
Minerals	2				
Overall			5		

Serving: 1 tbsp (.67 oz)   **Sweets**

Calories	6	(9.3 cal/oz)	Carbohydrate	10.79 g	(4% DV)
Fat Calories	0	(0% fat)	Dietary Fiber	.19 g	(1% DV)
Total Fat	0 g	(0% DV)	Protein	.19 g	(0% DV)
Saturated Fat	0 g	(0% DV)	Vitamin A	0 IU	(0% DV)
Poly Fat	0 g		Vitamin C	0 mg	(0% DV)
Mono Fat	0 g		Calcium	1.3 mg	(0% DV)
Cholesterol	0 mg	(0% DV)	Iron	0 mg	(0% DV)
Sodium	.2 mg	(0% DV)	Folate	.2 mcg	(0% DV)
Potassium	12.4 mg	(0% DV)	Beta Carotene	0 RE	

Ratings	Worst	Bad	Average	Good	Best
Weight Loss					10
LowCal Density				9	
Filling			7		
Energizing		4			
Fiber	2				
Vitamins	2				
Minerals	2				
Overall			7		

JUST RITE

Serving: 1 cup (1.54 oz)   **Cereal**

Calories	152	(98.6 cal/oz)	Carbohydrate	36.42 g	(12% DV)
Fat Calories	8	(5% fat)	Dietary Fiber	3.01 g	(12% DV)
Total Fat	.86 g	(1% DV)	Protein	4.73 g	(9% DV)
Saturated Fat	0 g	(0% DV)	Vitamin A	1137.4 IU	(23% DV)
Poly Fat	.43 g		Vitamin C	0 mg	(0% DV)
Mono Fat	.43 g		Calcium	10.8 mg	(1% DV)
Cholesterol	0 mg	(0% DV)	Iron	27.3 mg	(152% DV)
Sodium	288.1 mg	(12% DV)	Folate	4.7 mcg	(152% DV)
Potassium	98.5 mg	(3% DV)	Beta Carotene	0 RE	

Ratings	Worst	Bad	Average	Good	Best
Weight Loss				8	
LowCal Density		3			
Filling			5		
Energizing				8	
Fiber				8	
Vitamins					10
Minerals					10
Overall			6		

KIDNEY BEAN SALAD

Serving: 1 cup (8.25 oz)   **Salad**

Calories	356	(43.1 cal/oz)	Carbohydrate	48.05 g	(16% DV)
Fat Calories	125	(35% fat)	Dietary Fiber	9.24 g	(37% DV)
Total Fat	13.86 g	(21% DV)	Protein	13.86 g	(28% DV)
Saturated Fat	2.31 g	(12% DV)	Vitamin A	67 IU	(1% DV)
Poly Fat	6.93 g		Vitamin C	4.6 mg	(8% DV)
Mono Fat	2.31 g		Calcium	53.1 mg	(5% DV)
Cholesterol	0 mg	(0% DV)	Iron	4.6 mg	(26% DV)
Sodium	660.7 mg	(28% DV)	Folate	13.9 mcg	(49% DV)
Potassium	679.1 mg	(19% DV)	Beta Carotene	4.6 RE	

Ratings	Worst	Bad	Average	Good	Best
Weight Loss		3			
LowCal Density			6		
Filling				8	
Energizing				9	
Fiber					10
Vitamins			6		
Minerals				7	
Overall			6		

KING VITAMIN

Serving: 1 cup (.75 oz)   Cereal

Calories	85	(113.7 cal/oz)	Carbohydrate	17.83 g	(6% DV)
Fat Calories	11	(13% fat)	Dietary Fiber	.21 g	(1% DV)
Total Fat	1.26 g	(2% DV)	Protein	1.05 g	(2% DV)
Saturated Fat	.84 g	(4% DV)	Vitamin A	2387.7 IU	(48% DV)
Poly Fat	.21 g		Vitamin C	33.2 mg	(55% DV)
Mono Fat	.21 g		Calcium	1.7 mg	(0% DV)
Cholesterol	0 mg	(0% DV)	Iron	12.7 mg	(71% DV)
Sodium	161.5 mg	(7% DV)	Folate	1.1 mcg	(72% DV)
Potassium	25.8 mg	(1% DV)	Beta Carotene	0 RE	

Ratings	Worst	Bad	Average	Good	Best
Weight Loss					9
LowCal Density	2				
Filling		3			
Energizing			6		
Fiber	2				
Vitamins					10
Minerals				7	
Overall			5		

KIWI FRUIT, RAW

Serving: 1 fruit (2.71 oz)   Fruit

Calories	46	(17.1 cal/oz)	Carbohydrate	11.32 g	(4% DV)
Fat Calories	0	(0% fat)	Dietary Fiber	2.28 g	(9% DV)
Total Fat	0 g	(0% DV)	Protein	.76 g	(2% DV)
Saturated Fat	0 g	(0% DV)	Vitamin A	133 IU	(3% DV)
Poly Fat	0 g		Vitamin C	74.5 mg	(124% DV)
Mono Fat	0 g		Calcium	19.8 mg	(2% DV)
Cholesterol	0 mg	(0% DV)	Iron	.3 mg	(2% DV)
Sodium	3.8 mg	(0% DV)	Folate	.8 mcg	(7% DV)
Potassium	252.3 mg	(7% DV)	Beta Carotene	13.7 RE	

Ratings	Worst	Bad	Average	Good	Best
Weight Loss					10
LowCal Density				8	
Filling			6		
Energizing			5		
Fiber			6		
Vitamins				8	
Minerals		3			
Overall				8	

KIX

Serving: 1 cup (.68 oz)　　　　　　　　　　　　**Cereal**

Calories	74	(108.7 cal/oz)	Carbohydrate	15.69 g	(5% DV)
Fat Calories	3	(5% fat)	Dietary Fiber	.38 g	(2% DV)
Total Fat	.38 g	(1% DV)	Protein	1.71 g	(3% DV)
Saturated Fat	.19 g	(1% DV)	VItamin A	837.7 IU	(17% DV)
Poly Fat	.19 g		Vitamin C	10.1 mg	(17% DV)
Mono Fat	.19 g		Calcium	23.8 mg	(2% DV)
Cholesterol	0 mg	(0% DV)	Iron	5.4 mg	(30% DV)
Sodium	194.4 mg	(8% DV)	Folate	1.7 mcg	(17% DV)
Potassium	29.8 mg	(1% DV)	Beta Carotene	0 RE	

Ratings	Worst	Bad	Average	Good	Best
Weight Loss					9
LowCal Density	2				
Filling		3			
Energizing			5		
Fiber	2				
Vitamins				8	
Minerals			5		
Overall			5		

KNISH, CHEESE

Serving: 1 knish (2.14 oz)　　　　　　　　　　　　**Entree**

Calories	208	(97.3 cal/oz)	Carbohydrate	18.66 g	(6% DV)
Fat Calories	108	(52% fat)	Dietary Fiber	.6 g	(2% DV)
Total Fat	12 g	(18% DV)	Protein	6.6 g	(13% DV)
Saturated Fat	3 g	(15% DV)	VItamin A	606 IU	(12% DV)
Poly Fat	3 g		Vitamin C	0 mg	(0% DV)
Mono Fat	4.8 g		Calcium	24.6 mg	(2% DV)
Cholesterol	55.8 mg	(19% DV)	Iron	1.3 mg	(7% DV)
Sodium	204 mg	(8% DV)	Folate	6.6 mcg	(3% DV)
Potassium	61.8 mg	(2% DV)	Beta Carotene	10.8 RE	

Ratings	Worst	Bad	Average	Good	Best
Weight Loss			5		
LowCal Density		3			
Filling		3			
Energizing			6		
Fiber		3			
Vitamins		4			
Minerals		4			
Overall		4			

KOHLRABI, COOKED WITHOUT ADDED FAT

Serving: 1 cup (5.89 oz)   **Vegetable**

Calories	48	(8.1 cal/oz)	Carbohydrate	11.05 g	(4% DV)
Fat Calories	0	(0% fat)	Dietary Fiber	1.65 g	(7% DV)
Total Fat	0 g	(0% DV)	Protein	3.3 g	(7% DV)
Saturated Fat	0 g	(0% DV)	Vitamin A	57.8 IU	(1% DV)
Poly Fat	0 g		Vitamin C	89.1 mg	(148% DV)
Mono Fat	0 g		Calcium	41.3 mg	(4% DV)
Cholesterol	0 mg	(0% DV)	Iron	.7 mg	(4% DV)
Sodium	419.1 mg	(17% DV)	Folate	3.3 mcg	(5% DV)
Potassium	557.7 mg	(16% DV)	Beta Carotene	6.6 RE	

Ratings	Worst	Bad	Average	Good	Best
Weight Loss				9	
LowCal Density				9	
Filling			8		
Energizing		5			
Fiber		5			
Vitamins				9	
Minerals	4				
Overall			8		

KUNG PAO PORK

Serving: 1 cup (5.79 oz)   **Entree**

Calories	434	(75 cal/oz)	Carbohydrate	11.02 g	(4% DV)
Fat Calories	292	(67% fat)	Dietary Fiber	1.62 g	(6% DV)
Total Fat	32.4 g	(50% DV)	Protein	25.92 g	(52% DV)
Saturated Fat	6.48 g	(32% DV)	Vitamin A	895.9 IU	(18% DV)
Poly Fat	9.72 g		Vitamin C	9.7 mg	(16% DV)
Mono Fat	14.58 g		Calcium	48.6 mg	(5% DV)
Cholesterol	56.7 mg	(19% DV)	Iron	2 mg	(11% DV)
Sodium	975.2 mg	(41% DV)	Folate	25.9 mcg	(10% DV)
Potassium	533 mg	(15% DV)	Beta Carotene	89.1 RE	

Ratings	Worst	Bad	Average	Good	Best
Weight Loss	2				
LowCal Density		4			
Filling	3				
Energizing		5			
Fiber		5			
Vitamins				8	
Minerals			7		
Overall		4			

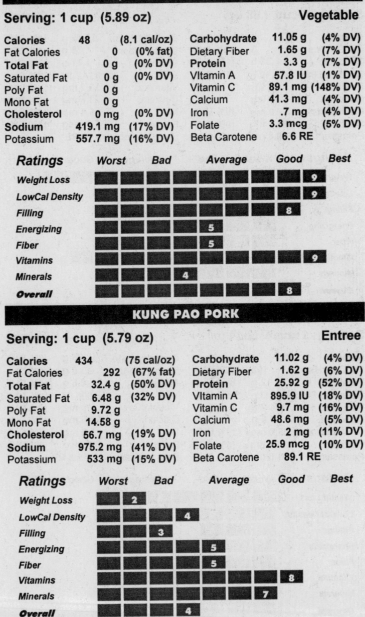

Edmund's Food Ratings

LAMB CHOP, COOKED, LEAN ONLY EATEN

Serving: 1 chop (2.79 oz)   **Meat**

Calories	183	(65.4 cal/oz)	Carbohydrate	0 g	(0% DV)
Fat Calories	91	(50% fat)	Dietary Fiber	0 g	(0% DV)
Total Fat	10.14 g	(16% DV)	Protein	21.84 g	(44% DV)
Saturated Fat	3.9 g	(19% DV)	VItamin A	0 IU	(0% DV)
Poly Fat	.78 g		Vitamin C	0 mg	(0% DV)
Mono Fat	3.9 g		Calcium	12.5 mg	(1% DV)
Cholesterol	70.2 mg	(23% DV)	Iron	1.7 mg	(9% DV)
Sodium	246.5 mg	(10% DV)	Folate	21.8 mcg	(4% DV)
Potassium	242.6 mg	(7% DV)	Beta Carotene	0 RE	

Ratings	Worst	Bad	Average	Good	Best
Weight Loss		4			
LowCal Density			5		
Filling	1				
Energizing	1				
Fiber	1				
Vitamins		4			
Minerals			6		
Overall		4			

LAMB OR MUTTON STEW, POTATOES & VEGETABLES

Serving: 1 cup (9 oz)   **Entree**

Calories	282	(31.4 cal/oz)	Carbohydrate	26.71 g	(9% DV)
Fat Calories	91	(32% fat)	Dietary Fiber	5.04 g	(20% DV)
Total Fat	10.08 g	(16% DV)	Protein	20.16 g	(40% DV)
Saturated Fat	5.04 g	(25% DV)	VItamin A	2663.6 IU	(53% DV)
Poly Fat	0 g		Vitamin C	7.6 mg	(13% DV)
Mono Fat	5.04 g		Calcium	32.8 mg	(3% DV)
Cholesterol	52.9 mg	(18% DV)	Iron	2.3 mg	(12% DV)
Sodium	1003 mg	(42% DV)	Folate	20.2 mcg	(8% DV)
Potassium	574.6 mg	(16% DV)	Beta Carotene	267.1 RE	

Ratings	Worst	Bad	Average	Good	Best
Weight Loss			6		
LowCal Density			7		
Filling			7		
Energizing			7		
Fiber					9
Vitamins			7		
Minerals			7		
Overall			7		

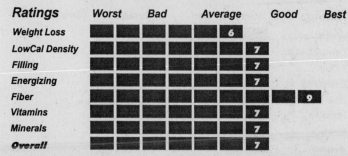

LAMB PATTY, COOKED

Serving: 1 patty (2.75 oz)   **Meat**

Calories	275	(100 cal/oz)	Carbohydrate	0 g	(0% DV)
Fat Calories	201	(73% fat)	Dietary Fiber	0 g	(0% DV)
Total Fat	22.33 g	(34% DV)	Protein	16.94 g	(34% DV)
Saturated Fat	10.01 g	(50% DV)	Vitamin A	0 IU	(0% DV)
Poly Fat	1.54 g		Vitamin C	0 mg	(0% DV)
Mono Fat	9.24 g		Calcium	6.9 mg	(1% DV)
Cholesterol	73.9 mg	(25% DV)	Iron	1.4 mg	(8% DV)
Sodium	219.5 mg	(9% DV)	Folate	16.9 mcg	(4% DV)
Potassium	188.7 mg	(5% DV)	Beta Carotene	0 RE	

Ratings	Worst	Bad	Average	Good	Best
Weight Loss	2				
LowCal Density	3				
Filling	1				
Energizing	1				
Fiber	1				
Vitamins	4				
Minerals	5				
Overall	2				

LAMB, ROAST, COOKED, LEAN ONLY EATEN

Serving: 1 piece (3.04 oz)   **Meat**

Calories	162	(53.4 cal/oz)	Carbohydrate	0 g	(0% DV)
Fat Calories	61	(38% fat)	Dietary Fiber	0 g	(0% DV)
Total Fat	6.8 g	(10% DV)	Protein	23.8 g	(48% DV)
Saturated Fat	2.55 g	(13% DV)	Vitamin A	0 IU	(0% DV)
Poly Fat	.85 g		Vitamin C	0 mg	(0% DV)
Mono Fat	2.55 g		Calcium	6.8 mg	(1% DV)
Cholesterol	75.7 mg	(25% DV)	Iron	1.8 mg	(10% DV)
Sodium	57.8 mg	(2% DV)	Folate	23.8 mcg	(5% DV)
Potassium	287.3 mg	(8% DV)	Beta Carotene	0 RE	

Ratings	Worst	Bad	Average	Good	Best
Weight Loss	5				
LowCal Density	6				
Filling	1				
Energizing	1				
Fiber	1				
Vitamins	5				
Minerals	6				
Overall	4				

LASAGNA WITH CHEESE & MEAT SAUCE

Serving: 1 Weight Watchers meal (11.14 oz)   **Entree**

Calories	359	(32.2 cal/oz)	Carbohydrate	38.38 g	(13% DV)
Fat Calories	112	(31% fat)	Dietary Fiber	3.12 g	(12% DV)
Total Fat	12.48 g	(19% DV)	Protein	21.84 g	(44% DV)
Saturated Fat	6.24 g	(31% DV)	Vitamin A	1741 IU	(35% DV)
Poly Fat	0 g		Vitamin C	37.4 mg	(62% DV)
Mono Fat	6.24 g		Calcium	240.2 mg	(24% DV)
Cholesterol	49.9 mg	(17% DV)	Iron	3.2 mg	(18% DV)
Sodium	755 mg	(31% DV)	Folate	21.8 mcg	(6% DV)
Potassium	689.5 mg	(20% DV)	Beta Carotene	146.6 RE	

Ratings	Worst	Bad	Average	Good	Best
Weight Loss			5		
LowCal Density				7	
Filling				8	
Energizing					9
Fiber				8	
Vitamins				8	
Minerals					9
Overall				7	

LASAGNA WITH CHEESE & MEAT SAUCE

Serving: 1 Healthy Choice meal (9.11 oz)   **Entree**

Calories	247	(27.2 cal/oz)	Carbohydrate	36.97 g	(12% DV)
Fat Calories	46	(19% fat)	Dietary Fiber	2.55 g	(10% DV)
Total Fat	5.1 g	(8% DV)	Protein	15.3 g	(31% DV)
Saturated Fat	2.55 g	(13% DV)	Vitamin A	839 IU	(17% DV)
Poly Fat	0 g		Vitamin C	28.1 mg	(47% DV)
Mono Fat	2.55 g		Calcium	135.2 mg	(14% DV)
Cholesterol	12.8 mg	(4% DV)	Iron	2 mg	(11% DV)
Sodium	466.7 mg	(19% DV)	Folate	15.3 mcg	(8% DV)
Potassium	484.5 mg	(14% DV)	Beta Carotene	79.1 RE	

Ratings	Worst	Bad	Average	Good	Best
Weight Loss			7		
LowCal Density				8	
Filling				8	
Energizing				8	
Fiber			7		
Vitamins			7		
Minerals			7		
Overall				8	

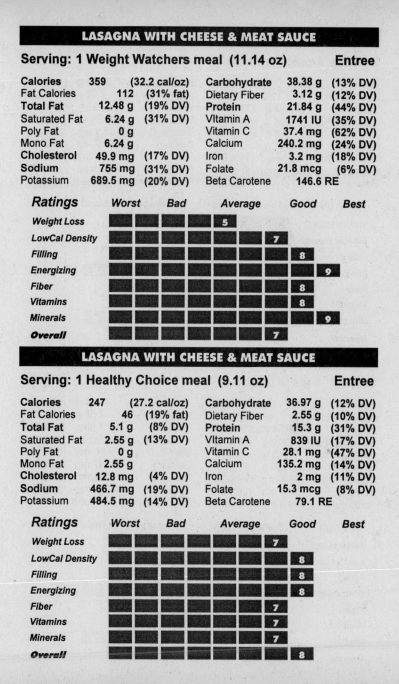

LASAGNA WITH MEAT, SPINACH NOODLES

Serving: 1 piece (approx 3½"x 4") (8.29 oz)   **Entree**

Calories	341	(41.1 cal/oz)	Carbohydrate	32.71 g	(11% DV)
Fat Calories	125	(37% fat)	Dietary Fiber	2.32 g	(9% DV)
Total Fat	13.92 g	(21% DV)	Protein	20.88 g	(42% DV)
Saturated Fat	6.96 g	(35% DV)	VItamin A	1146.1 IU	(23% DV)
Poly Fat	0 g		Vitamin C	13.9 mg	(23% DV)
Mono Fat	4.64 g		Calcium	257.5 mg	(26% DV)
Cholesterol	53.4 mg	(18% DV)	Iron	3.1 mg	(17% DV)
Sodium	877 mg	(37% DV)	Folate	20.9 mcg	(6% DV)
Potassium	417.6 mg	(12% DV)	Beta Carotene	90.5 RE	

Ratings	Worst	Bad	Average	Good	Best
Weight Loss			5		
LowCal Density			6		
Filling			6		
Energizing				8	
Fiber			6		
Vitamins			6		
Minerals				8	
Overall			6		

LASAGNA, MEATLESS

Serving: 1 piece (approx 3½"x 4") (9.14 oz)   **Entree**

Calories	351	(38.4 cal/oz)	Carbohydrate	45.31 g	(15% DV)
Fat Calories	92	(26% fat)	Dietary Fiber	2.56 g	(10% DV)
Total Fat	10.24 g	(16% DV)	Protein	17.92 g	(36% DV)
Saturated Fat	5.12 g	(26% DV)	VItamin A	1185.3 IU	(24% DV)
Poly Fat	0 g		Vitamin C	17.9 mg	(30% DV)
Mono Fat	2.56 g		Calcium	297 mg	(30% DV)
Cholesterol	35.8 mg	(12% DV)	Iron	2.9 mg	(16% DV)
Sodium	839.7 mg	(35% DV)	Folate	17.9 mcg	(5% DV)
Potassium	440.3 mg	(13% DV)	Beta Carotene	89.6 RE	

Ratings	Worst	Bad	Average	Good	Best
Weight Loss			5		
LowCal Density				7	
Filling				7	
Energizing					9
Fiber				7	
Vitamins				7	
Minerals				8	
Overall				7	

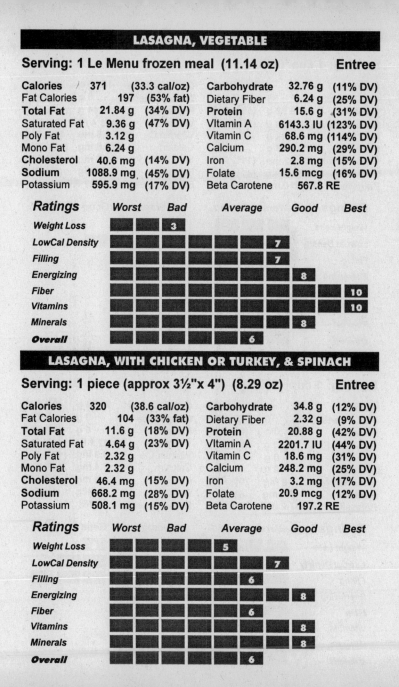

LASAGNA, VEGETABLE

Serving: 1 Le Menu frozen meal (11.14 oz)   **Entree**

Calories	371	(33.3 cal/oz)	Carbohydrate	32.76 g	(11% DV)
Fat Calories	197	(53% fat)	Dietary Fiber	6.24 g	(25% DV)
Total Fat	21.84 g	(34% DV)	Protein	15.6 g	(31% DV)
Saturated Fat	9.36 g	(47% DV)	Vitamin A	6143.3 IU	(123% DV)
Poly Fat	3.12 g		Vitamin C	68.6 mg	(114% DV)
Mono Fat	6.24 g		Calcium	290.2 mg	(29% DV)
Cholesterol	40.6 mg	(14% DV)	Iron	2.8 mg	(15% DV)
Sodium	1088.9 mg	(45% DV)	Folate	15.6 mcg	(16% DV)
Potassium	595.9 mg	(17% DV)	Beta Carotene	567.8 RE	

Ratings	Worst	Bad	Average	Good	Best
Weight Loss		3			
LowCal Density			7		
Filling			7		
Energizing				8	
Fiber					10
Vitamins					10
Minerals				8	
Overall			6		

LASAGNA, WITH CHICKEN OR TURKEY, & SPINACH

Serving: 1 piece (approx 3½"x 4") (8.29 oz)   **Entree**

Calories	320	(38.6 cal/oz)	Carbohydrate	34.8 g	(12% DV)
Fat Calories	104	(33% fat)	Dietary Fiber	2.32 g	(9% DV)
Total Fat	11.6 g	(18% DV)	Protein	20.88 g	(42% DV)
Saturated Fat	4.64 g	(23% DV)	Vitamin A	2201.7 IU	(44% DV)
Poly Fat	2.32 g		Vitamin C	18.6 mg	(31% DV)
Mono Fat	2.32 g		Calcium	248.2 mg	(25% DV)
Cholesterol	46.4 mg	(15% DV)	Iron	3.2 mg	(17% DV)
Sodium	668.2 mg	(28% DV)	Folate	20.9 mcg	(12% DV)
Potassium	508.1 mg	(15% DV)	Beta Carotene	197.2 RE	

Ratings	Worst	Bad	Average	Good	Best
Weight Loss		5			
LowCal Density			7		
Filling			6		
Energizing				8	
Fiber			6		
Vitamins				8	
Minerals				8	
Overall			6		

LEEK SOUP, CREAM OF, PREPARED WITH MILK

Serving: 1 cup (8.86 oz)   **Soup**

Calories	186	(21 cal/oz)	Carbohydrate	18.35 g	(6% DV)
Fat Calories	89	(48% fat)	Dietary Fiber	0 g	(0% DV)
Total Fat	9.92 g	(15% DV)	Protein	7.44 g	(15% DV)
Saturated Fat	4.96 g	(25% DV)	Vitamin A	451.4 IU	(9% DV)
Poly Fat	2.48 g		Vitamin C	2.5 mg	(4% DV)
Mono Fat	2.48 g		Calcium	178.6 mg	(18% DV)
Cholesterol	32.2 mg	(11% DV)	Iron	.7 mg	(4% DV)
Sodium	1004.4 mg	(42% DV)	Folate	7.4 mcg	(6% DV)
Potassium	310 mg	(9% DV)	Beta Carotene	34.7 RE	

Ratings	Worst	Bad	Average	Good	Best
Weight Loss		3			
LowCal Density				8	
Filling			6		
Energizing			6		
Fiber	1				
Vitamins		4			
Minerals			5		
Overall			5		

LEMONADE

Serving: 1 cup (8.86 oz)   **Beverage**

Calories	99	(11.2 cal/oz)	Carbohydrate	26.04 g	(9% DV)
Fat Calories	0	(0% fat)	Dietary Fiber	0 g	(0% DV)
Total Fat	0 g	(0% DV)	Protein	0 g	(0% DV)
Saturated Fat	0 g	(0% DV)	Vitamin A	52.1 IU	(1% DV)
Poly Fat	0 g		Vitamin C	9.9 mg	(17% DV)
Mono Fat	0 g		Calcium	7.4 mg	(1% DV)
Cholesterol	0 mg	(0% DV)	Iron	.4 mg	(2% DV)
Sodium	7.4 mg	(0% DV)	Folate	0 mcg	(1% DV)
Potassium	37.2 mg	(1% DV)	Beta Carotene	5 RE	

Ratings	Worst	Bad	Average	Good	Best
Weight Loss				8	
LowCal Density				9	
Filling					10
Energizing			7		
Fiber	1				
Vitamins		3			
Minerals	2				
Overall			7		

Edmund's Food Ratings

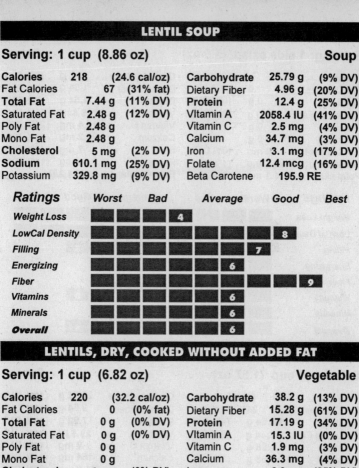

LENTIL SOUP

Serving: 1 cup (8.86 oz)   Soup

Calories	218	(24.6 cal/oz)	Carbohydrate	25.79 g	(9% DV)
Fat Calories	67	(31% fat)	Dietary Fiber	4.96 g	(20% DV)
Total Fat	7.44 g	(11% DV)	Protein	12.4 g	(25% DV)
Saturated Fat	2.48 g	(12% DV)	Vitamin A	2058.4 IU	(41% DV)
Poly Fat	2.48 g		Vitamin C	2.5 mg	(4% DV)
Mono Fat	2.48 g		Calcium	34.7 mg	(3% DV)
Cholesterol	5 mg	(2% DV)	Iron	3.1 mg	(17% DV)
Sodium	610.1 mg	(25% DV)	Folate	12.4 mcg	(16% DV)
Potassium	329.8 mg	(9% DV)	Beta Carotene	195.9 RE	

Ratings

	Worst	Bad	Average	Good	Best
Weight Loss		4			
LowCal Density				8	
Filling			7		
Energizing		6			
Fiber					9
Vitamins		6			
Minerals		6			
Overall		6			

LENTILS, DRY, COOKED WITHOUT ADDED FAT

Serving: 1 cup (6.82 oz)   Vegetable

Calories	220	(32.2 cal/oz)	Carbohydrate	38.2 g	(13% DV)
Fat Calories	0	(0% fat)	Dietary Fiber	15.28 g	(61% DV)
Total Fat	0 g	(0% DV)	Protein	17.19 g	(34% DV)
Saturated Fat	0 g	(0% DV)	Vitamin A	15.3 IU	(0% DV)
Poly Fat	0 g		Vitamin C	1.9 mg	(3% DV)
Mono Fat	0 g		Calcium	36.3 mg	(4% DV)
Cholesterol	0 mg	(0% DV)	Iron	6.3 mg	(35% DV)
Sodium	445 mg	(19% DV)	Folate	17.2 mcg	(86% DV)
Potassium	701 mg	(20% DV)	Beta Carotene	1.9 RE	

Ratings

	Worst	Bad	Average	Good	Best
Weight Loss		4			
LowCal Density			7		
Filling				9	
Energizing				9	
Fiber					10
Vitamins			8		
Minerals				9	
Overall			7		

LETTUCE, SALAD WITH ASSORTED VEGETABLES

Serving: 1 side salad (5.5 oz)   Salad

Calories	28	(5 cal/oz)	Carbohydrate	5.7 g	(2% DV)
Fat Calories	0	(0% fat)	Dietary Fiber	1.54 g	(6% DV)
Total Fat	0 g	(0% DV)	Protein	1.54 g	(3% DV)
Saturated Fat	0 g	(0% DV)	VItamin A	3746.8 IU	(75% DV)
Poly Fat	0 g		Vitamin C	15.4 mg	(26% DV)
Mono Fat	0 g		Calcium	26.2 mg	(3% DV)
Cholesterol	0 mg	(0% DV)	Iron	.7 mg	(4% DV)
Sodium	26.2 mg	(1% DV)	Folate	1.5 mcg	(14% DV)
Potassium	311.1 mg	(9% DV)	Beta Carotene	374.2 RE	

Ratings	Worst	Bad	Average	Good	Best
Weight Loss					10
LowCal Density					10
Filling				8	
Energizing	3				
Fiber			5		
Vitamins				8	
Minerals	3				
Overall				8	

LIFE (PLAIN & CINNAMON)

Serving: 1 cup (1.57 oz)   Cereal

Calories	167	(106.5 cal/oz)	Carbohydrate	29.22 g	(10% DV)
Fat Calories	24	(14% fat)	Dietary Fiber	2.64 g	(11% DV)
Total Fat	2.64 g	(4% DV)	Protein	7.92 g	(16% DV)
Saturated Fat	.44 g	(2% DV)	VItamin A	29.5 IU	(1% DV)
Poly Fat	.88 g		Vitamin C	.9 mg	(1% DV)
Mono Fat	.88 g		Calcium	154 mg	(15% DV)
Cholesterol	0 mg	(0% DV)	Iron	11.6 mg	(65% DV)
Sodium	229.2 mg	(10% DV)	Folate	7.9 mcg	(9% DV)
Potassium	150.5 mg	(4% DV)	Beta Carotene	3.1 RE	

Ratings	Worst	Bad	Average	Good	Best
Weight Loss				7	
LowCal Density	2				
Filling		4			
Energizing				7	
Fiber				7	
Vitamins					9
Minerals					9
Overall			5		

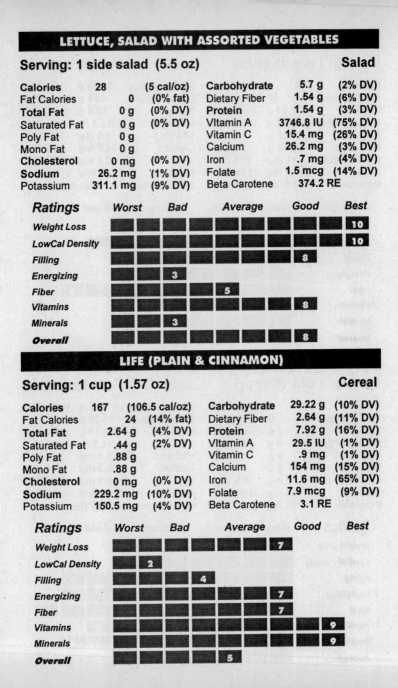

LIMA BEANS, & CORN, WITHOUT ADDED FAT

Serving: 1 cup (6.86 oz)   **Vegetable**

Calories	177	(25.8 cal/oz)	Carbohydrate	38.02 g	(13% DV)
Fat Calories	17	(10% fat)	Dietary Fiber	9.6 g	(38% DV)
Total Fat	1.92 g	(3% DV)	Protein	7.68 g	(15% DV)
Saturated Fat	0 g	(0% DV)	Vitamin A	441.6 IU	(9% DV)
Poly Fat	0 g		Vitamin C	11.5 mg	(19% DV)
Mono Fat	0 g		Calcium	28.8 mg	(3% DV)
Cholesterol	0 mg	(0% DV)	Iron	1.7 mg	(9% DV)
Sodium	520.3 mg	(22% DV)	Folate	7.7 mcg	(16% DV)
Potassium	505 mg	(14% DV)	Beta Carotene	44.2 RE	

Ratings	Worst	Bad	Average	Good	Best
Weight Loss			5		
LowCal Density				8	
Filling					9
Energizing					9
Fiber					10
Vitamins			6		
Minerals			5		
Overall				7	

LIMA BEANS, DRY, COOKED WITHOUT ADDED FAT

Serving: 1 cup (6.57 oz)   **Vegetable**

Calories	210	(31.9 cal/oz)	Carbohydrate	38.27 g	(13% DV)
Fat Calories	0	(0% fat)	Dietary Fiber	12.88 g	(52% DV)
Total Fat	0 g	(0% DV)	Protein	14.72 g	(29% DV)
Saturated Fat	0 g	(0% DV)	Vitamin A	0 IU	(0% DV)
Poly Fat	0 g		Vitamin C	0 mg	(0% DV)
Mono Fat	0 g		Calcium	31.3 mg	(3% DV)
Cholesterol	0 mg	(0% DV)	Iron	4.4 mg	(24% DV)
Sodium	428.7 mg	(18% DV)	Folate	14.7 mcg	(38% DV)
Potassium	929.2 mg	(27% DV)	Beta Carotene	0 RE	

Ratings	Worst	Bad	Average	Good	Best
Weight Loss			5		
LowCal Density			7		
Filling				9	
Energizing				9	
Fiber					10
Vitamins			5		
Minerals			7		
Overall			7		

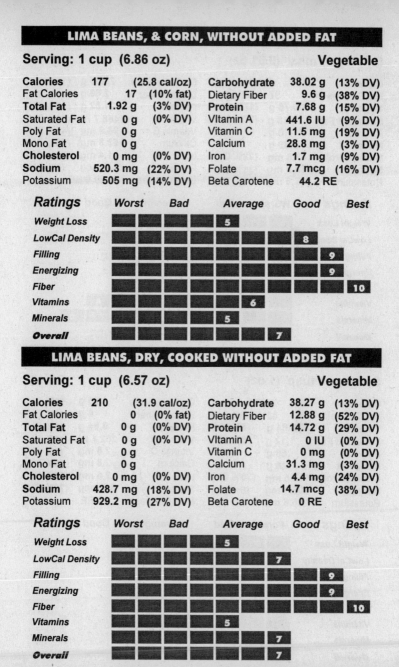

LINGUINI WITH VEGETABLES & SEAFOOD, WINE SAUCE

Serving: 1 meal (9.61 oz)   Entree

Calories	299	(31.1 cal/oz)	Carbohydrate	29.05 g	(10% DV)
Fat Calories	97	(32% fat)	Dietary Fiber	2.69 g	(11% DV)
Total Fat	10.76 g	(17% DV)	Protein	21.52 g	(43% DV)
Saturated Fat	5.38 g	(27% DV)	Vitamin A	1468.7 IU	(29% DV)
Poly Fat	0 g		Vitamin C	26.9 mg	(45% DV)
Mono Fat	2.69 g		Calcium	153.3 mg	(15% DV)
Cholesterol	67.3 mg	(22% DV)	Iron	11.4 mg	(63% DV)
Sodium	734.4 mg	(31% DV)	Folate	21.5 mcg	(9% DV)
Potassium	567.6 mg	(16% DV)	Beta Carotene	99.5 RE	

Ratings	Worst	Bad	Average	Good	Best
Weight Loss			5		
LowCal Density				7	
Filling				7	
Energizing				7	
Fiber				7	
Vitamins				8	
Minerals					9
Overall				7	

LIVER PASTE OR PATE, CHICKEN

Serving: 2 tbsp (1 oz)   Meat

Calories	56	(56.3 cal/oz)	Carbohydrate	1.85 g	(1% DV)
Fat Calories	33	(58% fat)	Dietary Fiber	0 g	(0% DV)
Total Fat	3.64 g	(6% DV)	Protein	3.64 g	(7% DV)
Saturated Fat	1.12 g	(6% DV)	Vitamin A	202.7 IU	(4% DV)
Poly Fat	.56 g		Vitamin C	2.8 mg	(5% DV)
Mono Fat	1.4 g		Calcium	2.8 mg	(0% DV)
Cholesterol	109.5 mg	(36% DV)	Iron	2.6 mg	(14% DV)
Sodium	108.1 mg	(5% DV)	Folate	3.6 mcg	(22% DV)
Potassium	26.6 mg	(1% DV)	Beta Carotene	0 RE	

Ratings	Worst	Bad	Average	Good	Best
Weight Loss			6		
LowCal Density			5		
Filling	1				
Energizing		3			
Fiber	1				
Vitamins			5		
Minerals		4			
Overall		4			

LIVERWURST

Serving: 1 slice (1 oz)   **Meat**

Calories	101	(100.5 cal/oz)	Carbohydrate	.87 g	(0% DV)
Fat Calories	81	(80% fat)	Dietary Fiber	0 g	(0% DV)
Total Fat	8.96 g	(14% DV)	Protein	3.92 g	(8% DV)
Saturated Fat	3.08 g	(15% DV)	Vitamin A	3934.3 IU	(79% DV)
Poly Fat	1.12 g		Vitamin C	2.8 mg	(5% DV)
Mono Fat	4.2 g		Calcium	2.5 mg	(0% DV)
Cholesterol	43.7 mg	(15% DV)	Iron	2.6 mg	(15% DV)
Sodium	320 mg	(13% DV)	Folate	3.9 mcg	(3% DV)
Potassium	55.7 mg	(2% DV)	Beta Carotene	0 RE	

Ratings	Worst	Bad	Average	Good	Best
Weight Loss		3			
LowCal Density	2				
Filling	1				
Energizing	2				
Fiber	1				
Vitamins					8
Minerals		4			
Overall		3			

LO MEIN WITH MEAT

Serving: 1 cup (7.14 oz)   **Entree**

Calories	286	(40.1 cal/oz)	Carbohydrate	31.4 g	(10% DV)
Fat Calories	90	(31% fat)	Dietary Fiber	2 g	(8% DV)
Total Fat	10 g	(15% DV)	Protein	16 g	(32% DV)
Saturated Fat	2 g	(10% DV)	Vitamin A	38 IU	(1% DV)
Poly Fat	4 g		Vitamin C	8 mg	(13% DV)
Mono Fat	2 g		Calcium	26 mg	(3% DV)
Cholesterol	30 mg	(10% DV)	Iron	2.1 mg	(12% DV)
Sodium	276 mg	(12% DV)	Folate	16 mcg	(10% DV)
Potassium	246 mg	(7% DV)	Beta Carotene	2 RE	

Ratings	Worst	Bad	Average	Good	Best
Weight Loss			6		
LowCal Density			6		
Filling			6		
Energizing				8	
Fiber			6		
Vitamins			6		
Minerals			6		
Overall			6		

LOBSTER BISQUE

Serving: 1 cup (8.86 oz)   **Soup**

Calories	273	(30.8 cal/oz)	Carbohydrate	12.65 g	(4% DV)
Fat Calories	134	(49% fat)	Dietary Fiber	0 g	(0% DV)
Total Fat	14.88 g	(23% DV)	Protein	19.84 g	(40% DV)
Saturated Fat	4.96 g	(25% DV)	Vitamin A	756.4 IU	(15% DV)
Poly Fat	2.48 g		Vitamin C	2.5 mg	(4% DV)
Mono Fat	4.96 g		Calcium	270.3 mg	(27% DV)
Cholesterol	71.9 mg	(24% DV)	Iron	.5 mg	(3% DV)
Sodium	858.1 mg	(36% DV)	Folate	19.8 mcg	(4% DV)
Potassium	538.2 mg	(15% DV)	Beta Carotene	14.9 RE	

Ratings	*Worst*	*Bad*	*Average*	*Good*	*Best*
Weight Loss	2				
LowCal Density				7	
Filling		5			
Energizing		5			
Fiber	1				
Vitamins		5			
Minerals				8	
Overall		5			

LOBSTER, BAKED OR BROILED

Serving: 1 tail (3.71 oz)   **Shellfish**

Calories	121	(32.5 cal/oz)	Carbohydrate	1.25 g	(0% DV)
Fat Calories	28	(23% fat)	Dietary Fiber	0 g	(0% DV)
Total Fat	3.12 g	(5% DV)	Protein	20.8 g	(42% DV)
Saturated Fat	2.08 g	(10% DV)	Vitamin A	183 IU	(4% DV)
Poly Fat	0 g		Vitamin C	0 mg	(0% DV)
Mono Fat	1.04 g		Calcium	62.4 mg	(6% DV)
Cholesterol	79 mg	(26% DV)	Iron	.4 mg	(2% DV)
Sodium	646.9 mg	(27% DV)	Folate	20.8 mcg	(3% DV)
Potassium	353.6 mg	(10% DV)	Beta Carotene	3.1 RE	

Ratings	*Worst*	*Bad*	*Average*	*Good*	*Best*
Weight Loss			6		
LowCal Density				7	
Filling	2				
Energizing	2				
Fiber	1				
Vitamins		3			
Minerals			6		
Overall		5			

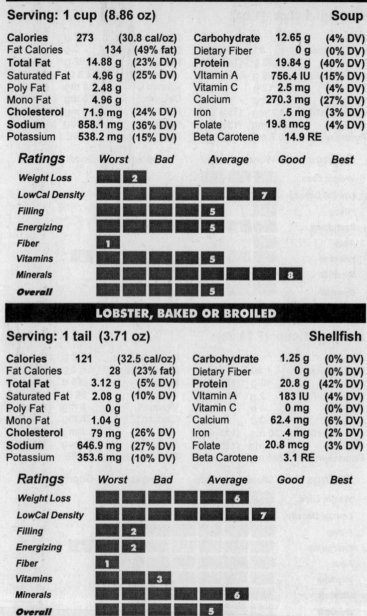

LUCKY CHARMS

Serving: 1 cup (1.14 oz)   **Cereal**

Calories	125	(109.5 cal/oz)	Carbohydrate	26.14 g	(9% DV)
Fat Calories	12	(9% fat)	Dietary Fiber	1.28 g	(5% DV)
Total Fat	1.28 g	(2% DV)	Protein	2.88 g	(6% DV)
Saturated Fat	.32 g	(2% DV)	VItamin A	1410.9 IU	(28% DV)
Poly Fat	.64 g		Vitamin C	17 mg	(28% DV)
Mono Fat	.32 g		Calcium	36.2 mg	(4% DV)
Cholesterol	0 mg	(0% DV)	Iron	5.1 mg	(28% DV)
Sodium	227.2 mg	(9% DV)	Folate	2.9 mcg	(28% DV)
Potassium	66.2 mg	(2% DV)	Beta Carotene	0 RE	

Ratings	Worst	Bad	Average	Good	Best
Weight Loss					8
LowCal Density	2				
Filling		4			
Energizing				7	
Fiber			5		
Vitamins					9
Minerals			6		
Overall			5		

MACADAMIA NUTS, ROASTED

Serving: 11 whole kernels (1 oz)   **Snack**

Calories	201	(201 cal/oz)	Carbohydrate	3.61 g	(1% DV)
Fat Calories	194	(97% fat)	Dietary Fiber	2.52 g	(10% DV)
Total Fat	21.56 g	(33% DV)	Protein	1.96 g	(4% DV)
Saturated Fat	3.08 g	(15% DV)	VItamin A	2.5 IU	(0% DV)
Poly Fat	.28 g		Vitamin C	0 mg	(0% DV)
Mono Fat	16.8 g		Calcium	12.6 mg	(1% DV)
Cholesterol	0 mg	(0% DV)	Iron	.5 mg	(3% DV)
Sodium	72.8 mg	(3% DV)	Folate	2 mcg	(1% DV)
Potassium	92.1 mg	(3% DV)	Beta Carotene	.3 RE	

Ratings	Worst	Bad	Average	Good	Best
Weight Loss	2				
LowCal Density	1				
Filling	1				
Energizing		3			
Fiber				7	
Vitamins		3			
Minerals		4			
Overall	2				

MACARONI & CHEESE

Serving: 1 diet meal (9.11 oz) **Entree**

Calories	314	(34.4 cal/oz)	Carbohydrate	40.54 g	(14% DV)
Fat Calories	92	(29% fat)	Dietary Fiber	2.55 g	(10% DV)
Total Fat	10.2 g	(16% DV)	Protein	15.3 g	(31% DV)
Saturated Fat	5.1 g	(25% DV)	Vitamin A	420.8 IU	(8% DV)
Poly Fat	0 g		Vitamin C	0 mg	(0% DV)
Mono Fat	2.55 g		Calcium	288.2 mg	(29% DV)
Cholesterol	30.6 mg	(10% DV)	Iron	1.9 mg	(11% DV)
Sodium	640.1 mg	(27% DV)	Folate	15.3 mcg	(3% DV)
Potassium	176 mg	(5% DV)	Beta Carotene	5.1 RE	

Ratings

	Worst	Bad	Average	Good	Best
Weight Loss			5		
LowCal Density			7		
Filling			7		
Energizing				9	
Fiber			7		
Vitamins		4			
Minerals				8	
Overall			6		

MACARONI & CHEESE, APPLES, VEGETABLES

Serving: 1 frozen meal (12.39 oz) **Entree**

Calories	420	(33.9 cal/oz)	Carbohydrate	55.52 g	(19% DV)
Fat Calories	156	(37% fat)	Dietary Fiber	3.47 g	(14% DV)
Total Fat	17.35 g	(27% DV)	Protein	13.88 g	(28% DV)
Saturated Fat	6.94 g	(35% DV)	Vitamin A	8310.7 IU	(166% DV)
Poly Fat	3.47 g		Vitamin C	6.9 mg	(12% DV)
Mono Fat	3.47 g		Calcium	267.2 mg	(27% DV)
Cholesterol	34.7 mg	(12% DV)	Iron	2.2 mg	(12% DV)
Sodium	1308.2 mg	(55% DV)	Folate	13.9 mcg	(9% DV)
Potassium	281.1 mg	(8% DV)	Beta Carotene	794.6 RE	

Ratings

	Worst	Bad	Average	Good	Best
Weight Loss		4			
LowCal Density			7		
Filling				9	
Energizing					10
Fiber			8		
Vitamins				9	
Minerals			8		
Overall			7		

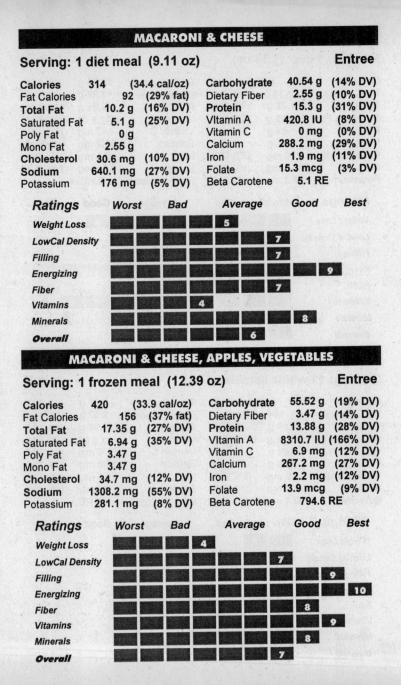

MACARONI OR NOODLES WITH CHEESE

Serving: 1 cup (8.68 oz)   **Entree**

Calories	505	(58.2 cal/oz)	Carbohydrate	45.68 g	(15% DV)
Fat Calories	241	(48% fat)	Dietary Fiber	2.43 g	(10% DV)
Total Fat	26.73 g	(41% DV)	Protein	19.44 g	(39% DV)
Saturated Fat	12.15 g	(61% DV)	VItamin A	1112.9 IU	(22% DV)
Poly Fat	4.86 g		Vitamin C	0 mg	(0% DV)
Mono Fat	9.72 g		Calcium	408.2 mg	(41% DV)
Cholesterol	53.5 mg	(18% DV)	Iron	2.3 mg	(13% DV)
Sodium	1057.1 mg	(44% DV)	Folate	19.4 mcg	(4% DV)
Potassium	272.2 mg	(8% DV)	Beta Carotene	29.2 RE	

Ratings	Worst	Bad	Average	Good	Best
Weight Loss		3			
LowCal Density			5		
Filling			6		
Energizing					9
Fiber				7	
Vitamins			5		
Minerals					9
Overall			5		

MACARONI SALAD WITH CHICKEN

Serving: 1 cup (6.32 oz)   **Salad**

Calories	304	(48.2 cal/oz)	Carbohydrate	29.38 g	(10% DV)
Fat Calories	112	(37% fat)	Dietary Fiber	1.77 g	(7% DV)
Total Fat	12.39 g	(19% DV)	Protein	17.7 g	(35% DV)
Saturated Fat	1.77 g	(9% DV)	VItamin A	168.2 IU	(3% DV)
Poly Fat	5.31 g		Vitamin C	10.6 mg	(18% DV)
Mono Fat	3.54 g		Calcium	30.1 mg	(3% DV)
Cholesterol	51.3 mg	(17% DV)	Iron	1.8 mg	(10% DV)
Sodium	821.3 mg	(34% DV)	Folate	17.7 mcg	(4% DV)
Potassium	235.4 mg	(7% DV)	Beta Carotene	8.9 RE	

Ratings	Worst	Bad	Average	Good	Best
Weight Loss		4			
LowCal Density			6		
Filling			5		
Energizing			7		
Fiber			6		
Vitamins			6		
Minerals			5		
Overall			5		

MACKEREL, BAKED OR BROILED

Serving: 1 piece (3.04 oz)   **Fish**

Calories	227	(74.7 cal/oz)	Carbohydrate	.34 g	(0% DV)
Fat Calories	145	(64% fat)	Dietary Fiber	0 g	(0% DV)
Total Fat	16.15 g	(25% DV)	Protein	18.7 g	(37% DV)
Saturated Fat	3.4 g	(17% DV)	Vitamin A	270.3 IU	(5% DV)
Poly Fat	5.1 g		Vitamin C	1.7 mg	(3% DV)
Mono Fat	5.1 g		Calcium	13.6 mg	(1% DV)
Cholesterol	69.7 mg	(23% DV)	Iron	1.6 mg	(9% DV)
Sodium	351.9 mg	(15% DV)	Folate	18.7 mcg	(0% DV)
Potassium	317.1 mg	(9% DV)	Beta Carotene	2.6 RE	

Ratings	Worst	Bad	Average	Good	Best
Weight Loss		3			
LowCal Density			4		
Filling	1				
Energizing	2				
Fiber	1				
Vitamins				6	
Minerals				6	
Overall		3			

MACKEREL, FLOURED OR BREADED, FRIED

Serving: 1 piece (3.04 oz)   **Fish**

Calories	278	(91.4 cal/oz)	Carbohydrate	6.72 g	(2% DV)
Fat Calories	176	(63% fat)	Dietary Fiber	0 g	(0% DV)
Total Fat	19.55 g	(30% DV)	Protein	17 g	(34% DV)
Saturated Fat	5.1 g	(25% DV)	Vitamin A	144.5 IU	(3% DV)
Poly Fat	5.95 g		Vitamin C	0 mg	(0% DV)
Mono Fat	6.8 g		Calcium	24.7 mg	(2% DV)
Cholesterol	76.5 mg	(26% DV)	Iron	1.8 mg	(10% DV)
Sodium	336.6 mg	(14% DV)	Folate	17 mcg	(1% DV)
Potassium	276.3 mg	(8% DV)	Beta Carotene	0 RE	

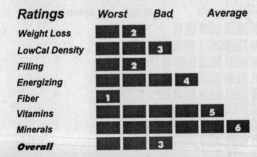

Ratings	Worst	Bad	Average	Good	Best
Weight Loss	2				
LowCal Density		3			
Filling	2				
Energizing			4		
Fiber	1				
Vitamins			5		
Minerals				6	
Overall		3			

MANGO, RAW

Serving: 1 mango (7.39 oz)   **Fruit**

Calories	135	(18.2 cal/oz)	Carbohydrate	35.19 g	(12% DV)
Fat Calories	0	(0% fat)	Dietary Fiber	4.14 g	(17% DV)
Total Fat	0 g	(0% DV)	Protein	2.07 g	(4% DV)
Saturated Fat	0 g	(0% DV)	VItamin A	8060.6 IU	(161% DV)
Poly Fat	0 g		Vitamin C	58 mg	(97% DV)
Mono Fat	0 g		Calcium	20.7 mg	(2% DV)
Cholesterol	0 mg	(0% DV)	Iron	.3 mg	(2% DV)
Sodium	4.1 mg	(0% DV)	Folate	2.1 mcg	(7% DV)
Potassium	322.9 mg	(9% DV)	Beta Carotene	805.2 RE	

Ratings	Worst	Bad	Average	Good	Best
Weight Loss				8	
LowCal Density				8	
Filling					10
Energizing				8	
Fiber				9	
Vitamins					10
Minerals		3			
Overall				8	

MANICOTTI, CHEESE-FILLED, TOMATO SAUCE

Serving: 1 diet meal (9.36 oz)   **Entree**

Calories	317	(33.9 cal/oz)	Carbohydrate	28.56 g	(10% DV)
Fat Calories	118	(37% fat)	Dietary Fiber	2.62 g	(10% DV)
Total Fat	13.1 g	(20% DV)	Protein	18.34 g	(37% DV)
Saturated Fat	7.86 g	(39% DV)	VItamin A	1150.2 IU	(23% DV)
Poly Fat	2.62 g		Vitamin C	21 mg	(35% DV)
Mono Fat	2.62 g		Calcium	419.2 mg	(42% DV)
Cholesterol	47.2 mg	(16% DV)	Iron	1.7 mg	(10% DV)
Sodium	809.6 mg	(34% DV)	Folate	18.3 mcg	(7% DV)
Potassium	393 mg	(11% DV)	Beta Carotene	76 RE	

Ratings	Worst	Bad	Average	Good	Best
Weight Loss			5		
LowCal Density				7	
Filling			6		
Energizing				7	
Fiber				7	
Vitamins			6		
Minerals					9
Overall			6		

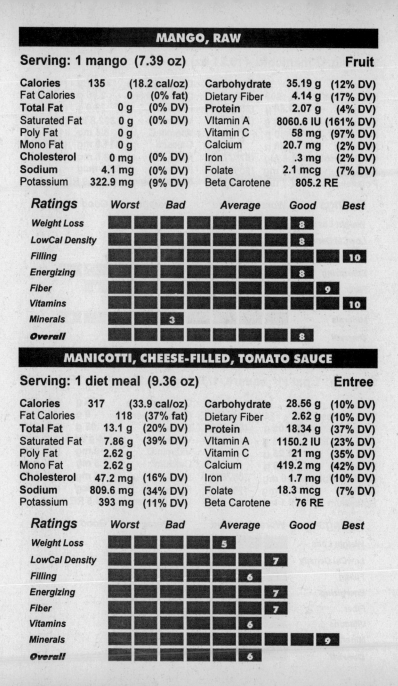

MANICOTTI, CHEESE-FILLED, WITH MEAT SAUCE

Serving: 2 manicotti (10.21 oz)   Entree

Calories	469	(45.9 cal/oz)	Carbohydrate	38.61 g	(13% DV)
Fat Calories	206	(44% fat)	Dietary Fiber	2.86 g	(11% DV)
Total Fat	22.88 g	(35% DV)	Protein	28.6 g	(57% DV)
Saturated Fat	11.44 g	(57% DV)	VItamin A	1392.8 IU	(28% DV)
Poly Fat	0 g		Vitamin C	8.6 mg	(14% DV)
Mono Fat	8.58 g		Calcium	411.8 mg	(41% DV)
Cholesterol	171.6 mg	(57% DV)	Iron	3.6 mg	(20% DV)
Sodium	1195.5 mg	(50% DV)	Folate	28.6 mcg	(9% DV)
Potassium	517.7 mg	(15% DV)	Beta Carotene	82.9 RE	

Ratings	Worst	Bad	Average	Good	Best
Weight Loss		3			
LowCal Density			6		
Filling			6		
Energizing					9
Fiber				8	
Vitamins			7		
Minerals					9
Overall			6		

MARGARINE, STICK, SALTED

Serving: 1 pat (1" square, 1/3" high) (.18 oz)   Fat & Oil

Calories	36	(199.7 cal/oz)	Carbohydrate	.05 g	(0% DV)
Fat Calories	36	(101% fat)	Dietary Fiber	0 g	(0% DV)
Total Fat	4.05 g	(6% DV)	Protein	.05 g	(0% DV)
Saturated Fat	.8 g	(4% DV)	VItamin A	209.9 IU	(4% DV)
Poly Fat	1.25 g		Vitamin C	0 mg	(0% DV)
Mono Fat	1.8 g		Calcium	1.5 mg	(0% DV)
Cholesterol	0 mg	(0% DV)	Iron	0 mg	(0% DV)
Sodium	47.2 mg	(2% DV)	Folate	.1 mcg	(0% DV)
Potassium	2.1 mg	(0% DV)	Beta Carotene	4.5 RE	

Ratings	Worst	Bad	Average	Good	Best
Weight Loss		3			
LowCal Density	1				
Filling	1				
Energizing		2			
Fiber	1				
Vitamins		2			
Minerals		2			
Overall		2			

MARGARINE-LIKE SPREAD, STICK, OR TUB

Serving: 1 tsp (.17 oz)   **Fat & Oil**

Calories	26	(152.5 cal/oz)	Carbohydrate	0 g	(0% DV)
Fat Calories	26	(102% fat)	Dietary Fiber	0 g	(0% DV)
Total Fat	2.93 g	(5% DV)	Protein	.05 g	(0% DV)
Saturated Fat	.62 g	(3% DV)	VItamin A	201.5 IU	(4% DV)
Poly Fat	.67 g		Vitamin C	0 mg	(0% DV)
Mono Fat	1.54 g		Calcium	1 mg	(0% DV)
Cholesterol	0 mg	(0% DV)	Iron	0 mg	(0% DV)
Sodium	47.7 mg	(2% DV)	Folate	.1 mcg	(0% DV)
Potassium	1.4 mg	(0% DV)	Beta Carotene	4.3 RE	

Ratings	Worst	Bad	Average	Good	Best
Weight Loss		3			
LowCal Density	1				
Filling	1				
Energizing	1				
Fiber	1				
Vitamins	2				
Minerals	2				
Overall	2				

MATZO BALL SOUP

Serving: 1 cup (8.61 oz)   **Soup**

Calories	118	(13.7 cal/oz)	Carbohydrate	9.64 g	(3% DV)
Fat Calories	43	(37% fat)	Dietary Fiber	0 g	(0% DV)
Total Fat	4.82 g	(7% DV)	Protein	7.23 g	(14% DV)
Saturated Fat	2.41 g	(12% DV)	VItamin A	81.9 IU	(2% DV)
Poly Fat	2.41 g		Vitamin C	0 mg	(0% DV)
Mono Fat	2.41 g		Calcium	16.9 mg	(2% DV)
Cholesterol	62.7 mg	(21% DV)	Iron	1.1 mg	(6% DV)
Sodium	730.2 mg	(30% DV)	Folate	7.2 mcg	(4% DV)
Potassium	188 mg	(5% DV)	Beta Carotene	0 RE	

Ratings	Worst	Bad	Average	Good	Best
Weight Loss			6		
LowCal Density					9
Filling			6		
Energizing		4			
Fiber	1				
Vitamins		4			
Minerals		4			
Overall			6		

MAYONNAISE, IMITATION

Serving: 1 tbsp (.54 oz)   **Fat & Oil**

Calories	35	(64.4 cal/oz)	Carbohydrate	2.4 g	(1% DV)
Fat Calories	26	(74% fat)	Dietary Fiber	0 g	(0% DV)
Total Fat	2.85 g	(4% DV)	Protein	0 g	(0% DV)
Saturated Fat	.45 g	(2% DV)	Vltamin A	0 IU	(0% DV)
Poly Fat	1.65 g		Vitamin C	0 mg	(0% DV)
Mono Fat	.75 g		Calcium	0 mg	(0% DV)
Cholesterol	3.6 mg	(1% DV)	Iron	0 mg	(0% DV)
Sodium	74.6 mg	(3% DV)	Folate	0 mcg	(0% DV)
Potassium	1.5 mg	(0% DV)	Beta Carotene	0 RE	

Ratings	Worst	Bad	Average	Good	Best
Weight Loss			4		
LowCal Density			5		
Filling	2				
Energizing		3			
Fiber	1				
Vitamins	2				
Minerals	2				
Overall		3			

MAYONNAISE, REGULAR

Serving: 1 tbsp (.49 oz)   **Fat & Oil**

Calories	99	(201.9 cal/oz)	Carbohydrate	.37 g	(0% DV)
Fat Calories	98	(99% fat)	Dietary Fiber	0 g	(0% DV)
Total Fat	10.9 g	(17% DV)	Protein	.14 g	(0% DV)
Saturated Fat	1.66 g	(8% DV)	Vltamin A	38.6 IU	(1% DV)
Poly Fat	5.66 g		Vitamin C	0 mg	(0% DV)
Mono Fat	3.17 g		Calcium	2.5 mg	(0% DV)
Cholesterol	8.1 mg	(3% DV)	Iron	.1 mg	(0% DV)
Sodium	78.4 mg	(3% DV)	Folate	.1 mcg	(0% DV)
Potassium	4.7 mg	(0% DV)	Beta Carotene	0 RE	

Ratings	Worst	Bad	Average	Good	Best
Weight Loss	1				
LowCal Density	1				
Filling	1				
Energizing		2			
Fiber	1				
Vitamins		3			
Minerals		2			
Overall	1				

MAYONNAISE-TYPE SALAD DRESSING, FAT-FREE

Serving: 1 tbsp (.57 oz) **Fat & Oil**

Calories	12	(21.1 cal/oz)	Carbohydrate	2.08 g	(1% DV)
Fat Calories	4	(36% fat)	Dietary Fiber	.64 g	(3% DV)
Total Fat	.48 g	(1% DV)	Protein	0 g	(0% DV)
Saturated Fat	0 g	(0% DV)	Vitamin A	0 IU	(0% DV)
Poly Fat	.32 g		Vitamin C	0 mg	(0% DV)
Mono Fat	.16 g		Calcium	0 mg	(0% DV)
Cholesterol	0 mg	(0% DV)	Iron	0 mg	(0% DV)
Sodium	190.1 mg	(8% DV)	Folate	0 mcg	(0% DV)
Potassium	15 mg	(0% DV)	Beta Carotene	0 RE	

Ratings	Worst	Bad	Average	Good	Best
Weight Loss				8	
LowCal Density				8	
Filling	2				
Energizing		3			
Fiber		3			
Vitamins	2				
Minerals	1				
Overall			6		

MEAT LOAF OR PATTIES, VEGETARIAN

Serving: 1 slice (2 oz) **Entree**

Calories	112	(56 cal/oz)	Carbohydrate	4.48 g	(1% DV)
Fat Calories	45	(41% fat)	Dietary Fiber	2.8 g	(11% DV)
Total Fat	5.04 g	(8% DV)	Protein	11.76 g	(24% DV)
Saturated Fat	.56 g	(3% DV)	Vitamin A	0 IU	(0% DV)
Poly Fat	2.8 g		Vitamin C	0 mg	(0% DV)
Mono Fat	1.12 g		Calcium	16.2 mg	(2% DV)
Cholesterol	0 mg	(0% DV)	Iron	1.2 mg	(7% DV)
Sodium	308 mg	(13% DV)	Folate	11.8 mcg	(11% DV)
Potassium	100.8 mg	(3% DV)	Beta Carotene	0 RE	

Ratings	Worst	Bad	Average	Good	Best
Weight Loss			7		
LowCal Density			5		
Filling	2				
Energizing		3			
Fiber				8	
Vitamins				8	
Minerals			5		
Overall			5		

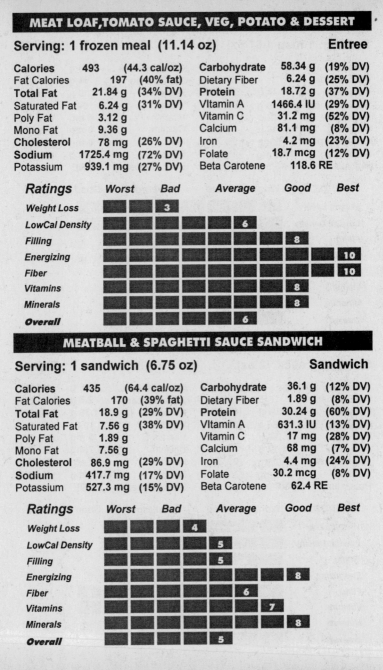

MEAT LOAF, TOMATO SAUCE, VEG, POTATO & DESSERT

Serving: 1 frozen meal (11.14 oz)   Entree

Calories	493	(44.3 cal/oz)	Carbohydrate	58.34 g	(19% DV)
Fat Calories	197	(40% fat)	Dietary Fiber	6.24 g	(25% DV)
Total Fat	21.84 g	(34% DV)	Protein	18.72 g	(37% DV)
Saturated Fat	6.24 g	(31% DV)	Vitamin A	1466.4 IU	(29% DV)
Poly Fat	3.12 g		Vitamin C	31.2 mg	(52% DV)
Mono Fat	9.36 g		Calcium	81.1 mg	(8% DV)
Cholesterol	78 mg	(26% DV)	Iron	4.2 mg	(23% DV)
Sodium	1725.4 mg	(72% DV)	Folate	18.7 mcg	(12% DV)
Potassium	939.1 mg	(27% DV)	Beta Carotene	118.6 RE	

Ratings	Worst	Bad	Average	Good	Best
Weight Loss		3			
LowCal Density			6		
Filling				8	
Energizing					10
Fiber					10
Vitamins				8	
Minerals				8	
Overall			6		

MEATBALL & SPAGHETTI SAUCE SANDWICH

Serving: 1 sandwich (6.75 oz)   Sandwich

Calories	435	(64.4 cal/oz)	Carbohydrate	36.1 g	(12% DV)
Fat Calories	170	(39% fat)	Dietary Fiber	1.89 g	(8% DV)
Total Fat	18.9 g	(29% DV)	Protein	30.24 g	(60% DV)
Saturated Fat	7.56 g	(38% DV)	Vitamin A	631.3 IU	(13% DV)
Poly Fat	1.89 g		Vitamin C	17 mg	(28% DV)
Mono Fat	7.56 g		Calcium	68 mg	(7% DV)
Cholesterol	86.9 mg	(29% DV)	Iron	4.4 mg	(24% DV)
Sodium	417.7 mg	(17% DV)	Folate	30.2 mcg	(8% DV)
Potassium	527.3 mg	(15% DV)	Beta Carotene	62.4 RE	

Ratings	Worst	Bad	Average	Good	Best
Weight Loss		4			
LowCal Density			5		
Filling			5		
Energizing				8	
Fiber			6		
Vitamins			7		
Minerals				8	
Overall			5		

MEATBALL, MEATLESS, VEGETARIAN

Serving: 1 meatball (.64 oz)   **Meat**

Calories	36	(56.3 cal/oz)	Carbohydrate	1.44 g	(0% DV)
Fat Calories	15	(41% fat)	Dietary Fiber	.9 g	(4% DV)
Total Fat	1.62 g	(2% DV)	Protein	3.78 g	(8% DV)
Saturated Fat	.18 g	(1% DV)	Vitamin A	0 IU	(0% DV)
Poly Fat	.9 g		Vitamin C	0 mg	(0% DV)
Mono Fat	.36 g		Calcium	5.2 mg	(1% DV)
Cholesterol	0 mg	(0% DV)	Iron	.4 mg	(2% DV)
Sodium	99 mg	(4% DV)	Folate	3.8 mcg	(4% DV)
Potassium	32.4 mg	(1% DV)	Beta Carotene	0 RE	

Ratings

	Worst	Bad	Average	Good	Best
Weight Loss				7	
LowCal Density			5		
Filling	2				
Energizing	2				
Fiber		4			
Vitamins			5		
Minerals		3			
Overall			5		

MELBA TOAST

Serving: 1 piece (.18 oz)   **Snack**

Calories	19	(108.1 cal/oz)	Carbohydrate	3.79 g	(1% DV)
Fat Calories	2	(12% fat)	Dietary Fiber	.35 g	(1% DV)
Total Fat	.25 g	(0% DV)	Protein	.6 g	(1% DV)
Saturated Fat	.05 g	(0% DV)	Vitamin A	0 IU	(0% DV)
Poly Fat	.05 g		Vitamin C	0 mg	(0% DV)
Mono Fat	.1 g		Calcium	5.4 mg	(1% DV)
Cholesterol	0 mg	(0% DV)	Iron	.1 mg	(1% DV)
Sodium	41.3 mg	(2% DV)	Folate	.6 mcg	(0% DV)
Potassium	11.3 mg	(0% DV)	Beta Carotene	0 RE	

Ratings

	Worst	Bad	Average	Good	Best
Weight Loss					9
LowCal Density	2				
Filling	2				
Energizing		3			
Fiber	2				
Vitamins	2				
Minerals	2				
Overall		4			

MEXICAN CASSEROLE, GROUND BEEF, BEANS, TOMATO

Serving: 1 cup (5.14 oz)   **Entree**

Calories	315	(61.4 cal/oz)	Carbohydrate	20.16 g	(7% DV)
Fat Calories	168	(53% fat)	Dietary Fiber	2.88 g	(12% DV)
Total Fat	18.72 g	(29% DV)	Protein	15.84 g	(32% DV)
Saturated Fat	7.2 g	(36% DV)	Vitamin A	485.3 IU	(10% DV)
Poly Fat	2.88 g		Vitamin C	4.3 mg	(7% DV)
Mono Fat	7.2 g		Calcium	100.8 mg	(10% DV)
Cholesterol	46.1 mg	(15% DV)	Iron	2.5 mg	(14% DV)
Sodium	309.6 mg	(13% DV)	Folate	15.8 mcg	(13% DV)
Potassium	400.3 mg	(11% DV)	Beta Carotene	43.2 RE	

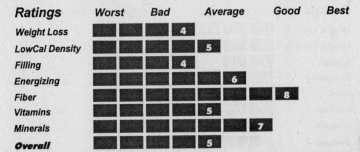

Ratings	Worst	Bad	Average	Good	Best
Weight Loss			4		
LowCal Density			5		
Filling			4		
Energizing			6		
Fiber				8	
Vitamins			5		
Minerals			7		
Overall			5		

MILK DESSERT, FROZEN, FAT FREE, WITH SIMPLESSE

Serving: 1 cup (6.39 oz)   **Dessert**

Calories	240	(37.5 cal/oz)	Carbohydrate	44.75 g	(15% DV)
Fat Calories	0	(0% fat)	Dietary Fiber	1.79 g	(7% DV)
Total Fat	0 g	(0% DV)	Protein	16.11 g	(32% DV)
Saturated Fat	0 g	(0% DV)	Vitamin A	111 IU	(2% DV)
Poly Fat	0 g		Vitamin C	1.8 mg	(3% DV)
Mono Fat	0 g		Calcium	186.2 mg	(19% DV)
Cholesterol	30.4 mg	(10% DV)	Iron	.3 mg	(1% DV)
Sodium	130.7 mg	(5% DV)	Folate	16.1 mcg	(3% DV)
Potassium	401 mg	(11% DV)	Beta Carotene	0 RE	

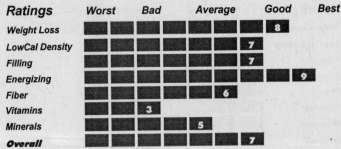

Ratings	Worst	Bad	Average	Good	Best
Weight Loss				8	
LowCal Density				7	
Filling				7	
Energizing					9
Fiber			6		
Vitamins		3			
Minerals			5		
Overall				7	

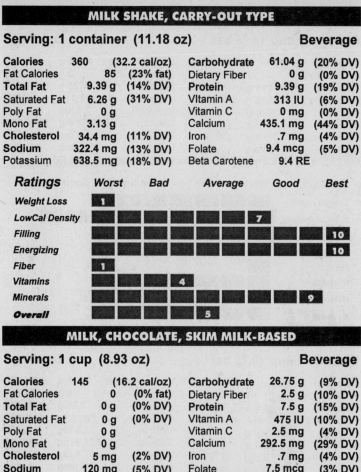

MILK SHAKE, CARRY-OUT TYPE

Serving: 1 container (11.18 oz)   **Beverage**

Calories	360	(32.2 cal/oz)	Carbohydrate	61.04 g	(20% DV)
Fat Calories	85	(23% fat)	Dietary Fiber	0 g	(0% DV)
Total Fat	9.39 g	(14% DV)	Protein	9.39 g	(19% DV)
Saturated Fat	6.26 g	(31% DV)	Vitamin A	313 IU	(6% DV)
Poly Fat	0 g		Vitamin C	0 mg	(0% DV)
Mono Fat	3.13 g		Calcium	435.1 mg	(44% DV)
Cholesterol	34.4 mg	(11% DV)	Iron	.7 mg	(4% DV)
Sodium	322.4 mg	(13% DV)	Folate	9.4 mcg	(5% DV)
Potassium	638.5 mg	(18% DV)	Beta Carotene	9.4 RE	

Ratings	Worst	Bad	Average	Good	Best
Weight Loss	1				
LowCal Density			7		
Filling					10
Energizing					10
Fiber	1				
Vitamins		4			
Minerals					9
Overall			5		

MILK, CHOCOLATE, SKIM MILK-BASED

Serving: 1 cup (8.93 oz)   **Beverage**

Calories	145	(16.2 cal/oz)	Carbohydrate	26.75 g	(9% DV)
Fat Calories	0	(0% fat)	Dietary Fiber	2.5 g	(10% DV)
Total Fat	0 g	(0% DV)	Protein	7.5 g	(15% DV)
Saturated Fat	0 g	(0% DV)	Vitamin A	475 IU	(10% DV)
Poly Fat	0 g		Vitamin C	2.5 mg	(4% DV)
Mono Fat	0 g		Calcium	292.5 mg	(29% DV)
Cholesterol	5 mg	(2% DV)	Iron	.7 mg	(4% DV)
Sodium	120 mg	(5% DV)	Folate	7.5 mcg	(3% DV)
Potassium	485 mg	(14% DV)	Beta Carotene	0 RE	

Ratings	Worst	Bad	Average	Good	Best
Weight Loss			6		
LowCal Density				9	
Filling				9	
Energizing			7		
Fiber			7		
Vitamins		4			
Minerals			7		
Overall			7		

MILK, COW'S, FLUID, 1% FAT

Serving: 1 cup (8.75 oz)   **Beverage**

Calories	103	(11.8 cal/oz)	Carbohydrate	11.76 g	(4% DV)
Fat Calories	22	(21% fat)	Dietary Fiber	0 g	(0% DV)
Total Fat	2.45 g	(4% DV)	Protein	7.35 g	(15% DV)
Saturated Fat	2.45 g	(12% DV)	Vitamin A	502.3 IU	(10% DV)
Poly Fat	0 g		Vitamin C	2.5 mg	(4% DV)
Mono Fat	0 g		Calcium	301.4 mg	(30% DV)
Cholesterol	9.8 mg	(3% DV)	Iron	.1 mg	(1% DV)
Sodium	125 mg	(5% DV)	Folate	7.4 mcg	(3% DV)
Potassium	382.2 mg	(11% DV)	Beta Carotene	2.5 RE	

Ratings	Worst	Bad	Average	Good	Best
Weight Loss			6		
LowCal Density					9
Filling			7		
Energizing		5			
Fiber	1				
Vitamins		4			
Minerals			7		
Overall			7		

MILK, COW'S, FLUID, 2% FAT

Serving: 1 cup (8.75 oz)   **Beverage**

Calories	123	(14 cal/oz)	Carbohydrate	11.76 g	(4% DV)
Fat Calories	44	(36% fat)	Dietary Fiber	0 g	(0% DV)
Total Fat	4.9 g	(8% DV)	Protein	7.35 g	(15% DV)
Saturated Fat	2.45 g	(12% DV)	Vitamin A	502.3 IU	(10% DV)
Poly Fat	0 g		Vitamin C	2.5 mg	(4% DV)
Mono Fat	2.45 g		Calcium	298.9 mg	(30% DV)
Cholesterol	19.6 mg	(7% DV)	Iron	.1 mg	(1% DV)
Sodium	122.5 mg	(5% DV)	Folate	7.4 mcg	(3% DV)
Potassium	377.3 mg	(11% DV)	Beta Carotene	4.9 RE	

Ratings	Worst	Bad	Average	Good	Best
Weight Loss		4			
LowCal Density					9
Filling			6		
Energizing		5			
Fiber	1				
Vitamins		4			
Minerals			7		
Overall			6		

MILK, COW'S, FLUID, SKIM OR NONFAT

Serving: 1 cup (8.75 oz)   **Beverage**

Calories	86	(9.8 cal/oz)	Carbohydrate	12.01 g	(4% DV)
Fat Calories	0	(0% fat)	Dietary Fiber	0 g	(0% DV)
Total Fat	0 g	(0% DV)	Protein	7.35 g	(15% DV)
Saturated Fat	0 g	(0% DV)	Vitamin A	499.8 IU	(10% DV)
Poly Fat	0 g		Vitamin C	2.5 mg	(4% DV)
Mono Fat	0 g		Calcium	301.4 mg	(30% DV)
Cholesterol	4.9 mg	(2% DV)	Iron	.1 mg	(1% DV)
Sodium	127.4 mg	(5% DV)	Folate	7.4 mcg	(3% DV)
Potassium	406.7 mg	(12% DV)	Beta Carotene	0 RE	

Ratings	Worst	Bad	Average	Good	Best
Weight Loss				8	
LowCal Density					9
Filling			7		
Energizing			5		
Fiber	1				
Vitamins		4			
Minerals				7	
Overall				7	

MILK, COW'S, FLUID, WHOLE

Serving: 1 cup (8.71 oz)   **Beverage**

Calories	149	(17.1 cal/oz)	Carbohydrate	11.47 g	(4% DV)
Fat Calories	66	(44% fat)	Dietary Fiber	0 g	(0% DV)
Total Fat	7.32 g	(11% DV)	Protein	7.32 g	(15% DV)
Saturated Fat	4.88 g	(24% DV)	Vitamin A	307.4 IU	(6% DV)
Poly Fat	0 g		Vitamin C	2.4 mg	(4% DV)
Mono Fat	2.44 g		Calcium	290.4 mg	(29% DV)
Cholesterol	34.2 mg	(11% DV)	Iron	.1 mg	(1% DV)
Sodium	119.6 mg	(5% DV)	Folate	7.3 mcg	(3% DV)
Potassium	370.9 mg	(11% DV)	Beta Carotene	7.3 RE	

Ratings	Worst	Bad	Average	Good	Best
Weight Loss	3				
LowCal Density				8	
Filling			6		
Energizing			5		
Fiber	1				
Vitamins		4			
Minerals				7	
Overall			5		

MILK, MALTED, UNFORTIFIED, MADE WITH MILK

Serving: 1 cup (8.39 oz)   **Beverage**

Calories	202	(24.1 cal/oz)	Carbohydrate	26.32 g	(9% DV)
Fat Calories	63	(31% fat)	Dietary Fiber	0 g	(0% DV)
Total Fat	7.05 g	(11% DV)	Protein	7.05 g	(14% DV)
Saturated Fat	4.7 g	(24% DV)	Vitamin A	289.1 IU	(6% DV)
Poly Fat	0 g		Vitamin C	2.4 mg	(4% DV)
Mono Fat	2.35 g		Calcium	270.3 mg	(27% DV)
Cholesterol	30.6 mg	(10% DV)	Iron	.5 mg	(3% DV)
Sodium	152.8 mg	(6% DV)	Folate	7.1 mcg	(4% DV)
Potassium	441.8 mg	(13% DV)	Beta Carotene	7.1 RE	

Ratings	Worst	Bad	Average	Good	Best
Weight Loss	2				
LowCal Density					8
Filling				7	
Energizing				7	
Fiber	1				
Vitamins			4		
Minerals				7	
Overall			5		

MIXED NUTS, DRY ROASTED

Serving: about 20 assorted (1 oz)   **Snack**

Calories	166	(166.3 cal/oz)	Carbohydrate	7.11 g	(2% DV)
Fat Calories	129	(77% fat)	Dietary Fiber	2.52 g	(10% DV)
Total Fat	14.28 g	(22% DV)	Protein	4.76 g	(10% DV)
Saturated Fat	1.96 g	(10% DV)	Vitamin A	4.2 IU	(0% DV)
Poly Fat	3.08 g		Vitamin C	0 mg	(0% DV)
Mono Fat	8.68 g		Calcium	19.6 mg	(2% DV)
Cholesterol	0 mg	(0% DV)	Iron	1 mg	(6% DV)
Sodium	187.3 mg	(8% DV)	Folate	4.8 mcg	(4% DV)
Potassium	167.2 mg	(5% DV)	Beta Carotene	.3 RE	

Ratings	Worst	Bad	Average	Good	Best
Weight Loss		3			
LowCal Density	1				
Filling	2				
Energizing			4		
Fiber				7	
Vitamins		3			
Minerals			5		
Overall		3			

280   **Edmund's Food Ratings**

MIXED NUTS, ROASTED, WITH PEANUTS

Serving: about 20 assorted (1 oz) **Snack**

Calories	173	(172.8 cal/oz)	Carbohydrate	5.99 g	(2% DV)
Fat Calories	141	(82% fat)	Dietary Fiber	2.52 g	(10% DV)
Total Fat	15.68 g	(24% DV)	Protein	4.76 g	(10% DV)
Saturated Fat	2.52 g	(13% DV)	Vitamin A	5.3 IU	(0% DV)
Poly Fat	3.64 g		Vitamin C	.3 mg	(0% DV)
Mono Fat	8.96 g		Calcium	30.2 mg	(3% DV)
Cholesterol	0 mg	(0% DV)	Iron	.9 mg	(5% DV)
Sodium	182.6 mg	(8% DV)	Folate	4.8 mcg	(6% DV)
Potassium	162.7 mg	(5% DV)	Beta Carotene	.6 RE	

Ratings	Worst	Bad	Average	Good	Best
Weight Loss		2			
LowCal Density	1				
Filling		2			
Energizing			3		
Fiber					7
Vitamins			4		
Minerals			5		
Overall			3		

MOO GOO GAI PAN

Serving: 1 cup (7.71 oz) **Entree**

Calories	281	(36.4 cal/oz)	Carbohydrate	11.88 g	(4% DV)
Fat Calories	175	(62% fat)	Dietary Fiber	2.16 g	(9% DV)
Total Fat	19.44 g	(30% DV)	Protein	15.12 g	(30% DV)
Saturated Fat	4.32 g	(22% DV)	Vitamin A	1317.6 IU	(26% DV)
Poly Fat	6.48 g		Vitamin C	34.6 mg	(58% DV)
Mono Fat	6.48 g		Calcium	129.6 mg	(13% DV)
Cholesterol	38.9 mg	(13% DV)	Iron	1.6 mg	(9% DV)
Sodium	326.2 mg	(14% DV)	Folate	15.1 mcg	(11% DV)
Potassium	475.2 mg	(14% DV)	Beta Carotene	103.7 RE	

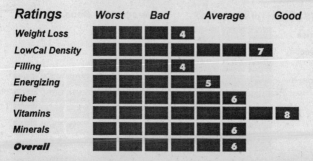

Ratings	Worst	Bad	Average	Good	Best
Weight Loss			4		
LowCal Density				7	
Filling			4		
Energizing			5		
Fiber			6		
Vitamins					8
Minerals			6		
Overall			6		

MOO SHI PORK

Serving: 1 cup (5.39 oz)　　　　　　　　　**Entree**

Calories	512	(95 cal/oz)	Carbohydrate	5.44 g	(2% DV)
Fat Calories	421	(82% fat)	Dietary Fiber	0 g	(0% DV)
Total Fat	46.81 g	(72% DV)	Protein	18.12 g	(36% DV)
Saturated Fat	7.55 g	(38% DV)	VItamin A	206.9 IU	(4% DV)
Poly Fat	24.16 g		Vitamin C	9.1 mg	(15% DV)
Mono Fat	12.08 g		Calcium	30.2 mg	(3% DV)
Cholesterol	172.1 mg	(57% DV)	Iron	1.4 mg	(8% DV)
Sodium	1020.8 mg	(43% DV)	Folate	18.1 mcg	(5% DV)
Potassium	327.7 mg	(9% DV)	Beta Carotene	1.5 RE	

Ratings	Worst	Bad	Average	Good	Best
Weight Loss	2				
LowCal Density	3				
Filling	2				
Energizing	3				
Fiber	1				
Vitamins			6		
Minerals			6		
Overall	3				

MUESLIX BRAN MUESLI

Serving: 1 cup (2.93 oz)　　　　　　　　　**Cereal**

Calories	262	(89.6 cal/oz)	Carbohydrate	63.14 g	(21% DV)
Fat Calories	22	(8% fat)	Dietary Fiber	12.3 g	(49% DV)
Total Fat	2.46 g	(4% DV)	Protein	8.2 g	(16% DV)
Saturated Fat	0 g	(0% DV)	VItamin A	2494.4 IU	(50% DV)
Poly Fat	.82 g		Vitamin C	.8 mg	(1% DV)
Mono Fat	.82 g		Calcium	55.8 mg	(6% DV)
Cholesterol	0 mg	(0% DV)	Iron	14.4 mg	(80% DV)
Sodium	205 mg	(9% DV)	Folate	8.2 mcg	(49% DV)
Potassium	467.4 mg	(13% DV)	Beta Carotene	0 RE	

Ratings	Worst	Bad	Average	Good	Best
Weight Loss			5		
LowCal Density	3				
Filling			6		
Energizing					10
Fiber					10
Vitamins					10
Minerals					10
Overall			6		

MUFFIN, BRAN

Serving: 1 muffin (2-5/8" dia) (1.79 oz)   **Bakery**

Calories	127	(71 cal/oz)	Carbohydrate	20.4 g	(7% DV)
Fat Calories	45	(35% fat)	Dietary Fiber	5.5 g	(22% DV)
Total Fat	5 g	(8% DV)	Protein	4.5 g	(9% DV)
Saturated Fat	1.5 g	(8% DV)	Vitamin A	77 IU	(2% DV)
Poly Fat	1 g		Vitamin C	0 mg	(0% DV)
Mono Fat	2 g		Calcium	105.5 mg	(11% DV)
Cholesterol	37.5 mg	(12% DV)	Iron	2.1 mg	(12% DV)
Sodium	176 mg	(7% DV)	Folate	4.5 mcg	(3% DV)
Potassium	270 mg	(8% DV)	Beta Carotene	.5 RE	

Ratings	Worst	Bad	Average	Good	Best
Weight Loss			5		
LowCal Density		4			
Filling		4			
Energizing			6		
Fiber					9
Vitamins		4			
Minerals				7	
Overall			5		

MUFFIN, BRAN WITH FRUIT, LOW FAT, NO CHOLESTEROL

Serving: 1 muffin (2-3/4" diameter) (2.07 oz)   **Bakery**

Calories	137	(66.1 cal/oz)	Carbohydrate	30.86 g	(10% DV)
Fat Calories	26	(19% fat)	Dietary Fiber	6.38 g	(26% DV)
Total Fat	2.9 g	(4% DV)	Protein	2.9 g	(6% DV)
Saturated Fat	.58 g	(3% DV)	Vitamin A	12.8 IU	(0% DV)
Poly Fat	1.16 g		Vitamin C	0 mg	(0% DV)
Mono Fat	1.16 g		Calcium	60.3 mg	(6% DV)
Cholesterol	9.3 mg	(3% DV)	Iron	1.3 mg	(7% DV)
Sodium	167 mg	(7% DV)	Folate	2.9 mcg	(1% DV)
Potassium	129.9 mg	(4% DV)	Beta Carotene	.6 RE	

Ratings	Worst	Bad	Average	Good	Best
Weight Loss			6		
LowCal Density			5		
Filling			5		
Energizing			7		
Fiber					10
Vitamins	3				
Minerals			5		
Overall			6		

MUFFIN, CARROT

Serving: 1 muffin (2-5/8" dia) (2.07 oz) **Bakery**

Calories	176	(85.2 cal/oz)	Carbohydrate	25.81 g	(9% DV)
Fat Calories	63	(36% fat)	Dietary Fiber	1.16 g	(5% DV)
Total Fat	6.96 g	(11% DV)	Protein	3.48 g	(7% DV)
Saturated Fat	1.16 g	(6% DV)	Vitamin A	2494 IU	(50% DV)
Poly Fat	3.48 g		Vitamin C	1.2 mg	(2% DV)
Mono Fat	1.74 g		Calcium	82.4 mg	(8% DV)
Cholesterol	18 mg	(6% DV)	Iron	1.2 mg	(7% DV)
Sodium	251.1 mg	(10% DV)	Folate	3.5 mcg	(2% DV)
Potassium	111.9 mg	(3% DV)	Beta Carotene	242.4 RE	

Ratings	Worst	Bad	Average	Good	Best
Weight Loss			4		
LowCal Density		3			
Filling			4		
Energizing				6	
Fiber			4		
Vitamins				6	
Minerals			4		
Overall			4		

MUFFIN, CHOCOLATE CHIP

Serving: 1 muffin (2-5/8" dia) (2.07 oz) **Bakery**

Calories	190	(91.9 cal/oz)	Carbohydrate	26.56 g	(9% DV)
Fat Calories	68	(36% fat)	Dietary Fiber	1.16 g	(5% DV)
Total Fat	7.54 g	(12% DV)	Protein	4.06 g	(8% DV)
Saturated Fat	2.9 g	(14% DV)	Vitamin A	63.8 IU	(1% DV)
Poly Fat	1.16 g		Vitamin C	0 mg	(0% DV)
Mono Fat	2.9 g		Calcium	74.2 mg	(7% DV)
Cholesterol	24.4 mg	(8% DV)	Iron	1.4 mg	(8% DV)
Sodium	185.6 mg	(8% DV)	Folate	4.1 mcg	(2% DV)
Potassium	91.6 mg	(3% DV)	Beta Carotene	.6 RE	

Ratings	Worst	Bad	Average	Good	Best
Weight Loss		3			
LowCal Density		3			
Filling			4		
Energizing				7	
Fiber			4		
Vitamins			4		
Minerals			4		
Overall			4		

MUFFIN, FRUIT AND/OR NUTS

Serving: 1 muffin (2-5/8" dia) (2.07 oz)   **Bakery**

Calories	165	(79.6 cal/oz)	Carbohydrate	25.35 g	(8% DV)
Fat Calories	47	(29% fat)	Dietary Fiber	.58 g	(2% DV)
Total Fat	5.22 g	(8% DV)	Protein	4.06 g	(8% DV)
Saturated Fat	1.74 g	(9% DV)	Vitamin A	84.1 IU	(2% DV)
Poly Fat	1.16 g		Vitamin C	0 mg	(0% DV)
Mono Fat	1.74 g		Calcium	81.2 mg	(8% DV)
Cholesterol	38.9 mg	(13% DV)	Iron	1.2 mg	(7% DV)
Sodium	326.5 mg	(14% DV)	Folate	4.1 mcg	(2% DV)
Potassium	71.3 mg	(2% DV)	Beta Carotene	1.2 RE	

Ratings	Worst	Bad	Average	Good	Best
Weight Loss				5	
LowCal Density			4		
Filling			4		
Energizing				6	
Fiber		3			
Vitamins			4		
Minerals			4		
Overall			4		

MUFFIN, FRUIT, REDUCED FAT, NO CHOLESTEROL

Serving: 1 muffin (2-5/8" dia) (2.07 oz)   **Bakery**

Calories	152	(73.4 cal/oz)	Carbohydrate	34.28 g	(11% DV)
Fat Calories	5	(3% fat)	Dietary Fiber	1.74 g	(7% DV)
Total Fat	.58 g	(1% DV)	Protein	3.48 g	(7% DV)
Saturated Fat	0 g	(0% DV)	Vitamin A	30.2 IU	(1% DV)
Poly Fat	0 g		Vitamin C	.6 mg	(1% DV)
Mono Fat	0 g		Calcium	77.7 mg	(8% DV)
Cholesterol	0 mg	(0% DV)	Iron	1.4 mg	(8% DV)
Sodium	251.7 mg	(10% DV)	Folate	3.5 mcg	(2% DV)
Potassium	60.9 mg	(2% DV)	Beta Carotene	.6 RE	

Ratings	Worst	Bad	Average	Good	Best
Weight Loss				7	
LowCal Density			4		
Filling			5		
Energizing				8	
Fiber			6		
Vitamins			4		
Minerals			5		
Overall			6		

MUFFIN, OATMEAL

Serving: 1 muffin (2-5/8" dia) (1.68 oz)   **Bakery**

Calories	112	(66.6 cal/oz)	Carbohydrate	17.39 g	(6% DV)
Fat Calories	30	(26% fat)	Dietary Fiber	.94 g	(4% DV)
Total Fat	**3.29 g**	**(5% DV)**	Protein	3.29 g	(7% DV)
Saturated Fat	.94 g	(5% DV)	Vitamin A	48.4 IU	(1% DV)
Poly Fat	.47 g		Vitamin C	0 mg	(0% DV)
Mono Fat	1.41 g		Calcium	68.6 mg	(7% DV)
Cholesterol	**18.3 mg**	**(6% DV)**	Iron	1 mg	(5% DV)
Sodium	**160.7 mg**	**(7% DV)**	Folate	3.3 mcg	(1% DV)
Potassium	58.3 mg	(2% DV)	Beta Carotene	.5 RE	

Ratings	Worst	Bad	Average	Good	Best
Weight Loss				6	
LowCal Density			5		
Filling		4			
Energizing				6	
Fiber		4			
Vitamins	3				
Minerals		4			
Overall			5		

MUFFIN, WHOLE WHEAT

Serving: 1 muffin (2-5/8" dia) (1.68 oz)   **Bakery**

Calories	142	(84.5 cal/oz)	Carbohydrate	20.02 g	(7% DV)
Fat Calories	51	(36% fat)	Dietary Fiber	2.35 g	(9% DV)
Total Fat	**5.64 g**	**(9% DV)**	Protein	3.76 g	(8% DV)
Saturated Fat	1.88 g	(9% DV)	Vitamin A	52.6 IU	(1% DV)
Poly Fat	1.41 g		Vitamin C	0 mg	(0% DV)
Mono Fat	2.35 g		Calcium	89.3 mg	(9% DV)
Cholesterol	**20.7 mg**	**(7% DV)**	Iron	.9 mg	(5% DV)
Sodium	**283.4 mg**	**(12% DV)**	Folate	3.8 mcg	(2% DV)
Potassium	119.4 mg	(3% DV)	Beta Carotene	.5 RE	

Ratings	Worst	Bad	Average	Good	Best
Weight Loss			5		
LowCal Density		3			
Filling		4			
Energizing				6	
Fiber				6	
Vitamins		3			
Minerals			5		
Overall			4		

MUNG BEANS, COOKED WITHOUT ADDED FAT

Serving: 1 cup (7.14 oz)   **Vegetable**

Calories	224	(31.4 cal/oz)	Carbohydrate	40.4 g	(13% DV)
Fat Calories	0	(0% fat)	Dietary Fiber	10 g	(40% DV)
Total Fat	0 g	(0% DV)	Protein	16 g	(32% DV)
Saturated Fat	0 g	(0% DV)	Vitamin A	62 IU	(1% DV)
Poly Fat	0 g		Vitamin C	2 mg	(3% DV)
Mono Fat	0 g		Calcium	76 mg	(8% DV)
Cholesterol	0 mg	(0% DV)	Iron	3.5 mg	(19% DV)
Sodium	464 mg	(19% DV)	Folate	16 mcg	(46% DV)
Potassium	564 mg	(16% DV)	Beta Carotene	6 RE	

Ratings	Worst	Bad	Average	Good	Best
Weight Loss		4			
LowCal Density			7		
Filling				9	
Energizing				9	
Fiber					10
Vitamins			6		
Minerals			7		
Overall			7		

MUSHROOM SOUP, CREAM OF, PREPARED WITH MILK

Serving: 1 cup (8.86 oz)   **Soup**

Calories	203	(23 cal/oz)	Carbohydrate	15.13 g	(5% DV)
Fat Calories	112	(55% fat)	Dietary Fiber	0 g	(0% DV)
Total Fat	12.4 g	(19% DV)	Protein	4.96 g	(10% DV)
Saturated Fat	4.96 g	(25% DV)	Vitamin A	153.8 IU	(3% DV)
Poly Fat	4.96 g		Vitamin C	2.5 mg	(4% DV)
Mono Fat	2.48 g		Calcium	178.6 mg	(18% DV)
Cholesterol	19.8 mg	(7% DV)	Iron	.6 mg	(3% DV)
Sodium	1076.3 mg	(45% DV)	Folate	5 mcg	(2% DV)
Potassium	270.3 mg	(8% DV)	Beta Carotene	0 RE	

Ratings	Worst	Bad	Average	Good	Best
Weight Loss	3				
LowCal Density				8	
Filling			6		
Energizing		5			
Fiber	1				
Vitamins		4			
Minerals		5			
Overall		5			

MUSHROOMS, BATTER-DIPPED, FRIED

Serving: 6 medium (3 oz)   **Vegetable**

Calories	177	(59.1 cal/oz)	Carbohydrate	9.91 g	(3% DV)
Fat Calories	129	(73% fat)	Dietary Fiber	.84 g	(3% DV)
Total Fat	14.28 g	(22% DV)	Protein	2.52 g	(5% DV)
Saturated Fat	2.52 g	(13% DV)	Vitamin A	42 IU	(1% DV)
Poly Fat	7.56 g		Vitamin C	1.7 mg	(3% DV)
Mono Fat	3.36 g		Calcium	64.7 mg	(6% DV)
Cholesterol	16.8 mg	(6% DV)	Iron	.9 mg	(5% DV)
Sodium	144.5 mg	(6% DV)	Folate	2.5 mcg	(2% DV)
Potassium	215.9 mg	(6% DV)	Beta Carotene	.8 RE	

Ratings	Worst	Bad	Average	Good	Best
Weight Loss	2				
LowCal Density				5	
Filling		3			
Energizing			4		
Fiber			4		
Vitamins			4		
Minerals			4		
Overall			4		

MUSHROOMS, COOKED WITHOUT ADDED FAT

Serving: 8 caps (1.68 oz)   **Vegetable**

Calories	13	(7.6 cal/oz)	Carbohydrate	2.4 g	(1% DV)
Fat Calories	0	(0% fat)	Dietary Fiber	.94 g	(4% DV)
Total Fat	0 g	(0% DV)	Protein	.94 g	(2% DV)
Saturated Fat	0 g	(0% DV)	Vitamin A	0 IU	(0% DV)
Poly Fat	0 g		Vitamin C	1.9 mg	(3% DV)
Mono Fat	0 g		Calcium	2.8 mg	(0% DV)
Cholesterol	0 mg	(0% DV)	Iron	.8 mg	(5% DV)
Sodium	109.5 mg	(5% DV)	Folate	.9 mcg	(2% DV)
Potassium	166.4 mg	(5% DV)	Beta Carotene	0 RE	

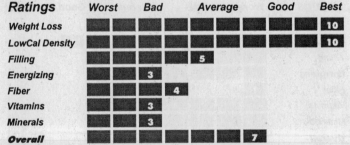

Ratings	Worst	Bad	Average	Good	Best
Weight Loss					10
LowCal Density					10
Filling			5		
Energizing		3			
Fiber		4			
Vitamins		3			
Minerals		3			
Overall				7	

MUSHROOMS, RAW

Serving: 1 medium (.64 oz)   **Vegetable**

Calories	5	(7 cal/oz)	Carbohydrate	.85 g	(0% DV)
Fat Calories	0	(0% fat)	Dietary Fiber	.18 g	(1% DV)
Total Fat	0 g	(0% DV)	Protein	.36 g	(1% DV)
Saturated Fat	0 g	(0% DV)	Vitamin A	0 IU	(0% DV)
Poly Fat	0 g		Vitamin C	.7 mg	(1% DV)
Mono Fat	0 g		Calcium	.9 mg	(0% DV)
Cholesterol	0 mg	(0% DV)	Iron	.2 mg	(1% DV)
Sodium	.7 mg	(0% DV)	Folate	.4 mcg	(1% DV)
Potassium	66.6 mg	(2% DV)	Beta Carotene	0 RE	

Ratings	Worst	Bad	Average	Good	Best
Weight Loss					10
LowCal Density					10
Filling		3			
Energizing	2				
Fiber	2				
Vitamins	2				
Minerals	2				
Overall				7	

MUSSELS, STEAMED OR POACHED

Serving: 1 cup (5.36 oz)   **Shellfish**

Calories	258	(48.1 cal/oz)	Carbohydrate	11.1 g	(4% DV)
Fat Calories	54	(21% fat)	Dietary Fiber	0 g	(0% DV)
Total Fat	6 g	(9% DV)	Protein	36 g	(72% DV)
Saturated Fat	1.5 g	(8% DV)	Vitamin A	432 IU	(9% DV)
Poly Fat	1.5 g		Vitamin C	18 mg	(30% DV)
Mono Fat	1.5 g		Calcium	73.5 mg	(7% DV)
Cholesterol	84 mg	(28% DV)	Iron	10.7 mg	(59% DV)
Sodium	729 mg	(30% DV)	Folate	36 mcg	(24% DV)
Potassium	672 mg	(19% DV)	Beta Carotene	0 RE	

Ratings	Worst	Bad	Average	Good	Best
Weight Loss		3			
LowCal Density			6		
Filling		4			
Energizing			5		
Fiber	1				
Vitamins				7	
Minerals					9
Overall			5		

NACHOS WITH BEEF, BEANS, CHEESE, SOUR CREAM

Serving: 1 cup (6.46 oz)   **Entree**

Calories	576	(89.1 cal/oz)	Carbohydrate	46.34 g	(15% DV)
Fat Calories	326	(57% fat)	Dietary Fiber	5.43 g	(22% DV)
Total Fat	36.2 g	(56% DV)	Protein	19.91 g	(40% DV)
Saturated Fat	14.48 g	(72% DV)	VItamin A	615.4 IU	(12% DV)
Poly Fat	3.62 g		Vitamin C	5.4 mg	(9% DV)
Mono Fat	16.29 g		Calcium	324 mg	(32% DV)
Cholesterol	57.9 mg	(19% DV)	Iron	2.6 mg	(14% DV)
Sodium	600.9 mg	(25% DV)	Folate	19.9 mcg	(19% DV)
Potassium	438 mg	(13% DV)	Beta Carotene	29 RE	

Ratings	Worst	Bad	Average	Good	Best
Weight Loss	2				
LowCal Density	3				
Filling			5		
Energizing					9
Fiber					9
Vitamins			6		
Minerals					9
Overall			5		

NACHOS WITH CHEESE, MEATLESS, NO BEANS

Serving: 1 cup (2.07 oz)   **Entree**

Calories	249	(120.5 cal/oz)	Carbohydrate	10.61 g	(4% DV)
Fat Calories	162	(65% fat)	Dietary Fiber	1.16 g	(5% DV)
Total Fat	17.98 g	(28% DV)	Protein	11.6 g	(23% DV)
Saturated Fat	9.86 g	(49% DV)	VItamin A	475.6 IU	(10% DV)
Poly Fat	1.16 g		Vitamin C	0 mg	(0% DV)
Mono Fat	6.38 g		Calcium	327.1 mg	(33% DV)
Cholesterol	44.1 mg	(15% DV)	Iron	.5 mg	(3% DV)
Sodium	345.1 mg	(14% DV)	Folate	11.6 mcg	(2% DV)
Potassium	73.1 mg	(2% DV)	Beta Carotene	11.6 RE	

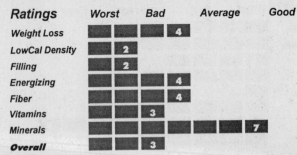

Ratings	Worst	Bad	Average	Good	Best
Weight Loss			4		
LowCal Density	2				
Filling	2				
Energizing			4		
Fiber			4		
Vitamins		3			
Minerals				7	
Overall		3			

NECTARINE, RAW

Serving: 1 fruit (2½" dia) (4.86 oz)

Fruit

Calories	67	(13.7 cal/oz)	Carbohydrate	16.05 g	(5% DV)
Fat Calories	0	(0% fat)	Dietary Fiber	2.72 g	(11% DV)
Total Fat	0 g	(0% DV)	Protein	1.36 g	(3% DV)
Saturated Fat	0 g	(0% DV)	Vitamin A	1001 IU	(20% DV)
Poly Fat	0 g		Vitamin C	6.8 mg	(11% DV)
Mono Fat	0 g		Calcium	6.8 mg	(1% DV)
Cholesterol	0 mg	(0% DV)	Iron	.2 mg	(1% DV)
Sodium	0 mg	(0% DV)	Folate	1.4 mcg	(1% DV)
Potassium	288.3 mg	(8% DV)	Beta Carotene	100.6 RE	

Ratings	Worst	Bad	Average	Good	Best
Weight Loss					9
LowCal Density					9
Filling				8	
Energizing			5		
Fiber				7	
Vitamins			5		
Minerals		3			
Overall				8	

NUT MIXTURE WITH DRIED FRUIT & SEEDS

Serving: 1 cup (5 oz)

Snack

Calories	701	(140.3 cal/oz)	Carbohydrate	54.88 g	(18% DV)
Fat Calories	454	(65% fat)	Dietary Fiber	9.8 g	(39% DV)
Total Fat	50.4 g	(78% DV)	Protein	22.4 g	(45% DV)
Saturated Fat	7 g	(35% DV)	Vitamin A	16.8 IU	(0% DV)
Poly Fat	21 g		Vitamin C	2.8 mg	(5% DV)
Mono Fat	21 g		Calcium	119 mg	(12% DV)
Cholesterol	0 mg	(0% DV)	Iron	3.9 mg	(22% DV)
Sodium	16.8 mg	(1% DV)	Folate	22.4 mcg	(30% DV)
Potassium	1006.6 mg	(29% DV)	Beta Carotene	1.4 RE	

Ratings	Worst	Bad	Average	Good	Best
Weight Loss	1				
LowCal Density	1				
Filling			5		
Energizing					10
Fiber					10
Vitamins				8	
Minerals				9	
Overall		4			

OATMEAL, COOKED

Serving: 1 cup (8.36 oz)

Cereal

Calories	145	(17.4 cal/oz)	Carbohydrate	25.27 g	(8% DV)
Fat Calories	21	(15% fat)	Dietary Fiber	4.68 g	(19% DV)
Total Fat	2.34 g	(4% DV)	Protein	7.02 g	(14% DV)
Saturated Fat	0 g	(0% DV)	Vitamin A	37.4 IU	(1% DV)
Poly Fat	0 g		Vitamin C	0 mg	(0% DV)
Mono Fat	0 g		Calcium	18.7 mg	(2% DV)
Cholesterol	0 mg	(0% DV)	Iron	1.6 mg	(9% DV)
Sodium	362.7 mg	(15% DV)	Folate	7 mcg	(2% DV)
Potassium	131 mg	(4% DV)	Beta Carotene	0 RE	

Ratings	Worst	Bad	Average	Good	Best
Weight Loss				7	
LowCal Density				8	
Filling					9
Energizing			6		
Fiber					9
Vitamins		4			
Minerals			6		
Overall				7	

OCEAN PERCH, BAKED OR BROILED

Serving: 1 piece (3.04 oz)

Fish

Calories	116	(38.3 cal/oz)	Carbohydrate	.34 g	(0% DV)
Fat Calories	38	(33% fat)	Dietary Fiber	0 g	(0% DV)
Total Fat	4.25 g	(7% DV)	Protein	18.7 g	(37% DV)
Saturated Fat	.85 g	(4% DV)	Vitamin A	166.6 IU	(3% DV)
Poly Fat	.85 g		Vitamin C	2.6 mg	(4% DV)
Mono Fat	1.7 g		Calcium	108 mg	(11% DV)
Cholesterol	41.7 mg	(14% DV)	Iron	.9 mg	(5% DV)
Sodium	336.6 mg	(14% DV)	Folate	18.7 mcg	(2% DV)
Potassium	276.3 mg	(8% DV)	Beta Carotene	2.6 RE	

Ratings	Worst	Bad	Average	Good	Best
Weight Loss			6		
LowCal Density			7		
Filling	1				
Energizing	2				
Fiber	1				
Vitamins		4			
Minerals			6		
Overall			5		

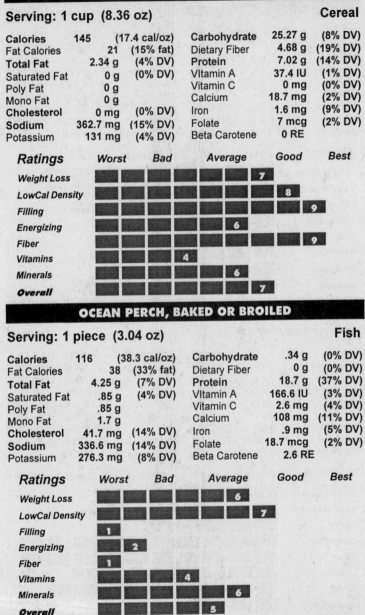

Edmund's Food Ratings

OCEAN PERCH, FLOURED OR BREADED, FRIED

Serving: 1 piece (3.04 oz)   **Fish**

Calories	187	(61.5 cal/oz)	Carbohydrate	6.72 g	(2% DV)
Fat Calories	92	(49% fat)	Dietary Fiber	0 g	(0% DV)
Total Fat	10.2 g	(16% DV)	Protein	17 g	(34% DV)
Saturated Fat	2.55 g	(13% DV)	VItamin A	57.8 IU	(1% DV)
Poly Fat	2.55 g		Vitamin C	.9 mg	(1% DV)
Mono Fat	4.25 g		Calcium	102 mg	(10% DV)
Cholesterol	53.6 mg	(18% DV)	Iron	1.2 mg	(7% DV)
Sodium	323.9 mg	(13% DV)	Folate	17 mcg	(3% DV)
Potassium	243.1 mg	(7% DV)	Beta Carotene	0 RE	

Ratings	Worst	Bad	Average	Good	Best
Weight Loss			4		
LowCal Density			5		
Filling	2				
Energizing			4		
Fiber	1				
Vitamins			4		
Minerals			5		
Overall			4		

OCTOPUS, COOKED

Serving: 1 piece (3.04 oz)   **Fish**

Calories	157	(51.7 cal/oz)	Carbohydrate	8.76 g	(3% DV)
Fat Calories	61	(39% fat)	Dietary Fiber	0 g	(0% DV)
Total Fat	6.8 g	(10% DV)	Protein	14.45 g	(29% DV)
Saturated Fat	1.7 g	(8% DV)	VItamin A	144.5 IU	(3% DV)
Poly Fat	1.7 g		Vitamin C	3.4 mg	(6% DV)
Mono Fat	2.55 g		Calcium	60.4 mg	(6% DV)
Cholesterol	60.4 mg	(20% DV)	Iron	4.9 mg	(27% DV)
Sodium	465.8 mg	(19% DV)	Folate	14.5 mcg	(4% DV)
Potassium	316.2 mg	(9% DV)	Beta Carotene	0 RE	

Ratings	Worst	Bad	Average	Good	Best
Weight Loss			4		
LowCal Density				6	
Filling		3			
Energizing			4		
Fiber	1				
Vitamins			4		
Minerals					7
Overall			4		

OKRA, COOKED WITHOUT ADDED FAT

Serving: 1 cup (6.57 oz)   **Vegetable**

Calories	63	(9.5 cal/oz)	Carbohydrate	11.78 g	(4% DV)
Fat Calories	0	(0% fat)	Dietary Fiber	5.52 g	(22% DV)
Total Fat	0 g	(0% DV)	Protein	3.68 g	(7% DV)
Saturated Fat	0 g	(0% DV)	Vitamin A	995.4 IU	(20% DV)
Poly Fat	0 g		Vitamin C	25.8 mg	(43% DV)
Mono Fat	0 g		Calcium	145.4 mg	(15% DV)
Cholesterol	0 mg	(0% DV)	Iron	1 mg	(6% DV)
Sodium	432.4 mg	(18% DV)	Folate	3.7 mcg	(44% DV)
Potassium	507.8 mg	(15% DV)	Beta Carotene	99.4 RE	

Ratings	Worst	Bad	Average	Good	Best
Weight Loss				9	
LowCal Density				9	
Filling				9	
Energizing			5		
Fiber				9	
Vitamins				8	
Minerals			6		
Overall				8	

OLIVE OIL

Serving: 1 tbsp (.48 oz)   **Fat & Oil**

Calories	119	(248.6 cal/oz)	Carbohydrate	0 g	(0% DV)
Fat Calories	122	(102% fat)	Dietary Fiber	0 g	(0% DV)
Total Fat	13.5 g	(21% DV)	Protein	0 g	(0% DV)
Saturated Fat	1.89 g	(9% DV)	Vitamin A	0 IU	(0% DV)
Poly Fat	1.08 g		Vitamin C	0 mg	(0% DV)
Mono Fat	9.99 g		Calcium	0 mg	(0% DV)
Cholesterol	0 mg	(0% DV)	Iron	.1 mg	(0% DV)
Sodium	0 mg	(0% DV)	Folate	0 mcg	(0% DV)
Potassium	0 mg	(0% DV)	Beta Carotene	0 RE	

Ratings	Worst	Bad	Average	Good	Best
Weight Loss	1				
LowCal Density	1				
Filling	1				
Energizing	1				
Fiber	1				
Vitamins		2			
Minerals		2			
Overall	1				

ONION RINGS, BATTER-DIPPED, FRIED

Serving: 1 fast food order (3.07 oz)   **Vegetable**

Calories	154	(50.1 cal/oz)	Carbohydrate	11.01 g	(4% DV)
Fat Calories	108	(70% fat)	Dietary Fiber	.86 g	(3% DV)
Total Fat	12.04 g	(19% DV)	Protein	1.72 g	(3% DV)
Saturated Fat	1.72 g	(9% DV)	VItamin A	33.5 IU	(1% DV)
Poly Fat	6.02 g		Vitamin C	2.6 mg	(4% DV)
Mono Fat	2.58 g		Calcium	61.1 mg	(6% DV)
Cholesterol	12.9 mg	(4% DV)	Iron	.4 mg	(2% DV)
Sodium	116.1 mg	(5% DV)	Folate	1.7 mcg	(2% DV)
Potassium	123 mg	(4% DV)	Beta Carotene	0 RE	

Ratings	Worst	Bad	Average	Good	Best
Weight Loss	2				
LowCal Density				6	
Filling			4		
Energizing			5		
Fiber			4		
Vitamins			4		
Minerals			4		
Overall			4		

ONION SOUP, FRENCH

Serving: 1 cup (8.61 oz)   **Soup**

Calories	58	(6.7 cal/oz)	Carbohydrate	8.19 g	(3% DV)
Fat Calories	22	(38% fat)	Dietary Fiber	0 g	(0% DV)
Total Fat	2.41 g	(4% DV)	Protein	4.82 g	(10% DV)
Saturated Fat	0 g	(0% DV)	VItamin A	0 IU	(0% DV)
Poly Fat	0 g		Vitamin C	2.4 mg	(4% DV)
Mono Fat	0 g		Calcium	26.5 mg	(3% DV)
Cholesterol	0 mg	(0% DV)	Iron	.7 mg	(4% DV)
Sodium	1053.2 mg	(44% DV)	Folate	4.8 mcg	(4% DV)
Potassium	67.5 mg	(2% DV)	Beta Carotene	0 RE	

Ratings	Worst	Bad	Average	Good	Best
Weight Loss				7	
LowCal Density					10
Filling				7	
Energizing			4		
Fiber	1				
Vitamins		3			
Minerals		3			
Overall				7	

ONION-FLAVORED RINGS

Serving: 10 rings (.36 oz) **Snack**

Calories	50	(138.9 cal/oz)	**Carbohydrate**	6.51 g	(2% DV)
Fat Calories	21	(41% fat)	Dietary Fiber	.4 g	(2% DV)
Total Fat	2.3 g	(4% DV)	**Protein**	.8 g	(2% DV)
Saturated Fat	.4 g	(2% DV)	VItamin A	12 IU	(0% DV)
Poly Fat	.3 g		Vitamin C	.2 mg	(0% DV)
Mono Fat	1.3 g		Calcium	2.9 mg	(0% DV)
Cholesterol	0 mg	(0% DV)	Iron	.4 mg	(2% DV)
Sodium	98.1 mg	(4% DV)	Folate	.8 mcg	(0% DV)
Potassium	14.3 mg	(0% DV)	Beta Carotene	1.2 RE	

Ratings	Worst	Bad	Average	Good	Best
Weight Loss					7
LowCal Density	1				
Filling	2				
Energizing			4		
Fiber		3			
Vitamins	2				
Minerals	2				
Overall		3			

ONIONS, MATURE, RAW

Serving: 1 slice (1/8" thick) (.5 oz) **Vegetable**

Calories	5	(10.6 cal/oz)	**Carbohydrate**	1.2 g	(0% DV)
Fat Calories	0	(0% fat)	Dietary Fiber	.28 g	(1% DV)
Total Fat	0 g	(0% DV)	**Protein**	.14 g	(0% DV)
Saturated Fat	0 g	(0% DV)	VItamin A	0 IU	(0% DV)
Poly Fat	0 g		Vitamin C	.8 mg	(1% DV)
Mono Fat	0 g		Calcium	2.8 mg	(0% DV)
Cholesterol	0 mg	(0% DV)	Iron	0 mg	(0% DV)
Sodium	.4 mg	(0% DV)	Folate	.1 mcg	(1% DV)
Potassium	22 mg	(1% DV)	Beta Carotene	0 RE	

Ratings	Worst	Bad	Average	Good	Best
Weight Loss					10
LowCal Density					9
Filling	2				
Energizing	2				
Fiber	2				
Vitamins	2				
Minerals	2				
Overall			6		

Edmund's Food Ratings

ONIONS, YOUNG GREEN, RAW

Serving: 1 medium (4-1/8" long) (.54 oz)   **Vegetable**

Calories	5	(8.9 cal/oz)	Carbohydrate	1.1 g	(0% DV)
Fat Calories	0	(0% fat)	Dietary Fiber	.3 g	(1% DV)
Total Fat	0 g	(0% DV)	Protein	.3 g	(1% DV)
Saturated Fat	0 g	(0% DV)	Vitamin A	57.8 IU	(1% DV)
Poly Fat	0 g		Vitamin C	2.9 mg	(5% DV)
Mono Fat	0 g		Calcium	10.8 mg	(1% DV)
Cholesterol	0 mg	(0% DV)	Iron	.2 mg	(1% DV)
Sodium	2.4 mg	(0% DV)	Folate	.3 mcg	(2% DV)
Potassium	41.4 mg	(1% DV)	Beta Carotene	5.9 RE	

Ratings	Worst	Bad	Average	Good	Best
Weight Loss					10
LowCal Density					9
Filling		3			
Energizing	2				
Fiber	2				
Vitamins		3			
Minerals	2				
Overall				7	

ORANGE JUICE, FROZEN, UNSWEETENED, + CALCIUM

Serving: 1 cup (8.89 oz)   **Beverage**

Calories	112	(12.6 cal/oz)	Carbohydrate	26.89 g	(9% DV)
Fat Calories	0	(0% fat)	Dietary Fiber	0 g	(0% DV)
Total Fat	0 g	(0% DV)	Protein	2.49 g	(5% DV)
Saturated Fat	0 g	(0% DV)	Vitamin A	194.2 IU	(4% DV)
Poly Fat	0 g		Vitamin C	97.1 mg	(162% DV)
Mono Fat	0 g		Calcium	301.3 mg	(30% DV)
Cholesterol	0 mg	(0% DV)	Iron	.3 mg	(1% DV)
Sodium	2.5 mg	(0% DV)	Folate	2.5 mcg	(27% DV)
Potassium	473.1 mg	(14% DV)	Beta Carotene	19.9 RE	

Ratings	Worst	Bad	Average	Good	Best
Weight Loss			7		
LowCal Density					9
Filling					10
Energizing			7		
Fiber	1				
Vitamins					9
Minerals		5			
Overall				8	

ORANGE JUICE, FROZEN, UNSWEETENED (RECONSTITUTED)

Serving: 1 cup (8.89 oz)   **Beverage**

Calories	112	(12.6 cal/oz)	Carbohydrate	26.89 g	(9% DV)
Fat Calories	0	(0% fat)	Dietary Fiber	0 g	(0% DV)
Total Fat	0 g	(0% DV)	Protein	2.49 g	(5% DV)
Saturated Fat	0 g	(0% DV)	Vitamin A	194.2 IU	(4% DV)
Poly Fat	0 g		Vitamin C	97.1 mg	(162% DV)
Mono Fat	0 g		Calcium	22.4 mg	(2% DV)
Cholesterol	0 mg	(0% DV)	Iron	.3 mg	(1% DV)
Sodium	2.5 mg	(0% DV)	Folate	2.5 mcg	(27% DV)
Potassium	473.1 mg	(14% DV)	Beta Carotene	19.9 RE	

Ratings	Worst	Bad	Average	Good	Best
Weight Loss				7	
LowCal Density				9	
Filling					10
Energizing				7	
Fiber	1				
Vitamins				9	
Minerals		3			
Overall				7	

ORANGE, RAW

Serving: 1 medium (2-5/8" dia) (4.68 oz)   **Fruit**

Calories	62	(13.2 cal/oz)	Carbohydrate	15.46 g	(5% DV)
Fat Calories	0	(0% fat)	Dietary Fiber	2.62 g	(10% DV)
Total Fat	0 g	(0% DV)	Protein	1.31 g	(3% DV)
Saturated Fat	0 g	(0% DV)	Vitamin A	268.6 IU	(5% DV)
Poly Fat	0 g		Vitamin C	69.4 mg	(116% DV)
Mono Fat	0 g		Calcium	52.4 mg	(5% DV)
Cholesterol	0 mg	(0% DV)	Iron	.1 mg	(1% DV)
Sodium	0 mg	(0% DV)	Folate	1.3 mcg	(10% DV)
Potassium	237.1 mg	(7% DV)	Beta Carotene	27.5 RE	

Ratings	Worst	Bad	Average	Good	Best
Weight Loss				9	
LowCal Density				9	
Filling				8	
Energizing			5		
Fiber				7	
Vitamins				8	
Minerals		3			
Overall				8	

OYSTER STEW

Serving: 1 cup (8.75 oz)   **Soup**

Calories	228	(26 cal/oz)	Carbohydrate	11.03 g	(4% DV)
Fat Calories	132	(58% fat)	Dietary Fiber	0 g	(0% DV)
Total Fat	14.7 g	(23% DV)	Protein	12.25 g	(24% DV)
Saturated Fat	9.8 g	(49% DV)	Vitamin A	725.2 IU	(15% DV)
Poly Fat	0 g		Vitamin C	4.9 mg	(8% DV)
Mono Fat	4.9 g		Calcium	240.1 mg	(24% DV)
Cholesterol	88.2 mg	(29% DV)	Iron	5.6 mg	(31% DV)
Sodium	850.2 mg	(35% DV)	Folate	12.3 mcg	(4% DV)
Potassium	445.9 mg	(13% DV)	Beta Carotene	12.3 RE	

Ratings   Worst   Bad   Average   Good   Best

Weight Loss	2
LowCal Density	8
Filling	5
Energizing	5
Fiber	1
Vitamins	5
Minerals	10
Overall	5

OYSTERS, CANNED

Serving: about 11 oysters (3.04 oz)   **Shellfish**

Calories	73	(24 cal/oz)	Carbohydrate	4.17 g	(1% DV)
Fat Calories	23	(31% fat)	Dietary Fiber	0 g	(0% DV)
Total Fat	2.55 g	(4% DV)	Protein	7.65 g	(15% DV)
Saturated Fat	.85 g	(4% DV)	Vitamin A	318.8 IU	(6% DV)
Poly Fat	.85 g		Vitamin C	5.1 mg	(8% DV)
Mono Fat	0 g		Calcium	47.6 mg	(5% DV)
Cholesterol	58.7 mg	(20% DV)	Iron	7.1 mg	(40% DV)
Sodium	119 mg	(5% DV)	Folate	7.7 mcg	(2% DV)
Potassium	243.1 mg	(7% DV)	Beta Carotene	0 RE	

Ratings   Worst   Bad   Average   Good   Best

Weight Loss	7
LowCal Density	8
Filling	3
Energizing	3
Fiber	1
Vitamins	5
Minerals	10
Overall	6

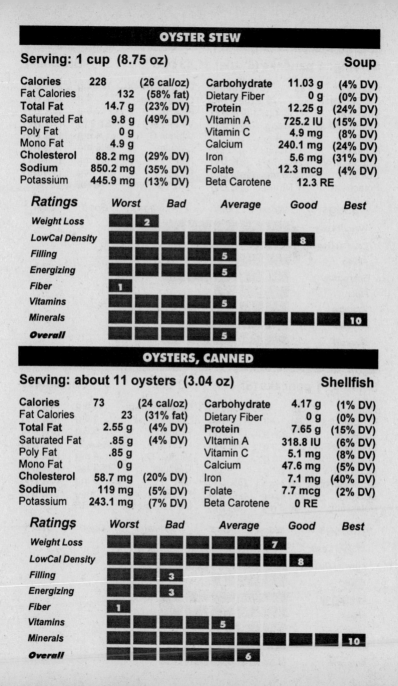

PANCAKES, PLAIN

Serving: 1 pancake (5" dia) (1.43 oz)   Breakfast

Calories	88	(61.5 cal/oz)	Carbohydrate	12.32 g	(4% DV)
Fat Calories	29	(33% fat)	Dietary Fiber	.4 g	(2% DV)
Total Fat	3.2 g	(5% DV)	Protein	2.8 g	(6% DV)
Saturated Fat	1.2 g	(6% DV)	Vitamin A	67.2 IU	(1% DV)
Poly Fat	.4 g		Vitamin C	.4 mg	(1% DV)
Mono Fat	1.2 g		Calcium	99.6 mg	(10% DV)
Cholesterol	26.4 mg	(9% DV)	Iron	.5 mg	(3% DV)
Sodium	228 mg	(10% DV)	Folate	2.8 mcg	(1% DV)
Potassium	70 mg	(2% DV)	Beta Carotene	.8 RE	

Ratings	Worst	Bad	Average	Good	Best
Weight Loss				7	
LowCal Density			5		
Filling		3			
Energizing			5		
Fiber		3			
Vitamins		3			
Minerals			4		
Overall			5		

PANCAKES, WHOLE WHEAT

Serving: 1 pancake (5" dia) (1.43 oz)   Breakfast

Calories	95	(66.6 cal/oz)	Carbohydrate	11.6 g	(4% DV)
Fat Calories	40	(42% fat)	Dietary Fiber	1.6 g	(6% DV)
Total Fat	4.4 g	(7% DV)	Protein	3.2 g	(6% DV)
Saturated Fat	1.2 g	(6% DV)	Vitamin A	64.4 IU	(1% DV)
Poly Fat	2 g		Vitamin C	.4 mg	(1% DV)
Mono Fat	1.2 g		Calcium	70.8 mg	(7% DV)
Cholesterol	25.2 mg	(8% DV)	Iron	.6 mg	(3% DV)
Sodium	208.4 mg	(9% DV)	Folate	3.2 mcg	(2% DV)
Potassium	95.2 mg	(3% DV)	Beta Carotene	.8 RE	

Ratings	Worst	Bad	Average	Good	Best
Weight Loss				6	
LowCal Density			5		
Filling		3			
Energizing			5		
Fiber			5		
Vitamins		3			
Minerals			4		
Overall			5		

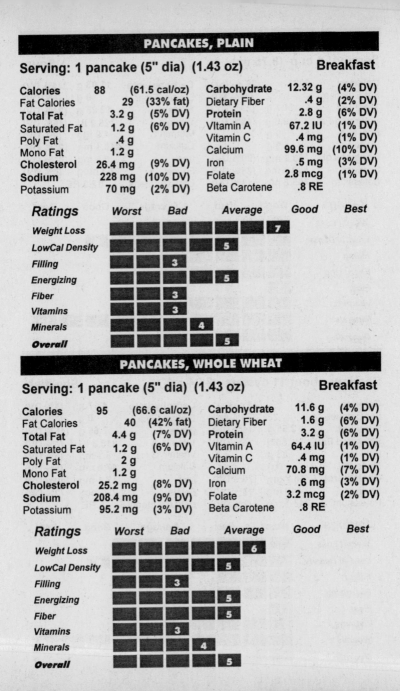

PANNETONE (ITALIAN-STYLE SWEETBREAD)

Serving: 1 slice (.96 oz)   **Bakery**

Calories	86	(89.7 cal/oz)	Carbohydrate	14.58 g	(5% DV)
Fat Calories	19	(23% fat)	Dietary Fiber	.81 g	(3% DV)
Total Fat	2.16 g	(3% DV)	Protein	2.16 g	(4% DV)
Saturated Fat	1.08 g	(5% DV)	Vitamin A	86.9 IU	(2% DV)
Poly Fat	.27 g		Vitamin C	.3 mg	(0% DV)
Mono Fat	.54 g		Calcium	16.2 mg	(2% DV)
Cholesterol	18.9 mg	(6% DV)	Iron	.8 mg	(4% DV)
Sodium	96.1 mg	(4% DV)	Folate	2.2 mcg	(6% DV)
Potassium	53.5 mg	(2% DV)	Beta Carotene	1.9 RE	

Ratings	Worst	Bad	Average	Good	Best
Weight Loss				7	
LowCal Density		3			
Filling		3			
Energizing			5		
Fiber		4			
Vitamins		3			
Minerals		3			
Overall			4		

PAPAYA, RAW

Serving: 1 medium (10.86 oz)   **Fruit**

Calories	119	(10.9 cal/oz)	Carbohydrate	29.79 g	(10% DV)
Fat Calories	0	(0% fat)	Dietary Fiber	6.08 g	(24% DV)
Total Fat	0 g	(0% DV)	Protein	3.04 g	(6% DV)
Saturated Fat	0 g	(0% DV)	Vitamin A	863.4 IU	(17% DV)
Poly Fat	0 g		Vitamin C	188.5 mg	(314% DV)
Mono Fat	0 g		Calcium	73 mg	(7% DV)
Cholesterol	0 mg	(0% DV)	Iron	.3 mg	(2% DV)
Sodium	9.1 mg	(0% DV)	Folate	3 mcg	(29% DV)
Potassium	781.3 mg	(22% DV)	Beta Carotene	85.1 RE	

Ratings	Worst	Bad	Average	Good	Best
Weight Loss				9	
LowCal Density				9	
Filling					10
Energizing			7		
Fiber					10
Vitamins					10
Minerals		4			
Overall				9	

PARSNIPS, COOKED WITHOUT ADDED FAT

Serving: 1 cup (5.57 oz)   **Vegetable**

Calories	126	(22.7 cal/oz)	Carbohydrate	30.26 g	(10% DV)
Fat Calories	0	(0% fat)	Dietary Fiber	6.24 g	(25% DV)
Total Fat	**0 g**	**(0% DV)**	Protein	1.56 g	(3% DV)
Saturated Fat	0 g	(0% DV)	Vitamin A	0 IU	(0% DV)
Poly Fat	0 g		Vitamin C	20.3 mg	(34% DV)
Mono Fat	0 g		Calcium	57.7 mg	(6% DV)
Cholesterol	**0 mg**	**(0% DV)**	Iron	.9 mg	(5% DV)
Sodium	**376 mg**	**(16% DV)**	Folate	1.6 mcg	(23% DV)
Potassium	569.4 mg	(16% DV)	Beta Carotene	0 RE	

Ratings	Worst	Bad	Average	Good	Best
Weight Loss				7	
LowCal Density				8	
Filling					9
Energizing				7	
Fiber					10
Vitamins			6		
Minerals			5		
Overall				8	

PASTA SALAD WITH MEAT

Serving: 1 cup (6.32 oz)   **Salad**

Calories	354	(56 cal/oz)	Carbohydrate	26.9 g	(9% DV)
Fat Calories	191	(54% fat)	Dietary Fiber	1.77 g	(7% DV)
Total Fat	**21.24 g**	**(33% DV)**	Protein	12.39 g	(25% DV)
Saturated Fat	5.31 g	(27% DV)	Vitamin A	3373.6 IU	(67% DV)
Poly Fat	8.85 g		Vitamin C	7.1 mg	(12% DV)
Mono Fat	7.08 g		Calcium	24.8 mg	(2% DV)
Cholesterol	**26.6 mg**	**(9% DV)**	Iron	1.8 mg	(10% DV)
Sodium	**1124 mg**	**(47% DV)**	Folate	12.4 mcg	(4% DV)
Potassium	224.8 mg	(6% DV)	Beta Carotene	334.5 RE	

Ratings	Worst	Bad	Average	Good	Best
Weight Loss		3			
LowCal Density			5		
Filling			5		
Energizing				7	
Fiber			6		
Vitamins				8	
Minerals			5		
Overall			5		

PASTA WITH PESTO SAUCE

Serving: 1 cup (4.36 oz)   **Entree**

Calories	348	(79.7 cal/oz)	Carbohydrate	27.57 g	(9% DV)
Fat Calories	209	(60% fat)	Dietary Fiber	2.44 g	(10% DV)
Total Fat	23.18 g	(36% DV)	Protein	10.98 g	(22% DV)
Saturated Fat	4.88 g	(24% DV)	VItamin A	267.2 IU	(5% DV)
Poly Fat	3.66 g		Vitamin C	2.4 mg	(4% DV)
Mono Fat	12.2 g		Calcium	185.4 mg	(19% DV)
Cholesterol	7.3 mg	(2% DV)	Iron	3.4 mg	(19% DV)
Sodium	176.9 mg	(7% DV)	Folate	11 mcg	(5% DV)
Potassium	194 mg	(6% DV)	Beta Carotene	23.2 RE	

Ratings	Worst	Bad	Average	Good	Best
Weight Loss	3				
LowCal Density	4				
Filling	4				
Energizing	7				
Fiber	7				
Vitamins	5				
Minerals	7				
Overall	4				

PASTRAMI SANDWICH

Serving: 1 sandwich (4.79 oz)   **Sandwich**

Calories	334	(69.7 cal/oz)	Carbohydrate	27.2 g	(9% DV)
Fat Calories	169	(51% fat)	Dietary Fiber	1.34 g	(5% DV)
Total Fat	18.76 g	(29% DV)	Protein	13.4 g	(27% DV)
Saturated Fat	6.7 g	(34% DV)	VItamin A	28.1 IU	(1% DV)
Poly Fat	1.34 g		Vitamin C	4 mg	(7% DV)
Mono Fat	9.38 g		Calcium	71 mg	(7% DV)
Cholesterol	52.3 mg	(17% DV)	Iron	2.6 mg	(15% DV)
Sodium	1341.3 mg	(56% DV)	Folate	13.4 mcg	(5% DV)
Potassium	241.2 mg	(7% DV)	Beta Carotene	2.7 RE	

Ratings	Worst	Bad	Average	Good	Best
Weight Loss	4				
LowCal Density	4				
Filling	5				
Energizing	7				
Fiber	5				
Vitamins	5				
Minerals	6				
Overall	5				

PEA SALAD WITH CHEESE

Serving: 1 cup (7.64 oz)   **Salad**

Calories	550	(72 cal/oz)	Carbohydrate	18.4 g	(6% DV)
Fat Calories	404	(74% fat)	Dietary Fiber	4.28 g	(17% DV)
Total Fat	44.94 g	(69% DV)	Protein	19.26 g	(39% DV)
Saturated Fat	12.84 g	(64% DV)	Vitamin A	1423.1 IU	(28% DV)
Poly Fat	17.12 g		Vitamin C	36.4 mg	(61% DV)
Mono Fat	12.84 g		Calcium	318.9 mg	(32% DV)
Cholesterol	137 mg	(46% DV)	Iron	2.3 mg	(13% DV)
Sodium	577.8 mg	(24% DV)	Folate	19.3 mcg	(19% DV)
Potassium	355.2 mg	(10% DV)	Beta Carotene	89.9 RE	

Ratings	Worst	Bad	Average	Good	Best
Weight Loss	1				
LowCal Density		4			
Filling		4			
Energizing			6		
Fiber					9
Vitamins					9
Minerals					9
Overall		4			

PEACH, RAW

Serving: 1 medium (2½" dia) (3.5 oz)   **Fruit**

Calories	42	(12 cal/oz)	Carbohydrate	10.88 g	(4% DV)
Fat Calories	0	(0% fat)	Dietary Fiber	1.96 g	(8% DV)
Total Fat	0 g	(0% DV)	Protein	.98 g	(2% DV)
Saturated Fat	0 g	(0% DV)	Vitamin A	524.3 IU	(10% DV)
Poly Fat	0 g		Vitamin C	6.9 mg	(11% DV)
Mono Fat	0 g		Calcium	4.9 mg	(0% DV)
Cholesterol	0 mg	(0% DV)	Iron	.1 mg	(1% DV)
Sodium	0 mg	(0% DV)	Folate	1 mcg	(1% DV)
Potassium	193.1 mg	(6% DV)	Beta Carotene	52.9 RE	

Ratings	Worst	Bad	Average	Good	Best
Weight Loss					10
LowCal Density				9	
Filling			7		
Energizing		4			
Fiber			6		
Vitamins		4			
Minerals	2				
Overall				8	

PEANUT BUTTER

Serving: 1 tbsp (.57 oz)   Snack

Calories	94	(165.1 cal/oz)	Carbohydrate	3.31 g	(1% DV)
Fat Calories	72	(77% fat)	Dietary Fiber	.96 g	(4% DV)
Total Fat	8 g	(12% DV)	Protein	4 g	(8% DV)
Saturated Fat	1.6 g	(8% DV)	VItamin A	0 IU	(0% DV)
Poly Fat	2.24 g		Vitamin C	0 mg	(0% DV)
Mono Fat	3.84 g		Calcium	5.4 mg	(1% DV)
Cholesterol	0 mg	(0% DV)	Iron	.3 mg	(2% DV)
Sodium	76.5 mg	(3% DV)	Folate	4 mcg	(3% DV)
Potassium	115.4 mg	(3% DV)	Beta Carotene	0 RE	

Ratings

	Worst	Bad	Average	Good	Best
Weight Loss			4		
LowCal Density	1				
Filling	1				
Energizing		3			
Fiber			4		
Vitamins			4		
Minerals			4		
Overall		3			

PEANUT BUTTER & JELLY SANDWICH

Serving: 1 sandwich (3.32 oz)   Sandwich

Calories	330	(99.4 cal/oz)	Carbohydrate	41.85 g	(14% DV)
Fat Calories	134	(41% fat)	Dietary Fiber	2.79 g	(11% DV)
Total Fat	14.88 g	(23% DV)	Protein	10.23 g	(20% DV)
Saturated Fat	2.79 g	(14% DV)	VItamin A	2.8 IU	(0% DV)
Poly Fat	4.65 g		Vitamin C	0 mg	(0% DV)
Mono Fat	6.51 g		Calcium	70.7 mg	(7% DV)
Cholesterol	.9 mg	(0% DV)	Iron	2 mg	(11% DV)
Sodium	417.6 mg	(17% DV)	Folate	10.2 mcg	(10% DV)
Potassium	253.9 mg	(7% DV)	Beta Carotene	0 RE	

Ratings

	Worst	Bad	Average	Good	Best
Weight Loss			5		
LowCal Density		3			
Filling			5		
Energizing					9
Fiber				7	
Vitamins			5		
Minerals			6		
Overall			5		

PEANUT OIL

Serving: 1 tbsp (.48 oz)   **Fat & Oil**

Calories	119	(248.6 cal/oz)	Carbohydrate	0 g	(0% DV)
Fat Calories	122	(102% fat)	Dietary Fiber	0 g	(0% DV)
Total Fat	13.5 g	(21% DV)	Protein	0 g	(0% DV)
Saturated Fat	2.29 g	(11% DV)	Vitamin A	0 IU	(0% DV)
Poly Fat	4.32 g		Vitamin C	0 mg	(0% DV)
Mono Fat	6.21 g		Calcium	0 mg	(0% DV)
Cholesterol	0 mg	(0% DV)	Iron	0 mg	(0% DV)
Sodium	0 mg	(0% DV)	Folate	0 mcg	(0% DV)
Potassium	0 mg	(0% DV)	Beta Carotene	0 RE	

Ratings	Worst	Bad	Average	Good	Best
Weight Loss	1				
LowCal Density	1				
Filling	1				
Energizing	1				
Fiber	1				
Vitamins		2			
Minerals	1				
Overall	1				

PEANUTS, DRY ROASTED, SALTED

Serving: about 28 nuts (1 oz)   **Snack**

Calories	164	(163.8 cal/oz)	Carbohydrate	6.02 g	(2% DV)
Fat Calories	126	(77% fat)	Dietary Fiber	2.24 g	(9% DV)
Total Fat	14 g	(22% DV)	Protein	6.72 g	(13% DV)
Saturated Fat	1.96 g	(10% DV)	Vitamin A	0 IU	(0% DV)
Poly Fat	4.48 g		Vitamin C	0 mg	(0% DV)
Mono Fat	7 g		Calcium	15.1 mg	(2% DV)
Cholesterol	0 mg	(0% DV)	Iron	.6 mg	(4% DV)
Sodium	227.6 mg	(9% DV)	Folate	6.7 mcg	(10% DV)
Potassium	184.2 mg	(5% DV)	Beta Carotene	0 RE	

Ratings	Worst	Bad	Average	Good	Best
Weight Loss			3		
LowCal Density	1				
Filling		2			
Energizing			4		
Fiber					6
Vitamins				5	
Minerals				5	
Overall			3		

PEANUTS, ROASTED, SALTED

Serving: about 32 nuts (1 oz)   **Snack**

Calories	163	(162.7 cal/oz)	Carbohydrate	5.29 g	(2% DV)
Fat Calories	123	(76% fat)	Dietary Fiber	2.52 g	(10% DV)
Total Fat	13.72 g	(21% DV)	Protein	7.28 g	(15% DV)
Saturated Fat	1.96 g	(10% DV)	Vltamin A	0 IU	(0% DV)
Poly Fat	4.48 g		Vitamin C	0 mg	(0% DV)
Mono Fat	6.72 g		Calcium	24.6 mg	(2% DV)
Cholesterol	0 mg	(0% DV)	Iron	.5 mg	(3% DV)
Sodium	121.2 mg	(5% DV)	Folate	7.3 mcg	(9% DV)
Potassium	191 mg	(5% DV)	Beta Carotene	0 RE	

Ratings	Worst	Bad	Average	Good	Best
Weight Loss		3			
LowCal Density	1				
Filling	2				
Energizing		3			
Fiber				7	
Vitamins			5		
Minerals			5		
Overall		3			

PEAR, RAW

Serving: 1 pear (5.93 oz)   **Fruit**

Calories	98	(16.5 cal/oz)	Carbohydrate	25.07 g	(8% DV)
Fat Calories	0	(0% fat)	Dietary Fiber	4.98 g	(20% DV)
Total Fat	0 g	(0% DV)	Protein	0 g	(0% DV)
Saturated Fat	0 g	(0% DV)	Vltamin A	33.2 IU	(1% DV)
Poly Fat	0 g		Vitamin C	6.6 mg	(11% DV)
Mono Fat	0 g		Calcium	18.3 mg	(2% DV)
Cholesterol	0 mg	(0% DV)	Iron	.4 mg	(2% DV)
Sodium	0 mg	(0% DV)	Folate	0 mcg	(3% DV)
Potassium	207.5 mg	(6% DV)	Beta Carotene	3.3 RE	

Ratings	Worst	Bad	Average	Good	Best
Weight Loss				9	
LowCal Density				9	
Filling				9	
Energizing			6		
Fiber				9	
Vitamins		4			
Minerals		3			
Overall				8	

PEAS & CARROTS, COOKED WITHOUT ADDED FAT

Serving: 1 cup (5.71 oz)   **Vegetable**

Calories	77	(13.5 cal/oz)	Carbohydrate	16.16 g	(5% DV)
Fat Calories	0	(0% fat)	Dietary Fiber	6.4 g	(26% DV)
Total Fat	0 g	(0% DV)	Protein	4.8 g	(10% DV)
Saturated Fat	0 g	(0% DV)	Vitamin A	12344 IU	(247% DV)
Poly Fat	0 g		Vitamin C	12.8 mg	(21% DV)
Mono Fat	0 g		Calcium	36.8 mg	(4% DV)
Cholesterol	0 mg	(0% DV)	Iron	1.5 mg	(8% DV)
Sodium	478.4 mg	(20% DV)	Folate	4.8 mcg	(10% DV)
Potassium	251.2 mg	(7% DV)	Beta Carotene	1233.6 RE	

Ratings	Worst	Bad	Average	Good	Best
Weight Loss				9	
LowCal Density				9	
Filling				9	
Energizing			5		
Fiber					10
Vitamins					10
Minerals			5		
Overall				9	

PEAS & ONIONS, COOKED WITHOUT ADDED FAT

Serving: 1 cup (6.43 oz)   **Vegetable**

Calories	81	(12.6 cal/oz)	Carbohydrate	15.48 g	(5% DV)
Fat Calories	0	(0% fat)	Dietary Fiber	5.4 g	(22% DV)
Total Fat	0 g	(0% DV)	Protein	5.4 g	(11% DV)
Saturated Fat	0 g	(0% DV)	Vitamin A	621 IU	(12% DV)
Poly Fat	0 g		Vitamin C	12.6 mg	(21% DV)
Mono Fat	0 g		Calcium	25.2 mg	(3% DV)
Cholesterol	0 mg	(0% DV)	Iron	1.7 mg	(9% DV)
Sodium	567 mg	(24% DV)	Folate	5.4 mcg	(9% DV)
Potassium	208.8 mg	(6% DV)	Beta Carotene	63 RE	

Ratings	Worst	Bad	Average	Good	Best
Weight Loss				9	
LowCal Density				9	
Filling				9	
Energizing			5		
Fiber				9	
Vitamins			6		
Minerals		4			
Overall				8	

PEAS, COWPEAS, FIELD PEAS, BLACKEYE (COOKED)

Serving: 1 cup (6.07 oz)　　　　　　　**Vegetable**

Calories	163	(26.9 cal/oz)	Carbohydrate	34.34 g	(11% DV)
Fat Calories	0	(0% fat)	Dietary Fiber	8.5 g	(34% DV)
Total Fat	0 g	(0% DV)	Protein	5.1 g	(10% DV)
Saturated Fat	0 g	(0% DV)	Vitamin A	1336.2 IU	(27% DV)
Poly Fat	0 g		Vitamin C	3.4 mg	(6% DV)
Mono Fat	0 g		Calcium	217.6 mg	(22% DV)
Cholesterol	0 mg	(0% DV)	Iron	1.9 mg	(10% DV)
Sodium	399.5 mg	(17% DV)	Folate	5.1 mcg	(54% DV)
Potassium	707.2 mg	(20% DV)	Beta Carotene	134.3 RE	

Ratings	Worst	Bad	Average	Good	Best
Weight Loss			6		
LowCal Density				8	
Filling				9	
Energizing				8	
Fiber					10
Vitamins			7		
Minerals			7		
Overall				8	

PEAS, GREEN, COOKED WITHOUT ADDED FAT

Serving: 1 cup (5.71 oz)　　　　　　　**Vegetable**

Calories	133	(23.3 cal/oz)	Carbohydrate	24.8 g	(8% DV)
Fat Calories	0	(0% fat)	Dietary Fiber	4.8 g	(19% DV)
Total Fat	0 g	(0% DV)	Protein	8 g	(16% DV)
Saturated Fat	0 g	(0% DV)	Vitamin A	948.8 IU	(19% DV)
Poly Fat	0 g		Vitamin C	22.4 mg	(37% DV)
Mono Fat	0 g		Calcium	43.2 mg	(4% DV)
Cholesterol	0 mg	(0% DV)	Iron	2.5 mg	(14% DV)
Sodium	374.4 mg	(16% DV)	Folate	8 mcg	(25% DV)
Potassium	430.4 mg	(12% DV)	Beta Carotene	96 RE	

Ratings	Worst	Bad	Average	Good	Best
Weight Loss			7		
LowCal Density				8	
Filling				8	
Energizing			6		
Fiber					9
Vitamins				8	
Minerals			6		
Overall				8	

PECANS

Serving: about 20 halves (1 oz)   **Snack**

Calories	187	(186.8 cal/oz)	Carbohydrate	5.1 g	(2% DV)
Fat Calories	171	(92% fat)	Dietary Fiber	1.96 g	(8% DV)
Total Fat	19.04 g	(29% DV)	Protein	2.24 g	(4% DV)
Saturated Fat	1.4 g	(7% DV)	VItamin A	35.8 IU	(1% DV)
Poly Fat	4.76 g		Vitamin C	.6 mg	(1% DV)
Mono Fat	11.76 g		Calcium	10.1 mg	(1% DV)
Cholesterol	0 mg	(0% DV)	Iron	.6 mg	(3% DV)
Sodium	.3 mg	(0% DV)	Folate	2.2 mcg	(3% DV)
Potassium	109.8 mg	(3% DV)	Beta Carotene	3.6 RE	

Ratings	Worst	Bad	Average	Good	Best
Weight Loss	2				
LowCal Density	1				
Filling	2				
Energizing	3				
Fiber				6	
Vitamins			4		
Minerals			5		
Overall	2				

PEPPER STEAK

Serving: 1 cup (7.75 oz)   **Entree**

Calories	332	(42.8 cal/oz)	Carbohydrate	5.42 g	(2% DV)
Fat Calories	195	(59% fat)	Dietary Fiber	0 g	(0% DV)
Total Fat	21.7 g	(33% DV)	Protein	28.21 g	(56% DV)
Saturated Fat	4.34 g	(22% DV)	VItamin A	193.1 IU	(4% DV)
Poly Fat	8.68 g		Vitamin C	19.5 mg	(33% DV)
Mono Fat	6.51 g		Calcium	28.2 mg	(3% DV)
Cholesterol	71.6 mg	(24% DV)	Iron	3.2 mg	(18% DV)
Sodium	648.8 mg	(27% DV)	Folate	28.2 mcg	(7% DV)
Potassium	555.5 mg	(16% DV)	Beta Carotene	19.5 RE	

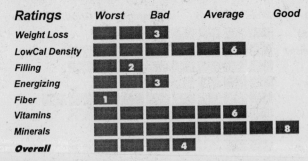

Ratings	Worst	Bad	Average	Good	Best
Weight Loss	3				
LowCal Density				6	
Filling	2				
Energizing	3				
Fiber	1				
Vitamins				6	
Minerals				8	
Overall			4		

PEPPER, SWEET, GREEN, RAW

Serving: 1 ring (3" dia, ¼" thick) (.36 oz)   Vegetable

Calories	3	(7.5 cal/oz)	Carbohydrate	.64 g	(0% DV)
Fat Calories	0	(0% fat)	Dietary Fiber	.2 g	(1% DV)
Total Fat	0 g	(0% DV)	**Protein**	.1 g	(0% DV)
Saturated Fat	0 g	(0% DV)	Vitamin A	63.2 IU	(1% DV)
Poly Fat	0 g		Vitamin C	8.9 mg	(15% DV)
Mono Fat	0 g		Calcium	.9 mg	(0% DV)
Cholesterol	0 mg	(0% DV)	Iron	.1 mg	(0% DV)
Sodium	.2 mg	(0% DV)	Folate	.1 mcg	(1% DV)
Potassium	17.7 mg	(1% DV)	Beta Carotene	6.3 RE	

Ratings	Worst	Bad	Average	Good	Best
Weight Loss					10
LowCal Density					10
Filling	2				
Energizing	2				
Fiber	2				
Vitamins	3				
Minerals	2				
Overall				7	

PEPPERCORN DRESSING

Serving: 1 tbsp (.48 oz)   Fat & Oil

Calories	76	(157.5 cal/oz)	Carbohydrate	.47 g	(0% DV)
Fat Calories	74	(97% fat)	Dietary Fiber	0 g	(0% DV)
Total Fat	8.17 g	(13% DV)	**Protein**	.13 g	(0% DV)
Saturated Fat	1.21 g	(6% DV)	Vitamin A	8.4 IU	(0% DV)
Poly Fat	4.42 g		Vitamin C	.1 mg	(0% DV)
Mono Fat	1.88 g		Calcium	3 mg	(0% DV)
Cholesterol	6.6 mg	(2% DV)	Iron	.1 mg	(0% DV)
Sodium	142.7 mg	(6% DV)	Folate	.1 mcg	(1% DV)
Potassium	23.6 mg	(1% DV)	Beta Carotene	.3 RE	

Ratings	Worst	Bad	Average	Good	Best
Weight Loss	2				
LowCal Density	1				
Filling	1				
Energizing	2				
Fiber	1				
Vitamins	2				
Minerals	2				
Overall	2				

PEPPERONI

Serving: 5 slices (1.07 oz)   **Meat**

Calories	149	(139.3 cal/oz)	Carbohydrate	.84 g	(0% DV)
Fat Calories	119	(80% fat)	Dietary Fiber	0 g	(0% DV)
Total Fat	13.2 g	(20% DV)	**Protein**	6.3 g	(13% DV)
Saturated Fat	4.8 g	(24% DV)	Vitamin A	0 IU	(0% DV)
Poly Fat	1.2 g		Vitamin C	0 mg	(0% DV)
Mono Fat	6.3 g		Calcium	3 mg	(0% DV)
Cholesterol	23.7 mg	(8% DV)	Iron	.4 mg	(2% DV)
Sodium	612 mg	(26% DV)	Folate	6.3 mcg	(0% DV)
Potassium	104.1 mg	(3% DV)	Beta Carotene	0 RE	

Ratings	Worst	Bad	Average	Good	Best
Weight Loss		3			
LowCal Density	1				
Filling	1				
Energizing	2				
Fiber	1				
Vitamins		3			
Minerals		3			
Overall	2				

PICKLED PIGS FEET, PORK

Serving: 1 foot (3.11 oz)   **Meat**

Calories	177	(56.8 cal/oz)	Carbohydrate	0 g	(0% DV)
Fat Calories	125	(71% fat)	Dietary Fiber	0 g	(0% DV)
Total Fat	13.92 g	(21% DV)	**Protein**	12.18 g	(24% DV)
Saturated Fat	5.22 g	(26% DV)	Vitamin A	0 IU	(0% DV)
Poly Fat	1.74 g		Vitamin C	0 mg	(0% DV)
Mono Fat	6.96 g		Calcium	27.8 mg	(3% DV)
Cholesterol	80 mg	(27% DV)	Iron	.5 mg	(3% DV)
Sodium	803 mg	(33% DV)	Folate	12.2 mcg	(1% DV)
Potassium	204.5 mg	(6% DV)	Beta Carotene	0 RE	

Ratings	Worst	Bad	Average	Good	Best
Weight Loss		3			
LowCal Density				5	
Filling	1				
Energizing	1				
Fiber	1				
Vitamins	2				
Minerals			4		
Overall		3			

PIE, APPLE, FRIED

Serving: 1 piece (3.07 oz)   **Dessert**

Calories	312	(101.7 cal/oz)	Carbohydrate	34.66 g	(12% DV)
Fat Calories	170	(55% fat)	Dietary Fiber	.86 g	(3% DV)
Total Fat	18.92 g	(29% DV)	Protein	2.58 g	(5% DV)
Saturated Fat	4.3 g	(21% DV)	VItamin A	24.1 IU	(0% DV)
Poly Fat	5.16 g		Vitamin C	.9 mg	(1% DV)
Mono Fat	7.74 g		Calcium	5.2 mg	(1% DV)
Cholesterol	0 mg	(0% DV)	Iron	1.1 mg	(6% DV)
Sodium	276.1 mg	(12% DV)	Folate	2.6 mcg	(1% DV)
Potassium	54.2 mg	(2% DV)	Beta Carotene	.9 RE	

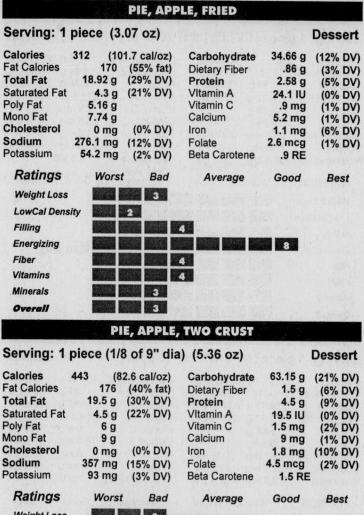

Ratings	Worst	Bad	Average	Good	Best
Weight Loss		3			
LowCal Density	2				
Filling			4		
Energizing					8
Fiber			4		
Vitamins			4		
Minerals		3			
Overall		3			

PIE, APPLE, TWO CRUST

Serving: 1 piece (1/8 of 9" dia) (5.36 oz)   **Dessert**

Calories	443	(82.6 cal/oz)	Carbohydrate	63.15 g	(21% DV)
Fat Calories	176	(40% fat)	Dietary Fiber	1.5 g	(6% DV)
Total Fat	19.5 g	(30% DV)	Protein	4.5 g	(9% DV)
Saturated Fat	4.5 g	(22% DV)	VItamin A	19.5 IU	(0% DV)
Poly Fat	6 g		Vitamin C	1.5 mg	(2% DV)
Mono Fat	9 g		Calcium	9 mg	(1% DV)
Cholesterol	0 mg	(0% DV)	Iron	1.8 mg	(10% DV)
Sodium	357 mg	(15% DV)	Folate	4.5 mcg	(2% DV)
Potassium	93 mg	(3% DV)	Beta Carotene	1.5 RE	

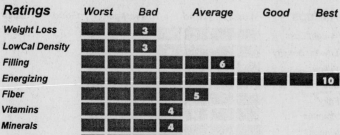

Ratings	Worst	Bad	Average	Good	Best
Weight Loss		3			
LowCal Density		3			
Filling			6		
Energizing					10
Fiber		5			
Vitamins		4			
Minerals		4			
Overall		4			

PIE, BANANA CREAM

Serving: 1 piece (1/8 of 9" dia) (5.14 oz)   **Dessert**

Calories	308	(60 cal/oz)	Carbohydrate	41.9 g	(14% DV)
Fat Calories	117	(38% fat)	Dietary Fiber	1.44 g	(6% DV)
Total Fat	12.96 g	(20% DV)	Protein	5.76 g	(12% DV)
Saturated Fat	4.32 g	(22% DV)	VItamin A	191.5 IU	(4% DV)
Poly Fat	2.88 g		Vitamin C	2.9 mg	(5% DV)
Mono Fat	5.76 g		Calcium	83.5 mg	(8% DV)
Cholesterol	67.7 mg	(23% DV)	Iron	1.2 mg	(7% DV)
Sodium	193 mg	(8% DV)	Folate	5.8 mcg	(4% DV)
Potassium	269.3 mg	(8% DV)	Beta Carotene	4.3 RE	

Ratings	Worst	Bad	Average	Good	Best
Weight Loss			5		
LowCal Density			5		
Filling			6		
Energizing					9
Fiber			5		
Vitamins		4			
Minerals			5		
Overall			5		

PIE, BLACK BOTTOM

Serving: 1 piece (1/8 of 9" dia) (3.54 oz)   **Dessert**

Calories	277	(78.3 cal/oz)	Carbohydrate	28.21 g	(9% DV)
Fat Calories	151	(55% fat)	Dietary Fiber	.99 g	(4% DV)
Total Fat	16.83 g	(26% DV)	Protein	4.95 g	(10% DV)
Saturated Fat	7.92 g	(40% DV)	VItamin A	626.7 IU	(13% DV)
Poly Fat	1.98 g		Vitamin C	0 mg	(0% DV)
Mono Fat	5.94 g		Calcium	74.3 mg	(7% DV)
Cholesterol	92.1 mg	(31% DV)	Iron	.9 mg	(5% DV)
Sodium	156.4 mg	(7% DV)	Folate	5 mcg	(2% DV)
Potassium	173.3 mg	(5% DV)	Beta Carotene	7.9 RE	

Ratings	Worst	Bad	Average	Good	Best
Weight Loss		4			
LowCal Density		4			
Filling		4			
Energizing				7	
Fiber		4			
Vitamins		4			
Minerals			5		
Overall		4			

PIE, BLUEBERRY, TWO CRUST

Serving: 1 piece (1/8 of 9" dia) (5.36 oz)   **Dessert**

Calories	404	(75.3 cal/oz)	Carbohydrate	56.85 g	(19% DV)
Fat Calories	162	(40% fat)	Dietary Fiber	3 g	(12% DV)
Total Fat	18 g	(28% DV)	Protein	3 g	(6% DV)
Saturated Fat	4.5 g	(22% DV)	Vitamin A	174 IU	(3% DV)
Poly Fat	4.5 g		Vitamin C	9 mg	(15% DV)
Mono Fat	7.5 g		Calcium	10.5 mg	(1% DV)
Cholesterol	0 mg	(0% DV)	Iron	1.6 mg	(9% DV)
Sodium	297 mg	(12% DV)	Folate	3 mcg	(2% DV)
Potassium	96 mg	(3% DV)	Beta Carotene	9 RE	

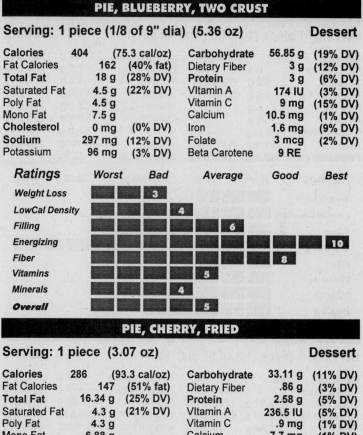

Ratings	Worst	Bad	Average	Good	Best
Weight Loss		3			
LowCal Density		4			
Filling			6		
Energizing					10
Fiber				8	
Vitamins			5		
Minerals		4			
Overall			5		

PIE, CHERRY, FRIED

Serving: 1 piece (3.07 oz)   **Dessert**

Calories	286	(93.3 cal/oz)	Carbohydrate	33.11 g	(11% DV)
Fat Calories	147	(51% fat)	Dietary Fiber	.86 g	(3% DV)
Total Fat	16.34 g	(25% DV)	Protein	2.58 g	(5% DV)
Saturated Fat	4.3 g	(21% DV)	Vitamin A	236.5 IU	(5% DV)
Poly Fat	4.3 g		Vitamin C	.9 mg	(1% DV)
Mono Fat	6.88 g		Calcium	7.7 mg	(1% DV)
Cholesterol	0 mg	(0% DV)	Iron	1.7 mg	(9% DV)
Sodium	24.1 mg	(1% DV)	Folate	2.6 mcg	(1% DV)
Potassium	61.9 mg	(2% DV)	Beta Carotene	23.2 RE	

Ratings	Worst	Bad	Average	Good	Best
Weight Loss		4			
LowCal Density		3			
Filling		4			
Energizing				8	
Fiber		4			
Vitamins		4			
Minerals		4			
Overall		4			

PIE, CHERRY, TWO CRUST

Serving: 1 piece (1/8 of 9" dia) (5.36 oz)   Dessert

Calories	396	(73.9 cal/oz)	Carbohydrate	54.45 g	(18% DV)
Fat Calories	176	(44% fat)	Dietary Fiber	1.5 g	(6% DV)
Total Fat	19.5 g	(30% DV)	Protein	4.5 g	(9% DV)
Saturated Fat	4.5 g	(22% DV)	Vitamin A	213 IU	(4% DV)
Poly Fat	4.5 g		Vitamin C	1.5 mg	(2% DV)
Mono Fat	9 g		Calcium	13.5 mg	(1% DV)
Cholesterol	0 mg	(0% DV)	Iron	1.7 mg	(10% DV)
Sodium	321 mg	(13% DV)	Folate	4.5 mcg	(2% DV)
Potassium	123 mg	(4% DV)	Beta Carotene	12 RE	

Ratings	Worst	Bad	Average	Good	Best
Weight Loss	3				
LowCal Density	4				
Filling	6				
Energizing					10
Fiber	5				
Vitamins	4				
Minerals	4				
Overall	5				

PIE, CHIFFON, NOT CHOCOLATE

Serving: 1 piece (1/8 of 9" dia) (3.54 oz)   Dessert

Calories	295	(83.3 cal/oz)	Carbohydrate	39.8 g	(13% DV)
Fat Calories	116	(39% fat)	Dietary Fiber	0 g	(0% DV)
Total Fat	12.87 g	(20% DV)	Protein	6.93 g	(14% DV)
Saturated Fat	2.97 g	(15% DV)	Vitamin A	206.9 IU	(4% DV)
Poly Fat	2.97 g		Vitamin C	5 mg	(8% DV)
Mono Fat	4.95 g		Calcium	20.8 mg	(2% DV)
Cholesterol	137.6 mg	(46% DV)	Iron	1.3 mg	(7% DV)
Sodium	179.2 mg	(7% DV)	Folate	6.9 mcg	(4% DV)
Potassium	70.3 mg	(2% DV)	Beta Carotene	0 RE	

Ratings	Worst	Bad	Average	Good	Best
Weight Loss	5				
LowCal Density	3				
Filling	5				
Energizing					9
Fiber	1				
Vitamins	4				
Minerals	4				
Overall	4				

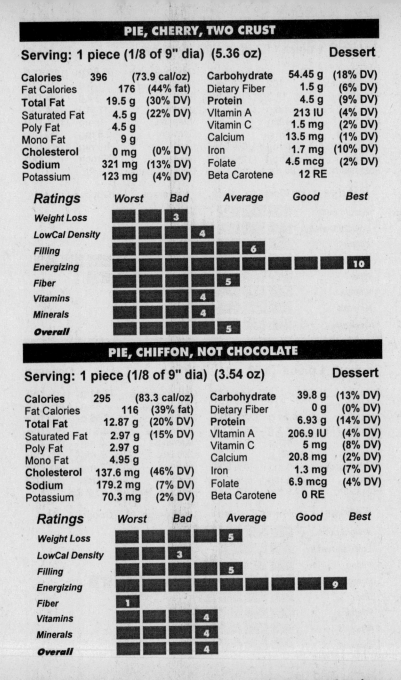

PIE, COCONUT CREAM

Serving: 1 piece (1/8 of 9" dia) (5.14 oz)　　　　**Dessert**

Calories	340	(66.1 cal/oz)	Carbohydrate	32.26 g	(11% DV)
Fat Calories	181	(53% fat)	Dietary Fiber	2.88 g	(12% DV)
Total Fat	20.16 g	(31% DV)	Protein	7.2 g	(14% DV)
Saturated Fat	10.08 g	(50% DV)	Vitamin A	220.3 IU	(4% DV)
Poly Fat	2.88 g		Vitamin C	1.4 mg	(2% DV)
Mono Fat	5.76 g		Calcium	108 mg	(11% DV)
Cholesterol	92.2 mg	(31% DV)	Iron	1.6 mg	(9% DV)
Sodium	236.2 mg	(10% DV)	Folate	7.2 mcg	(5% DV)
Potassium	233.3 mg	(7% DV)	Beta Carotene	2.9 RE	

Ratings	Worst	Bad	Average	Good	Best
Weight Loss		3			
LowCal Density			5		
Filling			5		
Energizing				8	
Fiber				8	
Vitamins			4		
Minerals			5		
Overall			5		

PIE, CUSTARD

Serving: 1 piece (1/8 of 9" dia) (4.86 oz)　　　　**Dessert**

Calories	282	(57.9 cal/oz)	Carbohydrate	30.46 g	(10% DV)
Fat Calories	135	(48% fat)	Dietary Fiber	0 g	(0% DV)
Total Fat	14.96 g	(23% DV)	Protein	6.8 g	(14% DV)
Saturated Fat	5.44 g	(27% DV)	Vitamin A	239.4 IU	(5% DV)
Poly Fat	2.72 g		Vitamin C	0 mg	(0% DV)
Mono Fat	5.44 g		Calcium	118.3 mg	(12% DV)
Cholesterol	97.9 mg	(33% DV)	Iron	1.1 mg	(6% DV)
Sodium	299.2 mg	(12% DV)	Folate	6.8 mcg	(3% DV)
Potassium	176.8 mg	(5% DV)	Beta Carotene	2.7 RE	

Ratings	Worst	Bad	Average	Good	Best
Weight Loss			4		
LowCal Density			5		
Filling			5		
Energizing				7	
Fiber	1				
Vitamins			4		
Minerals			5		
Overall			5		

PIE, LEMON MERINGUE

Serving: 1 piece (1/8 of 9" dia) (4.89 oz)   **Dessert**

Calories	340	(69.5 cal/oz)	Carbohydrate	48.22 g	(16% DV)
Fat Calories	136	(40% fat)	Dietary Fiber	0 g	(0% DV)
Total Fat	15.07 g	(23% DV)	Protein	4.11 g	(8% DV)
Saturated Fat	4.11 g	(21% DV)	Vitamin A	232.9 IU	(5% DV)
Poly Fat	4.11 g		Vitamin C	4.1 mg	(7% DV)
Mono Fat	6.85 g		Calcium	16.4 mg	(2% DV)
Cholesterol	94.5 mg	(32% DV)	Iron	1.2 mg	(7% DV)
Sodium	287.7 mg	(12% DV)	Folate	4.1 mcg	(3% DV)
Potassium	60.3 mg	(2% DV)	Beta Carotene	1.4 RE	

Ratings	Worst	Bad	Average	Good	Best
Weight Loss			4		
LowCal Density			4		
Filling			6		
Energizing					9
Fiber	1				
Vitamins			4		
Minerals			4		
Overall			4		

PIE, PEACH, TWO CRUST

Serving: 1 piece (1/8 of 9" dia) (5.36 oz)   **Dessert**

Calories	396	(73.9 cal/oz)	Carbohydrate	56.4 g	(19% DV)
Fat Calories	162	(41% fat)	Dietary Fiber	1.5 g	(6% DV)
Total Fat	18 g	(28% DV)	Protein	4.5 g	(9% DV)
Saturated Fat	4.5 g	(22% DV)	Vitamin A	369 IU	(7% DV)
Poly Fat	4.5 g		Vitamin C	4.5 mg	(8% DV)
Mono Fat	7.5 g		Calcium	9 mg	(1% DV)
Cholesterol	0 mg	(0% DV)	Iron	1.7 mg	(9% DV)
Sodium	292.5 mg	(12% DV)	Folate	4.5 mcg	(2% DV)
Potassium	180 mg	(5% DV)	Beta Carotene	37.5 RE	

Ratings	Worst	Bad	Average	Good	Best
Weight Loss		3			
LowCal Density			4		
Filling			6		
Energizing					10
Fiber			5		
Vitamins			5		
Minerals			4		
Overall			5		

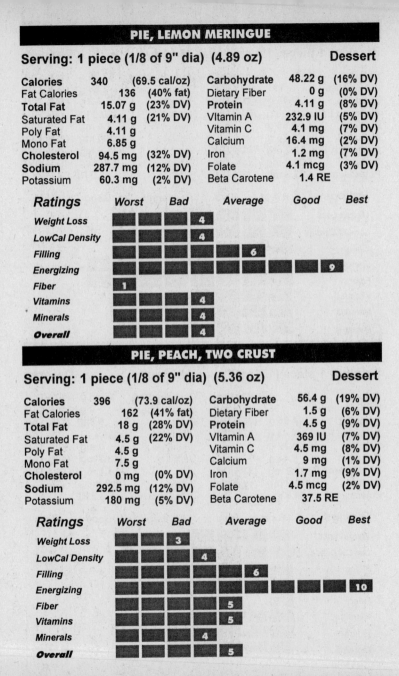

PIE, PECAN

Serving: 1 piece (1/8 of 9" dia) (4.07 oz)　　　**Dessert**

Calories	478	(117.4 cal/oz)	Carbohydrate	61.33 g	(20% DV)
Fat Calories	236	(49% fat)	Dietary Fiber	2.28 g	(9% DV)
Total Fat	26.22 g	(40% DV)	Protein	5.7 g	(11% DV)
Saturated Fat	4.56 g	(23% DV)	Vitamin A	112.9 IU	(2% DV)
Poly Fat	6.84 g		Vitamin C	0 mg	(0% DV)
Mono Fat	13.68 g		Calcium	27.4 mg	(3% DV)
Cholesterol	58.1 mg	(19% DV)	Iron	1.8 mg	(10% DV)
Sodium	240.5 mg	(10% DV)	Folate	5.7 mcg	(4% DV)
Potassium	145.9 mg	(4% DV)	Beta Carotene	2.3 RE	

Ratings	Worst	Bad	Average	Good	Best
Weight Loss	2				
LowCal Density	2				
Filling			5		
Energizing					10
Fiber			6		
Vitamins			5		
Minerals			5		
Overall		4			

PIE, PUDDING, FLAVORS OTHER THAN CHOCOLATE

Serving: 1 piece (1/8 of 9" dia) (5.14 oz)　　　**Dessert**

Calories	320	(62.2 cal/oz)	Carbohydrate	38.59 g	(13% DV)
Fat Calories	143	(45% fat)	Dietary Fiber	0 g	(0% DV)
Total Fat	15.84 g	(24% DV)	Protein	5.76 g	(12% DV)
Saturated Fat	5.76 g	(29% DV)	Vitamin A	118.1 IU	(2% DV)
Poly Fat	2.88 g		Vitamin C	1.4 mg	(2% DV)
Mono Fat	7.2 g		Calcium	118.1 mg	(12% DV)
Cholesterol	13 mg	(4% DV)	Iron	1.2 mg	(7% DV)
Sodium	385.9 mg	(16% DV)	Folate	5.8 mcg	(2% DV)
Potassium	171.4 mg	(5% DV)	Beta Carotene	2.9 RE	

Ratings	Worst	Bad	Average	Good	Best
Weight Loss		4			
LowCal Density			5		
Filling			5		
Energizing					9
Fiber	1				
Vitamins		4			
Minerals			5		
Overall			5		

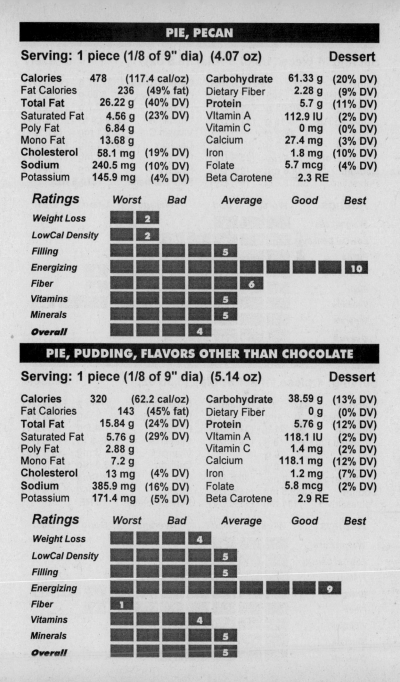

PIE, PUMPKIN

Serving: 1 piece (1/8 of 9" dia) (5.5 oz) **Dessert**

Calories	330	(59.9 cal/oz)	Carbohydrate	31.57 g	(11% DV)
Fat Calories	180	(55% fat)	Dietary Fiber	3.08 g	(12% DV)
Total Fat	20.02 g	(31% DV)	Protein	7.7 g	(15% DV)
Saturated Fat	6.16 g	(31% DV)	Vitamin A	13893.9 IU	(278% DV)
Poly Fat	4.62 g		Vitamin C	3.1 mg	(5% DV)
Mono Fat	7.7 g		Calcium	157.1 mg	(16% DV)
Cholesterol	75.5 mg	(25% DV)	Iron	2.1 mg	(12% DV)
Sodium	224.8 mg	(9% DV)	Folate	7.7 mcg	(5% DV)
Potassium	321.9 mg	(9% DV)	Beta Carotene	1370.6 RE	

Ratings	Worst	Bad	Average	Good	Best
Weight Loss		3			
LowCal Density			5		
Filling			5		
Energizing				8	
Fiber				8	
Vitamins					10
Minerals			6		
Overall			5		

PIE, RHUBARB, TWO CRUST

Serving: 1 piece (1/8 of 9" dia) (5.36 oz) **Dessert**

Calories	413	(77 cal/oz)	Carbohydrate	51.45 g	(17% DV)
Fat Calories	189	(46% fat)	Dietary Fiber	3 g	(12% DV)
Total Fat	21 g	(32% DV)	Protein	4.5 g	(9% DV)
Saturated Fat	6 g	(30% DV)	Vitamin A	55.5 IU	(1% DV)
Poly Fat	6 g		Vitamin C	3 mg	(5% DV)
Mono Fat	9 g		Calcium	133.5 mg	(13% DV)
Cholesterol	0 mg	(0% DV)	Iron	2.1 mg	(12% DV)
Sodium	349.5 mg	(15% DV)	Folate	4.5 mcg	(3% DV)
Potassium	111 mg	(3% DV)	Beta Carotene	6 RE	

Ratings	Worst	Bad	Average	Good	Best
Weight Loss		3			
LowCal Density		4			
Filling			6		
Energizing					10
Fiber				8	
Vitamins			5		
Minerals			5		
Overall			5		

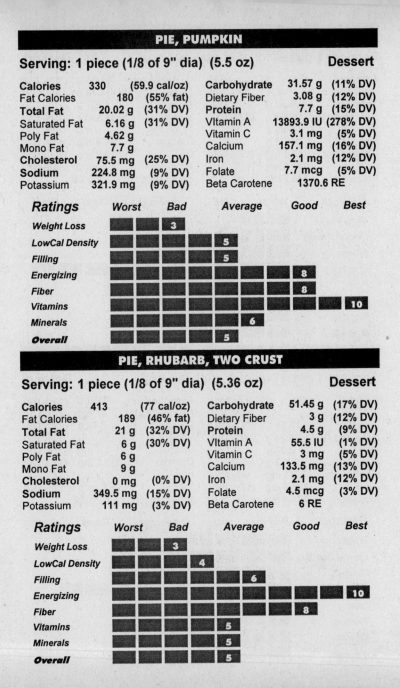

PIE, SOUR CREAM, RAISIN

Serving: 1 piece (1/8 of 9" dia) (5.14 oz)   Dessert

Calories	517	(100.6 cal/oz)	Carbohydrate	51.26 g	(17% DV)
Fat Calories	298	(58% fat)	Dietary Fiber	2.88 g	(12% DV)
Total Fat	33.12 g	(51% DV)	Protein	7.2 g	(14% DV)
Saturated Fat	12.96 g	(65% DV)	Vitamin A	682.6 IU	(14% DV)
Poly Fat	5.76 g		Vitamin C	1.4 mg	(2% DV)
Mono Fat	12.96 g		Calcium	95 mg	(10% DV)
Cholesterol	77.8 mg	(26% DV)	Iron	2.3 mg	(13% DV)
Sodium	354.2 mg	(15% DV)	Folate	7.2 mcg	(4% DV)
Potassium	345.6 mg	(10% DV)	Beta Carotene	15.8 RE	

Ratings	Worst	Bad	Average	Good	Best
Weight Loss	2				
LowCal Density	2				
Filling			5		
Energizing					10
Fiber				8	
Vitamins			5		
Minerals			6		
Overall		4			

PIE, STRAWBERRY, ONE CRUST

Serving: 1 piece (1/8 of 9" dia) (6 oz)   Dessert

Calories	388	(64.7 cal/oz)	Carbohydrate	56.28 g	(19% DV)
Fat Calories	151	(39% fat)	Dietary Fiber	3.36 g	(13% DV)
Total Fat	16.8 g	(26% DV)	Protein	3.36 g	(7% DV)
Saturated Fat	5.04 g	(25% DV)	Vitamin A	25.2 IU	(1% DV)
Poly Fat	5.04 g		Vitamin C	48.7 mg	(81% DV)
Mono Fat	6.72 g		Calcium	20.2 mg	(2% DV)
Cholesterol	0 mg	(0% DV)	Iron	1.8 mg	(10% DV)
Sodium	248.6 mg	(10% DV)	Folate	3.4 mcg	(4% DV)
Potassium	193.2 mg	(6% DV)	Beta Carotene	3.4 RE	

Ratings	Worst	Bad	Average	Good	Best
Weight Loss		3			
LowCal Density			5		
Filling			6		
Energizing					10
Fiber				8	
Vitamins			7		
Minerals		4			
Overall			5		

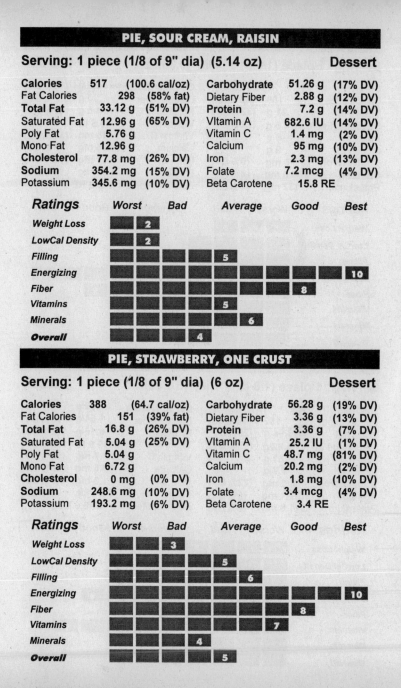

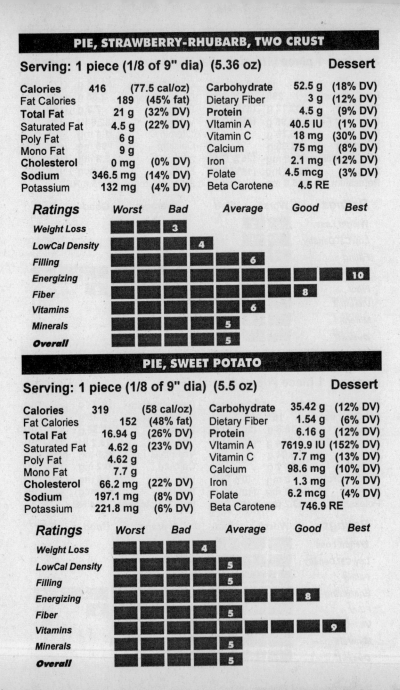

PIE, STRAWBERRY-RHUBARB, TWO CRUST

Serving: 1 piece (1/8 of 9" dia) (5.36 oz) Dessert

Calories	416	(77.5 cal/oz)	Carbohydrate	52.5 g	(18% DV)
Fat Calories	189	(45% fat)	Dietary Fiber	3 g	(12% DV)
Total Fat	21 g	(32% DV)	Protein	4.5 g	(9% DV)
Saturated Fat	4.5 g	(22% DV)	Vitamin A	40.5 IU	(1% DV)
Poly Fat	6 g		Vitamin C	18 mg	(30% DV)
Mono Fat	9 g		Calcium	75 mg	(8% DV)
Cholesterol	0 mg	(0% DV)	Iron	2.1 mg	(12% DV)
Sodium	346.5 mg	(14% DV)	Folate	4.5 mcg	(3% DV)
Potassium	132 mg	(4% DV)	Beta Carotene	4.5 RE	

Ratings	Worst	Bad	Average	Good	Best
Weight Loss	3				
LowCal Density		4			
Filling			6		
Energizing					10
Fiber				8	
Vitamins			6		
Minerals			5		
Overall			5		

PIE, SWEET POTATO

Serving: 1 piece (1/8 of 9" dia) (5.5 oz) Dessert

Calories	319	(58 cal/oz)	Carbohydrate	35.42 g	(12% DV)
Fat Calories	152	(48% fat)	Dietary Fiber	1.54 g	(6% DV)
Total Fat	16.94 g	(26% DV)	Protein	6.16 g	(12% DV)
Saturated Fat	4.62 g	(23% DV)	Vitamin A	7619.9 IU	(152% DV)
Poly Fat	4.62 g		Vitamin C	7.7 mg	(13% DV)
Mono Fat	7.7 g		Calcium	98.6 mg	(10% DV)
Cholesterol	66.2 mg	(22% DV)	Iron	1.3 mg	(7% DV)
Sodium	197.1 mg	(8% DV)	Folate	6.2 mcg	(4% DV)
Potassium	221.8 mg	(6% DV)	Beta Carotene	746.9 RE	

Ratings	Worst	Bad	Average	Good	Best
Weight Loss		4			
LowCal Density		5			
Filling		5			
Energizing				8	
Fiber		5			
Vitamins					9
Minerals		5			
Overall		5			

PIG IN A BLANKET (FRANKFURTER WRAPPED IN DOUGH)

Serving: 1 pig in blanket (3.04 oz)   **Sandwich**

Calories	278	(91.4 cal/oz)	Carbohydrate	14.62 g	(5% DV)
Fat Calories	191	(69% fat)	Dietary Fiber	0 g	(0% DV)
Total Fat	21.25 g	(33% DV)	Protein	7.65 g	(15% DV)
Saturated Fat	6.8 g	(34% DV)	Vitamin A	47.6 IU	(1% DV)
Poly Fat	3.4 g		Vitamin C	10.2 mg	(17% DV)
Mono Fat	9.35 g		Calcium	136.9 mg	(14% DV)
Cholesterol	22.1 mg	(7% DV)	Iron	1.2 mg	(7% DV)
Sodium	818.6 mg	(34% DV)	Folate	7.7 mcg	(1% DV)
Potassium	130.9 mg	(4% DV)	Beta Carotene	0 RE	

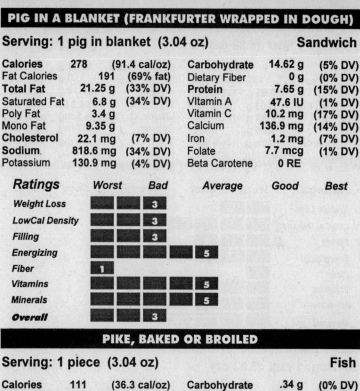

Ratings	Worst	Bad	Average	Good	Best
Weight Loss		3			
LowCal Density		3			
Filling		3			
Energizing			5		
Fiber	1				
Vitamins			5		
Minerals			5		
Overall		3			

PIKE, BAKED OR BROILED

Serving: 1 piece (3.04 oz)   **Fish**

Calories	111	(36.3 cal/oz)	Carbohydrate	.34 g	(0% DV)
Fat Calories	31	(28% fat)	Dietary Fiber	0 g	(0% DV)
Total Fat	3.4 g	(5% DV)	Protein	19.55 g	(39% DV)
Saturated Fat	.85 g	(4% DV)	Vitamin A	193.8 IU	(4% DV)
Poly Fat	.85 g		Vitamin C	4.3 mg	(7% DV)
Mono Fat	.85 g		Calcium	57.8 mg	(6% DV)
Cholesterol	39.1 mg	(13% DV)	Iron	.6 mg	(3% DV)
Sodium	300.9 mg	(13% DV)	Folate	19.6 mcg	(3% DV)
Potassium	262.7 mg	(8% DV)	Beta Carotene	2.6 RE	

Ratings	Worst	Bad	Average	Good	Best
Weight Loss				7	
LowCal Density				7	
Filling	1				
Energizing	2				
Fiber	1				
Vitamins			4		
Minerals			5		
Overall			5		

PIKE, BATTERED, FRIED

Serving: 1 fillet (5.39 oz)   **Fish**

Calories	307	(56.9 cal/oz)	Carbohydrate	10.12 g	(3% DV)
Fat Calories	149	(49% fat)	Dietary Fiber	0 g	(0% DV)
Total Fat	16.61 g	(26% DV)	Protein	27.18 g	(54% DV)
Saturated Fat	4.53 g	(23% DV)	VItamin A	104.2 IU	(2% DV)
Poly Fat	4.53 g		Vitamin C	4.5 mg	(8% DV)
Mono Fat	7.55 g		Calcium	108.7 mg	(11% DV)
Cholesterol	77 mg	(26% DV)	Iron	1.4 mg	(8% DV)
Sodium	140.4 mg	(6% DV)	Folate	27.2 mcg	(6% DV)
Potassium	373 mg	(11% DV)	Beta Carotene	0 RE	

Ratings	Worst	Bad	Average	Good	Best
Weight Loss	2				
LowCal Density			5		
Filling	3				
Energizing		4			
Fiber	1				
Vitamins			5		
Minerals				7	
Overall		4			

PINEAPPLE JUICE, UNSWEETENED

Serving: 1 cup (8.93 oz)   **Beverage**

Calories	140	(15.7 cal/oz)	Carbohydrate	34.5 g	(12% DV)
Fat Calories	0	(0% fat)	Dietary Fiber	0 g	(0% DV)
Total Fat	0 g	(0% DV)	Protein	0 g	(0% DV)
Saturated Fat	0 g	(0% DV)	VItamin A	12.5 IU	(0% DV)
Poly Fat	0 g		Vitamin C	27.5 mg	(46% DV)
Mono Fat	0 g		Calcium	42.5 mg	(4% DV)
Cholesterol	0 mg	(0% DV)	Iron	.7 mg	(4% DV)
Sodium	2.5 mg	(0% DV)	Folate	0 mcg	(14% DV)
Potassium	335 mg	(10% DV)	Beta Carotene	0 RE	

Ratings	Worst	Bad	Average	Good	Best
Weight Loss			6		
LowCal Density				9	
Filling					10
Energizing			8		
Fiber	1				
Vitamins			6		
Minerals		4			
Overall				7	

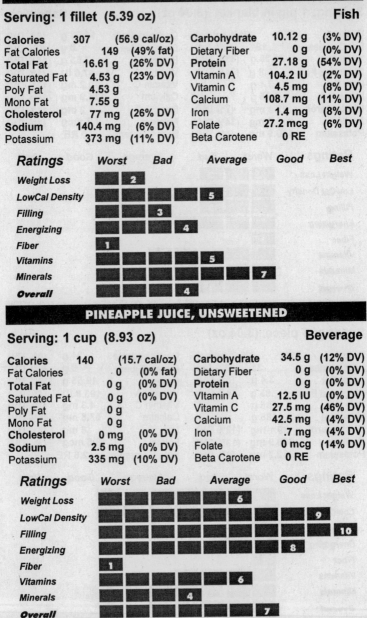

PINEAPPLE, RAW

Serving: 1 slice (3½" dia x ¾" thick) (3 oz)   **Fruit**

Calories	41	(13.7 cal/oz)	Carbohydrate	10.42 g	(3% DV)
Fat Calories	0	(0% fat)	Dietary Fiber	.84 g	(3% DV)
Total Fat	0 g	(0% DV)	Protein	0 g	(0% DV)
Saturated Fat	0 g	(0% DV)	Vltamin A	19.3 IU	(0% DV)
Poly Fat	0 g		Vitamin C	12.6 mg	(21% DV)
Mono Fat	0 g		Calcium	5.9 mg	(1% DV)
Cholesterol	0 mg	(0% DV)	Iron	.3 mg	(2% DV)
Sodium	.8 mg	(0% DV)	Folate	0 mcg	(2% DV)
Potassium	94.9 mg	(3% DV)	Beta Carotene	1.7 RE	

Ratings

	Worst	Bad	Average	Good	Best
Weight Loss					10
LowCal Density				9	
Filling			6		
Energizing		4			
Fiber		4			
Vitamins		4			
Minerals	2				
Overall				7	

PINK BEANS, DRY, COOKED WITHOUT ADDED FAT

Serving: 1 cup (6.04 oz)   **Vegetable**

Calories	250	(41.4 cal/oz)	Carbohydrate	46.98 g	(16% DV)
Fat Calories	0	(0% fat)	Dietary Fiber	8.45 g	(34% DV)
Total Fat	0 g	(0% DV)	Protein	15.21 g	(30% DV)
Saturated Fat	0 g	(0% DV)	Vltamin A	0 IU	(0% DV)
Poly Fat	0 g		Vitamin C	0 mg	(0% DV)
Mono Fat	0 g		Calcium	87.9 mg	(9% DV)
Cholesterol	0 mg	(0% DV)	Iron	3.9 mg	(22% DV)
Sodium	329.6 mg	(14% DV)	Folate	15.2 mcg	(71% DV)
Potassium	855.1 mg	(24% DV)	Beta Carotene	0 RE	

Ratings

	Worst	Bad	Average	Good	Best
Weight Loss		3			
LowCal Density			6		
Filling				8	
Energizing				9	
Fiber					10
Vitamins			7		
Minerals				8	
Overall			6		

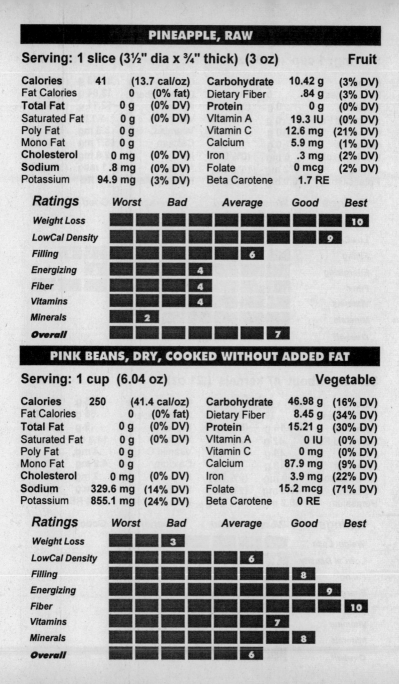

PINTO/CALICO/RED MEXICAN BEANS, DRY, COOKED

Serving: 1 cup (6.18 oz)   **Vegetable**

Calories	194	(31.4 cal/oz)	Carbohydrate	36.33 g	(12% DV)
Fat Calories	0	(0% fat)	Dietary Fiber	13.84 g	(55% DV)
Total Fat	0 g	(0% DV)	Protein	12.11 g	(24% DV)
Saturated Fat	0 g	(0% DV)	Vitamin A	1.7 IU	(0% DV)
Poly Fat	0 g		Vitamin C	3.5 mg	(6% DV)
Mono Fat	0 g		Calcium	65.7 mg	(7% DV)
Cholesterol	0 mg	(0% DV)	Iron	2.9 mg	(16% DV)
Sodium	372 mg	(15% DV)	Folate	12.1 mcg	(36% DV)
Potassium	570.9 mg	(16% DV)	Beta Carotene	0 RE	

Ratings	Worst	Bad	Average	Good	Best
Weight Loss			5		
LowCal Density				7	
Filling					9
Energizing				8	
Fiber					10
Vitamins			5		
Minerals				7	
Overall				7	

PISTACHIO NUTS, ROASTED, SALTED

Serving: about 47 kernels (.21 oz)   **Snack**

Calories	36	(173.1 cal/oz)	Carbohydrate	1.65 g	(1% DV)
Fat Calories	29	(79% fat)	Dietary Fiber	.66 g	(3% DV)
Total Fat	3.18 g	(5% DV)	Protein	.9 g	(2% DV)
Saturated Fat	.42 g	(2% DV)	Vitamin A	14.3 IU	(0% DV)
Poly Fat	.48 g		Vitamin C	.4 mg	(1% DV)
Mono Fat	2.16 g		Calcium	4.2 mg	(0% DV)
Cholesterol	0 mg	(0% DV)	Iron	.2 mg	(1% DV)
Sodium	46.8 mg	(2% DV)	Folate	.9 mcg	(1% DV)
Potassium	58.2 mg	(2% DV)	Beta Carotene	1.4 RE	

Ratings	Worst	Bad	Average	Good	Best
Weight Loss			5		
LowCal Density	1				
Filling	1				
Energizing		3			
Fiber		3			
Vitamins	2				
Minerals	2				
Overall		3			

PIZZA ROLLS

Serving: 1 miniature (.5 oz)   **Snack**

Calories	42	(84 cal/oz)	Carbohydrate	4.31 g	(1% DV)
Fat Calories	18	(42% fat)	Dietary Fiber	.28 g	(1% DV)
Total Fat	1.96 g	(3% DV)	Protein	1.82 g	(4% DV)
Saturated Fat	.7 g	(3% DV)	Vitamin A	62.4 IU	(1% DV)
Poly Fat	.28 g		Vitamin C	1.1 mg	(2% DV)
Mono Fat	.84 g		Calcium	25.9 mg	(3% DV)
Cholesterol	3.1 mg	(1% DV)	Iron	.3 mg	(2% DV)
Sodium	101.6 mg	(4% DV)	Folate	1.8 mcg	(1% DV)
Potassium	31.2 mg	(1% DV)	Beta Carotene	4.9 RE	

Ratings	Worst	Bad	Average	Good	Best
Weight Loss				7	
LowCal Density		3			
Filling	2				
Energizing		3			
Fiber	2				
Vitamins		3			
Minerals		3			
Overall			4		

PIZZA WITH MEAT

Serving: 1 piece (1/8 of 12" dia) (2.54 oz)   **Entree**

Calories	209	(82.2 cal/oz)	Carbohydrate	19.31 g	(6% DV)
Fat Calories	89	(43% fat)	Dietary Fiber	1.42 g	(6% DV)
Total Fat	9.94 g	(15% DV)	Protein	9.23 g	(18% DV)
Saturated Fat	4.26 g	(21% DV)	Vitamin A	358.6 IU	(7% DV)
Poly Fat	1.42 g		Vitamin C	6.4 mg	(11% DV)
Mono Fat	4.26 g		Calcium	147 mg	(15% DV)
Cholesterol	17.8 mg	(6% DV)	Iron	1.5 mg	(8% DV)
Sodium	525.4 mg	(22% DV)	Folate	9.2 mcg	(5% DV)
Potassium	167.6 mg	(5% DV)	Beta Carotene	27.7 RE	

Ratings	Worst	Bad	Average	Good	Best
Weight Loss				6	
LowCal Density		3			
Filling		4			
Energizing				6	
Fiber			5		
Vitamins			5		
Minerals				6	
Overall			5		

PIZZA WITH MEAT & VEGETABLES, LOWFAT, THIN CRUST

Serving: 1 piece (4.64 oz)   Entree

Calories	264	(56.9 cal/oz)	Carbohydrate	28.08 g	(9% DV)
Fat Calories	94	(35% fat)	Dietary Fiber	1.3 g	(5% DV)
Total Fat	10.4 g	(16% DV)	Protein	13 g	(26% DV)
Saturated Fat	3.9 g	(19% DV)	VItamin A	456.3 IU	(9% DV)
Poly Fat	1.3 g		Vitamin C	11.7 mg	(19% DV)
Mono Fat	3.9 g		Calcium	179.4 mg	(18% DV)
Cholesterol	18.2 mg	(6% DV)	Iron	2.1 mg	(11% DV)
Sodium	666.9 mg	(28% DV)	Folate	13 mcg	(7% DV)
Potassium	226.2 mg	(6% DV)	Beta Carotene	39 RE	

Ratings	Worst	Bad	Average	Good	Best
Weight Loss				6	
LowCal Density			5		
Filling			5		
Energizing				7	
Fiber			5		
Vitamins			6		
Minerals			6		
Overall			6		

PIZZA, CHEESE

Serving: 1 piece (1/8 of 12" dia) (2.25 oz)   Entree

Calories	163	(72.2 cal/oz)	Carbohydrate	19.09 g	(6% DV)
Fat Calories	57	(35% fat)	Dietary Fiber	1.26 g	(5% DV)
Total Fat	6.3 g	(10% DV)	Protein	7.56 g	(15% DV)
Saturated Fat	2.52 g	(13% DV)	VItamin A	360.4 IU	(7% DV)
Poly Fat	.63 g		Vitamin C	6.9 mg	(12% DV)
Mono Fat	2.52 g		Calcium	146.8 mg	(15% DV)
Cholesterol	9.5 mg	(3% DV)	Iron	1.3 mg	(7% DV)
Sodium	392.5 mg	(16% DV)	Folate	7.6 mcg	(5% DV)
Potassium	138.6 mg	(4% DV)	Beta Carotene	27.7 RE	

Ratings	Worst	Bad	Average	Good	Best
Weight Loss				7	
LowCal Density		4			
Filling		4			
Energizing			6		
Fiber			5		
Vitamins			5		
Minerals			5		
Overall			5		

PIZZABURGER (HAMBURGER,CHEESE,SAUCE) ON BUN

Serving: 1 pizzaburger (5.89 oz)   **Sandwich**

Calories	436	(74 cal/oz)	Carbohydrate	32.01 g	(11% DV)
Fat Calories	193	(44% fat)	Dietary Fiber	1.65 g	(7% DV)
Total Fat	21.45 g	(33% DV)	Protein	26.4 g	(53% DV)
Saturated Fat	9.9 g	(50% DV)	Vitamin A	529.7 IU	(11% DV)
Poly Fat	1.65 g		Vitamin C	3.3 mg	(5% DV)
Mono Fat	8.25 g		Calcium	206.3 mg	(21% DV)
Cholesterol	82.5 mg	(28% DV)	Iron	3.5 mg	(19% DV)
Sodium	823.4 mg	(34% DV)	Folate	26.4 mcg	(8% DV)
Potassium	382.8 mg	(11% DV)	Beta Carotene	33 RE	

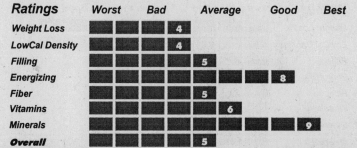

Ratings	Worst	Bad	Average	Good	Best
Weight Loss			4		
LowCal Density			4		
Filling			5		
Energizing				8	
Fiber			5		
Vitamins			6		
Minerals				9	
Overall			5		

PLANTAIN, RIPE, ROLLED IN FLOUR, FRIED

Serving: 1 piece (2½" long) (1.61 oz)   **Vegetable**

Calories	112	(69.6 cal/oz)	Carbohydrate	16.38 g	(5% DV)
Fat Calories	49	(43% fat)	Dietary Fiber	.9 g	(4% DV)
Total Fat	5.4 g	(8% DV)	Protein	.9 g	(2% DV)
Saturated Fat	.9 g	(5% DV)	Vitamin A	379.4 IU	(8% DV)
Poly Fat	3.15 g		Vitamin C	5.9 mg	(10% DV)
Mono Fat	1.35 g		Calcium	1.8 mg	(0% DV)
Cholesterol	0 mg	(0% DV)	Iron	.4 mg	(2% DV)
Sodium	1.8 mg	(0% DV)	Folate	.9 mcg	(1% DV)
Potassium	204.3 mg	(6% DV)	Beta Carotene	38.3 RE	

Ratings	Worst	Bad	Average	Good	Best
Weight Loss			5		
LowCal Density		4			
Filling		4			
Energizing			5		
Fiber		4			
Vitamins		4			
Minerals	3				
Overall		4			

PLUM, RAW

Serving: 1 plum (2-1/8" dia) (2.36 oz)   **Fruit**

Calories	36	(15.4 cal/oz)	Carbohydrate	8.58 g	(3% DV)
Fat Calories	6	(16% fat)	Dietary Fiber	1.32 g	(5% DV)
Total Fat	.66 g	(1% DV)	Protein	.66 g	(1% DV)
Saturated Fat	0 g	(0% DV)	Vitamin A	213.2 IU	(4% DV)
Poly Fat	0 g		Vitamin C	6.6 mg	(11% DV)
Mono Fat	0 g		Calcium	2.6 mg	(0% DV)
Cholesterol	0 mg	(0% DV)	Iron	.1 mg	(0% DV)
Sodium	0 mg	(0% DV)	Folate	.7 mcg	(0% DV)
Potassium	113.5 mg	(3% DV)	Beta Carotene	21.1 RE	

Ratings

	Worst	Bad	Average	Good	Best
Weight Loss					9
LowCal Density					9
Filling			5		
Energizing		4			
Fiber			5		
Vitamins		4			
Minerals	2				
Overall				7	

POLISH SAUSAGE

Serving: 1 link (3 oz)   **Meat**

Calories	260	(86.8 cal/oz)	Carbohydrate	1.76 g	(1% DV)
Fat Calories	204	(78% fat)	Dietary Fiber	0 g	(0% DV)
Total Fat	22.68 g	(35% DV)	Protein	10.92 g	(22% DV)
Saturated Fat	8.4 g	(42% DV)	Vitamin A	0 IU	(0% DV)
Poly Fat	2.52 g		Vitamin C	17.6 mg	(29% DV)
Mono Fat	10.92 g		Calcium	37 mg	(4% DV)
Cholesterol	56.3 mg	(19% DV)	Iron	1.2 mg	(7% DV)
Sodium	903.8 mg	(38% DV)	Folate	10.9 mcg	(1% DV)
Potassium	227.6 mg	(7% DV)	Beta Carotene	0 RE	

Ratings

	Worst	Bad	Average	Good	Best
Weight Loss	2				
LowCal Density		3			
Filling	1				
Energizing		3			
Fiber	1				
Vitamins			5		
Minerals			5		
Overall		3			

POMPANO, BAKED OR BROILED

Serving: 1 piece (3.04 oz)   **Fish**

Calories	216	(71 cal/oz)	Carbohydrate	.51 g	(0% DV)
Fat Calories	130	(60% fat)	Dietary Fiber	0 g	(0% DV)
Total Fat	14.45 g	(22% DV)	Protein	20.4 g	(41% DV)
Saturated Fat	4.25 g	(21% DV)	VItamin A	316.2 IU	(6% DV)
Poly Fat	2.55 g		Vitamin C	2.6 mg	(4% DV)
Mono Fat	4.25 g		Calcium	26.4 mg	(3% DV)
Cholesterol	54.4 mg	(18% DV)	Iron	.7 mg	(4% DV)
Sodium	499.8 mg	(21% DV)	Folate	20.4 mcg	(4% DV)
Potassium	423.3 mg	(12% DV)	Beta Carotene	4.3 RE	

Ratings	Worst	Bad	Average	Good	Best
Weight Loss		3			
LowCal Density			4		
Filling	1				
Energizing	2				
Fiber	1				
Vitamins					6
Minerals				5	
Overall		3			

POMPANO, BATTERED, FRIED

Serving: 1 piece (3.04 oz)   **Fish**

Calories	228	(74.9 cal/oz)	Carbohydrate	5.69 g	(2% DV)
Fat Calories	145	(64% fat)	Dietary Fiber	0 g	(0% DV)
Total Fat	16.15 g	(25% DV)	Protein	14.45 g	(29% DV)
Saturated Fat	5.1 g	(25% DV)	VItamin A	83.3 IU	(2% DV)
Poly Fat	3.4 g		Vitamin C	0 mg	(0% DV)
Mono Fat	5.95 g		Calcium	35.7 mg	(4% DV)
Cholesterol	51.9 mg	(17% DV)	Iron	.8 mg	(5% DV)
Sodium	97.8 mg	(4% DV)	Folate	14.5 mcg	(3% DV)
Potassium	298.4 mg	(9% DV)	Beta Carotene	0 RE	

Ratings	Worst	Bad	Average	Good	Best
Weight Loss		3			
LowCal Density			4		
Filling	2				
Energizing		3			
Fiber	1				
Vitamins				5	
Minerals				5	
Overall		3			

POPCORN, AIR-POPPED (NO BUTTER OR OIL ADDED)

Serving: 1 cup (.29 oz)   **Snack**

Calories	31	(105.4 cal/oz)	Carbohydrate	6.23 g	(2% DV)
Fat Calories	3	(9% fat)	Dietary Fiber	1.2 g	(5% DV)
Total Fat	.32 g	(0% DV)	Protein	.96 g	(2% DV)
Saturated Fat	.08 g	(0% DV)	VItamin A	15.7 IU	(0% DV)
Poly Fat	.16 g		Vitamin C	0 mg	(0% DV)
Mono Fat	.08 g		Calcium	.8 mg	(0% DV)
Cholesterol	0 mg	(0% DV)	Iron	.2 mg	(1% DV)
Sodium	.3 mg	(0% DV)	Folate	1 mcg	(0% DV)
Potassium	24.1 mg	(1% DV)	Beta Carotene	1.6 RE	

Ratings	Worst	Bad	Average	Good	Best
Weight Loss					9
LowCal Density	2				
Filling	2				
Energizing	4				
Fiber	5				
Vitamins	2				
Minerals	3				
Overall	4				

POPCORN, AIR-POPPED, BUTTERED

Serving: 1 cup (.46 oz)   **Snack**

Calories	63	(136.5 cal/oz)	Carbohydrate	6.98 g	(2% DV)
Fat Calories	33	(52% fat)	Dietary Fiber	1.3 g	(5% DV)
Total Fat	3.64 g	(6% DV)	Protein	1.17 g	(2% DV)
Saturated Fat	2.08 g	(10% DV)	VItamin A	139.2 IU	(3% DV)
Poly Fat	.26 g		Vitamin C	0 mg	(0% DV)
Mono Fat	1.04 g		Calcium	1.8 mg	(0% DV)
Cholesterol	8.7 mg	(3% DV)	Iron	.2 mg	(1% DV)
Sodium	55 mg	(2% DV)	Folate	1.2 mcg	(1% DV)
Potassium	28.1 mg	(1% DV)	Beta Carotene	5.1 RE	

Ratings	Worst	Bad	Average	Good	Best
Weight Loss	6				
LowCal Density	1				
Filling	2				
Energizing	4				
Fiber	5				
Vitamins	2				
Minerals	3				
Overall	3				

POPCORN, POPPED IN OIL, BUTTERED

Serving: 1 cup (.5 oz)   **Snack**

Calories	73	(145.9 cal/oz)	Carbohydrate	7.22 g	(2% DV)
Fat Calories	42	(57% fat)	Dietary Fiber	1.26 g	(5% DV)
Total Fat	4.62 g	(7% DV)	Protein	1.12 g	(2% DV)
Saturated Fat	1.26 g	(6% DV)	Vitamin A	61.6 IU	(1% DV)
Poly Fat	1.68 g		Vitamin C	0 mg	(0% DV)
Mono Fat	1.4 g		Calcium	1.5 mg	(0% DV)
Cholesterol	3.1 mg	(1% DV)	Iron	.4 mg	(2% DV)
Sodium	122.9 mg	(5% DV)	Folate	1.1 mcg	(1% DV)
Potassium	28.7 mg	(1% DV)	Beta Carotene	3.1 RE	

Ratings	Worst	Bad	Average	Good	Best
Weight Loss				5	
LowCal Density	1				
Filling	2				
Energizing			4		
Fiber			5		
Vitamins	2				
Minerals		3			
Overall		3			

POPOVER

Serving: 1 popover (1.11 oz)   **Bakery**

Calories	69	(62.6 cal/oz)	Carbohydrate	8.65 g	(3% DV)
Fat Calories	22	(32% fat)	Dietary Fiber	.31 g	(1% DV)
Total Fat	2.48 g	(4% DV)	Protein	2.79 g	(6% DV)
Saturated Fat	.93 g	(5% DV)	Vitamin A	75.6 IU	(2% DV)
Poly Fat	.31 g		Vitamin C	0 mg	(0% DV)
Mono Fat	.93 g		Calcium	28.8 mg	(3% DV)
Cholesterol	36.9 mg	(12% DV)	Iron	.6 mg	(3% DV)
Sodium	63.6 mg	(3% DV)	Folate	2.8 mcg	(1% DV)
Potassium	50.2 mg	(1% DV)	Beta Carotene	.6 RE	

Ratings	Worst	Bad	Average	Good	Best
Weight Loss					7
LowCal Density			5		
Filling		3			
Energizing			4		
Fiber	2				
Vitamins		3			
Minerals		3			
Overall			5		

PORCUPINE BALLS WITH TOMATO-BASED SAUCE

Serving: 1 ball (1.25 oz)   **Entree**

Calories	58	(46.2 cal/oz)	Carbohydrate	4.51 g	(2% DV)
Fat Calories	22	(38% fat)	Dietary Fiber	0 g	(0% DV)
Total Fat	2.45 g	(4% DV)	Protein	3.85 g	(8% DV)
Saturated Fat	1.05 g	(5% DV)	Vitamin A	58.5 IU	(1% DV)
Poly Fat	.35 g		Vitamin C	5.6 mg	(9% DV)
Mono Fat	1.05 g		Calcium	4.6 mg	(0% DV)
Cholesterol	12.6 mg	(4% DV)	Iron	.7 mg	(4% DV)
Sodium	166.6 mg	(7% DV)	Folate	3.9 mcg	(1% DV)
Potassium	72.5 mg	(2% DV)	Beta Carotene	6 RE	

Ratings	Worst	Bad	Average	Good	Best
Weight Loss				8	
LowCal Density			6		
Filling	2				
Energizing	3				
Fiber	1				
Vitamins	3				
Minerals	3				
Overall			5		

PORK & BEANS

Serving: 1 cup (9.04 oz)   **Vegetable**

Calories	248	(27.4 cal/oz)	Carbohydrate	49.08 g	(16% DV)
Fat Calories	23	(9% fat)	Dietary Fiber	15.18 g	(61% DV)
Total Fat	2.53 g	(4% DV)	Protein	12.65 g	(25% DV)
Saturated Fat	0 g	(0% DV)	Vitamin A	313.7 IU	(6% DV)
Poly Fat	0 g		Vitamin C	7.6 mg	(13% DV)
Mono Fat	0 g		Calcium	141.7 mg	(14% DV)
Cholesterol	17.7 mg	(6% DV)	Iron	8.3 mg	(46% DV)
Sodium	1113.2 mg	(46% DV)	Folate	12.7 mcg	(15% DV)
Potassium	759 mg	(22% DV)	Beta Carotene	30.4 RE	

Ratings	Worst	Bad	Average	Good	Best
Weight Loss	3				
LowCal Density				8	
Filling					10
Energizing				9	
Fiber					10
Vitamins			5		
Minerals					10
Overall			7		

PORK BACON, SMOKED OR CURED, COOKED

Serving: 1 slice (.29 oz)   **Meat**

Calories	46	(158.9 cal/oz)	Carbohydrate	.05 g	(0% DV)
Fat Calories	35	(77% fat)	Dietary Fiber	0 g	(0% DV)
Total Fat	3.92 g	(6% DV)	Protein	2.4 g	(5% DV)
Saturated Fat	1.36 g	(7% DV)	Vitamin A	0 IU	(0% DV)
Poly Fat	.48 g		Vitamin C	2.7 mg	(5% DV)
Mono Fat	1.92 g		Calcium	1 mg	(0% DV)
Cholesterol	6.8 mg	(2% DV)	Iron	.1 mg	(1% DV)
Sodium	127.7 mg	(5% DV)	Folate	2.4 mcg	(0% DV)
Potassium	38.9 mg	(1% DV)	Beta Carotene	0 RE	

Ratings	Worst	Bad	Average	Good	Best
Weight Loss			5		
LowCal Density	1				
Filling	1				
Energizing		2			
Fiber	1				
Vitamins			3		
Minerals		2			
Overall		2			

PORK BARBECUE OR SLOPPY JOE, ON BUN

Serving: 1 barbecue (6.64 oz)   **Sandwich**

Calories	346	(52.1 cal/oz)	Carbohydrate	38.69 g	(13% DV)
Fat Calories	84	(24% fat)	Dietary Fiber	3.72 g	(15% DV)
Total Fat	9.3 g	(14% DV)	Protein	24.18 g	(48% DV)
Saturated Fat	3.72 g	(19% DV)	Vitamin A	611.9 IU	(12% DV)
Poly Fat	1.86 g		Vitamin C	5.6 mg	(9% DV)
Mono Fat	5.58 g		Calcium	81.8 mg	(8% DV)
Cholesterol	52.1 mg	(17% DV)	Iron	2.9 mg	(16% DV)
Sodium	889.1 mg	(37% DV)	Folate	24.2 mcg	(7% DV)
Potassium	399.9 mg	(11% DV)	Beta Carotene	61.4 RE	

Ratings	Worst	Bad	Average	Good	Best
Weight Loss			6		
LowCal Density			6		
Filling			6		
Energizing				9	
Fiber				9	
Vitamins			7		
Minerals			7		
Overall			7		

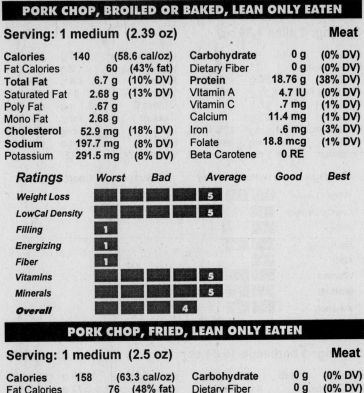

PORK CHOP, BROILED OR BAKED, LEAN ONLY EATEN

Serving: 1 medium (2.39 oz) — Meat

Calories	140	(58.6 cal/oz)	Carbohydrate	0 g	(0% DV)
Fat Calories	60	(43% fat)	Dietary Fiber	0 g	(0% DV)
Total Fat	6.7 g	(10% DV)	Protein	18.76 g	(38% DV)
Saturated Fat	2.68 g	(13% DV)	Vitamin A	4.7 IU	(0% DV)
Poly Fat	.67 g		Vitamin C	.7 mg	(1% DV)
Mono Fat	2.68 g		Calcium	11.4 mg	(1% DV)
Cholesterol	52.9 mg	(18% DV)	Iron	.6 mg	(3% DV)
Sodium	197.7 mg	(8% DV)	Folate	18.8 mcg	(1% DV)
Potassium	291.5 mg	(8% DV)	Beta Carotene	0 RE	

Ratings	Worst	Bad	Average	Good	Best
Weight Loss			5		
LowCal Density			5		
Filling	1				
Energizing	1				
Fiber	1				
Vitamins				5	
Minerals				5	
Overall			4		

PORK CHOP, FRIED, LEAN ONLY EATEN

Serving: 1 medium (2.5 oz) — Meat

Calories	158	(63.3 cal/oz)	Carbohydrate	0 g	(0% DV)
Fat Calories	76	(48% fat)	Dietary Fiber	0 g	(0% DV)
Total Fat	8.4 g	(13% DV)	Protein	20.3 g	(41% DV)
Saturated Fat	2.8 g	(14% DV)	Vitamin A	4.9 IU	(0% DV)
Poly Fat	.7 g		Vitamin C	.7 mg	(1% DV)
Mono Fat	3.5 g		Calcium	12.6 mg	(1% DV)
Cholesterol	54.6 mg	(18% DV)	Iron	.6 mg	(3% DV)
Sodium	207.9 mg	(9% DV)	Folate	20.3 mcg	(1% DV)
Potassium	310.1 mg	(9% DV)	Beta Carotene	0 RE	

Ratings	Worst	Bad	Average	Good	Best
Weight Loss		4			
LowCal Density			5		
Filling	1				
Energizing	1				
Fiber	1				
Vitamins				5	
Minerals				5	
Overall			4		

PORK PATTY, COOKED

Serving: 1 patty (3.04 oz)   **Meat**

Calories	246	(80.8 cal/oz)	Carbohydrate	0 g	(0% DV)
Fat Calories	161	(65% fat)	Dietary Fiber	0 g	(0% DV)
Total Fat	17.85 g	(27% DV)	Protein	19.55 g	(39% DV)
Saturated Fat	6.8 g	(34% DV)	Vltamin A	6.8 IU	(0% DV)
Poly Fat	1.7 g		Vitamin C	0 mg	(0% DV)
Mono Fat	7.65 g		Calcium	20.4 mg	(2% DV)
Cholesterol	75.7 mg	(25% DV)	Iron	1.1 mg	(6% DV)
Sodium	383.4 mg	(16% DV)	Folate	19.6 mcg	(1% DV)
Potassium	277.1 mg	(8% DV)	Beta Carotene	0 RE	

Ratings	Worst	Bad	Average	Good	Best
Weight Loss	2				
LowCal Density	3				
Filling	1				
Energizing	1				
Fiber	1				
Vitamins			5		
Minerals				6	
Overall	3				

PORK SANDWICH

Serving: 1 sandwich (4.86 oz)   **Sandwich**

Calories	314	(64.6 cal/oz)	Carbohydrate	24.62 g	(8% DV)
Fat Calories	86	(27% fat)	Dietary Fiber	1.36 g	(5% DV)
Total Fat	9.52 g	(15% DV)	Protein	28.56 g	(57% DV)
Saturated Fat	2.72 g	(14% DV)	Vltamin A	5.4 IU	(0% DV)
Poly Fat	1.36 g		Vitamin C	0 mg	(0% DV)
Mono Fat	4.08 g		Calcium	76.2 mg	(8% DV)
Cholesterol	74.8 mg	(25% DV)	Iron	2.4 mg	(13% DV)
Sodium	518.2 mg	(22% DV)	Folate	28.6 mcg	(5% DV)
Potassium	379.4 mg	(11% DV)	Beta Carotene	0 RE	

Ratings	Worst	Bad	Average	Good	Best
Weight Loss			6		
LowCal Density			5		
Filling			5		
Energizing			6		
Fiber			5		
Vitamins				7	
Minerals				7	
Overall			6		

PORK SKIN, RINDS, DEEP-FRIED

Serving: 1 bag (2.04 oz)   **Snack**

Calories	307	(150.3 cal/oz)	Carbohydrate	0 g	(0% DV)
Fat Calories	159	(52% fat)	Dietary Fiber	0 g	(0% DV)
Total Fat	17.67 g	(27% DV)	Protein	35.34 g	(71% DV)
Saturated Fat	6.27 g	(31% DV)	VItamin A	0 IU	(0% DV)
Poly Fat	1.71 g		Vitamin C	0 mg	(0% DV)
Mono Fat	7.98 g		Calcium	12.5 mg	(1% DV)
Cholesterol	54.7 mg	(18% DV)	Iron	.5 mg	(3% DV)
Sodium	1527.6 mg	(64% DV)	Folate	35.3 mcg	(0% DV)
Potassium	99.2 mg	(3% DV)	Beta Carotene	0 RE	

Ratings	Worst	Bad	Average	Good	Best
Weight Loss		2			
LowCal Density	1				
Filling	1				
Energizing	1				
Fiber	1				
Vitamins		2			
Minerals			3		
Overall		2			

PORK STEAK OR CUTLET, BATTERED, FRIED, LEAN ONLY

Serving: 1 steak (3.04 oz)   **Meat**

Calories	217	(71.3 cal/oz)	Carbohydrate	5.53 g	(2% DV)
Fat Calories	107	(49% fat)	Dietary Fiber	0 g	(0% DV)
Total Fat	11.9 g	(18% DV)	Protein	20.4 g	(41% DV)
Saturated Fat	3.4 g	(17% DV)	VItamin A	31.5 IU	(1% DV)
Poly Fat	1.7 g		Vitamin C	.9 mg	(1% DV)
Mono Fat	5.1 g		Calcium	40 mg	(4% DV)
Cholesterol	68 mg	(23% DV)	Iron	1.1 mg	(6% DV)
Sodium	255 mg	(11% DV)	Folate	20.4 mcg	(1% DV)
Potassium	282.2 mg	(8% DV)	Beta Carotene	0 RE	

Ratings	Worst	Bad	Average	Good	Best
Weight Loss		3			
LowCal Density			4		
Filling	2				
Energizing		3			
Fiber	1				
Vitamins				6	
Minerals				6	
Overall		3			

PORK STEAK OR CUTLET, LEAN ONLY EATEN

Serving: 1 small steak (4.57 oz)   **Meat**

Calories	311	(68.1 cal/oz)	Carbohydrate	0 g	(0% DV)
Fat Calories	150	(48% fat)	Dietary Fiber	0 g	(0% DV)
Total Fat	16.64 g	(26% DV)	Protein	38.4 g	(77% DV)
Saturated Fat	6.4 g	(32% DV)	Vitamin A	10.2 IU	(0% DV)
Poly Fat	1.28 g		Vitamin C	1.3 mg	(2% DV)
Mono Fat	7.68 g		Calcium	35.8 mg	(4% DV)
Cholesterol	128 mg	(43% DV)	Iron	2 mg	(11% DV)
Sodium	373.8 mg	(16% DV)	Folate	38.4 mcg	(1% DV)
Potassium	510.7 mg	(15% DV)	Beta Carotene	0 RE	

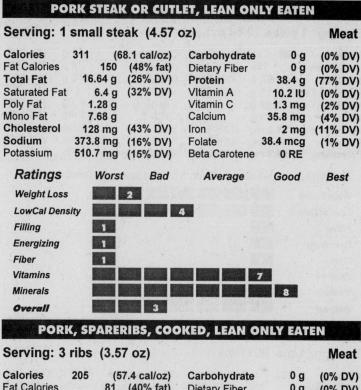

Ratings	Worst	Bad	Average	Good	Best
Weight Loss	2				
LowCal Density			4		
Filling	1				
Energizing	1				
Fiber	1				
Vitamins				7	
Minerals					8
Overall		3			

PORK, SPARERIBS, COOKED, LEAN ONLY EATEN

Serving: 3 ribs (3.57 oz)   **Meat**

Calories	205	(57.4 cal/oz)	Carbohydrate	0 g	(0% DV)
Fat Calories	81	(40% fat)	Dietary Fiber	0 g	(0% DV)
Total Fat	9 g	(14% DV)	Protein	28 g	(56% DV)
Saturated Fat	4 g	(20% DV)	Vitamin A	6 IU	(0% DV)
Poly Fat	1 g		Vitamin C	0 mg	(0% DV)
Mono Fat	4 g		Calcium	22 mg	(2% DV)
Cholesterol	71 mg	(24% DV)	Iron	1 mg	(5% DV)
Sodium	272 mg	(11% DV)	Folate	28 mcg	(0% DV)
Potassium	403 mg	(12% DV)	Beta Carotene	0 RE	

Ratings	Worst	Bad	Average	Good	Best
Weight Loss			4		
LowCal Density			5		
Filling	1				
Energizing	1				
Fiber	1				
Vitamins				6	
Minerals			5		
Overall			4		

PORK, TENDERLOIN, BAKED

Serving: 1 piece (3.04 oz)   **Meat**

Calories	147	(48.4 cal/oz)	Carbohydrate	0 g	(0% DV)
Fat Calories	46	(31% fat)	Dietary Fiber	0 g	(0% DV)
Total Fat	5.1 g	(8% DV)	Protein	23.8 g	(48% DV)
Saturated Fat	1.7 g	(8% DV)	Vitamin A	6 IU	(0% DV)
Poly Fat	.85 g		Vitamin C	0 mg	(0% DV)
Mono Fat	1.7 g		Calcium	5.1 mg	(1% DV)
Cholesterol	67.2 mg	(22% DV)	Iron	1.2 mg	(7% DV)
Sodium	46.8 mg	(2% DV)	Folate	23.8 mcg	(1% DV)
Potassium	368.1 mg	(11% DV)	Beta Carotene	0 RE	

Ratings

	Worst	Bad	Average	Good	Best
Weight Loss				6	
LowCal Density				6	
Filling	1				
Energizing	1				
Fiber	1				
Vitamins				6	
Minerals				6	
Overall			5		

POT PIE, VEGETARIAN

Serving: 1 pie (8.11 oz)   **Entree**

Calories	524	(64.7 cal/oz)	Carbohydrate	41.09 g	(14% DV)
Fat Calories	306	(58% fat)	Dietary Fiber	4.54 g	(18% DV)
Total Fat	34.05 g	(52% DV)	Protein	13.62 g	(27% DV)
Saturated Fat	9.08 g	(45% DV)	Vitamin A	6269.7 IU	(125% DV)
Poly Fat	9.08 g		Vitamin C	9.1 mg	(15% DV)
Mono Fat	13.62 g		Calcium	65.8 mg	(7% DV)
Cholesterol	20.4 mg	(7% DV)	Iron	2.9 mg	(16% DV)
Sodium	538 mg	(22% DV)	Folate	13.6 mcg	(10% DV)
Potassium	331.4 mg	(9% DV)	Beta Carotene	572 RE	

Ratings

	Worst	Bad	Average	Good	Best
Weight Loss	2				
LowCal Density			5		
Filling			6		
Energizing					9
Fiber					9
Vitamins					10
Minerals			6		
Overall			5		

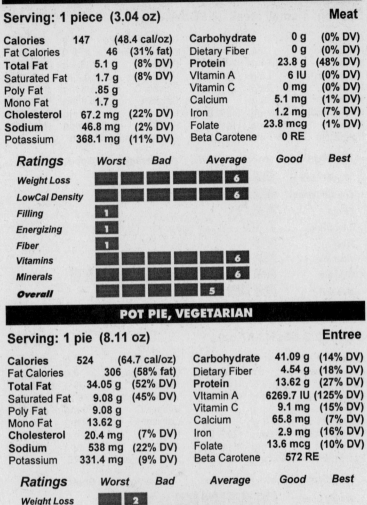

POTATO , SKINS, FRIED

Serving: 1 large (3-4¼" raw dia) (2.5 oz)　　　**Vegetable**

Calories	316	(126.6 cal/oz)	Carbohydrate	24.78 g	(8% DV)
Fat Calories	170	(54% fat)	Dietary Fiber	2.1 g	(8% DV)
Total Fat	18.9 g	(29% DV)	Protein	11.9 g	(24% DV)
Saturated Fat	7.7 g	(39% DV)	Vitamin A	187.6 IU	(4% DV)
Poly Fat	2.8 g		Vitamin C	15.4 mg	(26% DV)
Mono Fat	7.7 g		Calcium	144.2 mg	(14% DV)
Cholesterol	33.6 mg	(11% DV)	Iron	3.1 mg	(17% DV)
Sodium	401.8 mg	(17% DV)	Folate	11.9 mcg	(4% DV)
Potassium	452.2 mg	(13% DV)	Beta Carotene	3.5 RE	

Ratings	Worst	Bad	Average	Good	Best
Weight Loss	1				
LowCal Density	2				
Filling	3				
Energizing			6		
Fiber			6		
Vitamins				7	
Minerals				7	
Overall	3				

POTATO PANCAKE, FROZEN

Serving: 1 pancake (1.54 oz)　　　**Vegetable**

Calories	83	(53.6 cal/oz)	Carbohydrate	9.2 g	(3% DV)
Fat Calories	39	(47% fat)	Dietary Fiber	.86 g	(3% DV)
Total Fat	4.3 g	(7% DV)	Protein	2.15 g	(4% DV)
Saturated Fat	1.29 g	(6% DV)	Vitamin A	44.3 IU	(1% DV)
Poly Fat	.86 g		Vitamin C	6.9 mg	(11% DV)
Mono Fat	1.72 g		Calcium	7.3 mg	(1% DV)
Cholesterol	29.7 mg	(10% DV)	Iron	.5 mg	(3% DV)
Sodium	162.5 mg	(7% DV)	Folate	2.2 mcg	(2% DV)
Potassium	242.1 mg	(7% DV)	Beta Carotene	0 RE	

Ratings	Worst	Bad	Average	Good	Best
Weight Loss			5		
LowCal Density			6		
Filling	3				
Energizing		4			
Fiber		4			
Vitamins		4			
Minerals	3				
Overall			5		

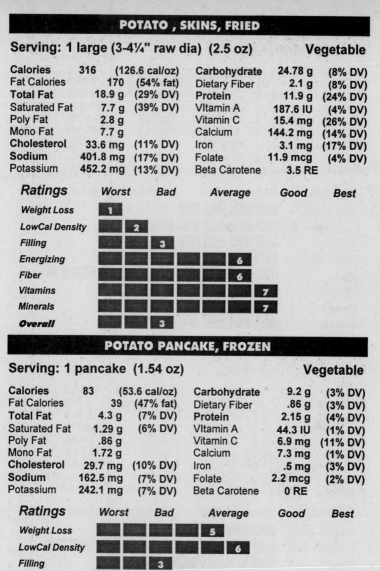

POTATO SALAD WITH EGG

Serving: 1 cup (6.89 oz)   **Salad**

Calories	270	(39.2 cal/oz)	Carbohydrate	29.53 g	(10% DV)
Fat Calories	139	(51% fat)	Dietary Fiber	3.86 g	(15% DV)
Total Fat	15.44 g	(24% DV)	Protein	5.79 g	(12% DV)
Saturated Fat	1.93 g	(10% DV)	Vitamin A	252.8 IU	(5% DV)
Poly Fat	7.72 g		Vitamin C	21.2 mg	(35% DV)
Mono Fat	3.86 g		Calcium	29 mg	(3% DV)
Cholesterol	100.4 mg	(33% DV)	Iron	.9 mg	(5% DV)
Sodium	638.8 mg	(27% DV)	Folate	5.8 mcg	(7% DV)
Potassium	573.2 mg	(16% DV)	Beta Carotene	9.7 RE	

Ratings	Worst	Bad	Average	Good	Best
Weight Loss		4			
LowCal Density			6		
Filling			6		
Energizing			7		
Fiber					9
Vitamins			6		
Minerals			5		
Overall			6		

POTATO SOUP, PREPARED WITH MILK

Serving: 1 cup (8.86 oz)   **Soup**

Calories	149	(16.8 cal/oz)	Carbohydrate	17.11 g	(6% DV)
Fat Calories	67	(45% fat)	Dietary Fiber	0 g	(0% DV)
Total Fat	7.44 g	(11% DV)	Protein	4.96 g	(10% DV)
Saturated Fat	4.96 g	(25% DV)	Vitamin A	443.9 IU	(9% DV)
Poly Fat	0 g		Vitamin C	2.5 mg	(4% DV)
Mono Fat	2.48 g		Calcium	166.2 mg	(17% DV)
Cholesterol	22.3 mg	(7% DV)	Iron	.6 mg	(3% DV)
Sodium	1061.4 mg	(44% DV)	Folate	5 mcg	(2% DV)
Potassium	322.4 mg	(9% DV)	Beta Carotene	29.8 RE	

Ratings	Worst	Bad	Average	Good	Best
Weight Loss		4			
LowCal Density					9
Filling			7		
Energizing			6		
Fiber	1				
Vitamins		4			
Minerals			5		
Overall			6		

POTATO, BAKED, PEEL EATEN, NO FAT ADDED

Serving: 1 medium (2¼-3" dia, raw) (4.36 oz)   Vegetable

Calories	132	(30.2 cal/oz)	Carbohydrate	30.62 g	(10% DV)
Fat Calories	0	(0% fat)	Dietary Fiber	2.44 g	(10% DV)
Total Fat	0 g	(0% DV)	Protein	2.44 g	(5% DV)
Saturated Fat	0 g	(0% DV)	Vitamin A	0 IU	(0% DV)
Poly Fat	0 g		Vitamin C	15.9 mg	(26% DV)
Mono Fat	0 g		Calcium	12.2 mg	(1% DV)
Cholesterol	0 mg	(0% DV)	Iron	1.7 mg	(9% DV)
Sodium	291.6 mg	(12% DV)	Folate	2.4 mcg	(3% DV)
Potassium	507.5 mg	(15% DV)	Beta Carotene	0 RE	

Ratings	Worst	Bad	Average	Good	Best
Weight Loss				7	
LowCal Density				7	
Filling				7	
Energizing				7	
Fiber				7	
Vitamins			5		
Minerals		4			
Overall				7	

POTATO, BOILED, WITHOUT PEEL, FAT ADDED

Serving: 1 medium (2¼-3" dia, raw) (4.54 oz)   Vegetable

Calories	138	(30.5 cal/oz)	Carbohydrate	24.38 g	(8% DV)
Fat Calories	34	(25% fat)	Dietary Fiber	2.54 g	(10% DV)
Total Fat	3.81 g	(6% DV)	Protein	2.54 g	(5% DV)
Saturated Fat	1.27 g	(6% DV)	Vitamin A	194.3 IU	(4% DV)
Poly Fat	1.27 g		Vitamin C	8.9 mg	(15% DV)
Mono Fat	1.27 g		Calcium	11.4 mg	(1% DV)
Cholesterol	0 mg	(0% DV)	Iron	.4 mg	(2% DV)
Sodium	337.8 mg	(14% DV)	Folate	2.5 mcg	(3% DV)
Potassium	401.3 mg	(11% DV)	Beta Carotene	3.8 RE	

Ratings	Worst	Bad	Average	Good	Best
Weight Loss			5		
LowCal Density				7	
Filling			6		
Energizing			6		
Fiber				7	
Vitamins			5		
Minerals		4			
Overall			6		

POTATO, CHIPS

Serving: 10 chips regular or rippled (.75 oz)   Snack

Calories	113	(150.1 cal/oz)	Carbohydrate	11.11 g	(4% DV)
Fat Calories	66	(59% fat)	Dietary Fiber	1.05 g	(4% DV)
Total Fat	7.35 g	(11% DV)	Protein	1.47 g	(3% DV)
Saturated Fat	2.31 g	(12% DV)	VItamin A	0 IU	(0% DV)
Poly Fat	2.52 g		Vitamin C	6.5 mg	(11% DV)
Mono Fat	2.1 g		Calcium	5 mg	(1% DV)
Cholesterol	0 mg	(0% DV)	Iron	.3 mg	(2% DV)
Sodium	124.7 mg	(5% DV)	Folate	1.5 mcg	(2% DV)
Potassium	267.8 mg	(8% DV)	Beta Carotene	0 RE	

Ratings	Worst	Bad	Average	Good	Best
Weight Loss			4		
LowCal Density	1				
Filling	2				
Energizing				5	
Fiber			4		
Vitamins			4		
Minerals		3			
Overall		3			

POTATO, CHIPS, RESTRUCTURED

Serving: approx 10 chips (.79 oz)   Snack

Calories	123	(155.4 cal/oz)	Carbohydrate	11.22 g	(4% DV)
Fat Calories	75	(61% fat)	Dietary Fiber	.88 g	(4% DV)
Total Fat	8.36 g	(13% DV)	Protein	1.32 g	(3% DV)
Saturated Fat	1.98 g	(10% DV)	VItamin A	0 IU	(0% DV)
Poly Fat	4.4 g		Vitamin C	1.8 mg	(3% DV)
Mono Fat	1.54 g		Calcium	5.3 mg	(1% DV)
Cholesterol	0 mg	(0% DV)	Iron	.3 mg	(2% DV)
Sodium	144.3 mg	(6% DV)	Folate	1.3 mcg	(0% DV)
Potassium	221.8 mg	(6% DV)	Beta Carotene	0 RE	

Ratings	Worst	Bad	Average	Good	Best
Weight Loss			4		
LowCal Density	1				
Filling	2				
Energizing				5	
Fiber			4		
Vitamins		3			
Minerals		3			
Overall		3			

POTATO, FRENCH FRIED, FROM FROZEN

Serving: 1 fast food order (3.04 oz)   **Vegetable**

Calories	263	(86.4 cal/oz)	Carbohydrate	32.81 g	(11% DV)
Fat Calories	122	(47% fat)	Dietary Fiber	2.55 g	(10% DV)
Total Fat	13.6 g	(21% DV)	Protein	3.4 g	(7% DV)
Saturated Fat	4.25 g	(21% DV)	Vitamin A	24.7 IU	(0% DV)
Poly Fat	1.7 g		Vitamin C	4.3 mg	(7% DV)
Mono Fat	6.8 g		Calcium	13.6 mg	(1% DV)
Cholesterol	1.7 mg	(1% DV)	Iron	1.2 mg	(6% DV)
Sodium	138.6 mg	(6% DV)	Folate	3.4 mcg	(7% DV)
Potassium	605.2 mg	(17% DV)	Beta Carotene	0 RE	

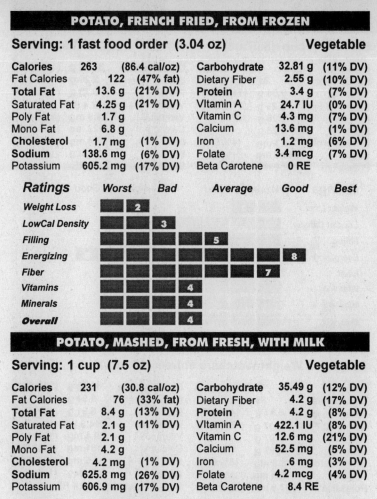

Ratings	Worst	Bad	Average	Good	Best
Weight Loss	2				
LowCal Density	3				
Filling			5		
Energizing				8	
Fiber				7	
Vitamins		4			
Minerals		4			
Overall		4			

POTATO, MASHED, FROM FRESH, WITH MILK

Serving: 1 cup (7.5 oz)   **Vegetable**

Calories	231	(30.8 cal/oz)	Carbohydrate	35.49 g	(12% DV)
Fat Calories	76	(33% fat)	Dietary Fiber	4.2 g	(17% DV)
Total Fat	8.4 g	(13% DV)	Protein	4.2 g	(8% DV)
Saturated Fat	2.1 g	(11% DV)	Vitamin A	422.1 IU	(8% DV)
Poly Fat	2.1 g		Vitamin C	12.6 mg	(21% DV)
Mono Fat	4.2 g		Calcium	52.5 mg	(5% DV)
Cholesterol	4.2 mg	(1% DV)	Iron	.6 mg	(3% DV)
Sodium	625.8 mg	(26% DV)	Folate	4.2 mcg	(4% DV)
Potassium	606.9 mg	(17% DV)	Beta Carotene	8.4 RE	

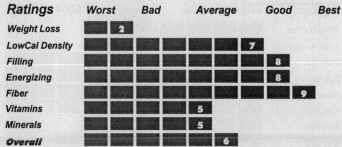

Ratings	Worst	Bad	Average	Good	Best
Weight Loss	2				
LowCal Density				7	
Filling				8	
Energizing				8	
Fiber					9
Vitamins			5		
Minerals			5		
Overall			6		

POTATO, SCALLOPED

Serving: 1 cup (8.07 oz)   **Vegetable**

Calories	235	(29.1 cal/oz)	Carbohydrate	34.35 g	(11% DV)
Fat Calories	81	(35% fat)	Dietary Fiber	2.26 g	(9% DV)
Total Fat	9.04 g	(14% DV)	Protein	6.78 g	(14% DV)
Saturated Fat	2.26 g	(11% DV)	VItamin A	377.4 IU	(8% DV)
Poly Fat	2.26 g		Vitamin C	24.9 mg	(41% DV)
Mono Fat	2.26 g		Calcium	122 mg	(12% DV)
Cholesterol	11.3 mg	(4% DV)	Iron	1.4 mg	(8% DV)
Sodium	743.5 mg	(31% DV)	Folate	6.8 mcg	(5% DV)
Potassium	949.2 mg	(27% DV)	Beta Carotene	9 RE	

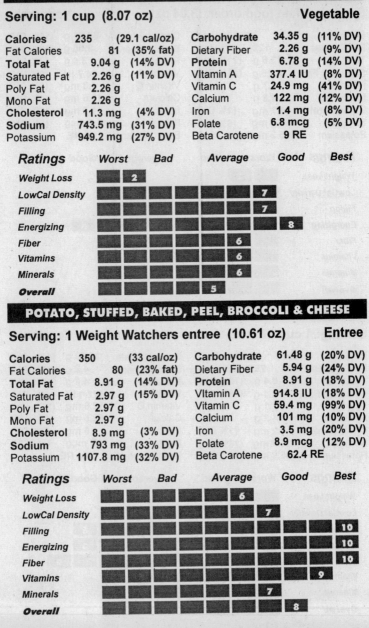

Ratings	Worst	Bad	Average	Good	Best
Weight Loss	2				
LowCal Density				7	
Filling				7	
Energizing				8	
Fiber			6		
Vitamins			6		
Minerals			6		
Overall			5		

POTATO, STUFFED, BAKED, PEEL, BROCCOLI & CHEESE

Serving: 1 Weight Watchers entree (10.61 oz)   **Entree**

Calories	350	(33 cal/oz)	Carbohydrate	61.48 g	(20% DV)
Fat Calories	80	(23% fat)	Dietary Fiber	5.94 g	(24% DV)
Total Fat	8.91 g	(14% DV)	Protein	8.91 g	(18% DV)
Saturated Fat	2.97 g	(15% DV)	VItamin A	914.8 IU	(18% DV)
Poly Fat	2.97 g		Vitamin C	59.4 mg	(99% DV)
Mono Fat	2.97 g		Calcium	101 mg	(10% DV)
Cholesterol	8.9 mg	(3% DV)	Iron	3.5 mg	(20% DV)
Sodium	793 mg	(33% DV)	Folate	8.9 mcg	(12% DV)
Potassium	1107.8 mg	(32% DV)	Beta Carotene	62.4 RE	

Ratings	Worst	Bad	Average	Good	Best
Weight Loss			6		
LowCal Density			7		
Filling					10
Energizing					10
Fiber					10
Vitamins				9	
Minerals			7		
Overall				8	

POTATO, STUFFED, BAKED, WITH PEEL, SOUR CREAM

Serving: 1 long type (10.14 oz)   Entree

Calories	406	(40.1 cal/oz)	Carbohydrate	57.08 g	(19% DV)
Fat Calories	153	(38% fat)	Dietary Fiber	5.68 g	(23% DV)
Total Fat	17.04 g	(26% DV)	Protein	5.68 g	(11% DV)
Saturated Fat	8.52 g	(43% DV)	VItamin A	710 IU	(14% DV)
Poly Fat	2.84 g		Vitamin C	28.4 mg	(47% DV)
Mono Fat	5.68 g		Calcium	96.6 mg	(10% DV)
Cholesterol	28.4 mg	(9% DV)	Iron	3 mg	(17% DV)
Sodium	596.4 mg	(25% DV)	Folate	5.7 mcg	(8% DV)
Potassium	994 mg	(28% DV)	Beta Carotene	17 RE	

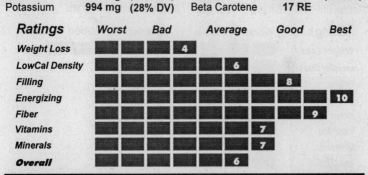

Ratings	Worst	Bad	Average	Good	Best
Weight Loss			4		
LowCal Density			6		
Filling				8	
Energizing					10
Fiber					9
Vitamins				7	
Minerals				7	
Overall			6		

POTATO, HASH BROWN, FROM FROZEN

Serving: 1 patty (2.36 oz)   Vegetable

Calories	143	(60.7 cal/oz)	Carbohydrate	18.41 g	(6% DV)
Fat Calories	65	(46% fat)	Dietary Fiber	1.32 g	(5% DV)
Total Fat	7.26 g	(11% DV)	Protein	1.98 g	(4% DV)
Saturated Fat	2.64 g	(13% DV)	VItamin A	0 IU	(0% DV)
Poly Fat	.66 g		Vitamin C	4 mg	(7% DV)
Mono Fat	3.3 g		Calcium	9.9 mg	(1% DV)
Cholesterol	0 mg	(0% DV)	Iron	1 mg	(5% DV)
Sodium	170.3 mg	(7% DV)	Folate	2 mcg	(1% DV)
Potassium	286.4 mg	(8% DV)	Beta Carotene	0 RE	

Ratings	Worst	Bad	Average	Good	Best
Weight Loss		3			
LowCal Density			5		
Filling		4			
Energizing			6		
Fiber			5		
Vitamins		4			
Minerals		3			
Overall		4			

PRETZELS, HARD

Serving: 10 bite-size pretzels (.43 oz)   **Snack**

Calories	46	(106.3 cal/oz)	Carbohydrate	9.5 g	(3% DV)
Fat Calories	4	(9% fat)	Dietary Fiber	.36 g	(1% DV)
Total Fat	.48 g	(1% DV)	Protein	1.08 g	(2% DV)
Saturated Fat	.12 g	(1% DV)	Vitamin A	0 IU	(0% DV)
Poly Fat	.12 g		Vitamin C	0 mg	(0% DV)
Mono Fat	.12 g		Calcium	4.3 mg	(0% DV)
Cholesterol	0 mg	(0% DV)	Iron	.5 mg	(3% DV)
Sodium	205.8 mg	(9% DV)	Folate	1.1 mcg	(2% DV)
Potassium	17.5 mg	(1% DV)	Beta Carotene	0 RE	

Ratings	Worst	Bad	Average	Good	Best
Weight Loss					9
LowCal Density	2				
Filling	2				
Energizing	4				
Fiber	2				
Vitamins	3				
Minerals	2				
Overall	4				

PRETZELS, SOFT

Serving: 1 pretzel (1.96 oz)   **Snack**

Calories	190	(97.1 cal/oz)	Carbohydrate	38.39 g	(13% DV)
Fat Calories	15	(8% fat)	Dietary Fiber	1.1 g	(4% DV)
Total Fat	1.65 g	(3% DV)	Protein	4.4 g	(9% DV)
Saturated Fat	.55 g	(3% DV)	Vitamin A	0 IU	(0% DV)
Poly Fat	0 g		Vitamin C	0 mg	(0% DV)
Mono Fat	.55 g		Calcium	12.7 mg	(1% DV)
Cholesterol	1.7 mg	(1% DV)	Iron	2.2 mg	(12% DV)
Sodium	772.2 mg	(32% DV)	Folate	4.4 mcg	(2% DV)
Potassium	48.4 mg	(1% DV)	Beta Carotene	0 RE	

Ratings	Worst	Bad	Average	Good	Best
Weight Loss			6		
LowCal Density	3				
Filling			5		
Energizing					9
Fiber		4			
Vitamins		4			
Minerals		4			
Overall			5		

PRODUCT 19

Serving: 1 cup (1.18 oz)　　　　　　　　**Cereal**

Calories	126	(106.6 cal/oz)	Carbohydrate	27.39 g	(9% DV)
Fat Calories	3	(2% fat)	Dietary Fiber	.66 g	(3% DV)
Total Fat	.33 g	(1% DV)	Protein	3.3 g	(7% DV)
Saturated Fat	0 g	(0% DV)	VItamin A	872.9 IU	(17% DV)
Poly Fat	0 g		Vitamin C	70 mg	(117% DV)
Mono Fat	0 g		Calcium	4 mg	(0% DV)
Cholesterol	0 mg	(0% DV)	Iron	21 mg	(116% DV)
Sodium	378.2 mg	(16% DV)	Folate	3.3 mcg	(116% DV)
Potassium	51.5 mg	(1% DV)	Beta Carotene	0 RE	

Ratings	Worst	Bad	Average	Good	Best
Weight Loss					9
LowCal Density	2				
Filling			4		
Energizing				7	
Fiber		3			
Vitamins					10
Minerals					10
Overall				6	

PRUNE JUICE

Serving: 1 cup (9.14 oz)　　　　　　　　**Beverage**

Calories	182	(19.9 cal/oz)	Carbohydrate	44.8 g	(15% DV)
Fat Calories	0	(0% fat)	Dietary Fiber	2.56 g	(10% DV)
Total Fat	0 g	(0% DV)	Protein	2.56 g	(5% DV)
Saturated Fat	0 g	(0% DV)	VItamin A	7.7 IU	(0% DV)
Poly Fat	0 g		Vitamin C	10.2 mg	(17% DV)
Mono Fat	0 g		Calcium	30.7 mg	(3% DV)
Cholesterol	0 mg	(0% DV)	Iron	3 mg	(17% DV)
Sodium	10.2 mg	(0% DV)	Folate	2.6 mcg	(0% DV)
Potassium	706.6 mg	(20% DV)	Beta Carotene	0 RE	

Ratings	Worst	Bad	Average	Good	Best
Weight Loss			5		
LowCal Density				8	
Filling					10
Energizing				9	
Fiber				7	
Vitamins		4			
Minerals			5		
Overall				7	

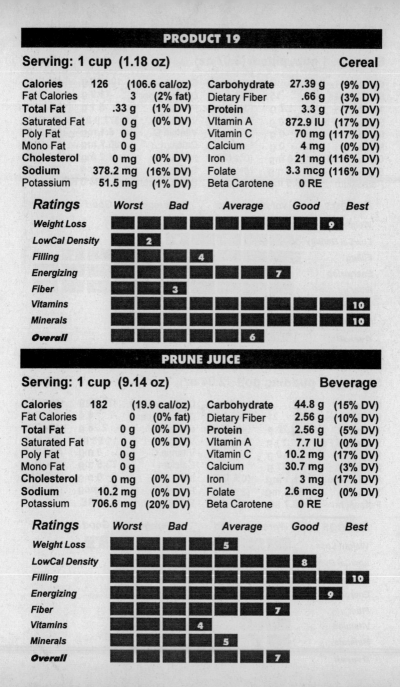

PRUNE, DRIED, UNCOOKED

Serving: 1 cup, pitted (6.07 oz)

Fruit

Calories	406	(66.9 cal/oz)	Carbohydrate	106.59 g	(36% DV)
Fat Calories	15	(4% fat)	Dietary Fiber	11.9 g	(48% DV)
Total Fat	1.7 g	(3% DV)	Protein	5.1 g	(10% DV)
Saturated Fat	0 g	(0% DV)	Vitamin A	3377.9 IU	(68% DV)
Poly Fat	0 g		Vitamin C	5.1 mg	(8% DV)
Mono Fat	0 g		Calcium	86.7 mg	(9% DV)
Cholesterol	0 mg	(0% DV)	Iron	4.2 mg	(23% DV)
Sodium	6.8 mg	(0% DV)	Folate	5.1 mcg	(2% DV)
Potassium	1266.5 mg	(36% DV)	Beta Carotene	338.3 RE	

Ratings	Worst	Bad	Average	Good	Best
Weight Loss	2				
LowCal Density			5		
Filling				9	
Energizing					10
Fiber					10
Vitamins			7		
Minerals			7		
Overall			6		

PUDDING POPS, FLAVORS OTHER THAN CHOCOLATE

Serving: 1 pudding pop (2.04 oz)

Dessert

Calories	91	(44.4 cal/oz)	Carbohydrate	15.28 g	(5% DV)
Fat Calories	21	(23% fat)	Dietary Fiber	0 g	(0% DV)
Total Fat	2.28 g	(4% DV)	Protein	2.28 g	(5% DV)
Saturated Fat	1.71 g	(9% DV)	Vitamin A	98 IU	(2% DV)
Poly Fat	0 g		Vitamin C	0 mg	(0% DV)
Mono Fat	.57 g		Calcium	73.5 mg	(7% DV)
Cholesterol	1.1 mg	(0% DV)	Iron	0 mg	(0% DV)
Sodium	60.4 mg	(3% DV)	Folate	2.3 mcg	(1% DV)
Potassium	78.7 mg	(2% DV)	Beta Carotene	0 RE	

Ratings	Worst	Bad	Average	Good	Best
Weight Loss				8	
LowCal Density			6		
Filling		4			
Energizing			5		
Fiber	1				
Vitamins	2				
Minerals		4			
Overall			5		

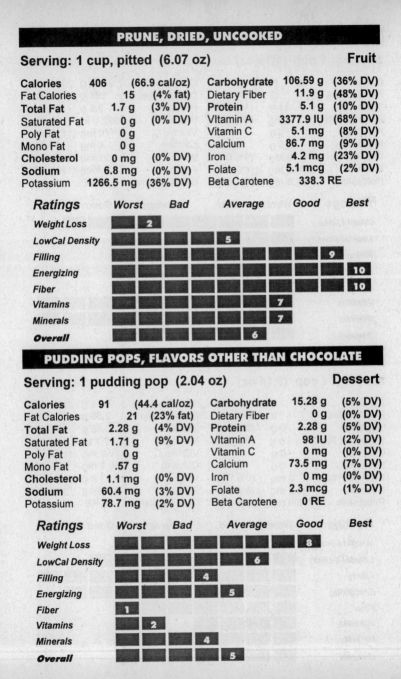

PUDDING, NOT CHOC, FROM DRY MIX WITH MILK

Serving: 1 cup (9.43 oz)   **Dessert**

Calories	298	(31.6 cal/oz)	Carbohydrate	50.42 g	(17% DV)
Fat Calories	71	(24% fat)	Dietary Fiber	0 g	(0% DV)
Total Fat	7.92 g	(12% DV)	Protein	7.92 g	(16% DV)
Saturated Fat	5.28 g	(26% DV)	Vitamin A	285.1 IU	(6% DV)
Poly Fat	0 g		Vitamin C	2.6 mg	(4% DV)
Mono Fat	2.64 g		Calcium	274.6 mg	(27% DV)
Cholesterol	31.7 mg	(11% DV)	Iron	.2 mg	(1% DV)
Sodium	588.7 mg	(25% DV)	Folate	7.9 mcg	(3% DV)
Potassium	348.5 mg	(10% DV)	Beta Carotene	7.9 RE	

Ratings	Worst	Bad	Average	Good	Best
Weight Loss				6	
LowCal Density				7	
Filling					9
Energizing					10
Fiber	1				
Vitamins		3			
Minerals				7	
Overall				7	

PUDDING, NOT CHOC, FROM DRY MIX WITH MILK, DIET

Serving: 1 cup (8.93 oz)   **Dessert**

Calories	168	(18.8 cal/oz)	Carbohydrate	23.5 g	(8% DV)
Fat Calories	45	(27% fat)	Dietary Fiber	0 g	(0% DV)
Total Fat	5 g	(8% DV)	Protein	7.5 g	(15% DV)
Saturated Fat	2.5 g	(12% DV)	Vitamin A	482.5 IU	(10% DV)
Poly Fat	0 g		Vitamin C	2.5 mg	(4% DV)
Mono Fat	2.5 g		Calcium	290 mg	(29% DV)
Cholesterol	17.5 mg	(6% DV)	Iron	.1 mg	(1% DV)
Sodium	582.5 mg	(24% DV)	Folate	7.5 mcg	(3% DV)
Potassium	367.5 mg	(10% DV)	Beta Carotene	5 RE	

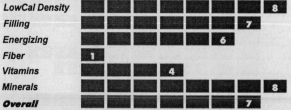

Ratings	Worst	Bad	Average	Good	Best
Weight Loss				7	
LowCal Density				8	
Filling				7	
Energizing			6		
Fiber	1				
Vitamins		4			
Minerals				8	
Overall				7	

PUFFS, FRIED, CRABMEAT & CREAM CHEESE FILLED

Serving: 1 puff (.82 oz)   **Entree**

Calories	81	(98.5 cal/oz)	Carbohydrate	7.45 g	(2% DV)
Fat Calories	39	(49% fat)	Dietary Fiber	.23 g	(1% DV)
Total Fat	4.37 g	(7% DV)	Protein	2.53 g	(5% DV)
Saturated Fat	2.3 g	(11% DV)	VItamin A	157.8 IU	(3% DV)
Poly Fat	.46 g		Vitamin C	0 mg	(0% DV)
Mono Fat	1.15 g		Calcium	12.9 mg	(1% DV)
Cholesterol	21.2 mg	(7% DV)	Iron	.6 mg	(3% DV)
Sodium	188.8 mg	(8% DV)	Folate	2.5 mcg	(1% DV)
Potassium	36.8 mg	(1% DV)	Beta Carotene	2.3 RE	

Ratings	Worst	Bad	Average	Good	Best
Weight Loss				7	
LowCal Density	3				
Filling	2				
Energizing	4				
Fiber	2				
Vitamins	3				
Minerals	3				
Overall	4				

PUMPKIN, COOKED WITHOUT ADDED FAT

Serving: 1 cup (8.75 oz)   **Vegetable**

Calories	64	(7.3 cal/oz)	Carbohydrate	15.93 g	(5% DV)
Fat Calories	0	(0% fat)	Dietary Fiber	4.9 g	(20% DV)
Total Fat	0 g	(0% DV)	Protein	2.45 g	(5% DV)
Saturated Fat	0 g	(0% DV)	VItamin A	3506 IU	(70% DV)
Poly Fat	0 g		Vitamin C	17.2 mg	(29% DV)
Mono Fat	0 g		Calcium	49 mg	(5% DV)
Cholesterol	0 mg	(0% DV)	Iron	1.9 mg	(10% DV)
Sodium	568.4 mg	(24% DV)	Folate	2.5 mcg	(7% DV)
Potassium	744.8 mg	(21% DV)	Beta Carotene	350.4 RE	

Ratings	Worst	Bad	Average	Good	Best
Weight Loss					9
LowCal Density					10
Filling					10
Energizing			5		
Fiber					9
Vitamins				8	
Minerals			5		
Overall					9

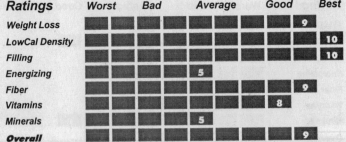

352   **Edmund's Food Ratings**

QUAKER OAT SQUARES

Serving: 1 cup (2.04 oz)   **Cereal**

Calories	201	(98.6 cal/oz)	Carbohydrate	42.24 g	(14% DV)
Fat Calories	36	(18% fat)	Dietary Fiber	3.99 g	(16% DV)
Total Fat	3.99 g	(6% DV)	Protein	7.98 g	(16% DV)
Saturated Fat	.57 g	(3% DV)	VItamin A	2513.1 IU	(50% DV)
Poly Fat	1.71 g		Vitamin C	0 mg	(0% DV)
Mono Fat	1.71 g		Calcium	29.6 mg	(3% DV)
Cholesterol	0 mg	(0% DV)	Iron	10.1 mg	(56% DV)
Sodium	321.5 mg	(13% DV)	Folate	8 mcg	(60% DV)
Potassium	201.2 mg	(6% DV)	Beta Carotene	0 RE	

Ratings	Worst	Bad	Average	Good	Best
Weight Loss				6	
LowCal Density		3			
Filling			5		
Energizing					9
Fiber					9
Vitamins					10
Minerals					9
Overall				6	

QUESADILLA WITH CHEESE, MEATLESS

Serving: 1 cup (3.39 oz)   **Entree**

Calories	350	(103.1 cal/oz)	Carbohydrate	36.29 g	(12% DV)
Fat Calories	154	(44% fat)	Dietary Fiber	1.9 g	(8% DV)
Total Fat	17.1 g	(26% DV)	Protein	11.4 g	(23% DV)
Saturated Fat	6.65 g	(33% DV)	VItamin A	514 IU	(10% DV)
Poly Fat	3.8 g		Vitamin C	5.7 mg	(10% DV)
Mono Fat	6.65 g		Calcium	216.6 mg	(22% DV)
Cholesterol	23.8 mg	(8% DV)	Iron	2.3 mg	(13% DV)
Sodium	448.4 mg	(19% DV)	Folate	11.4 mcg	(2% DV)
Potassium	115 mg	(3% DV)	Beta Carotene	32.3 RE	

Ratings	Worst	Bad	Average	Good	Best
Weight Loss		4			
LowCal Density	2				
Filling		4			
Energizing				8	
Fiber			6		
Vitamins			5		
Minerals				7	
Overall		4			

QUICHE WITH MEAT, POULTRY OR FISH

Serving: 1 piece (1/8 of 9" dia) (6.86 oz)　　Entree

Calories	555	(80.9 cal/oz)	Carbohydrate	21.7 g	(7% DV)
Fat Calories	380	(69% fat)	Dietary Fiber	0 g	(0% DV)
Total Fat	42.24 g	(65% DV)	Protein	21.12 g	(42% DV)
Saturated Fat	19.2 g	(96% DV)	Vitamin A	998.4 IU	(20% DV)
Poly Fat	5.76 g		Vitamin C	3.8 mg	(6% DV)
Mono Fat	15.36 g		Calcium	218.9 mg	(22% DV)
Cholesterol	222.7 mg	(74% DV)	Iron	2.1 mg	(11% DV)
Sodium	599 mg	(25% DV)	Folate	21.1 mcg	(5% DV)
Potassium	295.7 mg	(8% DV)	Beta Carotene	5.8 RE	

Ratings	Worst	Bad	Average	Good	Best
Weight Loss	2				
LowCal Density	3				
Filling	4				
Energizing			6		
Fiber	1				
Vitamins			6		
Minerals			7		
Overall	3				

RADISH, RAW

Serving: 1 large (1" to 1¼" dia) (.32 oz)　　Vegetable

Calories	2	(4.8 cal/oz)	Carbohydrate	.32 g	(0% DV)
Fat Calories	1	(53% fat)	Dietary Fiber	.18 g	(1% DV)
Total Fat	.09 g	(0% DV)	Protein	.09 g	(0% DV)
Saturated Fat	0 g	(0% DV)	Vitamin A	.7 IU	(0% DV)
Poly Fat	0 g		Vitamin C	2.1 mg	(3% DV)
Mono Fat	0 g		Calcium	1.9 mg	(0% DV)
Cholesterol	0 mg	(0% DV)	Iron	0 mg	(0% DV)
Sodium	2.2 mg	(0% DV)	Folate	.1 mcg	(1% DV)
Potassium	20.9 mg	(1% DV)	Beta Carotene	.1 RE	

Ratings	Worst	Bad	Average	Good	Best
Weight Loss				7	
LowCal Density					10
Filling	2				
Energizing	2				
Fiber	2				
Vitamins	2				
Minerals	2				
Overall			6		

RAISIN BRAN

Serving: 1 cup (2 oz)   **Cereal**

Calories	174	(87.1 cal/oz)	Carbohydrate	42.73 g	(14% DV)
Fat Calories	10	(6% fat)	Dietary Fiber	7.28 g	(29% DV)
Total Fat	1.12 g	(2% DV)	Protein	5.6 g	(11% DV)
Saturated Fat	0 g	(0% DV)	VItamin A	1490.2 IU	(30% DV)
Poly Fat	.56 g		Vitamin C	0 mg	(0% DV)
Mono Fat	0 g		Calcium	21.8 mg	(2% DV)
Cholesterol	0 mg	(0% DV)	Iron	21.5 mg	(119% DV)
Sodium	341.6 mg	(14% DV)	Folate	5.6 mcg	(41% DV)
Potassium	304.1 mg	(9% DV)	Beta Carotene	0 RE	

Ratings	Worst	Bad	Average	Good	Best
Weight Loss				7	
LowCal Density		3			
Filling			5		
Energizing					9
Fiber					10
Vitamins					9
Minerals					10
Overall				6	

RAISINS

Serving: 1 cup (5.18 oz)   **Fruit**

Calories	435	(84 cal/oz)	Carbohydrate	114.7 g	(38% DV)
Fat Calories	0	(0% fat)	Dietary Fiber	7.25 g	(29% DV)
Total Fat	0 g	(0% DV)	Protein	4.35 g	(9% DV)
Saturated Fat	0 g	(0% DV)	VItamin A	11.6 IU	(0% DV)
Poly Fat	0 g		Vitamin C	4.4 mg	(7% DV)
Mono Fat	0 g		Calcium	71.1 mg	(7% DV)
Cholesterol	0 mg	(0% DV)	Iron	3 mg	(17% DV)
Sodium	17.4 mg	(1% DV)	Folate	4.4 mcg	(1% DV)
Potassium	1089 mg	(31% DV)	Beta Carotene	1.5 RE	

Ratings	Worst	Bad	Average	Good	Best
Weight Loss	2				
LowCal Density		3			
Filling				8	
Energizing					10
Fiber					10
Vitamins		4			
Minerals			6		
Overall			5		

RAPESEED OIL

Serving: 1 tbsp (.49 oz)   Fat & Oil

Calories	120	(245.3 cal/oz)	**Carbohydrate**	0 g	(0% DV)
Fat Calories	122	(102% fat)	Dietary Fiber	0 g	(0% DV)
Total Fat	13.6 g	(21% DV)	**Protein**	0 g	(0% DV)
Saturated Fat	.95 g	(5% DV)	VItamin A	0 IU	(0% DV)
Poly Fat	4.49 g		Vitamin C	0 mg	(0% DV)
Mono Fat	7.62 g		Calcium	0 mg	(0% DV)
Cholesterol	0 mg	(0% DV)	Iron	0 mg	(0% DV)
Sodium	0 mg	(0% DV)	Folate	0 mcg	(0% DV)
Potassium	0 mg	(0% DV)	Beta Carotene	0 RE	

Ratings	Worst	Bad	Average	Good	Best
Weight Loss	1				
LowCal Density	1				
Filling	1				
Energizing	1				
Fiber	1				
Vitamins			3		
Minerals	1				
Overall	1				

RASPBERRIES, RAW

Serving: 1 cup (4.39 oz)   Fruit

Calories	60	(13.7 cal/oz)	**Carbohydrate**	14.27 g	(5% DV)
Fat Calories	11	(18% fat)	Dietary Fiber	6.15 g	(25% DV)
Total Fat	1.23 g	(2% DV)	**Protein**	1.23 g	(2% DV)
Saturated Fat	0 g	(0% DV)	VItamin A	159.9 IU	(3% DV)
Poly Fat	0 g		Vitamin C	30.8 mg	(51% DV)
Mono Fat	0 g		Calcium	27.1 mg	(3% DV)
Cholesterol	0 mg	(0% DV)	Iron	.7 mg	(4% DV)
Sodium	0 mg	(0% DV)	Folate	1.2 mcg	(8% DV)
Potassium	187 mg	(5% DV)	Beta Carotene	16 RE	

Ratings	Worst	Bad	Average	Good	Best
Weight Loss				9	
LowCal Density				9	
Filling				8	
Energizing			5		
Fiber					10
Vitamins			6		
Minerals		4			
Overall				8	

RATATOUILLE

Serving: 1 cup (7.64 oz)   **Entree**

Calories	150	(19.6 cal/oz)	Carbohydrate	11.34 g	(4% DV)
Fat Calories	116	(77% fat)	Dietary Fiber	4.28 g	(17% DV)
Total Fat	12.84 g	(20% DV)	Protein	2.14 g	(4% DV)
Saturated Fat	2.14 g	(11% DV)	Vitamin A	584.2 IU	(12% DV)
Poly Fat	2.14 g		Vitamin C	19.3 mg	(32% DV)
Mono Fat	8.56 g		Calcium	34.2 mg	(3% DV)
Cholesterol	0 mg	(0% DV)	Iron	.9 mg	(5% DV)
Sodium	440.8 mg	(18% DV)	Folate	2.1 mcg	(7% DV)
Potassium	468.7 mg	(13% DV)	Beta Carotene	57.8 RE	

Ratings

	Worst	Bad	Average	Good	Best
Weight Loss		4			
LowCal Density				8	
Filling			6		
Energizing		5			
Fiber					9
Vitamins			6		
Minerals		4			
Overall			6		

RAVIOLI, CHEESE-FILLED, WITH TOMATO SAUCE

Serving: 1 diet meal (9.11 oz)   **Entree**

Calories	281	(30.8 cal/oz)	Carbohydrate	30.6 g	(10% DV)
Fat Calories	92	(33% fat)	Dietary Fiber	2.55 g	(10% DV)
Total Fat	10.2 g	(16% DV)	Protein	17.85 g	(36% DV)
Saturated Fat	5.1 g	(25% DV)	Vitamin A	1494.3 IU	(30% DV)
Poly Fat	0 g		Vitamin C	30.6 mg	(51% DV)
Mono Fat	2.55 g		Calcium	339.2 mg	(34% DV)
Cholesterol	33.2 mg	(11% DV)	Iron	2 mg	(11% DV)
Sodium	1040.4 mg	(43% DV)	Folate	17.9 mcg	(5% DV)
Potassium	466.7 mg	(13% DV)	Beta Carotene	122.4 RE	

Ratings

	Worst	Bad	Average	Good	Best
Weight Loss			6		
LowCal Density			7		
Filling			7		
Energizing			7		
Fiber			7		
Vitamins				8	
Minerals				8	
Overall			7		

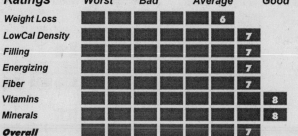

RAVIOLI, MEAT-FILLED, WITH TOMATO OR MEAT SAUCE

Serving: 1 cup (8.93 oz)   **Entree**

Calories	388	(43.4 cal/oz)	Carbohydrate	36.5 g	(12% DV)
Fat Calories	158	(41% fat)	Dietary Fiber	2.5 g	(10% DV)
Total Fat	17.5 g	(27% DV)	Protein	20 g	(40% DV)
Saturated Fat	5 g	(25% DV)	Vitamin A	1230 IU	(25% DV)
Poly Fat	2.5 g		Vitamin C	22.5 mg	(38% DV)
Mono Fat	7.5 g		Calcium	65 mg	(6% DV)
Cholesterol	167.5 mg	(56% DV)	Iron	4.1 mg	(22% DV)
Sodium	1237.5 mg	(52% DV)	Folate	20 mcg	(7% DV)
Potassium	517.5 mg	(15% DV)	Beta Carotene	90 RE	

Ratings	Worst	Bad	Average	Good	Best
Weight Loss		4			
LowCal Density			6		
Filling			6		
Energizing				8	
Fiber			7		
Vitamins				8	
Minerals			7		
Overall			6		

RED KIDNEY BEANS, DRY, WITHOUT ADDED FAT

Serving: 1 cup cooked (6.14 oz)   **Vegetable**

Calories	217	(35.3 cal/oz)	Carbohydrate	39.04 g	(13% DV)
Fat Calories	0	(0% fat)	Dietary Fiber	8.6 g	(34% DV)
Total Fat	0 g	(0% DV)	Protein	15.48 g	(31% DV)
Saturated Fat	0 g	(0% DV)	Vitamin A	0 IU	(0% DV)
Poly Fat	0 g		Vitamin C	1.7 mg	(3% DV)
Mono Fat	0 g		Calcium	48.2 mg	(5% DV)
Cholesterol	0 mg	(0% DV)	Iron	5 mg	(28% DV)
Sodium	400.8 mg	(17% DV)	Folate	15.5 mcg	(55% DV)
Potassium	689.7 mg	(20% DV)	Beta Carotene	0 RE	

Ratings	Worst	Bad	Average	Good	Best
Weight Loss		4			
LowCal Density			7		
Filling				8	
Energizing				9	
Fiber					10
Vitamins			6		
Minerals				8	
Overall			7		

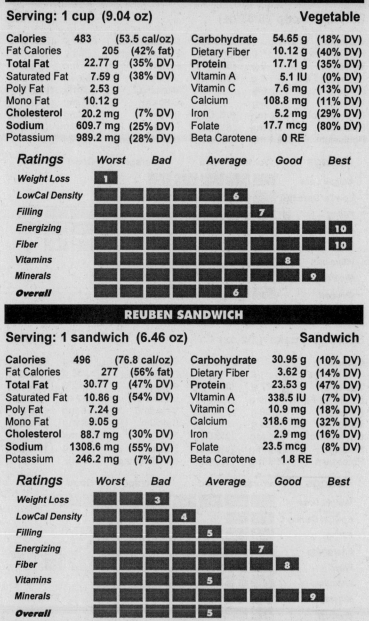

REFRIED BEANS

Serving: 1 cup (9.04 oz) **Vegetable**

Calories	483	(53.5 cal/oz)	Carbohydrate	54.65 g	(18% DV)
Fat Calories	205	(42% fat)	Dietary Fiber	10.12 g	(40% DV)
Total Fat	22.77 g	(35% DV)	Protein	17.71 g	(35% DV)
Saturated Fat	7.59 g	(38% DV)	Vitamin A	5.1 IU	(0% DV)
Poly Fat	2.53 g		Vitamin C	7.6 mg	(13% DV)
Mono Fat	10.12 g		Calcium	108.8 mg	(11% DV)
Cholesterol	20.2 mg	(7% DV)	Iron	5.2 mg	(29% DV)
Sodium	609.7 mg	(25% DV)	Folate	17.7 mcg	(80% DV)
Potassium	989.2 mg	(28% DV)	Beta Carotene	0 RE	

Ratings Worst Bad Average Good Best

Rating	Score
Weight Loss	1
LowCal Density	6
Filling	7
Energizing	10
Fiber	10
Vitamins	8
Minerals	9
Overall	6

REUBEN SANDWICH

Serving: 1 sandwich (6.46 oz) **Sandwich**

Calories	496	(76.8 cal/oz)	Carbohydrate	30.95 g	(10% DV)
Fat Calories	277	(56% fat)	Dietary Fiber	3.62 g	(14% DV)
Total Fat	30.77 g	(47% DV)	Protein	23.53 g	(47% DV)
Saturated Fat	10.86 g	(54% DV)	Vitamin A	338.5 IU	(7% DV)
Poly Fat	7.24 g		Vitamin C	10.9 mg	(18% DV)
Mono Fat	9.05 g		Calcium	318.6 mg	(32% DV)
Cholesterol	88.7 mg	(30% DV)	Iron	2.9 mg	(16% DV)
Sodium	1308.6 mg	(55% DV)	Folate	23.5 mcg	(8% DV)
Potassium	246.2 mg	(7% DV)	Beta Carotene	1.8 RE	

Ratings Worst Bad Average Good Best

Rating	Score
Weight Loss	3
LowCal Density	4
Filling	5
Energizing	7
Fiber	8
Vitamins	5
Minerals	9
Overall	5

RHUBARB, COOKED OR CANNED

Serving: 1 cup (8.57 oz)   **Fruit**

Calories	278	(32.5 cal/oz)	Carbohydrate	74.88 g	(25% DV)
Fat Calories	0	(0% fat)	Dietary Fiber	4.8 g	(19% DV)
Total Fat	0 g	(0% DV)	Protein	0 g	(0% DV)
Saturated Fat	0 g	(0% DV)	Vitamin A	165.6 IU	(3% DV)
Poly Fat	0 g		Vitamin C	7.2 mg	(12% DV)
Mono Fat	0 g		Calcium	348 mg	(35% DV)
Cholesterol	0 mg	(0% DV)	Iron	.5 mg	(3% DV)
Sodium	2.4 mg	(0% DV)	Folate	0 mcg	(3% DV)
Potassium	230.4 mg	(7% DV)	Beta Carotene	16.8 RE	

Ratings	Worst	Bad	Average	Good	Best
Weight Loss			5		
LowCal Density				7	
Filling					10
Energizing					10
Fiber					9
Vitamins		4			
Minerals			6		
Overall				7	

RICE CAKE

Serving: 1 cake (.32 oz)   **Snack**

Calories	35	(108.8 cal/oz)	Carbohydrate	7.33 g	(2% DV)
Fat Calories	2	(7% fat)	Dietary Fiber	.36 g	(1% DV)
Total Fat	.27 g	(0% DV)	Protein	.72 g	(1% DV)
Saturated Fat	.09 g	(0% DV)	Vitamin A	3.7 IU	(0% DV)
Poly Fat	.09 g		Vitamin C	0 mg	(0% DV)
Mono Fat	.09 g		Calcium	1 mg	(0% DV)
Cholesterol	0 mg	(0% DV)	Iron	.1 mg	(1% DV)
Sodium	29.3 mg	(1% DV)	Folate	.7 mcg	(0% DV)
Potassium	26.1 mg	(1% DV)	Beta Carotene	0 RE	

Ratings	Worst	Bad	Average	Good	Best
Weight Loss					9
LowCal Density	2				
Filling	2				
Energizing		4			
Fiber	2				
Vitamins	2				
Minerals		3			
Overall		4			

RICE DESSERT OR SALAD WITH FRUIT

Serving: 1 cup (5.54 oz)   **Salad**

Calories	274	(49.5 cal/oz)	Carbohydrate	34.72 g	(12% DV)
Fat Calories	126	(46% fat)	Dietary Fiber	1.55 g	(6% DV)
Total Fat	13.95 g	(21% DV)	Protein	3.1 g	(6% DV)
Saturated Fat	9.3 g	(47% DV)	Vitamin A	578.2 IU	(12% DV)
Poly Fat	0 g		Vitamin C	7.8 mg	(13% DV)
Mono Fat	4.65 g		Calcium	34.1 mg	(3% DV)
Cholesterol	52.7 mg	(18% DV)	Iron	.8 mg	(4% DV)
Sodium	21.7 mg	(1% DV)	Folate	3.1 mcg	(2% DV)
Potassium	107 mg	(3% DV)	Beta Carotene	6.2 RE	

Ratings	Worst	Bad	Average	Good	Best
Weight Loss		4			
LowCal Density			6		
Filling			6		
Energizing				8	
Fiber			5		
Vitamins			5		
Minerals		4			
Overall			5		

RICE KRISPIES

Serving: 1 cup (.96 oz)   **Cereal**

Calories	107	(111.1 cal/oz)	Carbohydrate	23.6 g	(8% DV)
Fat Calories	2	(2% fat)	Dietary Fiber	.27 g	(1% DV)
Total Fat	.27 g	(0% DV)	Protein	1.89 g	(4% DV)
Saturated Fat	0 g	(0% DV)	Vitamin A	714.2 IU	(14% DV)
Poly Fat	0 g		Vitamin C	14.3 mg	(24% DV)
Mono Fat	0 g		Calcium	3.8 mg	(0% DV)
Cholesterol	0 mg	(0% DV)	Iron	1.7 mg	(9% DV)
Sodium	324 mg	(14% DV)	Folate	1.9 mcg	(24% DV)
Potassium	28.1 mg	(1% DV)	Beta Carotene	0 RE	

Ratings	Worst	Bad	Average	Good	Best
Weight Loss					9
LowCal Density	2				
Filling		3			
Energizing			6		
Fiber	2				
Vitamins					9
Minerals		4			
Overall			5		

RICE PILAF

Serving: 1 cup (7.36 oz)　　　　　**Entree**

Calories	268	(36.4 cal/oz)	Carbohydrate	46.14 g	(15% DV)
Fat Calories	56	(21% fat)	Dietary Fiber	2.06 g	(8% DV)
Total Fat	6.18 g	(10% DV)	Protein	4.12 g	(8% DV)
Saturated Fat	2.06 g	(10% DV)	Vitamin A	335.8 IU	(7% DV)
Poly Fat	2.06 g		Vitamin C	0 mg	(0% DV)
Mono Fat	2.06 g		Calcium	26.8 mg	(3% DV)
Cholesterol	0 mg	(0% DV)	Iron	2.4 mg	(14% DV)
Sodium	754 mg	(31% DV)	Folate	4.1 mcg	(2% DV)
Potassium	107.1 mg	(3% DV)	Beta Carotene	6.2 RE	

Ratings

	Worst	Bad	Average	Good	Best
Weight Loss			7		
LowCal Density			7		
Filling				8	
Energizing					9
Fiber			6		
Vitamins			5		
Minerals			5		
Overall				7	

RICE WITH BEANS

Serving: 1 cup (8.54 oz)　　　　　**Entree**

Calories	318	(37.2 cal/oz)	Carbohydrate	62.62 g	(21% DV)
Fat Calories	0	(0% fat)	Dietary Fiber	7.17 g	(29% DV)
Total Fat	0 g	(0% DV)	Protein	14.34 g	(29% DV)
Saturated Fat	0 g	(0% DV)	Vitamin A	0 IU	(0% DV)
Poly Fat	0 g		Vitamin C	0 mg	(0% DV)
Mono Fat	0 g		Calcium	126.7 mg	(13% DV)
Cholesterol	0 mg	(0% DV)	Iron	5.9 mg	(33% DV)
Sodium	662 mg	(28% DV)	Folate	14.3 mcg	(26% DV)
Potassium	752.9 mg	(22% DV)	Beta Carotene	0 RE	

Ratings

	Worst	Bad	Average	Good	Best
Weight Loss				8	
LowCal Density			7		
Filling					10
Energizing					10
Fiber					10
Vitamins			5		
Minerals				8	
Overall				8	

RICE, BROWN, COOKED WITHOUT ADDED FAT

Serving: 1 cup, cooked, hot (6.96 oz)   **Entree**

Calories	232	(33.3 cal/oz)	Carbohydrate	49.73 g	(17% DV)
Fat Calories	18	(8% fat)	Dietary Fiber	3.9 g	(16% DV)
Total Fat	1.95 g	(3% DV)	Protein	5.85 g	(12% DV)
Saturated Fat	0 g	(0% DV)	VItamin A	0 IU	(0% DV)
Poly Fat	0 g		Vitamin C	0 mg	(0% DV)
Mono Fat	0 g		Calcium	23.4 mg	(2% DV)
Cholesterol	0 mg	(0% DV)	Iron	1.2 mg	(6% DV)
Sodium	549.9 mg	(23% DV)	Folate	5.9 mcg	(2% DV)
Potassium	136.5 mg	(4% DV)	Beta Carotene	0 RE	

Ratings	Worst	Bad	Average	Good	Best
Weight Loss				8	
LowCal Density			7		
Filling					9
Energizing					9
Fiber					9
Vitamins		4			
Minerals			6		
Overall				8	

RICE, FLAVORED, WHITE & WILD

Serving: 1 cup (6.5 oz)   **Entree**

Calories	173	(26.6 cal/oz)	Carbohydrate	31.12 g	(10% DV)
Fat Calories	33	(19% fat)	Dietary Fiber	1.82 g	(7% DV)
Total Fat	3.64 g	(6% DV)	Protein	5.46 g	(11% DV)
Saturated Fat	0 g	(0% DV)	VItamin A	147.4 IU	(3% DV)
Poly Fat	1.82 g		Vitamin C	0 mg	(0% DV)
Mono Fat	1.82 g		Calcium	51 mg	(5% DV)
Cholesterol	0 mg	(0% DV)	Iron	1.5 mg	(8% DV)
Sodium	671.6 mg	(28% DV)	Folate	5.5 mcg	(2% DV)
Potassium	134.7 mg	(4% DV)	Beta Carotene	3.6 RE	

Ratings	Worst	Bad	Average	Good	Best
Weight Loss				8	
LowCal Density				8	
Filling				7	
Energizing				8	
Fiber			6		
Vitamins		4			
Minerals			5		
Overall				7	

Serving: 1 cup (5.93 oz)　　　　　　　　**Entree**

Calories	264	(44.5 cal/oz)	Carbohydrate	33.86 g	(11% DV)
Fat Calories	105	(40% fat)	Dietary Fiber	1.66 g	(7% DV)
Total Fat	11.62 g	(18% DV)	Protein	4.98 g	(10% DV)
Saturated Fat	1.66 g	(8% DV)	Vitamin A	94.6 IU	(2% DV)
Poly Fat	6.64 g		Vitamin C	3.3 mg	(6% DV)
Mono Fat	3.32 g		Calcium	29.9 mg	(3% DV)
Cholesterol	43.2 mg	(14% DV)	Iron	1.8 mg	(10% DV)
Sodium	285.5 mg	(12% DV)	Folate	5 mcg	(5% DV)
Potassium	134.5 mg	(4% DV)	Beta Carotene	3.3 RE	

Ratings	Worst	Bad	Average	Good	Best
Weight Loss			5		
LowCal Density			6		
Filling			6		
Energizing				8	
Fiber			5		
Vitamins			5		
Minerals			5		
Overall			6		

Serving: 1 cup (.5 oz)　　　　　　　　**Cereal**

Calories	56	(112.6 cal/oz)	Carbohydrate	12.57 g	(4% DV)
Fat Calories	1	(2% fat)	Dietary Fiber	.28 g	(1% DV)
Total Fat	.14 g	(0% DV)	Protein	.84 g	(2% DV)
Saturated Fat	0 g	(0% DV)	Vitamin A	0 IU	(0% DV)
Poly Fat	0 g		Vitamin C	0 mg	(0% DV)
Mono Fat	0 g		Calcium	.8 mg	(0% DV)
Cholesterol	0 mg	(0% DV)	Iron	.2 mg	(1% DV)
Sodium	.4 mg	(0% DV)	Folate	.8 mcg	(1% DV)
Potassium	15.8 mg	(0% DV)	Beta Carotene	0 RE	

Ratings	Worst	Bad	Average	Good	Best
Weight Loss					9
LowCal Density	2				
Filling	2				
Energizing			5		
Fiber	2				
Vitamins	2				
Minerals	2				
Overall		4			

RICE, WHITE, REGULAR, COOKED WITHOUT ADDED FAT

Serving: 1 cup, cooked (7.32 oz)   Entree

Calories	262	(35.8 cal/oz)	Carbohydrate	56.79 g	(19% DV)
Fat Calories	0	(0% fat)	Dietary Fiber	0 g	(0% DV)
Total Fat	0 g	(0% DV)	Protein	6.15 g	(12% DV)
Saturated Fat	0 g	(0% DV)	VItamin A	0 IU	(0% DV)
Poly Fat	0 g		Vitamin C	0 mg	(0% DV)
Mono Fat	0 g		Calcium	22.6 mg	(2% DV)
Cholesterol	0 mg	(0% DV)	Iron	2.2 mg	(12% DV)
Sodium	701.1 mg	(29% DV)	Folate	6.2 mcg	(2% DV)
Potassium	80 mg	(2% DV)	Beta Carotene	0 RE	

Ratings	Worst	Bad	Average	Good	Best
Weight Loss				8	
LowCal Density			7		
Filling					9
Energizing					10
Fiber	1				
Vitamins			5		
Minerals			5		
Overall				7	

RICE, WILD, 100%, COOKED WITHOUT ADDED FAT

Serving: 1 cup, cooked (4.64 oz)   Entree

Calories	118	(25.5 cal/oz)	Carbohydrate	24.7 g	(8% DV)
Fat Calories	0	(0% fat)	Dietary Fiber	1.3 g	(5% DV)
Total Fat	0 g	(0% DV)	Protein	5.2 g	(10% DV)
Saturated Fat	0 g	(0% DV)	VItamin A	6.5 IU	(0% DV)
Poly Fat	0 g		Vitamin C	0 mg	(0% DV)
Mono Fat	0 g		Calcium	9.1 mg	(1% DV)
Cholesterol	0 mg	(0% DV)	Iron	.6 mg	(4% DV)
Sodium	477.1 mg	(20% DV)	Folate	5.2 mcg	(6% DV)
Potassium	133.9 mg	(4% DV)	Beta Carotene	0 RE	

Ratings	Worst	Bad	Average	Good	Best
Weight Loss				9	
LowCal Density				8	
Filling			7		
Energizing			6		
Fiber			5		
Vitamins		3			
Minerals			5		
Overall				7	

ROAST BEEF SANDWICH

Serving: 1 Arby's regular (5.25 oz) — **Sandwich**

Calories	370	(70.6 cal/oz)	Carbohydrate	26.75 g	(9% DV)
Fat Calories	132	(36% fat)	Dietary Fiber	1.47 g	(6% DV)
Total Fat	14.7 g	(23% DV)	Protein	29.4 g	(59% DV)
Saturated Fat	5.88 g	(29% DV)	Vitamin A	0 IU	(0% DV)
Poly Fat	1.47 g		Vitamin C	0 mg	(0% DV)
Mono Fat	5.88 g		Calcium	72 mg	(7% DV)
Cholesterol	75 mg	(25% DV)	Iron	4 mg	(22% DV)
Sodium	577.7 mg	(24% DV)	Folate	29.4 mcg	(7% DV)
Potassium	410.1 mg	(12% DV)	Beta Carotene	0 RE	

Ratings	Worst	Bad	Average	Good	Best
Weight Loss			5		
LowCal Density		4			
Filling			5		
Energizing				7	
Fiber			5		
Vitamins			5		
Minerals					9
Overall			5		

ROAST BEEF SANDWICH, WITH GRAVY

Serving: 1 sandwich (7.93 oz) — **Sandwich**

Calories	386	(48.7 cal/oz)	Carbohydrate	28.86 g	(10% DV)
Fat Calories	140	(36% fat)	Dietary Fiber	2.22 g	(9% DV)
Total Fat	15.54 g	(24% DV)	Protein	31.08 g	(62% DV)
Saturated Fat	6.66 g	(33% DV)	Vitamin A	0 IU	(0% DV)
Poly Fat	0 g		Vitamin C	0 mg	(0% DV)
Mono Fat	6.66 g		Calcium	71 mg	(7% DV)
Cholesterol	71 mg	(24% DV)	Iron	4.3 mg	(24% DV)
Sodium	1016.8 mg	(42% DV)	Folate	31.1 mcg	(6% DV)
Potassium	446.2 mg	(13% DV)	Beta Carotene	0 RE	

Ratings	Worst	Bad	Average	Good	Best
Weight Loss			5		
LowCal Density			6		
Filling			5		
Energizing				7	
Fiber			6		
Vitamins			5		
Minerals					9
Overall			6		

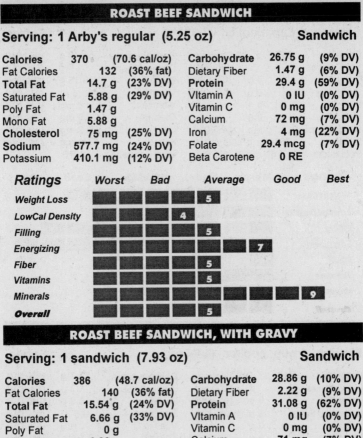

ROE, STURGEON

Serving: 1 tbsp (.57 oz)   **Fish**

Calories	40	(70.7 cal/oz)	Carbohydrate	.64 g	(0% DV)
Fat Calories	26	(64% fat)	Dietary Fiber	0 g	(0% DV)
Total Fat	2.88 g	(4% DV)	Protein	4 g	(8% DV)
Saturated Fat	.64 g	(3% DV)	Vitamin A	298.9 IU	(6% DV)
Poly Fat	1.12 g		Vitamin C	0 mg	(0% DV)
Mono Fat	.8 g		Calcium	44 mg	(4% DV)
Cholesterol	94.1 mg	(31% DV)	Iron	1.9 mg	(11% DV)
Sodium	240 mg	(10% DV)	Folate	4 mcg	(2% DV)
Potassium	29 mg	(1% DV)	Beta Carotene	0 RE	

Ratings	Worst	Bad	Average	Good	Best
Weight Loss				6	
LowCal Density			4		
Filling	1				
Energizing	2				
Fiber	1				
Vitamins			4		
Minerals			5		
Overall			4		

ROLL, HARD

Serving: 1 medium (1.79 oz)   **Bread**

Calories	156	(87.2 cal/oz)	Carbohydrate	29.75 g	(10% DV)
Fat Calories	14	(9% fat)	Dietary Fiber	1 g	(4% DV)
Total Fat	1.5 g	(2% DV)	Protein	5 g	(10% DV)
Saturated Fat	.5 g	(2% DV)	Vitamin A	0 IU	(0% DV)
Poly Fat	.5 g		Vitamin C	0 mg	(0% DV)
Mono Fat	.5 g		Calcium	50 mg	(5% DV)
Cholesterol	0 mg	(0% DV)	Iron	1.4 mg	(8% DV)
Sodium	312.5 mg	(13% DV)	Folate	5 mcg	(4% DV)
Potassium	48.5 mg	(1% DV)	Beta Carotene	0 RE	

Ratings	Worst	Bad	Average	Good	Best
Weight Loss			5		
LowCal Density		3			
Filling			4		
Energizing					7
Fiber			4		
Vitamins			4		
Minerals			4		
Overall			4		

ROLL, HOME RECIPE OR PURCHASED AT A BAKERY

Serving: 1 roll (1.29 oz)   **Bread**

Calories	123	(95.4 cal/oz)	Carbohydrate	20.27 g	(7% DV)
Fat Calories	29	(24% fat)	Dietary Fiber	.72 g	(3% DV)
Total Fat	3.24 g	(5% DV)	Protein	3.24 g	(6% DV)
Saturated Fat	1.08 g	(5% DV)	Vitamin A	28.4 IU	(1% DV)
Poly Fat	.72 g		Vitamin C	0 mg	(0% DV)
Mono Fat	1.08 g		Calcium	18 mg	(2% DV)
Cholesterol	11.2 mg	(4% DV)	Iron	1.2 mg	(6% DV)
Sodium	155.2 mg	(6% DV)	Folate	3.2 mcg	(4% DV)
Potassium	50.4 mg	(1% DV)	Beta Carotene	.4 RE	

Ratings	Worst	Bad	Average	Good	Best
Weight Loss				5	
LowCal Density		3			
Filling		3			
Energizing				6	
Fiber		3			
Vitamins		4			
Minerals		4			
Overall		4			

ROLL, MULTIGRAIN

Serving: 1 roll (1 oz)   **Bread**

Calories	80	(79.5 cal/oz)	Carbohydrate	13.89 g	(5% DV)
Fat Calories	15	(19% fat)	Dietary Fiber	1.4 g	(6% DV)
Total Fat	1.68 g	(3% DV)	Protein	2.8 g	(6% DV)
Saturated Fat	.56 g	(3% DV)	Vitamin A	24.9 IU	(0% DV)
Poly Fat	.28 g		Vitamin C	0 mg	(0% DV)
Mono Fat	.56 g		Calcium	18.8 mg	(2% DV)
Cholesterol	9.8 mg	(3% DV)	Iron	.7 mg	(4% DV)
Sodium	135.2 mg	(6% DV)	Folate	2.8 mcg	(4% DV)
Potassium	85.4 mg	(2% DV)	Beta Carotene	.3 RE	

Ratings	Worst	Bad	Average	Good	Best
Weight Loss					7
LowCal Density			4		
Filling		3			
Energizing			5		
Fiber			5		
Vitamins		3			
Minerals		4			
Overall			5		

ROLL, OATMEAL

Serving: 1 roll (1 oz)   **Bread**

Calories	80	(79.5 cal/oz)	Carbohydrate	12.88 g	(4% DV)
Fat Calories	18	(22% fat)	Dietary Fiber	.84 g	(3% DV)
Total Fat	1.96 g	(3% DV)	Protein	2.52 g	(5% DV)
Saturated Fat	.56 g	(3% DV)	Vitamin A	18.2 IU	(0% DV)
Poly Fat	.56 g		Vitamin C	0 mg	(0% DV)
Mono Fat	.84 g		Calcium	11.8 mg	(1% DV)
Cholesterol	5.6 mg	(2% DV)	Iron	.8 mg	(4% DV)
Sodium	107.8 mg	(4% DV)	Folate	2.5 mcg	(3% DV)
Potassium	40.6 mg	(1% DV)	Beta Carotene	.3 RE	

Ratings	Worst	Bad	Average	Good	Best
Weight Loss				6	
LowCal Density			4		
Filling		3			
Energizing			5		
Fiber			4		
Vitamins		3			
Minerals		3			
Overall			4		

ROLL, PUMPERNICKEL

Serving: 1 roll (1 oz)   **Bread**

Calories	78	(77.6 cal/oz)	Carbohydrate	14.78 g	(5% DV)
Fat Calories	8	(10% fat)	Dietary Fiber	1.4 g	(6% DV)
Total Fat	.84 g	(1% DV)	Protein	3.08 g	(6% DV)
Saturated Fat	.28 g	(1% DV)	Vitamin A	0 IU	(0% DV)
Poly Fat	.28 g		Vitamin C	0 mg	(0% DV)
Mono Fat	.28 g		Calcium	18.8 mg	(2% DV)
Cholesterol	0 mg	(0% DV)	Iron	.8 mg	(4% DV)
Sodium	159.3 mg	(7% DV)	Folate	3.1 mcg	(2% DV)
Potassium	58.2 mg	(2% DV)	Beta Carotene	0 RE	

Ratings	Worst	Bad	Average	Good	Best
Weight Loss				8	
LowCal Density		4			
Filling		3			
Energizing			5		
Fiber			5		
Vitamins		3			
Minerals		4			
Overall			5		

ROLL, WHITE, SOFT

Serving: 1 roll (1 oz)   **Bread**

Calories	83	(83.4 cal/oz)	Carbohydrate	14.84 g	(5% DV)
Fat Calories	15	(18% fat)	Dietary Fiber	.56 g	(2% DV)
Total Fat	1.68 g	(3% DV)	Protein	2.24 g	(4% DV)
Saturated Fat	.28 g	(1% DV)	Vitamin A	0 IU	(0% DV)
Poly Fat	.28 g		Vitamin C	0 mg	(0% DV)
Mono Fat	.84 g		Calcium	28 mg	(3% DV)
Cholesterol	0 mg	(0% DV)	Iron	.8 mg	(4% DV)
Sodium	141.7 mg	(6% DV)	Folate	2.2 mcg	(3% DV)
Potassium	26.6 mg	(1% DV)	Beta Carotene	0 RE	

Ratings	Worst	Bad	Average	Good	Best
Weight Loss					7
LowCal Density		3			
Filling		3			
Energizing			5		
Fiber		3			
Vitamins		3			
Minerals		3			
Overall			4		

ROLL, WHOLE WHEAT, 100%

Serving: 1 roll (1 oz)   **Bread**

Calories	72	(72 cal/oz)	Carbohydrate	14.64 g	(5% DV)
Fat Calories	8	(11% fat)	Dietary Fiber	1.68 g	(7% DV)
Total Fat	.84 g	(1% DV)	Protein	2.8 g	(6% DV)
Saturated Fat	.28 g	(1% DV)	Vitamin A	0 IU	(0% DV)
Poly Fat	.28 g		Vitamin C	0 mg	(0% DV)
Mono Fat	.28 g		Calcium	29.7 mg	(3% DV)
Cholesterol	0 mg	(0% DV)	Iron	.7 mg	(4% DV)
Sodium	157.9 mg	(7% DV)	Folate	2.8 mcg	(4% DV)
Potassium	81.8 mg	(2% DV)	Beta Carotene	0 RE	

Ratings	Worst	Bad	Average	Good	Best
Weight Loss					8
LowCal Density			4		
Filling		3			
Energizing			5		
Fiber			5		
Vitamins		3			
Minerals			4		
Overall			5		

RUSSIAN DRESSING

Serving: 1 tbsp (.55 oz)   Fat & Oil

Calories	76	(137.4 cal/oz)	Carbohydrate	1.59 g	(1% DV)
Fat Calories	70	(93% fat)	Dietary Fiber	0 g	(0% DV)
Total Fat	7.8 g	(12% DV)	Protein	.31 g	(1% DV)
Saturated Fat	1.07 g	(5% DV)	Vitamin A	105.6 IU	(2% DV)
Poly Fat	4.44 g		Vitamin C	.9 mg	(2% DV)
Mono Fat	1.84 g		Calcium	2.9 mg	(0% DV)
Cholesterol	2.8 mg	(1% DV)	Iron	.1 mg	(0% DV)
Sodium	132.8 mg	(6% DV)	Folate	.3 mcg	(0% DV)
Potassium	24 mg	(1% DV)	Beta Carotene	0 RE	

Ratings	Worst	Bad	Average	Good	Best
Weight Loss	2				
LowCal Density	1				
Filling	1				
Energizing	3				
Fiber	1				
Vitamins	3				
Minerals	2				
Overall	2				

RUSSIAN DRESSING, LOW-CALORIE

Serving: 1 tbsp (.58 oz)   Fat & Oil

Calories	23	(39.4 cal/oz)	Carbohydrate	4.47 g	(1% DV)
Fat Calories	6	(26% fat)	Dietary Fiber	0 g	(0% DV)
Total Fat	.65 g	(1% DV)	Protein	.16 g	(0% DV)
Saturated Fat	.16 g	(1% DV)	Vitamin A	9.1 IU	(0% DV)
Poly Fat	.32 g		Vitamin C	1 mg	(2% DV)
Mono Fat	.16 g		Calcium	3.1 mg	(0% DV)
Cholesterol	1 mg	(0% DV)	Iron	.1 mg	(1% DV)
Sodium	140.6 mg	(6% DV)	Folate	.2 mcg	(0% DV)
Potassium	25.4 mg	(1% DV)	Beta Carotene	0 RE	

Ratings	Worst	Bad	Average	Good	Best
Weight Loss				8	
LowCal Density			6		
Filling	2				
Energizing	3				
Fiber	1				
Vitamins	2				
Minerals	2				
Overall			5		

RUTABAGA, COOKED WITHOUT ADDED FAT

Serving: 1 cup (6.07 oz)   Vegetable

Calories	58	(9.5 cal/oz)	Carbohydrate	13.09 g	(4% DV)
Fat Calories	0	(0% fat)	Dietary Fiber	3.4 g	(14% DV)
Total Fat	0 g	(0% DV)	Protein	1.7 g	(3% DV)
Saturated Fat	0 g	(0% DV)	Vitamin A	0 IU	(0% DV)
Poly Fat	0 g		Vitamin C	37.4 mg	(62% DV)
Mono Fat	0 g		Calcium	71.4 mg	(7% DV)
Cholesterol	0 mg	(0% DV)	Iron	.8 mg	(4% DV)
Sodium	423.3 mg	(18% DV)	Folate	1.7 mcg	(6% DV)
Potassium	484.5 mg	(14% DV)	Beta Carotene	0 RE	

Ratings	Worst	Bad	Average	Good	Best
Weight Loss					9
LowCal Density					9
Filling					9
Energizing			5		
Fiber				8	
Vitamins			6		
Minerals			5		
Overall				8	

SAFFLOWER OIL

Serving: 1 tbsp (.49 oz)   Fat & Oil

Calories	120	(245.3 cal/oz)	Carbohydrate	0 g	(0% DV)
Fat Calories	122	(102% fat)	Dietary Fiber	0 g	(0% DV)
Total Fat	13.6 g	(21% DV)	Protein	0 g	(0% DV)
Saturated Fat	1.22 g	(6% DV)	Vitamin A	0 IU	(0% DV)
Poly Fat	10.2 g		Vitamin C	0 mg	(0% DV)
Mono Fat	1.63 g		Calcium	0 mg	(0% DV)
Cholesterol	0 mg	(0% DV)	Iron	0 mg	(0% DV)
Sodium	0 mg	(0% DV)	Folate	0 mcg	(0% DV)
Potassium	0 mg	(0% DV)	Beta Carotene	0 RE	

Ratings	Worst	Bad	Average	Good	Best
Weight Loss	1				
LowCal Density	1				
Filling	1				
Energizing	1				
Fiber	1				
Vitamins		3			
Minerals	1				
Overall	1				

SALAD GREENS, MIXED, RAW

Serving: 1 cup, shredded or chopped (1.96 oz)   **Salad**

Calories	9	(4.8 cal/oz)	Carbohydrate	1.65 g	(1% DV)
Fat Calories	0	(0% fat)	Dietary Fiber	1.1 g	(4% DV)
Total Fat	0 g	(0% DV)	Protein	1.1 g	(2% DV)
Saturated Fat	0 g	(0% DV)	Vitamin A	1495.5 IU	(30% DV)
Poly Fat	0 g		Vitamin C	8.8 mg	(15% DV)
Mono Fat	0 g		Calcium	30.3 mg	(3% DV)
Cholesterol	0 mg	(0% DV)	Iron	.7 mg	(4% DV)
Sodium	13.8 mg	(1% DV)	Folate	1.1 mcg	(16% DV)
Potassium	174.4 mg	(5% DV)	Beta Carotene	149.6 RE	

Ratings	Worst	Bad	Average	Good	Best
Weight Loss					10
LowCal Density					10
Filling			5		
Energizing		3			
Fiber		4			
Vitamins			6		
Minerals		3			
Overall				8	

SALAMI, BEEF

Serving: 1 slice (.82 oz)   **Meat**

Calories	60	(73.5 cal/oz)	Carbohydrate	.64 g	(0% DV)
Fat Calories	43	(72% fat)	Dietary Fiber	0 g	(0% DV)
Total Fat	4.83 g	(7% DV)	Protein	3.45 g	(7% DV)
Saturated Fat	2.07 g	(10% DV)	Vitamin A	0 IU	(0% DV)
Poly Fat	.23 g		Vitamin C	3.9 mg	(7% DV)
Mono Fat	2.07 g		Calcium	2.1 mg	(0% DV)
Cholesterol	15 mg	(5% DV)	Iron	.5 mg	(3% DV)
Sodium	270.5 mg	(11% DV)	Folate	3.5 mcg	(0% DV)
Potassium	51.5 mg	(1% DV)	Beta Carotene	0 RE	

Ratings	Worst	Bad	Average	Good	Best
Weight Loss			5		
LowCal Density		4			
Filling	1				
Energizing	2				
Fiber	1				
Vitamins		3			
Minerals		3			
Overall		3			

SALISBURY STEAK WITH GRAVY

Serving: 1 steak (4.61 oz)   **Entree**

Calories	217	(47 cal/oz)	Carbohydrate	6.84 g	(2% DV)
Fat Calories	128	(59% fat)	Dietary Fiber	0 g	(0% DV)
Total Fat	14.19 g	(22% DV)	Protein	16.77 g	(34% DV)
Saturated Fat	5.16 g	(26% DV)	Vitamin A	15.5 IU	(0% DV)
Poly Fat	0 g		Vitamin C	1.3 mg	(2% DV)
Mono Fat	6.45 g		Calcium	28.4 mg	(3% DV)
Cholesterol	59.3 mg	(20% DV)	Iron	2 mg	(11% DV)
Sodium	785.6 mg	(33% DV)	Folate	16.8 mcg	(2% DV)
Potassium	285.1 mg	(8% DV)	Beta Carotene	0 RE	

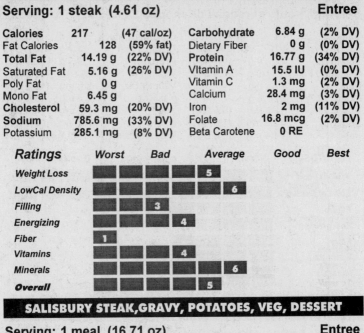

Ratings — Worst | Bad | Average | Good | Best

- Weight Loss: 5
- LowCal Density: 6
- Filling: 3
- Energizing: 4
- Fiber: 1
- Vitamins: 4
- Minerals: 6
- Overall: 5

SALISBURY STEAK, GRAVY, POTATOES, VEG, DESSERT

Serving: 1 meal (16.71 oz)   **Entree**

Calories	908	(54.3 cal/oz)	Carbohydrate	69.26 g	(23% DV)
Fat Calories	421	(46% fat)	Dietary Fiber	9.36 g	(37% DV)
Total Fat	46.8 g	(72% DV)	Protein	56.16 g	(112% DV)
Saturated Fat	18.72 g	(94% DV)	Vitamin A	4900 IU	(98% DV)
Poly Fat	4.68 g		Vitamin C	9.4 mg	(16% DV)
Mono Fat	18.72 g		Calcium	103 mg	(10% DV)
Cholesterol	145.1 mg	(48% DV)	Iron	9.1 mg	(51% DV)
Sodium	1595.9 mg	(66% DV)	Folate	56.2 mcg	(28% DV)
Potassium	1432.1 mg	(41% DV)	Beta Carotene	491.4 RE	

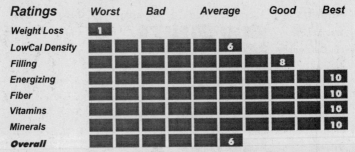

Ratings — Worst | Bad | Average | Good | Best

- Weight Loss: 1
- LowCal Density: 6
- Filling: 8
- Energizing: 10
- Fiber: 10
- Vitamins: 10
- Minerals: 10
- Overall: 6

SALMON, BAKED OR BROILED

Serving: 1 piece (3.04 oz)   **Fish**

Calories	146	(48.1 cal/oz)	Carbohydrate	.34 g	(0% DV)
Fat Calories	61	(42% fat)	Dietary Fiber	0 g	(0% DV)
Total Fat	6.8 g	(10% DV)	Protein	20.4 g	(41% DV)
Saturated Fat	.85 g	(4% DV)	Vitamin A	259.3 IU	(5% DV)
Poly Fat	2.55 g		Vitamin C	1.7 mg	(3% DV)
Mono Fat	2.55 g		Calcium	15.3 mg	(2% DV)
Cholesterol	52.7 mg	(18% DV)	Iron	.8 mg	(4% DV)
Sodium	382.5 mg	(16% DV)	Folate	20.4 mcg	(1% DV)
Potassium	336.6 mg	(10% DV)	Beta Carotene	3.4 RE	

Ratings	Worst	Bad	Average	Good	Best
Weight Loss				5	
LowCal Density				6	
Filling	1				
Energizing	2				
Fiber	1				
Vitamins				5	
Minerals				5	
Overall			4		

SALMON, BATTERED, FRIED

Serving: 1 piece (3.04 oz)   **Fish**

Calories	193	(63.5 cal/oz)	Carbohydrate	5.69 g	(2% DV)
Fat Calories	107	(56% fat)	Dietary Fiber	0 g	(0% DV)
Total Fat	11.9 g	(18% DV)	Protein	16.15 g	(32% DV)
Saturated Fat	2.55 g	(13% DV)	Vitamin A	88.4 IU	(2% DV)
Poly Fat	3.4 g		Vitamin C	0 mg	(0% DV)
Mono Fat	4.25 g		Calcium	28.9 mg	(3% DV)
Cholesterol	53.6 mg	(18% DV)	Iron	1 mg	(5% DV)
Sodium	99.5 mg	(4% DV)	Folate	16.2 mcg	(1% DV)
Potassium	256.7 mg	(7% DV)	Beta Carotene	0 RE	

Ratings	Worst	Bad	Average	Good	Best
Weight Loss			4		
LowCal Density				5	
Filling	2				
Energizing		3			
Fiber	1				
Vitamins				5	
Minerals				5	
Overall			4		

SALSA

Serving: 1 cup (9.25 oz)   **Sauce**

Calories	57	(6.2 cal/oz)	Carbohydrate	12.95 g	(4% DV)
Fat Calories	0	(0% fat)	Dietary Fiber	5.18 g	(21% DV)
Total Fat	0 g	(0% DV)	Protein	2.59 g	(5% DV)
Saturated Fat	0 g	(0% DV)	Vitamin A	1919.2 IU	(38% DV)
Poly Fat	0 g		Vitamin C	51.8 mg	(86% DV)
Mono Fat	0 g		Calcium	119.1 mg	(12% DV)
Cholesterol	0 mg	(0% DV)	Iron	1.9 mg	(10% DV)
Sodium	670.8 mg	(28% DV)	Folate	2.6 mcg	(9% DV)
Potassium	479.2 mg	(14% DV)	Beta Carotene	191.7 RE	

Ratings	Worst	Bad	Average	Good	Best
Weight Loss					9
LowCal Density					10
Filling					10
Energizing			5		
Fiber					9
Vitamins					9
Minerals			5		
Overall					9

SAUERKRAUT, COOKED WITHOUT ADDED FAT

Serving: 1 cup (5.07 oz)   **Vegetable**

Calories	27	(5.3 cal/oz)	Carbohydrate	6.11 g	(2% DV)
Fat Calories	0	(0% fat)	Dietary Fiber	4.26 g	(17% DV)
Total Fat	0 g	(0% DV)	Protein	1.42 g	(3% DV)
Saturated Fat	0 g	(0% DV)	Vitamin A	25.6 IU	(1% DV)
Poly Fat	0 g		Vitamin C	18.5 mg	(31% DV)
Mono Fat	0 g		Calcium	42.6 mg	(4% DV)
Cholesterol	0 mg	(0% DV)	Iron	2.1 mg	(12% DV)
Sodium	938.6 mg	(39% DV)	Folate	1.4 mcg	(8% DV)
Potassium	241.4 mg	(7% DV)	Beta Carotene	2.8 RE	

Ratings	Worst	Bad	Average	Good	Best
Weight Loss					10
LowCal Density					10
Filling					10
Energizing		4			
Fiber					9
Vitamins			5		
Minerals		4			
Overall					9

SAUSAGE & FRENCH TOAST

Serving: 1 frozen meal (6.57 oz)   **Breakfast**

Calories	432	(65.8 cal/oz)	**Carbohydrate**	33.67 g	(11% DV)
Fat Calories	199	(46% fat)	Dietary Fiber	1.84 g	(7% DV)
Total Fat	22.08 g	(34% DV)	**Protein**	22.08 g	(44% DV)
Saturated Fat	7.36 g	(37% DV)	VItamin A	274.2 IU	(5% DV)
Poly Fat	3.68 g		Vitamin C	1.8 mg	(3% DV)
Mono Fat	9.2 g		Calcium	152.7 mg	(15% DV)
Cholesterol	250.2 mg	(83% DV)	Iron	2.8 mg	(16% DV)
Sodium	1074.6 mg	(45% DV)	Folate	22.1 mcg	(11% DV)
Potassium	371.7 mg	(11% DV)	Beta Carotene	0 RE	

Ratings	Worst	Bad	Average	Good	Best
Weight Loss	2				
LowCal Density			5		
Filling			5		
Energizing				8	
Fiber			6		
Vitamins			7		
Minerals			7		
Overall			5		

SAUSAGE & PANCAKES

Serving: 1 frozen meal (6.07 oz)   **Breakfast**

Calories	476	(78.4 cal/oz)	**Carbohydrate**	46.75 g	(16% DV)
Fat Calories	230	(48% fat)	Dietary Fiber	1.7 g	(7% DV)
Total Fat	25.5 g	(39% DV)	**Protein**	15.3 g	(31% DV)
Saturated Fat	6.8 g	(34% DV)	VItamin A	627.3 IU	(13% DV)
Poly Fat	5.1 g		Vitamin C	1.7 mg	(3% DV)
Mono Fat	10.2 g		Calcium	90.1 mg	(9% DV)
Cholesterol	90.1 mg	(30% DV)	Iron	2.6 mg	(14% DV)
Sodium	1196.8 mg	(50% DV)	Folate	15.3 mcg	(4% DV)
Potassium	294.1 mg	(8% DV)	Beta Carotene	11.9 RE	

Ratings	Worst	Bad	Average	Good	Best
Weight Loss	1				
LowCal Density		4			
Filling			5		
Energizing					9
Fiber			6		
Vitamins			6		
Minerals			6		
Overall		4			

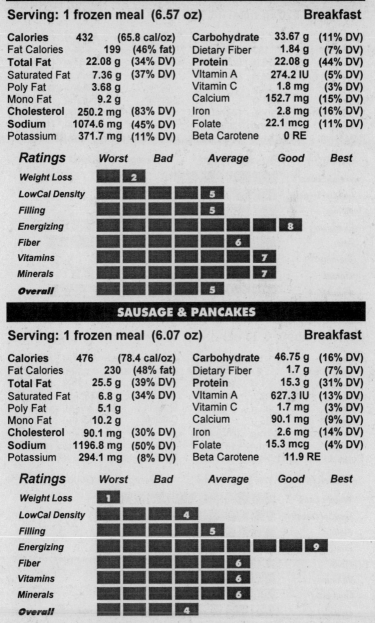

SCALLOPS WITH POTATOES, VEGETABLE

Serving: 1 frozen meal (8.11 oz)   **Entree**

Calories	413	(50.9 cal/oz)	Carbohydrate	38.82 g	(13% DV)
Fat Calories	163	(40% fat)	Dietary Fiber	4.54 g	(18% DV)
Total Fat	18.16 g	(28% DV)	Protein	24.97 g	(50% DV)
Saturated Fat	4.54 g	(23% DV)	Vitamin A	469.9 IU	(9% DV)
Poly Fat	4.54 g		Vitamin C	13.6 mg	(23% DV)
Mono Fat	6.81 g		Calcium	65.8 mg	(7% DV)
Cholesterol	61.3 mg	(20% DV)	Iron	2.5 mg	(14% DV)
Sodium	610.6 mg	(25% DV)	Folate	25 mcg	(16% DV)
Potassium	733.2 mg	(21% DV)	Beta Carotene	38.6 RE	

Ratings	Worst	Bad	Average	Good	Best
Weight Loss		4			
LowCal Density			6		
Filling			6		
Energizing					9
Fiber					9
Vitamins				7	
Minerals				8	
Overall			6		

SCALLOPS, BAKED OR BROILED

Serving: about 6 (3 oz)   **Shellfish**

Calories	113	(37.7 cal/oz)	Carbohydrate	2.47 g	(1% DV)
Fat Calories	31	(27% fat)	Dietary Fiber	0 g	(0% DV)
Total Fat	3.4 g	(5% DV)	Protein	17 g	(34% DV)
Saturated Fat	.85 g	(4% DV)	Vitamin A	178.5 IU	(4% DV)
Poly Fat	.85 g		Vitamin C	2.6 mg	(4% DV)
Mono Fat	.85 g		Calcium	25.5 mg	(3% DV)
Cholesterol	34 mg	(11% DV)	Iron	.3 mg	(2% DV)
Sodium	434.4 mg	(18% DV)	Folate	17 mcg	(4% DV)
Potassium	331.5 mg	(9% DV)	Beta Carotene	2.6 RE	

Ratings	Worst	Bad	Average	Good	Best
Weight Loss			6		
LowCal Density			7		
Filling	2				
Energizing		3			
Fiber	1				
Vitamins		4			
Minerals			6		
Overall			5		

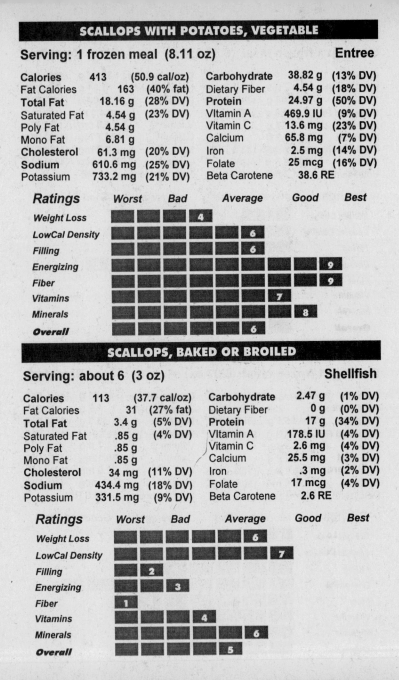

SCALLOPS, FLOURED OR BREADED, FRIED

Serving: about 5 (3 oz)   **Shellfish**

Calories	183	(60.9 cal/oz)	Carbohydrate	8.59 g	(3% DV)
Fat Calories	84	(46% fat)	Dietary Fiber	0 g	(0% DV)
Total Fat	9.35 g	(14% DV)	Protein	15.3 g	(31% DV)
Saturated Fat	2.55 g	(13% DV)	Vitamin A	68.9 IU	(1% DV)
Poly Fat	2.55 g		Vitamin C	1.7 mg	(3% DV)
Mono Fat	3.4 g		Calcium	34.9 mg	(3% DV)
Cholesterol	45.9 mg	(15% DV)	Iron	.7 mg	(4% DV)
Sodium	394.4 mg	(16% DV)	Folate	15.3 mcg	(4% DV)
Potassium	283.1 mg	(8% DV)	Beta Carotene	0 RE	

Ratings	Worst	Bad	Average	Good	Best
Weight Loss		3			
LowCal Density			5		
Filling		3			
Energizing			4		
Fiber	1				
Vitamins			4		
Minerals			5		
Overall			4		

SCRAMBLED EGG, FROM CHOLESTEROL-FREE MIXTURE

Serving: 1 cup, cooked (5.46 oz)   **Breakfast**

Calories	278	(51 cal/oz)	Carbohydrate	5.51 g	(2% DV)
Fat Calories	179	(64% fat)	Dietary Fiber	0 g	(0% DV)
Total Fat	19.89 g	(31% DV)	Protein	19.89 g	(40% DV)
Saturated Fat	3.06 g	(15% DV)	Vitamin A	2347 IU	(47% DV)
Poly Fat	10.71 g		Vitamin C	0 mg	(0% DV)
Mono Fat	4.59 g		Calcium	127 mg	(13% DV)
Cholesterol	3.1 mg	(1% DV)	Iron	3.4 mg	(19% DV)
Sodium	347.3 mg	(14% DV)	Folate	19.9 mcg	(5% DV)
Potassium	370.3 mg	(11% DV)	Beta Carotene	234.1 RE	

Ratings	Worst	Bad	Average	Good	Best
Weight Loss	2				
LowCal Density				6	
Filling	2				
Energizing		3			
Fiber	1				
Vitamins				6	
Minerals				6	
Overall			4		

SCRAMBLED EGGS, BACON, HOME FRIED POTATOES

Serving: 1 frozen meal (5.32 oz)   **Breakfast**

Calories	353	(66.4 cal/oz)	**Carbohydrate**	16.24 g	(5% DV)
Fat Calories	228	(65% fat)	Dietary Fiber	1.49 g	(6% DV)
Total Fat	25.33 g	(39% DV)	**Protein**	16.39 g	(33% DV)
Saturated Fat	8.94 g	(45% DV)	VItamin A	533.4 IU	(11% DV)
Poly Fat	2.98 g		Vitamin C	8.9 mg	(15% DV)
Mono Fat	10.43 g		Calcium	65.6 mg	(7% DV)
Cholesterol	292 mg	(97% DV)	Iron	2 mg	(11% DV)
Sodium	661.6 mg	(28% DV)	Folate	16.4 mcg	(7% DV)
Potassium	424.7 mg	(12% DV)	Beta Carotene	3 RE	

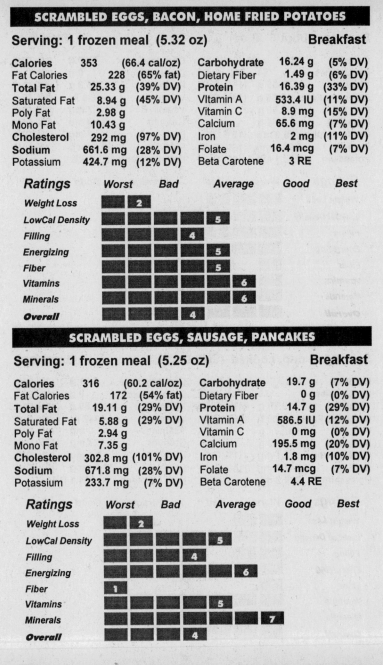

Ratings	Worst	Bad	Average	Good	Best
Weight Loss	2				
LowCal Density			5		
Filling			4		
Energizing			5		
Fiber			5		
Vitamins				6	
Minerals				6	
Overall			4		

SCRAMBLED EGGS, SAUSAGE, PANCAKES

Serving: 1 frozen meal (5.25 oz)   **Breakfast**

Calories	316	(60.2 cal/oz)	**Carbohydrate**	19.7 g	(7% DV)
Fat Calories	172	(54% fat)	Dietary Fiber	0 g	(0% DV)
Total Fat	19.11 g	(29% DV)	**Protein**	14.7 g	(29% DV)
Saturated Fat	5.88 g	(29% DV)	VItamin A	586.5 IU	(12% DV)
Poly Fat	2.94 g		Vitamin C	0 mg	(0% DV)
Mono Fat	7.35 g		Calcium	195.5 mg	(20% DV)
Cholesterol	302.8 mg	(101% DV)	Iron	1.8 mg	(10% DV)
Sodium	671.8 mg	(28% DV)	Folate	14.7 mcg	(7% DV)
Potassium	233.7 mg	(7% DV)	Beta Carotene	4.4 RE	

Ratings	Worst	Bad	Average	Good	Best
Weight Loss	2				
LowCal Density			5		
Filling			4		
Energizing			6		
Fiber	1				
Vitamins			5		
Minerals				7	
Overall			4		

SCRAMBLED EGGS, SAUSAGE, HASH BROWN POTATO

Serving: 1 frozen meal (6.32 oz)   **Breakfast**

Calories	420	(66.4 cal/oz)	Carbohydrate	18.94 g	(6% DV)
Fat Calories	287	(68% fat)	Dietary Fiber	1.77 g	(7% DV)
Total Fat	31.86 g	(49% DV)	Protein	15.93 g	(32% DV)
Saturated Fat	8.85 g	(44% DV)	VItamin A	339.8 IU	(7% DV)
Poly Fat	7.08 g		Vitamin C	3.5 mg	(6% DV)
Mono Fat	12.39 g		Calcium	60.2 mg	(6% DV)
Cholesterol	256.7 mg	(86% DV)	Iron	2.1 mg	(11% DV)
Sodium	842.5 mg	(35% DV)	Folate	15.9 mcg	(6% DV)
Potassium	463.7 mg	(13% DV)	Beta Carotene	0 RE	

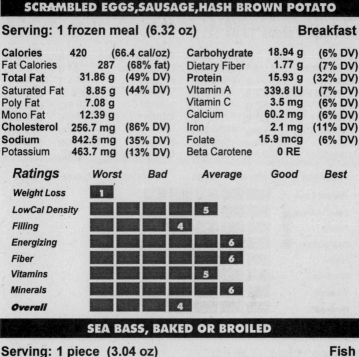

Ratings	Worst	Bad	Average	Good	Best
Weight Loss	1				
LowCal Density			5		
Filling		4			
Energizing			6		
Fiber			6		
Vitamins			5		
Minerals			6		
Overall		4			

SEA BASS, BAKED OR BROILED

Serving: 1 piece (3.04 oz)   **Fish**

Calories	127	(41.7 cal/oz)	Carbohydrate	.34 g	(0% DV)
Fat Calories	46	(36% fat)	Dietary Fiber	0 g	(0% DV)
Total Fat	5.1 g	(8% DV)	Protein	18.7 g	(37% DV)
Saturated Fat	.85 g	(4% DV)	VItamin A	325.6 IU	(7% DV)
Poly Fat	1.7 g		Vitamin C	1.7 mg	(3% DV)
Mono Fat	1.7 g		Calcium	11.9 mg	(1% DV)
Cholesterol	41.7 mg	(14% DV)	Iron	.3 mg	(2% DV)
Sodium	383.4 mg	(16% DV)	Folate	18.7 mcg	(1% DV)
Potassium	267.8 mg	(8% DV)	Beta Carotene	3.4 RE	

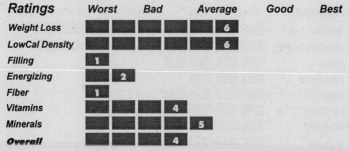

Ratings	Worst	Bad	Average	Good	Best
Weight Loss			6		
LowCal Density			6		
Filling	1				
Energizing	2				
Fiber	1				
Vitamins		4			
Minerals			5		
Overall		4			

SEA BASS, FLOURED OR BREADED, FRIED

Serving: 1 piece (3.04 oz)   **Fish**

Calories	180	(59.3 cal/oz)	Carbohydrate	8.07 g	(3% DV)
Fat Calories	69	(38% fat)	Dietary Fiber	.85 g	(3% DV)
Total Fat	7.65 g	(12% DV)	Protein	18.7 g	(37% DV)
Saturated Fat	1.7 g	(8% DV)	VItamin A	138.6 IU	(3% DV)
Poly Fat	1.7 g		Vitamin C	0 mg	(0% DV)
Mono Fat	3.4 g		Calcium	40.8 mg	(4% DV)
Cholesterol	54.4 mg	(18% DV)	Iron	1.3 mg	(7% DV)
Sodium	361.3 mg	(15% DV)	Folate	18.7 mcg	(3% DV)
Potassium	431 mg	(12% DV)	Beta Carotene	0 RE	

Ratings	Worst	Bad	Average	Good	Best
Weight Loss			5		
LowCal Density			5		
Filling		3			
Energizing			4		
Fiber			4		
Vitamins		3			
Minerals			5		
Overall			4		

SEAFOOD GARDEN SALAD, WITH TOMATOES & CARROTS

Serving: 1 cup (3.39 oz)   **Salad**

Calories	43	(12.6 cal/oz)	Carbohydrate	2.47 g	(1% DV)
Fat Calories	9	(20% fat)	Dietary Fiber	.95 g	(4% DV)
Total Fat	.95 g	(1% DV)	Protein	6.65 g	(13% DV)
Saturated Fat	0 g	(0% DV)	VItamin A	1563.7 IU	(31% DV)
Poly Fat	0 g		Vitamin C	8.6 mg	(14% DV)
Mono Fat	0 g		Calcium	35.2 mg	(4% DV)
Cholesterol	37.1 mg	(12% DV)	Iron	.8 mg	(5% DV)
Sodium	78.9 mg	(3% DV)	Folate	6.7 mcg	(8% DV)
Potassium	207.1 mg	(6% DV)	Beta Carotene	155.8 RE	

Ratings	Worst	Bad	Average	Good	Best
Weight Loss					9
LowCal Density					9
Filling			4		
Energizing		3			
Fiber			4		
Vitamins			5		
Minerals			4		
Overall				7	

SEAFOOD NEWBURG, RICE, VEGETABLE

Serving: 1 frozen meal (10.64 oz)   **Entree**

Calories	286	(26.9 cal/oz)	Carbohydrate	34.27 g	(11% DV)
Fat Calories	80	(28% fat)	Dietary Fiber	2.98 g	(12% DV)
Total Fat	8.94 g	(14% DV)	Protein	14.9 g	(30% DV)
Saturated Fat	5.96 g	(30% DV)	Vitamin A	736.1 IU	(15% DV)
Poly Fat	0 g		Vitamin C	6 mg	(10% DV)
Mono Fat	2.98 g		Calcium	80.5 mg	(8% DV)
Cholesterol	80.5 mg	(27% DV)	Iron	1.9 mg	(10% DV)
Sodium	1248.6 mg	(52% DV)	Folate	14.9 mcg	(4% DV)
Potassium	321.8 mg	(9% DV)	Beta Carotene	44.7 RE	

Ratings	Worst	Bad	Average	Good	Best
Weight Loss			6		
LowCal Density				8	
Filling				8	
Energizing				8	
Fiber				8	
Vitamins			5		
Minerals			6		
Overall				7	

SESAME BUTTER (TAHINI) (MADE FROM KERNELS)

Serving: 1 tbsp (.54 oz)   **Snack**

Calories	89	(164.4 cal/oz)	Carbohydrate	3.23 g	(1% DV)
Fat Calories	72	(81% fat)	Dietary Fiber	.75 g	(3% DV)
Total Fat	7.95 g	(12% DV)	Protein	2.55 g	(5% DV)
Saturated Fat	1.05 g	(5% DV)	Vitamin A	10.1 IU	(0% DV)
Poly Fat	3.45 g		Vitamin C	.6 mg	(1% DV)
Mono Fat	3 g		Calcium	21.2 mg	(2% DV)
Cholesterol	0 mg	(0% DV)	Iron	.7 mg	(4% DV)
Sodium	5.3 mg	(0% DV)	Folate	2.6 mcg	(4% DV)
Potassium	68.9 mg	(2% DV)	Beta Carotene	1.1 RE	

Ratings	Worst	Bad	Average	Good	Best
Weight Loss		4			
LowCal Density	1				
Filling	1				
Energizing		3			
Fiber		3			
Vitamins		4			
Minerals		4			
Overall		3			

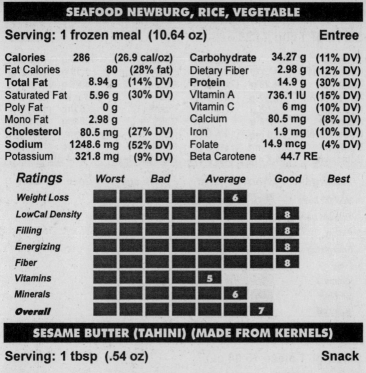

SEVEN-LAYER SALAD

Serving: 1 cup (4.25 oz)   **Salad**

Calories	200	(47 cal/oz)	Carbohydrate	12.85 g	(4% DV)
Fat Calories	129	(64% fat)	Dietary Fiber	1.19 g	(5% DV)
Total Fat	14.28 g	(22% DV)	Protein	5.95 g	(12% DV)
Saturated Fat	3.57 g	(18% DV)	Vitamin A	447.4 IU	(9% DV)
Poly Fat	5.95 g		Vitamin C	9.5 mg	(16% DV)
Mono Fat	4.76 g		Calcium	73.8 mg	(7% DV)
Cholesterol	55.9 mg	(19% DV)	Iron	.8 mg	(4% DV)
Sodium	334.4 mg	(14% DV)	Folate	6 mcg	(10% DV)
Potassium	154.7 mg	(4% DV)	Beta Carotene	27.4 RE	

Ratings	Worst	Bad	Average	Good	Best
Weight Loss			4		
LowCal Density				6	
Filling			4		
Energizing			5		
Fiber			4		
Vitamins			5		
Minerals			4		
Overall			5		

SHARK, BAKED OR BROILED

Serving: 1 piece (3.04 oz)   **Fish**

Calories	152	(50.1 cal/oz)	Carbohydrate	.34 g	(0% DV)
Fat Calories	61	(40% fat)	Dietary Fiber	0 g	(0% DV)
Total Fat	6.8 g	(10% DV)	Protein	21.25 g	(42% DV)
Saturated Fat	1.7 g	(8% DV)	Vitamin A	327.3 IU	(7% DV)
Poly Fat	2.55 g		Vitamin C	1.7 mg	(3% DV)
Mono Fat	2.55 g		Calcium	34.9 mg	(3% DV)
Cholesterol	51 mg	(17% DV)	Iron	.8 mg	(5% DV)
Sodium	340.9 mg	(14% DV)	Folate	21.3 mcg	(1% DV)
Potassium	164.1 mg	(5% DV)	Beta Carotene	2.6 RE	

Ratings	Worst	Bad	Average	Good	Best
Weight Loss			5		
LowCal Density				6	
Filling	1				
Energizing	2				
Fiber	1				
Vitamins			4		
Minerals			5		
Overall			4		

SHERBET, ALL FLAVORS

Serving: 1 cup (6.89 oz)   **Dessert**

Calories	270	(39.2 cal/oz)	Carbohydrate	58.67 g	(20% DV)
Fat Calories	35	(13% fat)	Dietary Fiber	0 g	(0% DV)
Total Fat	3.86 g	(6% DV)	Protein	1.93 g	(4% DV)
Saturated Fat	1.93 g	(10% DV)	Vitamin A	185.3 IU	(4% DV)
Poly Fat	0 g		Vitamin C	3.9 mg	(6% DV)
Mono Fat	1.93 g		Calcium	104.2 mg	(10% DV)
Cholesterol	13.5 mg	(5% DV)	Iron	.3 mg	(2% DV)
Sodium	88.8 mg	(4% DV)	Folate	1.9 mcg	(3% DV)
Potassium	198.8 mg	(6% DV)	Beta Carotene	3.9 RE	

Ratings	Worst	Bad	Average	Good	Best
Weight Loss				7	
LowCal Density			6		
Filling				8	
Energizing					10
Fiber	1				
Vitamins		3			
Minerals			5		
Overall			6		

SHREDDED WHEAT, 100%

Serving: 1 rectangular biscuit (.86 oz)   **Cereal**

Calories	85	(99.3 cal/oz)	Carbohydrate	19.15 g	(6% DV)
Fat Calories	4	(5% fat)	Dietary Fiber	2.4 g	(10% DV)
Total Fat	.48 g	(1% DV)	Protein	2.64 g	(5% DV)
Saturated Fat	0 g	(0% DV)	Vitamin A	0 IU	(0% DV)
Poly Fat	.24 g		Vitamin C	0 mg	(0% DV)
Mono Fat	0 g		Calcium	9.6 mg	(1% DV)
Cholesterol	0 mg	(0% DV)	Iron	.9 mg	(5% DV)
Sodium	1.4 mg	(0% DV)	Folate	2.6 mcg	(3% DV)
Potassium	82.6 mg	(2% DV)	Beta Carotene	0 RE	

Ratings	Worst	Bad	Average	Good	Best
Weight Loss					9
LowCal Density		3			
Filling		3			
Energizing			6		
Fiber				7	
Vitamins		3			
Minerals			4		
Overall			5		

SHRIMP & NOODLES IN TOMATO-BASED SAUCE

Serving: 1 Healthy Choice meal (10.64 oz)   Entree

Calories	232	(21.8 cal/oz)	Carbohydrate	43.21 g	(14% DV)
Fat Calories	27	(12% fat)	Dietary Fiber	2.98 g	(12% DV)
Total Fat	2.98 g	(5% DV)	Protein	11.92 g	(24% DV)
Saturated Fat	0 g	(0% DV)	Vitamin A	1975.7 IU	(40% DV)
Poly Fat	0 g		Vitamin C	71.5 mg	(119% DV)
Mono Fat	0 g		Calcium	44.7 mg	(4% DV)
Cholesterol	74.5 mg	(25% DV)	Iron	2.7 mg	(15% DV)
Sodium	223.5 mg	(9% DV)	Folate	11.9 mcg	(5% DV)
Potassium	417.2 mg	(12% DV)	Beta Carotene	187.7 RE	

Ratings	Worst	Bad	Average	Good	Best
Weight Loss				8	
LowCal Density				8	
Filling					10
Energizing				9	
Fiber				8	
Vitamins				9	
Minerals			6		
Overall				8	

SHRIMP & PASTA GARDEN SALAD

Serving: 1 fast food order (9.32 oz)   Salad

Calories	167	(17.9 cal/oz)	Carbohydrate	15.4 g	(5% DV)
Fat Calories	47	(28% fat)	Dietary Fiber	2.61 g	(10% DV)
Total Fat	5.22 g	(8% DV)	Protein	13.05 g	(26% DV)
Saturated Fat	0 g	(0% DV)	Vitamin A	1892.3 IU	(38% DV)
Poly Fat	2.61 g		Vitamin C	20.9 mg	(35% DV)
Mono Fat	2.61 g		Calcium	57.4 mg	(6% DV)
Cholesterol	73.1 mg	(24% DV)	Iron	2.4 mg	(13% DV)
Sodium	373.2 mg	(16% DV)	Folate	13.1 mcg	(18% DV)
Potassium	412.4 mg	(12% DV)	Beta Carotene	185.3 RE	

Ratings	Worst	Bad	Average	Good	Best
Weight Loss			6		
LowCal Density				8	
Filling			7		
Energizing		5			
Fiber			7		
Vitamins				8	
Minerals			6		
Overall			7		

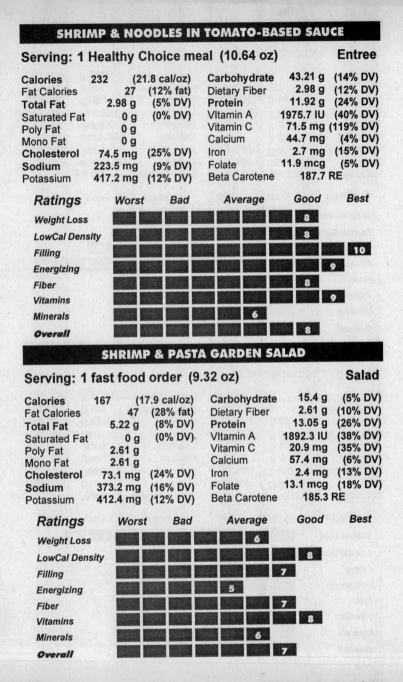

SHRIMP COCKTAIL (WITH COCKTAIL SAUCE)

Serving: 4 shrimp with sauce (3.29 oz)   **Entree**

Calories	78	(23.8 cal/oz)	Carbohydrate	7.73 g	(3% DV)
Fat Calories	8	(11% fat)	Dietary Fiber	1.84 g	(7% DV)
Total Fat	.92 g	(1% DV)	Protein	10.12 g	(20% DV)
Saturated Fat	0 g	(0% DV)	VItamin A	241 IU	(5% DV)
Poly Fat	0 g		Vitamin C	10.1 mg	(17% DV)
Mono Fat	0 g		Calcium	34 mg	(3% DV)
Cholesterol	69 mg	(23% DV)	Iron	1.4 mg	(8% DV)
Sodium	396.5 mg	(17% DV)	Folate	10.1 mcg	(6% DV)
Potassium	221.7 mg	(6% DV)	Beta Carotene	22.1 RE	

Ratings	Worst	Bad	Average	Good	Best
Weight Loss					9
LowCal Density				8	
Filling			5		
Energizing		4			
Fiber				6	
Vitamins			5		
Minerals			5		
Overall				7	

SHRIMP CREOLE, RICE, PEPPERS

Serving: 1 diet meal (10.14 oz)   **Entree**

Calories	250	(24.6 cal/oz)	Carbohydrate	46.58 g	(16% DV)
Fat Calories	26	(10% fat)	Dietary Fiber	2.84 g	(11% DV)
Total Fat	2.84 g	(4% DV)	Protein	8.52 g	(17% DV)
Saturated Fat	0 g	(0% DV)	VItamin A	744.1 IU	(15% DV)
Poly Fat	0 g		Vitamin C	51.1 mg	(85% DV)
Mono Fat	0 g		Calcium	42.6 mg	(4% DV)
Cholesterol	39.8 mg	(13% DV)	Iron	2.9 mg	(16% DV)
Sodium	823.6 mg	(34% DV)	Folate	8.5 mcg	(5% DV)
Potassium	394.8 mg	(11% DV)	Beta Carotene	73.8 RE	

Ratings	Worst	Bad	Average	Good	Best
Weight Loss				8	
LowCal Density				8	
Filling					10
Energizing				9	
Fiber				8	
Vitamins				8	
Minerals			6		
Overall				8	

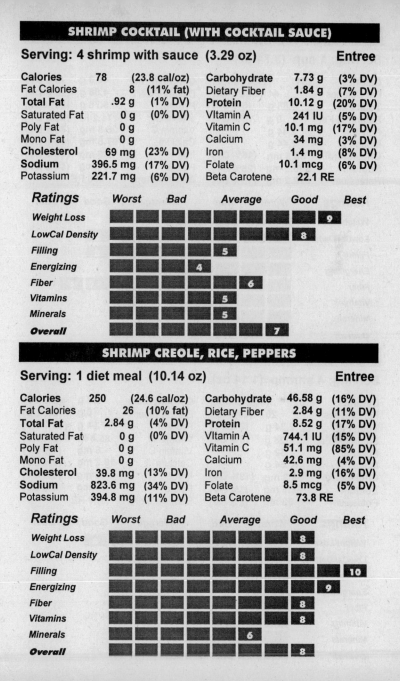

SHRIMP GUMBO

Serving: 1 cup (8.71 oz)   **Soup**

Calories	151	(17.4 cal/oz)	Carbohydrate	18.3 g	(6% DV)
Fat Calories	44	(29% fat)	Dietary Fiber	4.88 g	(20% DV)
Total Fat	4.88 g	(8% DV)	Protein	9.76 g	(20% DV)
Saturated Fat	0 g	(0% DV)	Vitamin A	1171.2 IU	(23% DV)
Poly Fat	2.44 g		Vitamin C	26.8 mg	(45% DV)
Mono Fat	2.44 g		Calcium	97.6 mg	(10% DV)
Cholesterol	48.8 mg	(16% DV)	Iron	2.8 mg	(15% DV)
Sodium	590.5 mg	(25% DV)	Folate	9.8 mcg	(15% DV)
Potassium	522.2 mg	(15% DV)	Beta Carotene	100 RE	

Ratings

	Worst	Bad	Average	Good	Best
Weight Loss			5		
LowCal Density				8	
Filling				8	
Energizing			6		
Fiber					9
Vitamins			7		
Minerals			6		
Overall			7		

SHRIMP SCAMPI

Serving: 4 shrimp (1.14 oz)   **Entree**

Calories	52	(45.2 cal/oz)	Carbohydrate	.32 g	(0% DV)
Fat Calories	20	(39% fat)	Dietary Fiber	0 g	(0% DV)
Total Fat	2.24 g	(3% DV)	Protein	7.04 g	(14% DV)
Saturated Fat	1.28 g	(6% DV)	Vitamin A	85.4 IU	(2% DV)
Poly Fat	.32 g		Vitamin C	.6 mg	(1% DV)
Mono Fat	.64 g		Calcium	18.2 mg	(2% DV)
Cholesterol	56.3 mg	(19% DV)	Iron	.8 mg	(5% DV)
Sodium	68.5 mg	(3% DV)	Folate	7 mcg	(0% DV)
Potassium	63 mg	(2% DV)	Beta Carotene	1.9 RE	

Ratings

	Worst	Bad	Average	Good	Best
Weight Loss				8	
LowCal Density			6		
Filling	1				
Energizing	2				
Fiber	1				
Vitamins		3			
Minerals		4			
Overall			5		

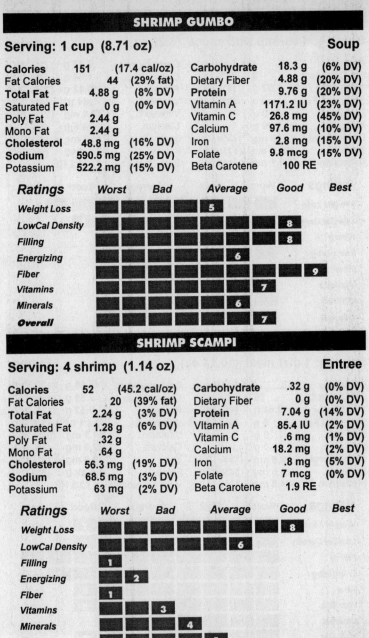

SHRIMP, FLOURED, BREADED, OR BATTERED, FRIED

Serving: about 8 medium (3.04 oz)   **Shellfish**

Calories	209	(68.8 cal/oz)	Carbohydrate	10.29 g	(3% DV)
Fat Calories	92	(44% fat)	Dietary Fiber	0 g	(0% DV)
Total Fat	10.2 g	(16% DV)	Protein	17.85 g	(36% DV)
Saturated Fat	2.55 g	(13% DV)	Vltamin A	192.1 IU	(4% DV)
Poly Fat	2.55 g		Vitamin C	.9 mg	(1% DV)
Mono Fat	4.25 g		Calcium	51 mg	(5% DV)
Cholesterol	156.4 mg	(52% DV)	Iron	2.5 mg	(14% DV)
Sodium	388.5 mg	(16% DV)	Folate	17.9 mcg	(2% DV)
Potassium	163.2 mg	(5% DV)	Beta Carotene	0 RE	

Ratings	Worst	Bad	Average	Good	Best
Weight Loss		3			
LowCal Density		4			
Filling		3			
Energizing		4			
Fiber	1				
Vitamins		4			
Minerals			6		
Overall		4			

SHRIMP, STEAMED OR BOILED

Serving: 14 large (3 oz)   **Shellfish**

Calories	118	(39.4 cal/oz)	Carbohydrate	1.02 g	(0% DV)
Fat Calories	15	(13% fat)	Dietary Fiber	0 g	(0% DV)
Total Fat	1.7 g	(3% DV)	Protein	22.95 g	(46% DV)
Saturated Fat	0 g	(0% DV)	Vltamin A	181.1 IU	(4% DV)
Poly Fat	.85 g		Vitamin C	1.7 mg	(3% DV)
Mono Fat	0 g		Calcium	57.8 mg	(6% DV)
Cholesterol	170 mg	(57% DV)	Iron	2.4 mg	(14% DV)
Sodium	141.1 mg	(6% DV)	Folate	23 mcg	(1% DV)
Potassium	144.5 mg	(4% DV)	Beta Carotene	0 RE	

Ratings	Worst	Bad	Average	Good	Best
Weight Loss				7	
LowCal Density				7	
Filling	1				
Energizing	2				
Fiber	1				
Vitamins			4		
Minerals			6		
Overall			5		

Serving: 1 piece (.54 oz)   **Fish**

Calories	25	(46.9 cal/oz)	Carbohydrate	.09 g	(0% DV)
Fat Calories	11	(43% fat)	Dietary Fiber	0 g	(0% DV)
Total Fat	1.2 g	(2% DV)	Protein	3.45 g	(7% DV)
Saturated Fat	.3 g	(1% DV)	Vitamin A	46.5 IU	(1% DV)
Poly Fat	.45 g		Vitamin C	.5 mg	(1% DV)
Mono Fat	.45 g		Calcium	12 mg	(1% DV)
Cholesterol	13.5 mg	(4% DV)	Iron	.2 mg	(1% DV)
Sodium	87.3 mg	(4% DV)	Folate	3.5 mcg	(0% DV)
Potassium	57.3 mg	(2% DV)	Beta Carotene	.8 RE	

Ratings	Worst	Bad	Average	Good	Best
Weight Loss				8	
LowCal Density			6		
Filling	1				
Energizing	2				
Fiber	1				
Vitamins	2				
Minerals	3				
Overall	5				

Serving: 1 smelt (.57 oz)   **Fish**

Calories	40	(70.2 cal/oz)	Carbohydrate	1.94 g	(1% DV)
Fat Calories	19	(47% fat)	Dietary Fiber	.16 g	(1% DV)
Total Fat	2.08 g	(3% DV)	Protein	3.36 g	(7% DV)
Saturated Fat	.48 g	(2% DV)	Vitamin A	15.4 IU	(0% DV)
Poly Fat	.48 g		Vitamin C	0 mg	(0% DV)
Mono Fat	.8 g		Calcium	13.8 mg	(1% DV)
Cholesterol	16.6 mg	(6% DV)	Iron	.3 mg	(2% DV)
Sodium	85.8 mg	(4% DV)	Folate	3.4 mcg	(0% DV)
Potassium	51.8 mg	(1% DV)	Beta Carotene	0 RE	

Ratings	Worst	Bad	Average	Good	Best
Weight Loss				7	
LowCal Density		4			
Filling	1				
Energizing	3				
Fiber	2				
Vitamins	2				
Minerals	3				
Overall	4				

SNAILS, COOKED (ESCARGOT)

Serving: about 6 (1 oz)   **Shellfish**

Calories	37	(37.2 cal/oz)	Carbohydrate	.67 g	(0% DV)
Fat Calories	10	(27% fat)	Dietary Fiber	0 g	(0% DV)
Total Fat	1.12 g	(2% DV)	Protein	5.6 g	(11% DV)
Saturated Fat	.56 g	(3% DV)	Vitamin A	57.1 IU	(1% DV)
Poly Fat	0 g		Vitamin C	0 mg	(0% DV)
Mono Fat	.28 g		Calcium	3.6 mg	(0% DV)
Cholesterol	19 mg	(6% DV)	Iron	1.2 mg	(7% DV)
Sodium	31.4 mg	(1% DV)	Folate	5.6 mcg	(0% DV)
Potassium	130.5 mg	(4% DV)	Beta Carotene	.8 RE	

Ratings	Worst	Bad	Average	Good	Best
Weight Loss				8	
LowCal Density				7	
Filling	1				
Energizing	2				
Fiber	1				
Vitamins	3				
Minerals			5		
Overall			5		

SNOW CONE, SLURPIE

Serving: 1 slurpie (11.14 oz)   **Dessert**

Calories	243	(21.8 cal/oz)	Carbohydrate	101.71 g	(34% DV)
Fat Calories	0	(0% fat)	Dietary Fiber	0 g	(0% DV)
Total Fat	0 g	(0% DV)	Protein	0 g	(0% DV)
Saturated Fat	0 g	(0% DV)	Vitamin A	0 IU	(0% DV)
Poly Fat	0 g		Vitamin C	3.1 mg	(5% DV)
Mono Fat	0 g		Calcium	6.2 mg	(1% DV)
Cholesterol	0 mg	(0% DV)	Iron	.5 mg	(3% DV)
Sodium	68.6 mg	(3% DV)	Folate	0 mcg	(0% DV)
Potassium	9.4 mg	(0% DV)	Beta Carotene	0 RE	

Ratings	Worst	Bad	Average	Good	Best
Weight Loss				8	
LowCal Density				8	
Filling					10
Energizing					10
Fiber	1				
Vitamins	2				
Minerals	2				
Overall			7		

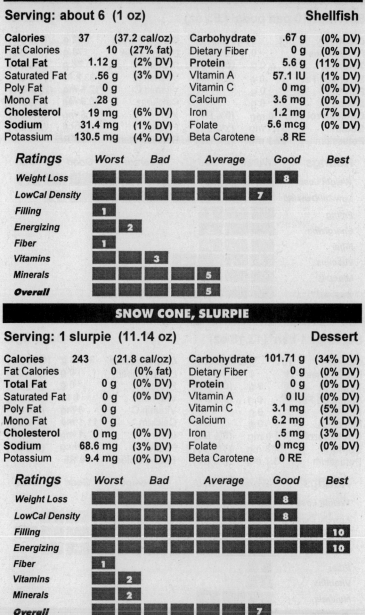

SNOWPEA (PEA POD), COOKED WITHOUT ADDED FAT

Serving: 10 pea pods (.93 oz)　　　　　　　**Vegetable**

Calories	11	(11.7 cal/oz)	**Carbohydrate**	1.82 g	(1% DV)
Fat Calories	0	(0% fat)	Dietary Fiber	.78 g	(3% DV)
Total Fat	0 g	(0% DV)	**Protein**	.78 g	(2% DV)
Saturated Fat	0 g	(0% DV)	Vitamin A	33.8 IU	(1% DV)
Poly Fat	0 g		Vitamin C	12.5 mg	(21% DV)
Mono Fat	0 g		Calcium	10.9 mg	(1% DV)
Cholesterol	0 mg	(0% DV)	Iron	.5 mg	(3% DV)
Sodium	61.1 mg	(3% DV)	Folate	.8 mcg	(2% DV)
Potassium	62.1 mg	(2% DV)	Beta Carotene	3.4 RE	

Ratings	Worst	Bad	Average	Good	Best
Weight Loss					10
LowCal Density					9
Filling		3			
Energizing		3			
Fiber		3			
Vitamins		4			
Minerals		3			
Overall				7	

SOFT DRINK

Serving: 1 can (13.18 oz)　　　　　　　**Beverage**

Calories	151	(11.5 cal/oz)	**Carbohydrate**	38.38 g	(13% DV)
Fat Calories	0	(0% fat)	Dietary Fiber	0 g	(0% DV)
Total Fat	0 g	(0% DV)	**Protein**	0 g	(0% DV)
Saturated Fat	0 g	(0% DV)	Vitamin A	0 IU	(0% DV)
Poly Fat	0 g		Vitamin C	0 mg	(0% DV)
Mono Fat	0 g		Calcium	11.1 mg	(1% DV)
Cholesterol	0 mg	(0% DV)	Iron	.1 mg	(1% DV)
Sodium	14.8 mg	(1% DV)	Folate	0 mcg	(0% DV)
Potassium	3.7 mg	(0% DV)	Beta Carotene	0 RE	

Ratings	Worst	Bad	Average	Good	Best
Weight Loss			6		
LowCal Density					9
Filling					10
Energizing					9
Fiber	1				
Vitamins	1				
Minerals		3			
Overall				7	

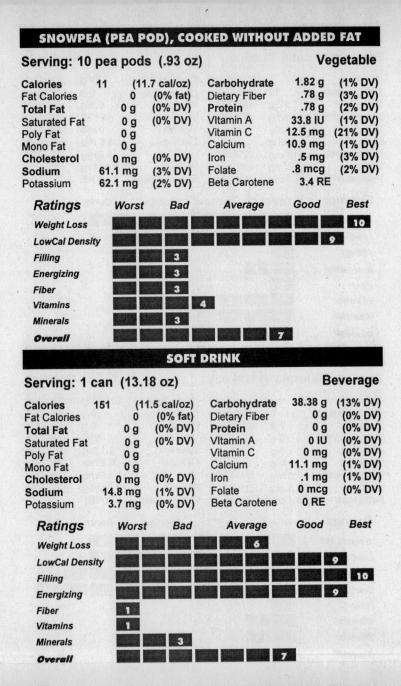

SOFT DRINK, SUGAR-FREE

Serving: 1 can (12.68 oz)   **Beverage**

Calories	4	(.3 cal/oz)	Carbohydrate	.35 g	(0% DV)
Fat Calories	0	(0% fat)	Dietary Fiber	0 g	(0% DV)
Total Fat	0 g	(0% DV)	Protein	0 g	(0% DV)
Saturated Fat	0 g	(0% DV)	VItamin A	0 IU	(0% DV)
Poly Fat	0 g		Vitamin C	0 mg	(0% DV)
Mono Fat	0 g		Calcium	14.2 mg	(1% DV)
Cholesterol	0 mg	(0% DV)	Iron	.1 mg	(1% DV)
Sodium	21.3 mg	(1% DV)	Folate	0 mcg	(0% DV)
Potassium	0 mg	(0% DV)	Beta Carotene	0 RE	

Ratings	Worst	Bad	Average	Good	Best
Weight Loss					10
LowCal Density					10
Filling				7	
Energizing	2				
Fiber	1				
Vitamins	2				
Minerals	3				
Overall				7	

SOFT TACO WITH BEEF, CHEESE, & LETTUCE

Serving: 1 Taco Bell (3.29 oz)   **Entree**

Calories	247	(75.2 cal/oz)	Carbohydrate	18.68 g	(6% DV)
Fat Calories	108	(43% fat)	Dietary Fiber	.92 g	(4% DV)
Total Fat	11.96 g	(18% DV)	Protein	15.64 g	(31% DV)
Saturated Fat	4.6 g	(23% DV)	VItamin A	129.7 IU	(3% DV)
Poly Fat	.92 g		Vitamin C	0 mg	(0% DV)
Mono Fat	4.6 g		Calcium	99.4 mg	(10% DV)
Cholesterol	43.2 mg	(14% DV)	Iron	2.1 mg	(12% DV)
Sodium	552 mg	(23% DV)	Folate	15.6 mcg	(4% DV)
Potassium	191.4 mg	(5% DV)	Beta Carotene	4.6 RE	

Ratings	Worst	Bad	Average	Good	Best
Weight Loss			5		
LowCal Density		4			
Filling		4			
Energizing			6		
Fiber		4			
Vitamins			5		
Minerals			6		
Overall			5		

SOLE WITH VEGETABLES

Serving: 1 diet meal (8.61 oz) Entree

Calories	215	(24.9 cal/oz)	Carbohydrate	13.5 g	(4% DV)
Fat Calories	22	(10% fat)	Dietary Fiber	2.41 g	(10% DV)
Total Fat	2.41 g	(4% DV)	Protein	33.74 g	(67% DV)
Saturated Fat	0 g	(0% DV)	Vitamin A	74.7 IU	(1% DV)
Poly Fat	0 g		Vitamin C	36.2 mg	(60% DV)
Mono Fat	0 g		Calcium	67.5 mg	(7% DV)
Cholesterol	77.1 mg	(26% DV)	Iron	1.6 mg	(9% DV)
Sodium	1761.7 mg	(73% DV)	Folate	33.7 mcg	(15% DV)
Potassium	768.8 mg	(22% DV)	Beta Carotene	2.4 RE	

Ratings	Worst	Bad	Average	Good	Best
Weight Loss				8	
LowCal Density				8	
Filling			5		
Energizing			5		
Fiber				7	
Vitamins				8	
Minerals				7	
Overall				7	

SOPAIPILLA WITH SYRUP OR HONEY

Serving: 1 sopaipilla (1½"x 1½") (.43 oz) Dessert

Calories	42	(98.5 cal/oz)	Carbohydrate	6.06 g	(2% DV)
Fat Calories	17	(41% fat)	Dietary Fiber	.12 g	(0% DV)
Total Fat	1.92 g	(3% DV)	Protein	.48 g	(1% DV)
Saturated Fat	.48 g	(2% DV)	Vitamin A	0 IU	(0% DV)
Poly Fat	.48 g		Vitamin C	0 mg	(0% DV)
Mono Fat	.84 g		Calcium	9.4 mg	(1% DV)
Cholesterol	0 mg	(0% DV)	Iron	.2 mg	(1% DV)
Sodium	74.5 mg	(3% DV)	Folate	.5 mcg	(0% DV)
Potassium	6.6 mg	(0% DV)	Beta Carotene	0 RE	

Ratings	Worst	Bad	Average	Good	Best
Weight Loss				8	
LowCal Density		3			
Filling	2				
Energizing			4		
Fiber	2				
Vitamins	2				
Minerals	2				
Overall			4		

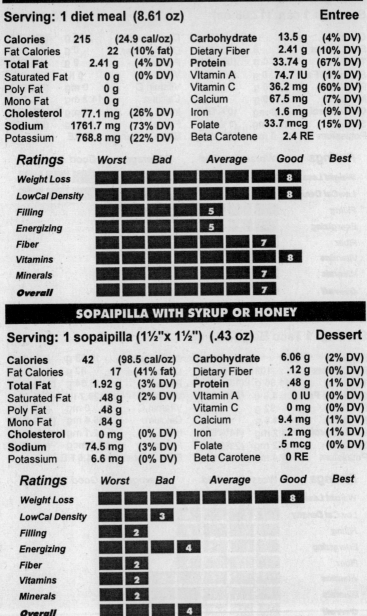

SORBET, FRUIT, NONCITRUS FLAVOR

Serving: 1 cup (7.14 oz)   **Dessert**

Calories	140	(19.6 cal/oz)	Carbohydrate	33.4 g	(11% DV)
Fat Calories	0	(0% fat)	Dietary Fiber	0 g	(0% DV)
Total Fat	0 g	(0% DV)	Protein	2 g	(4% DV)
Saturated Fat	0 g	(0% DV)	Vitamin A	0 IU	(0% DV)
Poly Fat	0 g		Vitamin C	0 mg	(0% DV)
Mono Fat	0 g		Calcium	4 mg	(0% DV)
Cholesterol	0 mg	(0% DV)	Iron	.1 mg	(0% DV)
Sodium	92 mg	(4% DV)	Folate	2 mcg	(0% DV)
Potassium	4 mg	(0% DV)	Beta Carotene	0 RE	

Ratings	Worst	Bad	Average	Good	Best
Weight Loss					9
LowCal Density				8	
Filling					9
Energizing				8	
Fiber	1				
Vitamins	1				
Minerals		2			
Overall				7	

SOUR CREAM

Serving: 1 cup (8.21 oz)   **Fat & Oil**

Calories	492	(60 cal/oz)	Carbohydrate	9.89 g	(3% DV)
Fat Calories	435	(88% fat)	Dietary Fiber	0 g	(0% DV)
Total Fat	48.3 g	(74% DV)	Protein	6.9 g	(14% DV)
Saturated Fat	29.9 g	(149% DV)	Vitamin A	1817 IU	(36% DV)
Poly Fat	2.3 g		Vitamin C	2.3 mg	(4% DV)
Mono Fat	13.8 g		Calcium	266.8 mg	(27% DV)
Cholesterol	101.2 mg	(34% DV)	Iron	.1 mg	(1% DV)
Sodium	121.9 mg	(5% DV)	Folate	6.9 mcg	(6% DV)
Potassium	331.2 mg	(9% DV)	Beta Carotene	48.3 RE	

Ratings	Worst	Bad	Average	Good	Best
Weight Loss	1				
LowCal Density			5		
Filling		3			
Energizing			4		
Fiber	1				
Vitamins			5		
Minerals			6		
Overall		3			

SOY NUTS

Serving: 1 package (4.82 oz) **Snack**

Calories	612	(126.9 cal/oz)	Carbohydrate	41.31 g	(14% DV)
Fat Calories	292	(48% fat)	Dietary Fiber	5.4 g	(22% DV)
Total Fat	32.4 g	(50% DV)	Protein	49.95 g	(100% DV)
Saturated Fat	4.05 g	(20% DV)	Vitamin A	270 IU	(5% DV)
Poly Fat	17.55 g		Vitamin C	2.7 mg	(5% DV)
Mono Fat	8.1 g		Calcium	186.3 mg	(19% DV)
Cholesterol	0 mg	(0% DV)	Iron	6 mg	(33% DV)
Sodium	5.4 mg	(0% DV)	Folate	50 mcg	(76% DV)
Potassium	1984.5 mg	(57% DV)	Beta Carotene	27 RE	

Ratings	Worst	Bad	Average	Good	Best
Weight Loss	1				
LowCal Density	2				
Filling		4			
Energizing				9	
Fiber				9	
Vitamins				7	
Minerals					10
Overall		4			

SOY SAUCE

Serving: 1 tbsp (.64 oz) **Sauce**

Calories	10	(14.9 cal/oz)	Carbohydrate	1.53 g	(1% DV)
Fat Calories	0	(0% fat)	Dietary Fiber	0 g	(0% DV)
Total Fat	0 g	(0% DV)	Protein	.9 g	(2% DV)
Saturated Fat	0 g	(0% DV)	Vitamin A	0 IU	(0% DV)
Poly Fat	0 g		Vitamin C	0 mg	(0% DV)
Mono Fat	0 g		Calcium	3.1 mg	(0% DV)
Cholesterol	0 mg	(0% DV)	Iron	.4 mg	(2% DV)
Sodium	1028.7 mg	(43% DV)	Folate	.9 mcg	(1% DV)
Potassium	32.4 mg	(1% DV)	Beta Carotene	0 RE	

Ratings	Worst	Bad	Average	Good	Best
Weight Loss					10
LowCal Density				9	
Filling	2				
Energizing		3			
Fiber	1				
Vitamins	2				
Minerals	2				
Overall			6		

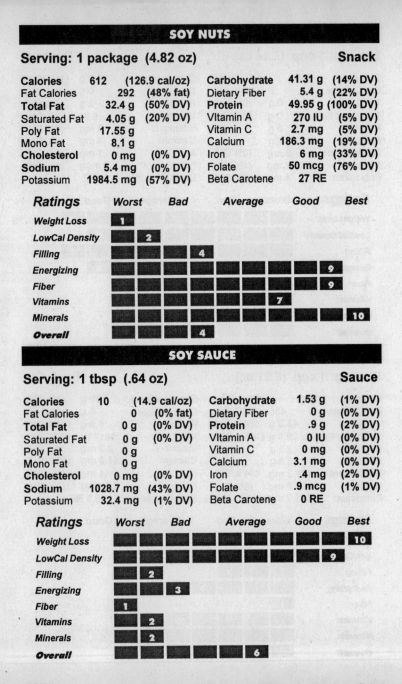

SOYBEAN OIL

Serving: 1 tbsp (.49 oz)   **Fat & Oil**

Calories	120	(245.3 cal/oz)	Carbohydrate	0 g	(0% DV)
Fat Calories	122	(102% fat)	Dietary Fiber	0 g	(0% DV)
Total Fat	13.6 g	(21% DV)	Protein	0 g	(0% DV)
Saturated Fat	1.9 g	(9% DV)	Vitamin A	0 IU	(0% DV)
Poly Fat	7.89 g		Vitamin C	0 mg	(0% DV)
Mono Fat	3.13 g		Calcium	0 mg	(0% DV)
Cholesterol	0 mg	(0% DV)	Iron	0 mg	(0% DV)
Sodium	0 mg	(0% DV)	Folate	0 mcg	(0% DV)
Potassium	0 mg	(0% DV)	Beta Carotene	0 RE	

Ratings	Worst	Bad	Average	Good	Best
Weight Loss	1				
LowCal Density	1				
Filling	1				
Energizing	1				
Fiber	1				
Vitamins	2				
Minerals	1				
Overall	1				

SOYBEANS (COOKED WITHOUT ADDED FAT)

Serving: 1 cup (6.43 oz)   **Vegetable**

Calories	310	(48.2 cal/oz)	Carbohydrate	17.82 g	(6% DV)
Fat Calories	146	(47% fat)	Dietary Fiber	7.2 g	(29% DV)
Total Fat	16.2 g	(25% DV)	Protein	30.6 g	(61% DV)
Saturated Fat	1.8 g	(9% DV)	Vitamin A	16.2 IU	(0% DV)
Poly Fat	9 g		Vitamin C	3.6 mg	(6% DV)
Mono Fat	3.6 g		Calcium	183.6 mg	(18% DV)
Cholesterol	0 mg	(0% DV)	Iron	9.2 mg	(51% DV)
Sodium	417.6 mg	(17% DV)	Folate	30.6 mcg	(24% DV)
Potassium	921.6 mg	(26% DV)	Beta Carotene	1.8 RE	

Ratings	Worst	Bad	Average	Good	Best
Weight Loss	1				
LowCal Density				6	
Filling			5		
Energizing				6	
Fiber					10
Vitamins			5		
Minerals					9
Overall			5		

SOYBURGER

Serving: 1 patty (2.5 oz)   **Sandwich**

Calories	140	(56 cal/oz)	Carbohydrate	5.6 g	(2% DV)
Fat Calories	57	(40% fat)	Dietary Fiber	3.5 g	(14% DV)
Total Fat	6.3 g	(10% DV)	Protein	14.7 g	(29% DV)
Saturated Fat	.7 g	(3% DV)	Vitamin A	0 IU	(0% DV)
Poly Fat	3.5 g		Vitamin C	0 mg	(0% DV)
Mono Fat	1.4 g		Calcium	20.3 mg	(2% DV)
Cholesterol	0 mg	(0% DV)	Iron	1.5 mg	(8% DV)
Sodium	385 mg	(16% DV)	Folate	14.7 mcg	(14% DV)
Potassium	126 mg	(4% DV)	Beta Carotene	0 RE	

Ratings

	Worst	Bad	Average	Good	Best
Weight Loss				7	
LowCal Density			5		
Filling		3			
Energizing		3			
Fiber				8	
Vitamins					9
Minerals			5		
Overall				6	

SOYBURGER WITH CHEESE

Serving: 1 sandwich (5 oz)   **Sandwich**

Calories	328	(65.5 cal/oz)	Carbohydrate	30.66 g	(10% DV)
Fat Calories	113	(35% fat)	Dietary Fiber	4.2 g	(17% DV)
Total Fat	12.6 g	(19% DV)	Protein	21 g	(42% DV)
Saturated Fat	4.2 g	(21% DV)	Vitamin A	228.2 IU	(5% DV)
Poly Fat	4.2 g		Vitamin C	1.4 mg	(2% DV)
Mono Fat	4.2 g		Calcium	151.2 mg	(15% DV)
Cholesterol	12.6 mg	(4% DV)	Iron	2.8 mg	(16% DV)
Sodium	966 mg	(40% DV)	Folate	21 mcg	(18% DV)
Potassium	219.8 mg	(6% DV)	Beta Carotene	11.2 RE	

Ratings

	Worst	Bad	Average	Good	Best
Weight Loss			5		
LowCal Density			5		
Filling			5		
Energizing				7	
Fiber					9
Vitamins					9
Minerals				8	
Overall				6	

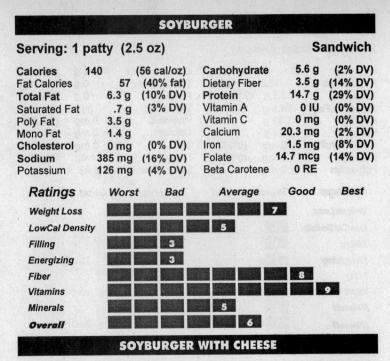

SPAGHETTI & MEATBALLS, VEGETABLE, DESSERT

Serving: 1 frozen meal (12.64 oz)　　　Entree

Calories	365	(28.8 cal/oz)	Carbohydrate	56.64 g	(19% DV)
Fat Calories	96	(26% fat)	Dietary Fiber	7.08 g	(28% DV)
Total Fat	10.62 g	(16% DV)	Protein	14.16 g	(28% DV)
Saturated Fat	3.54 g	(18% DV)	VItamin A	1635.5 IU	(33% DV)
Poly Fat	0 g		Vitamin C	31.9 mg	(53% DV)
Mono Fat	3.54 g		Calcium	95.6 mg	(10% DV)
Cholesterol	21.2 mg	(7% DV)	Iron	3.3 mg	(18% DV)
Sodium	1012.4 mg	(42% DV)	Folate	14.2 mcg	(12% DV)
Potassium	587.6 mg	(17% DV)	Beta Carotene	141.6 RE	

Ratings	Worst	Bad	Average	Good	Best
Weight Loss			5		
LowCal Density				8	
Filling					10
Energizing					10
Fiber					10
Vitamins				8	
Minerals			7		
Overall				8	

SPANAKOPITTA

Serving: 3 cubic inch (1.29 oz)　　　Entree

Calories	74	(57.5 cal/oz)	Carbohydrate	3.78 g	(1% DV)
Fat Calories	49	(66% fat)	Dietary Fiber	.36 g	(1% DV)
Total Fat	5.4 g	(8% DV)	Protein	2.88 g	(6% DV)
Saturated Fat	2.52 g	(13% DV)	VItamin A	1105.6 IU	(22% DV)
Poly Fat	.36 g		Vitamin C	3.2 mg	(5% DV)
Mono Fat	2.16 g		Calcium	58.7 mg	(6% DV)
Cholesterol	30.2 mg	(10% DV)	Iron	.7 mg	(4% DV)
Sodium	148 mg	(6% DV)	Folate	2.9 mcg	(7% DV)
Potassium	106.6 mg	(3% DV)	Beta Carotene	98.3 RE	

Ratings	Worst	Bad	Average	Good	Best
Weight Loss			6		
LowCal Density			5		
Filling	2				
Energizing		3			
Fiber	2				
Vitamins			5		
Minerals		4			
Overall		4			

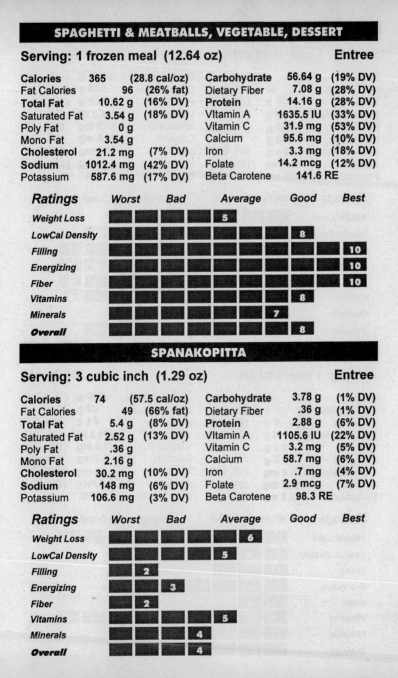

SPANISH RICE

Serving: 1 cup (8.68 oz)   **Entree**

Calories	216	(24.9 cal/oz)	Carbohydrate	41.31 g	(14% DV)
Fat Calories	44	(20% fat)	Dietary Fiber	4.86 g	(19% DV)
Total Fat	4.86 g	(7% DV)	Protein	4.86 g	(10% DV)
Saturated Fat	0 g	(0% DV)	VItamin A	1156.7 IU	(23% DV)
Poly Fat	2.43 g		Vitamin C	38.9 mg	(65% DV)
Mono Fat	2.43 g		Calcium	70.5 mg	(7% DV)
Cholesterol	0 mg	(0% DV)	Iron	2.4 mg	(14% DV)
Sodium	323.2 mg	(13% DV)	Folate	4.9 mcg	(5% DV)
Potassium	541.9 mg	(15% DV)	Beta Carotene	114.2 RE	

Ratings	Worst	Bad	Average	Good	Best
Weight Loss				7	
LowCal Density				8	
Filling					9
Energizing					9
Fiber					9
Vitamins				8	
Minerals			5		
Overall				8	

SPECIAL K

Serving: 1 cup (.82 oz)   **Cereal**

Calories	90	(109.4 cal/oz)	Carbohydrate	17.27 g	(6% DV)
Fat Calories	0	(0% fat)	Dietary Fiber	.23 g	(1% DV)
Total Fat	0 g	(0% DV)	Protein	4.6 g	(9% DV)
Saturated Fat	0 g	(0% DV)	VItamin A	608.4 IU	(12% DV)
Poly Fat	0 g		Vitamin C	12.2 mg	(20% DV)
Mono Fat	0 g		Calcium	6.7 mg	(1% DV)
Cholesterol	0 mg	(0% DV)	Iron	3.7 mg	(20% DV)
Sodium	215.1 mg	(9% DV)	Folate	4.6 mcg	(20% DV)
Potassium	39.8 mg	(1% DV)	Beta Carotene	0 RE	

Ratings	Worst	Bad	Average	Good	Best
Weight Loss					9
LowCal Density	2				
Filling		3			
Energizing			6		
Fiber	2				
Vitamins					9
Minerals			6		
Overall			5		

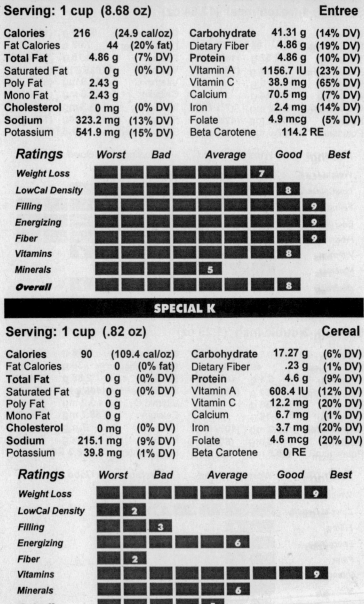

SPINACH SALAD, NO DRESSING

Serving: 1 cup (2.64 oz) — **Salad**

Calories	89	(33.6 cal/oz)	Carbohydrate	9.69 g	(3% DV)
Fat Calories	33	(38% fat)	Dietary Fiber	1.48 g	(6% DV)
Total Fat	3.7 g	(6% DV)	Protein	4.44 g	(9% DV)
Saturated Fat	.74 g	(4% DV)	Vitamin A	2237 IU	(45% DV)
Poly Fat	.74 g		Vitamin C	9.6 mg	(16% DV)
Mono Fat	1.48 g		Calcium	51.1 mg	(5% DV)
Cholesterol	60.7 mg	(20% DV)	Iron	1.6 mg	(9% DV)
Sodium	156.9 mg	(7% DV)	Folate	4.4 mcg	(19% DV)
Potassium	276.8 mg	(8% DV)	Beta Carotene	216.1 RE	

Ratings	Worst	Bad	Average	Good	Best
Weight Loss				7	
LowCal Density				7	
Filling		4			
Energizing		4			
Fiber			5		
Vitamins				7	
Minerals			5		
Overall			6		

SPINACH SOUFFLE

Serving: 1 cup (3.57 oz) — **Vegetable**

Calories	130	(36.4 cal/oz)	Carbohydrate	7.2 g	(2% DV)
Fat Calories	81	(62% fat)	Dietary Fiber	1 g	(4% DV)
Total Fat	9 g	(14% DV)	Protein	5 g	(10% DV)
Saturated Fat	3 g	(15% DV)	Vitamin A	2353 IU	(47% DV)
Poly Fat	2 g		Vitamin C	3 mg	(5% DV)
Mono Fat	4 g		Calcium	99 mg	(10% DV)
Cholesterol	100 mg	(33% DV)	Iron	.9 mg	(5% DV)
Sodium	189 mg	(8% DV)	Folate	5 mcg	(10% DV)
Potassium	173 mg	(5% DV)	Beta Carotene	198 RE	

Ratings	Worst	Bad	Average	Good	Best
Weight Loss	3				
LowCal Density				7	
Filling	3				
Energizing		4			
Fiber		4			
Vitamins				6	
Minerals			5		
Overall			5		

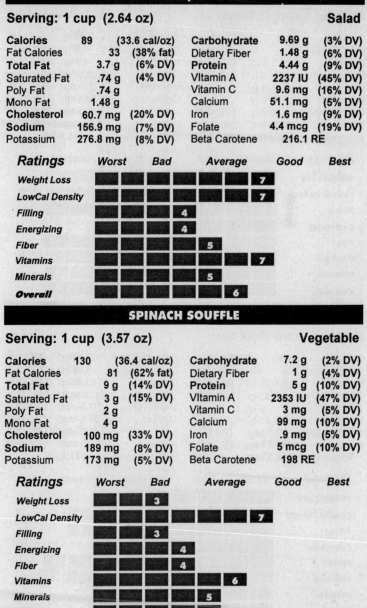

SPINACH, COOKED, FAT NOT ADDED IN COOKING

Serving: 1 cup (6.79 oz)   **Vegetable**

Calories	44	(6.4 cal/oz)	Carbohydrate	7.03 g	(2% DV)
Fat Calories	0	(0% fat)	Dietary Fiber	3.8 g	(15% DV)
Total Fat	0 g	(0% DV)	Protein	5.7 g	(11% DV)
Saturated Fat	0 g	(0% DV)	Vitamin A	15467.9 IU	(309% DV)
Poly Fat	0 g		Vitamin C	19 mg	(32% DV)
Mono Fat	0 g		Calcium	256.5 mg	(26% DV)
Cholesterol	0 mg	(0% DV)	Iron	6.7 mg	(37% DV)
Sodium	571.9 mg	(24% DV)	Folate	5.7 mcg	(69% DV)
Potassium	879.7 mg	(25% DV)	Beta Carotene	1546.6 RE	

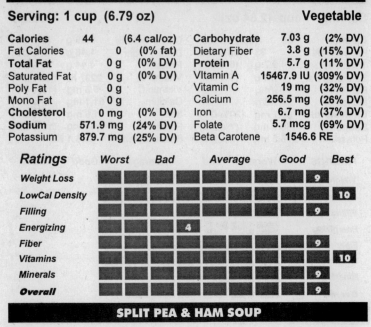

Ratings	Worst	Bad	Average	Good	Best
Weight Loss				9	
LowCal Density					10
Filling				9	
Energizing		4			
Fiber				9	
Vitamins					10
Minerals				9	
Overall				9	

SPLIT PEA & HAM SOUP

Serving: 1 cup (9.04 oz)   **Soup**

Calories	195	(21.6 cal/oz)	Carbohydrate	28.34 g	(9% DV)
Fat Calories	46	(23% fat)	Dietary Fiber	5.06 g	(20% DV)
Total Fat	5.06 g	(8% DV)	Protein	12.65 g	(25% DV)
Saturated Fat	2.53 g	(13% DV)	Vitamin A	5135.9 IU	(103% DV)
Poly Fat	0 g		Vitamin C	7.6 mg	(13% DV)
Mono Fat	2.53 g		Calcium	35.4 mg	(4% DV)
Cholesterol	7.6 mg	(3% DV)	Iron	2.3 mg	(12% DV)
Sodium	1017.1 mg	(42% DV)	Folate	12.7 mcg	(1% DV)
Potassium	321.3 mg	(9% DV)	Beta Carotene	513.6 RE	

Ratings	Worst	Bad	Average	Good	Best
Weight Loss			5		
LowCal Density				8	
Filling				8	
Energizing			7		
Fiber					9
Vitamins				8	
Minerals			7		
Overall			7		

SQUASH, SUMMER, BREADED OR BATTERED, FRIED

Serving: 6 slices (3 oz)   **Vegetable**

Calories	126	(42 cal/oz)	Carbohydrate	7.14 g	(2% DV)
Fat Calories	91	(72% fat)	Dietary Fiber	.84 g	(3% DV)
Total Fat	10.08 g	(16% DV)	Protein	1.68 g	(3% DV)
Saturated Fat	1.68 g	(8% DV)	Vitamin A	195.7 IU	(4% DV)
Poly Fat	5.04 g		Vitamin C	4.2 mg	(7% DV)
Mono Fat	2.52 g		Calcium	52.9 mg	(5% DV)
Cholesterol	11.8 mg	(4% DV)	Iron	.5 mg	(3% DV)
Sodium	103.3 mg	(4% DV)	Folate	1.7 mcg	(3% DV)
Potassium	173 mg	(5% DV)	Beta Carotene	16.8 RE	

Ratings	Worst	Bad	Average	Good	Best
Weight Loss		3			
LowCal Density				6	
Filling		3			
Energizing		4			
Fiber		4			
Vitamins		4			
Minerals		4			
Overall		4			

SQUASH, SUMMER, COOKED WITHOUT ADDED FAT

Serving: 1 cup (6.43 oz)   **Vegetable**

Calories	36	(5.6 cal/oz)	Carbohydrate	7.74 g	(3% DV)
Fat Calories	0	(0% fat)	Dietary Fiber	1.8 g	(7% DV)
Total Fat	0 g	(0% DV)	Protein	1.8 g	(4% DV)
Saturated Fat	0 g	(0% DV)	Vitamin A	513 IU	(10% DV)
Poly Fat	0 g		Vitamin C	9 mg	(15% DV)
Mono Fat	0 g		Calcium	48.6 mg	(5% DV)
Cholesterol	0 mg	(0% DV)	Iron	.6 mg	(4% DV)
Sodium	417.6 mg	(17% DV)	Folate	1.8 mcg	(9% DV)
Potassium	343.8 mg	(10% DV)	Beta Carotene	52.2 RE	

Ratings	Worst	Bad	Average	Good	Best
Weight Loss					10
LowCal Density					10
Filling					9
Energizing		4			
Fiber			6		
Vitamins			5		
Minerals			5		
Overall				8	

SQUASH, WINTER, BAKED, FAT & SUGAR ADDED

Serving: ½ acorn squash (5.89 oz) **Vegetable**

Calories	101	(17.1 cal/oz)	Carbohydrate	16.83 g	(6% DV)
Fat Calories	30	(30% fat)	Dietary Fiber	4.95 g	(20% DV)
Total Fat	3.3 g	(5% DV)	Protein	1.65 g	(3% DV)
Saturated Fat	0 g	(0% DV)	Vitamin A	5751.9 IU	(115% DV)
Poly Fat	1.65 g		Vitamin C	14.9 mg	(25% DV)
Mono Fat	1.65 g		Calcium	23.1 mg	(2% DV)
Cholesterol	0 mg	(0% DV)	Iron	.5 mg	(3% DV)
Sodium	394.4 mg	(16% DV)	Folate	1.7 mcg	(11% DV)
Potassium	688.1 mg	(20% DV)	Beta Carotene	562.7 RE	

Ratings	Worst	Bad	Average	Good	Best
Weight Loss			6		
LowCal Density				8	
Filling				8	
Energizing			5		
Fiber					9
Vitamins					9
Minerals		3			
Overall				7	

SQUASH, WINTER, MASHED, NO FAT OR SUGAR ADDED

Serving: 1 cup (8.57 oz) **Vegetable**

Calories	94	(10.9 cal/oz)	Carbohydrate	20.88 g	(7% DV)
Fat Calories	22	(23% fat)	Dietary Fiber	7.2 g	(29% DV)
Total Fat	2.4 g	(4% DV)	Protein	2.4 g	(5% DV)
Saturated Fat	0 g	(0% DV)	Vitamin A	8486.4 IU	(170% DV)
Poly Fat	0 g		Vitamin C	24 mg	(40% DV)
Mono Fat	0 g		Calcium	33.6 mg	(3% DV)
Cholesterol	0 mg	(0% DV)	Iron	.8 mg	(4% DV)
Sodium	556.8 mg	(23% DV)	Folate	2.4 mcg	(17% DV)
Potassium	1041.6 mg	(30% DV)	Beta Carotene	849.6 RE	

Ratings	Worst	Bad	Average	Good	Best
Weight Loss			6		
LowCal Density				9	
Filling					10
Energizing			6		
Fiber					10
Vitamins					10
Minerals		4			
Overall				8	

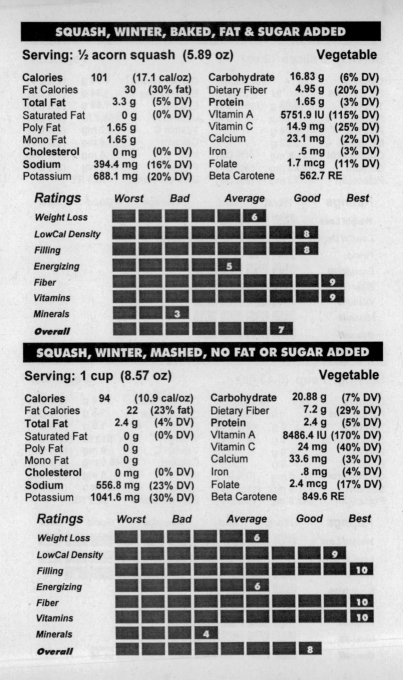

SQUID, BAKED, BROILED (CALAMARY)

Serving: 1 piece (3.04 oz)   **Fish**

Calories	117	(38.6 cal/oz)	Carbohydrate	3.15 g	(1% DV)
Fat Calories	38	(33% fat)	Dietary Fiber	0 g	(0% DV)
Total Fat	4.25 g	(7% DV)	Protein	16.15 g	(32% DV)
Saturated Fat	.85 g	(4% DV)	Vitamin A	163.2 IU	(3% DV)
Poly Fat	1.7 g		Vitamin C	4.3 mg	(7% DV)
Mono Fat	.85 g		Calcium	34 mg	(3% DV)
Cholesterol	238.9 mg	(80% DV)	Iron	.7 mg	(4% DV)
Sodium	314.5 mg	(13% DV)	Folate	16.2 mcg	(1% DV)
Potassium	253.3 mg	(7% DV)	Beta Carotene	2.6 RE	

Ratings	Worst	Bad	Average	Good	Best
Weight Loss			6		
LowCal Density				7	
Filling	2				
Energizing	3				
Fiber	1				
Vitamins		4			
Minerals			6		
Overall			5		

SQUID, BREADED, FRIED (CALAMARY)

Serving: 1 piece (3.04 oz)   **Fish**

Calories	166	(54.5 cal/oz)	Carbohydrate	9.52 g	(3% DV)
Fat Calories	61	(37% fat)	Dietary Fiber	0 g	(0% DV)
Total Fat	6.8 g	(10% DV)	Protein	15.3 g	(31% DV)
Saturated Fat	1.7 g	(8% DV)	Vitamin A	56.1 IU	(1% DV)
Poly Fat	1.7 g		Vitamin C	3.4 mg	(6% DV)
Mono Fat	2.55 g		Calcium	42.5 mg	(4% DV)
Cholesterol	215.9 mg	(72% DV)	Iron	1 mg	(6% DV)
Sodium	309.4 mg	(13% DV)	Folate	15.3 mcg	(2% DV)
Potassium	228.7 mg	(7% DV)	Beta Carotene	0 RE	

Ratings	Worst	Bad	Average	Good	Best
Weight Loss			5		
LowCal Density			6		
Filling	3				
Energizing	4				
Fiber	1				
Vitamins		4			
Minerals			6		
Overall			5		

Serving: 1 Arby's Philly Beef 'N Swiss (7.29 oz) Sandwich

Calories	494	(67.7 cal/oz)	Carbohydrate	38.76 g	(13% DV)
Fat Calories	184	(37% fat)	Dietary Fiber	2.04 g	(8% DV)
Total Fat	20.4 g	(31% DV)	Protein	36.72 g	(73% DV)
Saturated Fat	8.16 g	(41% DV)	VItamin A	289.7 IU	(6% DV)
Poly Fat	2.04 g		Vitamin C	14.3 mg	(24% DV)
Mono Fat	8.16 g		Calcium	248.9 mg	(25% DV)
Cholesterol	93.8 mg	(31% DV)	Iron	4.8 mg	(27% DV)
Sodium	628.3 mg	(26% DV)	Folate	36.7 mcg	(9% DV)
Potassium	387.6 mg	(11% DV)	Beta Carotene	10.2 RE	

Ratings	Worst	Bad	Average	Good	Best
Weight Loss		4			
LowCal Density			5		
Filling			5		
Energizing					9
Fiber			6		
Vitamins			6		
Minerals					9
Overall			5		

Serving: 1 cup (8.71 oz)   **Entree**

Calories	434	(49.9 cal/oz)	Carbohydrate	12.2 g	(4% DV)
Fat Calories	176	(40% fat)	Dietary Fiber	0 g	(0% DV)
Total Fat	19.52 g	(30% DV)	Protein	51.24 g	(102% DV)
Saturated Fat	4.88 g	(24% DV)	VItamin A	31.7 IU	(1% DV)
Poly Fat	2.44 g		Vitamin C	14.6 mg	(24% DV)
Mono Fat	7.32 g		Calcium	26.8 mg	(3% DV)
Cholesterol	148.8 mg	(50% DV)	Iron	6.3 mg	(35% DV)
Sodium	1507.9 mg	(63% DV)	Folate	51.2 mcg	(9% DV)
Potassium	585.6 mg	(17% DV)	Beta Carotene	2.4 RE	

Ratings	Worst	Bad	Average	Good	Best
Weight Loss	3				
LowCal Density			6		
Filling		4			
Energizing			5		
Fiber	1				
Vitamins			6		
Minerals					9
Overall			5		

STEW, VEGETARIAN

Serving: 1 cup (8.54 oz)   **Entree**

Calories	287	(33.6 cal/oz)	Carbohydrate	16.73 g	(6% DV)
Fat Calories	65	(22% fat)	Dietary Fiber	2.39 g	(10% DV)
Total Fat	7.17 g	(11% DV)	Protein	40.63 g	(81% DV)
Saturated Fat	0 g	(0% DV)	VItamin A	0 IU	(0% DV)
Poly Fat	2.39 g		Vitamin C	0 mg	(0% DV)
Mono Fat	2.39 g		Calcium	74.1 mg	(7% DV)
Cholesterol	0 mg	(0% DV)	Iron	3.1 mg	(17% DV)
Sodium	956 mg	(40% DV)	Folate	40.6 mcg	(62% DV)
Potassium	286.8 mg	(8% DV)	Beta Carotene	0 RE	

Ratings	Worst	Bad	Average	Good	Best
Weight Loss			6		
LowCal Density			7		
Filling		5			
Energizing		5			
Fiber			6		
Vitamins					10
Minerals				9	
Overall			7		

STRAWBERRIES, FROZEN

Serving: 1 cup (9.11 oz)   **Fruit**

Calories	222	(24.4 cal/oz)	Carbohydrate	59.93 g	(20% DV)
Fat Calories	0	(0% fat)	Dietary Fiber	5.1 g	(20% DV)
Total Fat	0 g	(0% DV)	Protein	2.55 g	(5% DV)
Saturated Fat	0 g	(0% DV)	VItamin A	66.3 IU	(1% DV)
Poly Fat	0 g		Vitamin C	102 mg	(170% DV)
Mono Fat	0 g		Calcium	28.1 mg	(3% DV)
Cholesterol	0 mg	(0% DV)	Iron	1.4 mg	(8% DV)
Sodium	5.1 mg	(0% DV)	Folate	2.6 mcg	(6% DV)
Potassium	249.9 mg	(7% DV)	Beta Carotene	7.7 RE	

Ratings	Worst	Bad	Average	Good	Best
Weight Loss			6		
LowCal Density				8	
Filling					10
Energizing					10
Fiber				9	
Vitamins				9	
Minerals		4			
Overall				8	

STRAWBERRIES, RAW

Serving: 1 cup, whole (5.14 oz)   Fruit

Calories	43	(8.4 cal/oz)	Carbohydrate	10.08 g	(3% DV)
Fat Calories	0	(0% fat)	Dietary Fiber	4.32 g	(17% DV)
Total Fat	0 g	(0% DV)	Protein	1.44 g	(3% DV)
Saturated Fat	0 g	(0% DV)	VItamin A	38.9 IU	(1% DV)
Poly Fat	0 g		Vitamin C	82.1 mg	(137% DV)
Mono Fat	0 g		Calcium	20.2 mg	(2% DV)
Cholesterol	0 mg	(0% DV)	Iron	.6 mg	(3% DV)
Sodium	1.4 mg	(0% DV)	Folate	1.4 mcg	(6% DV)
Potassium	239 mg	(7% DV)	Beta Carotene	4.3 RE	

Ratings	Worst	Bad	Average	Good	Best
Weight Loss					10
LowCal Density				9	
Filling				9	
Energizing		4			
Fiber				9	
Vitamins				8	
Minerals		3			
Overall				8	

STRUDEL, APPLE

Serving: 1 piece (2" - 2½" square) (2.29 oz)   Dessert

Calories	156	(68.2 cal/oz)	Carbohydrate	31.55 g	(11% DV)
Fat Calories	29	(18% fat)	Dietary Fiber	1.28 g	(5% DV)
Total Fat	3.2 g	(5% DV)	Protein	1.92 g	(4% DV)
Saturated Fat	.64 g	(3% DV)	VItamin A	169 IU	(3% DV)
Poly Fat	1.28 g		Vitamin C	1.9 mg	(3% DV)
Mono Fat	1.28 g		Calcium	14.7 mg	(1% DV)
Cholesterol	9 mg	(3% DV)	Iron	.8 mg	(4% DV)
Sodium	74.9 mg	(3% DV)	Folate	1.9 mcg	(1% DV)
Potassium	118.4 mg	(3% DV)	Beta Carotene	4.5 RE	

Ratings	Worst	Bad	Average	Good	Best
Weight Loss				8	
LowCal Density		4			
Filling			5		
Energizing				8	
Fiber			5		
Vitamins		3			
Minerals		3			
Overall			6		

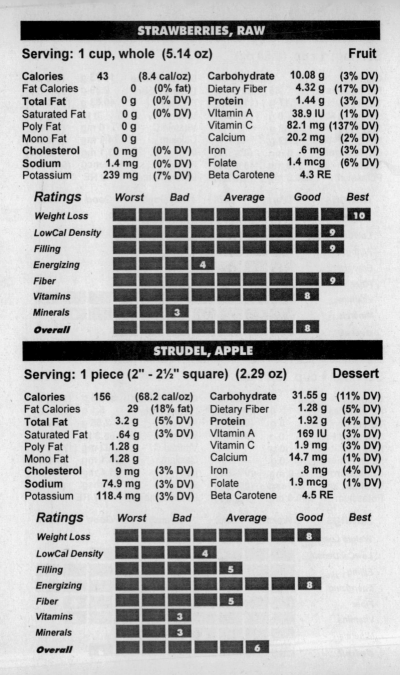

STUFFED CABBAGE, MEAT & TOMATO SAUCE

Serving: 1 diet meal (10.89 oz)   Entree

Calories	247	(22.7 cal/oz)	Carbohydrate	22.27 g	(7% DV)
Fat Calories	82	(33% fat)	Dietary Fiber	3.05 g	(12% DV)
Total Fat	9.15 g	(14% DV)	Protein	15.25 g	(30% DV)
Saturated Fat	3.05 g	(15% DV)	Vitamin A	3263.5 IU	(65% DV)
Poly Fat	0 g		Vitamin C	30.5 mg	(51% DV)
Mono Fat	3.05 g		Calcium	48.8 mg	(5% DV)
Cholesterol	48.8 mg	(16% DV)	Iron	2.1 mg	(12% DV)
Sodium	692.4 mg	(29% DV)	Folate	15.3 mcg	(8% DV)
Potassium	591.7 mg	(17% DV)	Beta Carotene	326.4 RE	

Ratings	Worst	Bad	Average	Good	Best
Weight Loss			6		
LowCal Density				8	
Filling			7		
Energizing			6		
Fiber				8	
Vitamins					9
Minerals			7		
Overall			7		

STUFFED GREEN PEPPER

Serving: 1 diet meal (11.89 oz)   Entree

Calories	303	(25.5 cal/oz)	Carbohydrate	31.3 g	(10% DV)
Fat Calories	90	(30% fat)	Dietary Fiber	3.33 g	(13% DV)
Total Fat	9.99 g	(15% DV)	Protein	23.31 g	(47% DV)
Saturated Fat	3.33 g	(17% DV)	Vitamin A	2694 IU	(54% DV)
Poly Fat	0 g		Vitamin C	129.9 mg	(216% DV)
Mono Fat	3.33 g		Calcium	36.6 mg	(4% DV)
Cholesterol	76.6 mg	(26% DV)	Iron	2.6 mg	(15% DV)
Sodium	1581.8 mg	(66% DV)	Folate	23.3 mcg	(10% DV)
Potassium	809.2 mg	(23% DV)	Beta Carotene	269.7 RE	

Ratings	Worst	Bad	Average	Good	Best
Weight Loss			6		
LowCal Density				8	
Filling				8	
Energizing				8	
Fiber				8	
Vitamins					10
Minerals			7		
Overall				8	

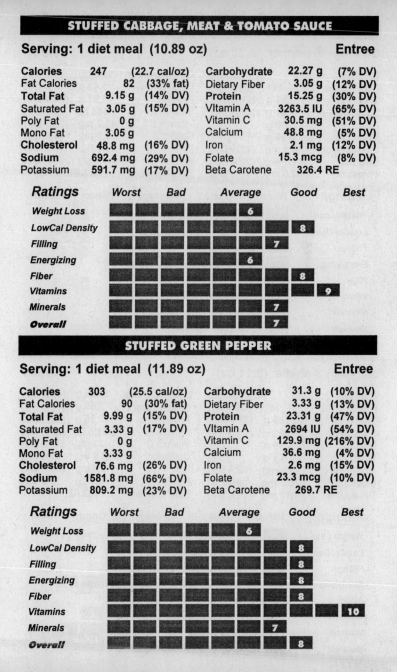

STUFFED PEPPER, WITH RICE & MEAT

Serving: ½ pepper (5.32 oz) **Entree**

Calories	222	(41.7 cal/oz)	Carbohydrate	14.01 g	(5% DV)
Fat Calories	121	(54% fat)	Dietary Fiber	1.49 g	(6% DV)
Total Fat	13.41 g	(21% DV)	Protein	11.92 g	(24% DV)
Saturated Fat	4.47 g	(22% DV)	VItamin A	453 IU	(9% DV)
Poly Fat	0 g		Vitamin C	43.2 mg	(72% DV)
Mono Fat	5.96 g		Calcium	35.8 mg	(4% DV)
Cholesterol	68.5 mg	(23% DV)	Iron	1.7 mg	(9% DV)
Sodium	941.7 mg	(39% DV)	Folate	11.9 mcg	(5% DV)
Potassium	302.5 mg	(9% DV)	Beta Carotene	38.7 RE	

Ratings	Worst	Bad	Average	Good	Best
Weight Loss			5		
LowCal Density			6		
Filling		4			
Energizing			5		
Fiber			5		
Vitamins				7	
Minerals			6		
Overall			5		

STUFFED SHELLS, CHEESE-FILLED, WITH MEAT SAUCE

Serving: 3 shells (9.11 oz) **Entree**

Calories	413	(45.3 cal/oz)	Carbohydrate	38.25 g	(13% DV)
Fat Calories	161	(39% fat)	Dietary Fiber	2.55 g	(10% DV)
Total Fat	17.85 g	(27% DV)	Protein	22.95 g	(46% DV)
Saturated Fat	10.2 g	(51% DV)	VItamin A	1481.6 IU	(30% DV)
Poly Fat	0 g		Vitamin C	23 mg	(38% DV)
Mono Fat	5.1 g		Calcium	323.9 mg	(32% DV)
Cholesterol	155.6 mg	(52% DV)	Iron	3.5 mg	(19% DV)
Sodium	670.7 mg	(28% DV)	Folate	23 mcg	(8% DV)
Potassium	510 mg	(15% DV)	Beta Carotene	102 RE	

Ratings	Worst	Bad	Average	Good	Best
Weight Loss		4			
LowCal Density			6		
Filling			6		
Energizing					9
Fiber			7		
Vitamins				8	
Minerals					9
Overall			6		

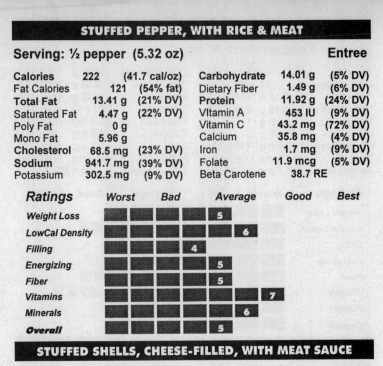

STUFFED SHELLS, CHEESE-FILLED, WITH TOMATO SAUCE

Serving: 3 shells (9.11 oz)   **Entree**

Calories	383	(42 cal/oz)	Carbohydrate	38.76 g	(13% DV)
Fat Calories	138	(36% fat)	Dietary Fiber	2.55 g	(10% DV)
Total Fat	15.3 g	(24% DV)	Protein	20.4 g	(41% DV)
Saturated Fat	7.65 g	(38% DV)	Vltamin A	1315.8 IU	(26% DV)
Poly Fat	0 g		Vitamin C	10.2 mg	(17% DV)
Mono Fat	5.1 g		Calcium	344.3 mg	(34% DV)
Cholesterol	147.9 mg	(49% DV)	Iron	3.1 mg	(17% DV)
Sodium	1134.8 mg	(47% DV)	Folate	20.4 mcg	(8% DV)
Potassium	451.4 mg	(13% DV)	Beta Carotene	81.6 RE	

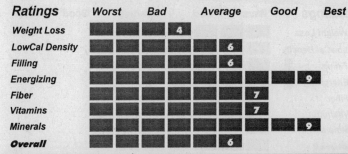

Ratings	Worst	Bad	Average	Good	Best
Weight Loss			4		
LowCal Density				6	
Filling				6	
Energizing					9
Fiber				7	
Vitamins				7	
Minerals					9
Overall				6	

SUBMARINE, COLD CUT SANDWICH, BUN, WITH LETTUCE

Serving: 1 submarine (7.07 oz)   **Sandwich**

Calories	560	(79.3 cal/oz)	Carbohydrate	34.25 g	(11% DV)
Fat Calories	339	(60% fat)	Dietary Fiber	1.98 g	(8% DV)
Total Fat	37.62 g	(58% DV)	Protein	21.78 g	(44% DV)
Saturated Fat	15.84 g	(79% DV)	Vltamin A	431.6 IU	(9% DV)
Poly Fat	3.96 g		Vitamin C	17.8 mg	(30% DV)
Mono Fat	15.84 g		Calcium	243.5 mg	(24% DV)
Cholesterol	73.3 mg	(24% DV)	Iron	3.1 mg	(17% DV)
Sodium	1578.1 mg	(66% DV)	Folate	21.8 mcg	(10% DV)
Potassium	289.1 mg	(8% DV)	Beta Carotene	17.8 RE	

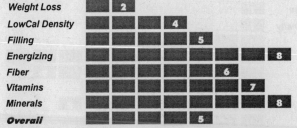

Ratings	Worst	Bad	Average	Good	Best
Weight Loss	2				
LowCal Density		4			
Filling			5		
Energizing				8	
Fiber			6		
Vitamins				7	
Minerals				8	
Overall			5		

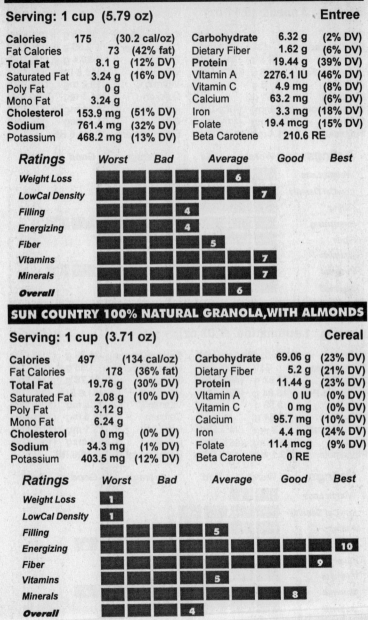

SUKIYAKI

Serving: 1 cup (5.79 oz)   **Entree**

Calories	175	(30.2 cal/oz)	Carbohydrate	6.32 g	(2% DV)
Fat Calories	73	(42% fat)	Dietary Fiber	1.62 g	(6% DV)
Total Fat	8.1 g	(12% DV)	Protein	19.44 g	(39% DV)
Saturated Fat	3.24 g	(16% DV)	VItamin A	2276.1 IU	(46% DV)
Poly Fat	0 g		Vitamin C	4.9 mg	(8% DV)
Mono Fat	3.24 g		Calcium	63.2 mg	(6% DV)
Cholesterol	153.9 mg	(51% DV)	Iron	3.3 mg	(18% DV)
Sodium	761.4 mg	(32% DV)	Folate	19.4 mcg	(15% DV)
Potassium	468.2 mg	(13% DV)	Beta Carotene	210.6 RE	

Ratings	Worst	Bad	Average	Good	Best
Weight Loss				6	
LowCal Density				7	
Filling			4		
Energizing			4		
Fiber			5		
Vitamins				7	
Minerals				7	
Overall				6	

SUN COUNTRY 100% NATURAL GRANOLA, WITH ALMONDS

Serving: 1 cup (3.71 oz)   **Cereal**

Calories	497	(134 cal/oz)	Carbohydrate	69.06 g	(23% DV)
Fat Calories	178	(36% fat)	Dietary Fiber	5.2 g	(21% DV)
Total Fat	19.76 g	(30% DV)	Protein	11.44 g	(23% DV)
Saturated Fat	2.08 g	(10% DV)	VItamin A	0 IU	(0% DV)
Poly Fat	3.12 g		Vitamin C	0 mg	(0% DV)
Mono Fat	6.24 g		Calcium	95.7 mg	(10% DV)
Cholesterol	0 mg	(0% DV)	Iron	4.4 mg	(24% DV)
Sodium	34.3 mg	(1% DV)	Folate	11.4 mcg	(9% DV)
Potassium	403.5 mg	(12% DV)	Beta Carotene	0 RE	

Ratings	Worst	Bad	Average	Good	Best
Weight Loss	1				
LowCal Density	1				
Filling			5		
Energizing					10
Fiber					9
Vitamins			5		
Minerals				8	
Overall		4			

SUNFLOWER OIL

Serving: 1 tbsp (.49 oz)   **Fat & Oil**

Calories	120	(245.3 cal/oz)	Carbohydrate	0 g	(0% DV)
Fat Calories	122	(102% fat)	Dietary Fiber	0 g	(0% DV)
Total Fat	13.6 g	(21% DV)	Protein	0 g	(0% DV)
Saturated Fat	1.36 g	(7% DV)	Vitamin A	0 IU	(0% DV)
Poly Fat	8.98 g		Vitamin C	0 mg	(0% DV)
Mono Fat	2.72 g		Calcium	0 mg	(0% DV)
Cholesterol	0 mg	(0% DV)	Iron	0 mg	(0% DV)
Sodium	0 mg	(0% DV)	Folate	0 mcg	(0% DV)
Potassium	0 mg	(0% DV)	Beta Carotene	0 RE	

Ratings	Worst	Bad	Average	Good	Best
Weight Loss	1				
LowCal Density	1				
Filling	1				
Energizing	1				
Fiber	1				
Vitamins				4	
Minerals	1				
Overall	1				

SUNFLOWER SEEDS, HULLED, ROASTED, SALTED

Serving: 40 seeds (1 oz)   **Snack**

Calories	185	(184.5 cal/oz)	Carbohydrate	4.41 g	(1% DV)
Fat Calories	154	(83% fat)	Dietary Fiber	2.1 g	(8% DV)
Total Fat	17.1 g	(26% DV)	Protein	6.3 g	(13% DV)
Saturated Fat	1.8 g	(9% DV)	Vitamin A	15.3 IU	(0% DV)
Poly Fat	11.4 g		Vitamin C	.3 mg	(0% DV)
Mono Fat	3.3 g		Calcium	16.8 mg	(2% DV)
Cholesterol	0 mg	(0% DV)	Iron	2 mg	(11% DV)
Sodium	180.9 mg	(8% DV)	Folate	6.3 mcg	(18% DV)
Potassium	144.9 mg	(4% DV)	Beta Carotene	1.5 RE	

Ratings	Worst	Bad	Average	Good	Best
Weight Loss		2			
LowCal Density	1				
Filling		2			
Energizing			3		
Fiber					6
Vitamins					6
Minerals					7
Overall			3		

SUSHI, WITH VEGETABLES & FISH

Serving: 1 piece (.93 oz)   **Entree**

Calories	37	(40 cal/oz)	Carbohydrate	7.54 g	(3% DV)
Fat Calories	0	(0% fat)	Dietary Fiber	.26 g	(1% DV)
Total Fat	0 g	(0% DV)	Protein	1.3 g	(3% DV)
Saturated Fat	0 g	(0% DV)	VItamin A	267.5 IU	(5% DV)
Poly Fat	0 g		Vitamin C	.5 mg	(1% DV)
Mono Fat	0 g		Calcium	4.2 mg	(0% DV)
Cholesterol	1.8 mg	(1% DV)	Iron	.4 mg	(2% DV)
Sodium	53.8 mg	(2% DV)	Folate	1.3 mcg	(1% DV)
Potassium	33.8 mg	(1% DV)	Beta Carotene	26.8 RE	

Ratings	Worst	Bad	Average	Good	Best
Weight Loss					10
LowCal Density			6		
Filling		3			
Energizing			4		
Fiber	2				
Vitamins		3			
Minerals	2				
Overall			6		

SWEDISH MEATBALLS, GRAVY, NOODLES

Serving: 1 diet meal (9.21 oz)   **Entree**

Calories	302	(32.8 cal/oz)	Carbohydrate	28.12 g	(9% DV)
Fat Calories	93	(31% fat)	Dietary Fiber	2.58 g	(10% DV)
Total Fat	10.32 g	(16% DV)	Protein	25.8 g	(52% DV)
Saturated Fat	2.58 g	(13% DV)	VItamin A	49 IU	(1% DV)
Poly Fat	2.58 g		Vitamin C	2.6 mg	(4% DV)
Mono Fat	2.58 g		Calcium	54.2 mg	(5% DV)
Cholesterol	41.3 mg	(14% DV)	Iron	3.7 mg	(20% DV)
Sodium	670.8 mg	(28% DV)	Folate	25.8 mcg	(8% DV)
Potassium	381.8 mg	(11% DV)	Beta Carotene	2.6 RE	

Ratings	Worst	Bad	Average	Good	Best
Weight Loss			6		
LowCal Density				7	
Filling			6		
Energizing				7	
Fiber				7	
Vitamins			5		
Minerals				7	
Overall			6		

SWEDISH MEATBALLS, SAUCE, NOODLES, VEGETABLE

Serving: 1 meal (8.61 oz)   **Entree**

Calories	270	(31.4 cal/oz)	Carbohydrate	32.29 g	(11% DV)
Fat Calories	65	(24% fat)	Dietary Fiber	2.41 g	(10% DV)
Total Fat	7.23 g	(11% DV)	**Protein**	16.87 g	(34% DV)
Saturated Fat	2.41 g	(12% DV)	VItamin A	7760.2 IU	(155% DV)
Poly Fat	2.41 g		Vitamin C	2.4 mg	(4% DV)
Mono Fat	2.41 g		Calcium	306.1 mg	(31% DV)
Cholesterol	33.7 mg	(11% DV)	Iron	1.7 mg	(10% DV)
Sodium	771.2 mg	(32% DV)	Folate	16.9 mcg	(6% DV)
Potassium	614.6 mg	(18% DV)	Beta Carotene	720.6 RE	

Ratings	Worst	Bad	Average	Good	Best
Weight Loss			6		
LowCal Density			7		
Filling			7		
Energizing				8	
Fiber			7		
Vitamins					9
Minerals				8	
Overall			7		

SWEET & SOUR PORK WITH RICE

Serving: 1 cup (8.71 oz)   **Entree**

Calories	268	(30.8 cal/oz)	Carbohydrate	39.77 g	(13% DV)
Fat Calories	66	(25% fat)	Dietary Fiber	2.44 g	(10% DV)
Total Fat	7.32 g	(11% DV)	Protein	12.2 g	(24% DV)
Saturated Fat	2.44 g	(12% DV)	VItamin A	207.4 IU	(4% DV)
Poly Fat	2.44 g		Vitamin C	14.6 mg	(24% DV)
Mono Fat	2.44 g		Calcium	29.3 mg	(3% DV)
Cholesterol	29.3 mg	(10% DV)	Iron	1.8 mg	(10% DV)
Sodium	907.7 mg	(38% DV)	Folate	12.2 mcg	(2% DV)
Potassium	319.6 mg	(9% DV)	Beta Carotene	19.5 RE	

Ratings	Worst	Bad	Average	Good	Best
Weight Loss			6		
LowCal Density			7		
Filling				8	
Energizing					9
Fiber			7		
Vitamins			6		
Minerals		5			
Overall			7		

SWEET POTATO, CANDIED

Serving: 1 cup (7 oz)   Vegetable

Calories	294	(42 cal/oz)	Carbohydrate	56.45 g	(19% DV)
Fat Calories	71	(24% fat)	Dietary Fiber	3.92 g	(16% DV)
Total Fat	7.84 g	(12% DV)	Protein	1.96 g	(4% DV)
Saturated Fat	1.96 g	(10% DV)	Vltamin A	11322.9 IU	(226% DV)
Poly Fat	1.96 g		Vitamin C	19.6 mg	(33% DV)
Mono Fat	3.92 g		Calcium	47 mg	(5% DV)
Cholesterol	0 mg	(0% DV)	Iron	1.9 mg	(11% DV)
Sodium	497.8 mg	(21% DV)	Folate	2 mcg	(3% DV)
Potassium	415.5 mg	(12% DV)	Beta Carotene	1103.5 RE	

Ratings	Worst	Bad	Average	Good	Best
Weight Loss	2				
LowCal Density			6		
Filling				8	
Energizing					10
Fiber					9
Vitamins					10
Minerals			5		
Overall			6		

SWEET POTATO, ROASTED OR BAKED

Serving: 1 cup (7.14 oz)   Vegetable

Calories	254	(35.6 cal/oz)	Carbohydrate	46.6 g	(16% DV)
Fat Calories	54	(21% fat)	Dietary Fiber	6 g	(24% DV)
Total Fat	6 g	(9% DV)	Protein	4 g	(8% DV)
Saturated Fat	2 g	(10% DV)	Vltamin A	42116 IU	(842% DV)
Poly Fat	2 g		Vitamin C	48 mg	(80% DV)
Mono Fat	2 g		Calcium	56 mg	(6% DV)
Cholesterol	0 mg	(0% DV)	Iron	.9 mg	(5% DV)
Sodium	310 mg	(13% DV)	Folate	4 mcg	(11% DV)
Potassium	670 mg	(19% DV)	Beta Carotene	4184 RE	

Ratings	Worst	Bad	Average	Good	Best
Weight Loss	2				
LowCal Density				7	
Filling				8	
Energizing				9	
Fiber					10
Vitamins					10
Minerals			5		
Overall			6		

SWEET ROLL, CINNAMON BUN, FROSTED

Serving: 1 medium (1.96 oz)   **Bakery**

Calories	185	(94.6 cal/oz)	Carbohydrate	30.91 g	(10% DV)
Fat Calories	50	(27% fat)	Dietary Fiber	.55 g	(2% DV)
Total Fat	5.5 g	(8% DV)	Protein	3.85 g	(8% DV)
Saturated Fat	1.1 g	(6% DV)	Vitamin A	100.7 IU	(2% DV)
Poly Fat	1.1 g		Vitamin C	0 mg	(0% DV)
Mono Fat	2.75 g		Calcium	46.2 mg	(5% DV)
Cholesterol	14.3 mg	(5% DV)	Iron	.9 mg	(5% DV)
Sodium	193.1 mg	(8% DV)	Folate	3.9 mcg	(3% DV)
Potassium	54.5 mg	(2% DV)	Beta Carotene	1.7 RE	

Ratings	Worst	Bad	Average	Good	Best
Weight Loss		4			
LowCal Density	3				
Filling		4			
Energizing				7	
Fiber	3				
Vitamins		4			
Minerals		4			
Overall		4			

SWEET ROLL, MEXICAN, PAN DULCE, NO TOPPING

Serving: 1 roll (2.46 oz)   **Bakery**

Calories	214	(87 cal/oz)	Carbohydrate	38.71 g	(13% DV)
Fat Calories	37	(17% fat)	Dietary Fiber	1.38 g	(6% DV)
Total Fat	4.14 g	(6% DV)	Protein	4.83 g	(10% DV)
Saturated Fat	1.38 g	(7% DV)	Vitamin A	50.4 IU	(1% DV)
Poly Fat	1.38 g		Vitamin C	0 mg	(0% DV)
Mono Fat	2.07 g		Calcium	9.7 mg	(1% DV)
Cholesterol	33.8 mg	(11% DV)	Iron	1.8 mg	(10% DV)
Sodium	94.5 mg	(4% DV)	Folate	4.8 mcg	(7% DV)
Potassium	58 mg	(2% DV)	Beta Carotene	0 RE	

Ratings	Worst	Bad	Average	Good	Best
Weight Loss		4			
LowCal Density	3				
Filling			5		
Energizing					9
Fiber			5		
Vitamins		4			
Minerals		4			
Overall		4			

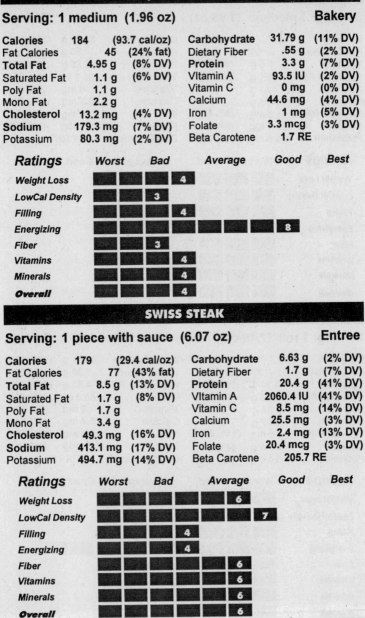

SWEET ROLL, WITH FRUIT, FROSTED

Serving: 1 medium (1.96 oz)   **Bakery**

Calories	184	(93.7 cal/oz)	Carbohydrate	31.79 g	(11% DV)
Fat Calories	45	(24% fat)	Dietary Fiber	.55 g	(2% DV)
Total Fat	4.95 g	(8% DV)	Protein	3.3 g	(7% DV)
Saturated Fat	1.1 g	(6% DV)	Vitamin A	93.5 IU	(2% DV)
Poly Fat	1.1 g		Vitamin C	0 mg	(0% DV)
Mono Fat	2.2 g		Calcium	44.6 mg	(4% DV)
Cholesterol	13.2 mg	(4% DV)	Iron	1 mg	(5% DV)
Sodium	179.3 mg	(7% DV)	Folate	3.3 mcg	(3% DV)
Potassium	80.3 mg	(2% DV)	Beta Carotene	1.7 RE	

Ratings	Worst	Bad	Average	Good	Best
Weight Loss			4		
LowCal Density		3			
Filling			4		
Energizing					8
Fiber		3			
Vitamins			4		
Minerals			4		
Overall			4		

SWISS STEAK

Serving: 1 piece with sauce (6.07 oz)   **Entree**

Calories	179	(29.4 cal/oz)	Carbohydrate	6.63 g	(2% DV)
Fat Calories	77	(43% fat)	Dietary Fiber	1.7 g	(7% DV)
Total Fat	8.5 g	(13% DV)	Protein	20.4 g	(41% DV)
Saturated Fat	1.7 g	(8% DV)	Vitamin A	2060.4 IU	(41% DV)
Poly Fat	1.7 g		Vitamin C	8.5 mg	(14% DV)
Mono Fat	3.4 g		Calcium	25.5 mg	(3% DV)
Cholesterol	49.3 mg	(16% DV)	Iron	2.4 mg	(13% DV)
Sodium	413.1 mg	(17% DV)	Folate	20.4 mcg	(3% DV)
Potassium	494.7 mg	(14% DV)	Beta Carotene	205.7 RE	

Ratings	Worst	Bad	Average	Good	Best
Weight Loss				6	
LowCal Density				7	
Filling			4		
Energizing			4		
Fiber				6	
Vitamins				6	
Minerals				6	
Overall				6	

SWISS STEAK, WITH GRAVY, MEATLESS, VEGETARIAN

Serving: 1 steak (3.29 oz)   **Entree**

Calories	182	(55.4 cal/oz)	Carbohydrate	8.46 g	(3% DV)
Fat Calories	83	(45% fat)	Dietary Fiber	3.68 g	(15% DV)
Total Fat	9.2 g	(14% DV)	Protein	15.64 g	(31% DV)
Saturated Fat	1.84 g	(9% DV)	Vitamin A	0 IU	(0% DV)
Poly Fat	5.52 g		Vitamin C	0 mg	(0% DV)
Mono Fat	1.84 g		Calcium	23 mg	(2% DV)
Cholesterol	0 mg	(0% DV)	Iron	1.7 mg	(9% DV)
Sodium	620.1 mg	(26% DV)	Folate	15.6 mcg	(14% DV)
Potassium	136.2 mg	(4% DV)	Beta Carotene	0 RE	

Ratings	Worst	Bad	Average	Good	Best
Weight Loss				6	
LowCal Density			5		
Filling		3			
Energizing			4		
Fiber					8
Vitamins					8
Minerals			6		
Overall			5		

SWORDFISH, BAKED OR BROILED

Serving: 1 piece (5.07 oz)   **Fish**

Calories	253	(49.9 cal/oz)	Carbohydrate	.57 g	(0% DV)
Fat Calories	102	(40% fat)	Dietary Fiber	0 g	(0% DV)
Total Fat	11.36 g	(17% DV)	Protein	34.08 g	(68% DV)
Saturated Fat	2.84 g	(14% DV)	Vitamin A	444.5 IU	(9% DV)
Poly Fat	2.84 g		Vitamin C	4.3 mg	(7% DV)
Mono Fat	4.26 g		Calcium	9.9 mg	(1% DV)
Cholesterol	66.7 mg	(22% DV)	Iron	1.4 mg	(8% DV)
Sodium	678.8 mg	(28% DV)	Folate	34.1 mcg	(1% DV)
Potassium	502.7 mg	(14% DV)	Beta Carotene	5.7 RE	

Ratings	Worst	Bad	Average	Good	Best
Weight Loss		4			
LowCal Density			6		
Filling	1				
Energizing	2				
Fiber	1				
Vitamins				7	
Minerals				7	
Overall		4			

SWORDFISH, FLOURED OR BREADED, FRIED

Serving: 1 piece (3.04 oz)   **Fish**

Calories	209	(68.8 cal/oz)	Carbohydrate	6.72 g	(2% DV)
Fat Calories	107	(51% fat)	Dietary Fiber	0 g	(0% DV)
Total Fat	11.9 g	(18% DV)	Protein	17.85 g	(36% DV)
Saturated Fat	3.4 g	(17% DV)	VItamin A	112.2 IU	(2% DV)
Poly Fat	2.55 g		Vitamin C	.9 mg	(1% DV)
Mono Fat	5.1 g		Calcium	17.9 mg	(2% DV)
Cholesterol	51 mg	(17% DV)	Iron	1.1 mg	(6% DV)
Sodium	336.6 mg	(14% DV)	Folate	17.9 mcg	(1% DV)
Potassium	255 mg	(7% DV)	Beta Carotene	0 RE	

Ratings	Worst	Bad	Average	Good	Best
Weight Loss			4		
LowCal Density			4		
Filling	2				
Energizing			4		
Fiber	1				
Vitamins				5	
Minerals				5	
Overall			4		

TABBOULEH

Serving: 1 cup (5.71 oz)   **Entree**

Calories	187	(32.8 cal/oz)	Carbohydrate	16.96 g	(6% DV)
Fat Calories	115	(62% fat)	Dietary Fiber	4.8 g	(19% DV)
Total Fat	12.8 g	(20% DV)	Protein	3.2 g	(6% DV)
Saturated Fat	1.6 g	(8% DV)	VItamin A	1668.8 IU	(33% DV)
Poly Fat	1.6 g		Vitamin C	52.8 mg	(88% DV)
Mono Fat	9.6 g		Calcium	54.4 mg	(5% DV)
Cholesterol	0 mg	(0% DV)	Iron	2.4 mg	(13% DV)
Sodium	641.6 mg	(27% DV)	Folate	3.2 mcg	(15% DV)
Potassium	336 mg	(10% DV)	Beta Carotene	166.4 RE	

Ratings	Worst	Bad	Average	Good	Best
Weight Loss			5		
LowCal Density				7	
Filling			6		
Energizing			5		
Fiber					9
Vitamins				8	
Minerals			5		
Overall			6		

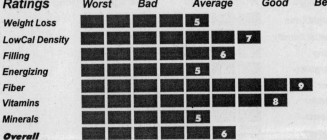

TACO OR TOSTADA SALAD, BEEF & CHEESE, CORN CHIPS

Serving: 1 salad (8.29 oz)   Salad

Calories	385	(46.5 cal/oz)	Carbohydrate	21.11 g	(7% DV)
Fat Calories	230	(60% fat)	Dietary Fiber	2.32 g	(9% DV)
Total Fat	25.52 g	(39% DV)	Protein	20.88 g	(42% DV)
Saturated Fat	9.28 g	(46% DV)	Vitamin A	3795.5 IU	(76% DV)
Poly Fat	4.64 g		Vitamin C	20.9 mg	(35% DV)
Mono Fat	9.28 g		Calcium	155.4 mg	(16% DV)
Cholesterol	69.6 mg	(23% DV)	Iron	2.6 mg	(14% DV)
Sodium	661.2 mg	(28% DV)	Folate	20.9 mcg	(12% DV)
Potassium	593.9 mg	(17% DV)	Beta Carotene	368.9 RE	

Ratings	Worst	Bad	Average	Good	Best
Weight Loss	2				
LowCal Density				6	
Filling			5		
Energizing				6	
Fiber				6	
Vitamins					8
Minerals					8
Overall			5		

TACO OR TOSTADA, BEEF, CHEESE, LETTUCE, TOMATO

Serving: 1 taco or tostada (2.96 oz)   Sandwich

Calories	179	(60.6 cal/oz)	Carbohydrate	12.53 g	(4% DV)
Fat Calories	90	(50% fat)	Dietary Fiber	2.49 g	(10% DV)
Total Fat	9.96 g	(15% DV)	Protein	10.79 g	(22% DV)
Saturated Fat	4.15 g	(21% DV)	Vitamin A	325.4 IU	(7% DV)
Poly Fat	.83 g		Vitamin C	5 mg	(8% DV)
Mono Fat	4.15 g		Calcium	88.8 mg	(9% DV)
Cholesterol	32.4 mg	(11% DV)	Iron	1.3 mg	(7% DV)
Sodium	297.1 mg	(12% DV)	Folate	10.8 mcg	(5% DV)
Potassium	224.1 mg	(6% DV)	Beta Carotene	26.6 RE	

Ratings	Worst	Bad	Average	Good	Best
Weight Loss				6	
LowCal Density			5		
Filling		4			
Energizing			5		
Fiber				7	
Vitamins			5		
Minerals				6	
Overall			5		

TACO OR TOSTADA,CHICKEN,CHEESE,LETTUCE,TOMATO

Serving: 1 Taco Bell Chicken Taco (2.89 oz)   Sandwich

Calories	152	(52.7 cal/oz)	Carbohydrate	12.8 g	(4% DV)
Fat Calories	58	(38% fat)	Dietary Fiber	2.43 g	(10% DV)
Total Fat	6.48 g	(10% DV)	Protein	10.53 g	(21% DV)
Saturated Fat	2.43 g	(12% DV)	VItamin A	346.7 IU	(7% DV)
Poly Fat	.81 g		Vitamin C	4.9 mg	(8% DV)
Mono Fat	2.43 g		Calcium	92.3 mg	(9% DV)
Cholesterol	30 mg	(10% DV)	Iron	.9 mg	(5% DV)
Sodium	301.3 mg	(13% DV)	Folate	10.5 mcg	(5% DV)
Potassium	181.4 mg	(5% DV)	Beta Carotene	26.7 RE	

Ratings	Worst	Bad	Average	Good	Best
Weight Loss				7	
LowCal Density				6	
Filling		4			
Energizing			5		
Fiber				7	
Vitamins			5		
Minerals			5		
Overall				6	

TAMALE WITH MEAT

Serving: 1 tamale (2.5 oz)   Entree

Calories	183	(73.1 cal/oz)	Carbohydrate	16.03 g	(5% DV)
Fat Calories	88	(48% fat)	Dietary Fiber	2.8 g	(11% DV)
Total Fat	9.8 g	(15% DV)	Protein	7 g	(14% DV)
Saturated Fat	3.5 g	(18% DV)	VItamin A	168 IU	(3% DV)
Poly Fat	1.4 g		Vitamin C	3.5 mg	(6% DV)
Mono Fat	4.2 g		Calcium	32.2 mg	(3% DV)
Cholesterol	23.8 mg	(8% DV)	Iron	1.9 mg	(10% DV)
Sodium	228.9 mg	(10% DV)	Folate	7 mcg	(1% DV)
Potassium	154 mg	(4% DV)	Beta Carotene	16.1 RE	

Ratings	Worst	Bad	Average	Good	Best
Weight Loss			6		
LowCal Density		4			
Filling		4			
Energizing			5		
Fiber					8
Vitamins			5		
Minerals			5		
Overall			5		

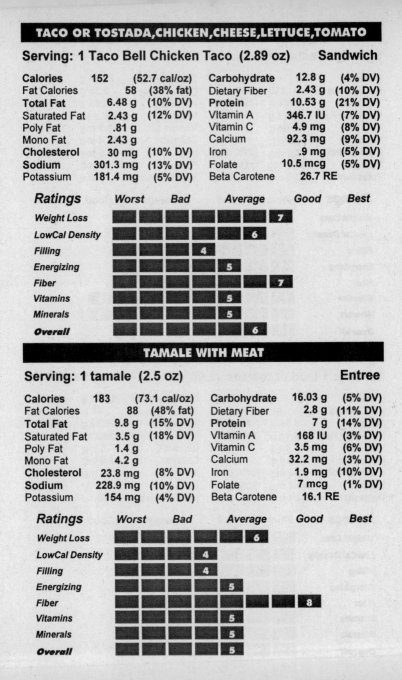

TAMALE, SWEET, WITH FRUIT

Serving: 1 tamale (1.75 oz)   **Dessert**

Calories	133	(76.2 cal/oz)	Carbohydrate	21.07 g	(7% DV)
Fat Calories	49	(36% fat)	Dietary Fiber	1.96 g	(8% DV)
Total Fat	5.39 g	(8% DV)	Protein	1.47 g	(3% DV)
Saturated Fat	1.47 g	(7% DV)	Vitamin A	8.3 IU	(0% DV)
Poly Fat	1.47 g		Vitamin C	1 mg	(2% DV)
Mono Fat	2.45 g		Calcium	26.5 mg	(3% DV)
Cholesterol	0 mg	(0% DV)	Iron	1.2 mg	(7% DV)
Sodium	101.9 mg	(4% DV)	Folate	1.5 mcg	(1% DV)
Potassium	89.2 mg	(3% DV)	Beta Carotene	1 RE	

Ratings	Worst	Bad	Average	Good	Best
Weight Loss				7	
LowCal Density		4			
Filling		4			
Energizing			6		
Fiber			6		
Vitamins		4			
Minerals		4			
Overall			5		

TANGELO, RAW

Serving: 1 medium (2½" dia) (3.39 oz)   **Fruit**

Calories	45	(13.2 cal/oz)	Carbohydrate	11.21 g	(4% DV)
Fat Calories	0	(0% fat)	Dietary Fiber	1.9 g	(8% DV)
Total Fat	0 g	(0% DV)	Protein	.95 g	(2% DV)
Saturated Fat	0 g	(0% DV)	Vitamin A	194.8 IU	(4% DV)
Poly Fat	0 g		Vitamin C	50.4 mg	(84% DV)
Mono Fat	0 g		Calcium	38 mg	(4% DV)
Cholesterol	0 mg	(0% DV)	Iron	.1 mg	(1% DV)
Sodium	0 mg	(0% DV)	Folate	1 mcg	(7% DV)
Potassium	172 mg	(5% DV)	Beta Carotene	20 RE	

Ratings	Worst	Bad	Average	Good	Best
Weight Loss					10
LowCal Density				9	
Filling			7		
Energizing		5			
Fiber			6		
Vitamins			7		
Minerals	3				
Overall				8	

TANGERINE JUICE

Serving: 1 cup (8.89 oz)   Beverage

Calories	125	(14 cal/oz)	Carbohydrate	29.88 g	(10% DV)
Fat Calories	0	(0% fat)	Dietary Fiber	0 g	(0% DV)
Total Fat	0 g	(0% DV)	Protein	2.49 g	(5% DV)
Saturated Fat	0 g	(0% DV)	VItamin A	1045.8 IU	(21% DV)
Poly Fat	0 g		Vitamin C	54.8 mg	(91% DV)
Mono Fat	0 g		Calcium	44.8 mg	(4% DV)
Cholesterol	0 mg	(0% DV)	Iron	.5 mg	(3% DV)
Sodium	2.5 mg	(0% DV)	Folate	2.5 mcg	(3% DV)
Potassium	443.2 mg	(13% DV)	Beta Carotene	104.6 RE	

Ratings	Worst	Bad	Average	Good	Best
Weight Loss			7		
LowCal Density				9	
Filling					10
Energizing			7		
Fiber	1				
Vitamins				8	
Minerals		4			
Overall			7		

TANGERINE, RAW

Serving: 1 medium (2-3/8" dia) (3 oz)   Fruit

Calories	37	(12.3 cal/oz)	Carbohydrate	9.41 g	(3% DV)
Fat Calories	0	(0% fat)	Dietary Fiber	.84 g	(3% DV)
Total Fat	0 g	(0% DV)	Protein	.84 g	(2% DV)
Saturated Fat	0 g	(0% DV)	VItamin A	772.8 IU	(15% DV)
Poly Fat	0 g		Vitamin C	26 mg	(43% DV)
Mono Fat	0 g		Calcium	11.8 mg	(1% DV)
Cholesterol	0 mg	(0% DV)	Iron	.1 mg	(0% DV)
Sodium	.8 mg	(0% DV)	Folate	.8 mcg	(4% DV)
Potassium	131.9 mg	(4% DV)	Beta Carotene	77.3 RE	

Ratings	Worst	Bad	Average	Good	Best
Weight Loss					10
LowCal Density				9	
Filling			6		
Energizing		4			
Fiber		4			
Vitamins			6		
Minerals	2				
Overall			7		

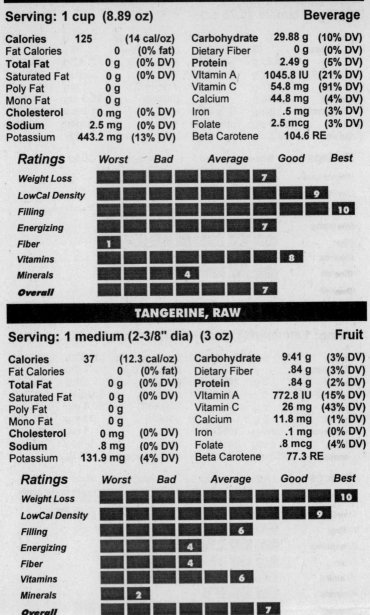

TARTAR SAUCE

Serving: 1 tbsp (.51 oz)   **Sauce**

Calories	74	(145.4 cal/oz)	Carbohydrate	2.03 g	(1% DV)
Fat Calories	67	(91% fat)	Dietary Fiber	0 g	(0% DV)
Total Fat	7.49 g	(12% DV)	Protein	.14 g	(0% DV)
Saturated Fat	1.15 g	(6% DV)	Vitamin A	52.9 IU	(1% DV)
Poly Fat	3.89 g		Vitamin C	.1 mg	(0% DV)
Mono Fat	2.16 g		Calcium	3.6 mg	(0% DV)
Cholesterol	5.6 mg	(2% DV)	Iron	.1 mg	(1% DV)
Sodium	102.7 mg	(4% DV)	Folate	.1 mcg	(0% DV)
Potassium	6.2 mg	(0% DV)	Beta Carotene	2 RE	

Ratings	Worst	Bad	Average	Good	Best
Weight Loss		3			
LowCal Density	1				
Filling	1				
Energizing		3			
Fiber	1				
Vitamins	2				
Minerals	2				
Overall	2				

TEA

Serving: 1 mug (8.57 oz)   **Beverage**

Calories	2	(.3 cal/oz)	Carbohydrate	.72 g	(0% DV)
Fat Calories	0	(0% fat)	Dietary Fiber	0 g	(0% DV)
Total Fat	0 g	(0% DV)	Protein	0 g	(0% DV)
Saturated Fat	0 g	(0% DV)	Vitamin A	0 IU	(0% DV)
Poly Fat	0 g		Vitamin C	0 mg	(0% DV)
Mono Fat	0 g		Calcium	0 mg	(0% DV)
Cholesterol	0 mg	(0% DV)	Iron	.1 mg	(0% DV)
Sodium	7.2 mg	(0% DV)	Folate	0 mcg	(3% DV)
Potassium	88.8 mg	(3% DV)	Beta Carotene	0 RE	

Ratings	Worst	Bad	Average	Good	Best
Weight Loss					10
LowCal Density					10
Filling					10
Energizing	2				
Fiber	1				
Vitamins	2				
Minerals	2				
Overall				8	

TEA, FROM POWDERED INSTANT, LOW-CAL SWEETENER

Serving: 1 mug (8.75 oz)   **Beverage**

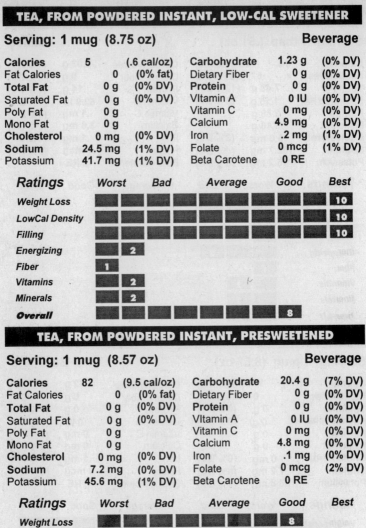

Calories	5	(.6 cal/oz)	Carbohydrate	1.23 g	(0% DV)
Fat Calories	0	(0% fat)	Dietary Fiber	0 g	(0% DV)
Total Fat	0 g	(0% DV)	Protein	0 g	(0% DV)
Saturated Fat	0 g	(0% DV)	Vitamin A	0 IU	(0% DV)
Poly Fat	0 g		Vitamin C	0 mg	(0% DV)
Mono Fat	0 g		Calcium	4.9 mg	(0% DV)
Cholesterol	0 mg	(0% DV)	Iron	.2 mg	(1% DV)
Sodium	24.5 mg	(1% DV)	Folate	0 mcg	(1% DV)
Potassium	41.7 mg	(1% DV)	Beta Carotene	0 RE	

Ratings	Worst	Bad	Average	Good	Best
Weight Loss					10
LowCal Density					10
Filling					10
Energizing	2				
Fiber	1				
Vitamins	2				
Minerals	2				
Overall				8	

TEA, FROM POWDERED INSTANT, PRESWEETENED

Serving: 1 mug (8.57 oz)   **Beverage**

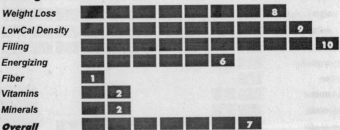

Calories	82	(9.5 cal/oz)	Carbohydrate	20.4 g	(7% DV)
Fat Calories	0	(0% fat)	Dietary Fiber	0 g	(0% DV)
Total Fat	0 g	(0% DV)	Protein	0 g	(0% DV)
Saturated Fat	0 g	(0% DV)	Vitamin A	0 IU	(0% DV)
Poly Fat	0 g		Vitamin C	0 mg	(0% DV)
Mono Fat	0 g		Calcium	4.8 mg	(0% DV)
Cholesterol	0 mg	(0% DV)	Iron	.1 mg	(0% DV)
Sodium	7.2 mg	(0% DV)	Folate	0 mcg	(2% DV)
Potassium	45.6 mg	(1% DV)	Beta Carotene	0 RE	

Ratings	Worst	Bad	Average	Good	Best
Weight Loss				8	
LowCal Density					9
Filling					10
Energizing				6	
Fiber	1				
Vitamins	2				
Minerals	2				
Overall				7	

TEMPURA, VEGETABLE

Serving: 1 cup (2.25 oz)   **Vegetable**

Calories	101	(44.8 cal/oz)	Carbohydrate	9.01 g	(3% DV)
Fat Calories	57	(56% fat)	Dietary Fiber	.63 g	(3% DV)
Total Fat	6.3 g	(10% DV)	Protein	2.52 g	(5% DV)
Saturated Fat	1.26 g	(6% DV)	Vitamin A	1340.6 IU	(27% DV)
Poly Fat	2.52 g		Vitamin C	2.5 mg	(4% DV)
Mono Fat	1.89 g		Calcium	15.1 mg	(2% DV)
Cholesterol	41 mg	(14% DV)	Iron	.8 mg	(4% DV)
Sodium	19.5 mg	(1% DV)	Folate	2.5 mcg	(4% DV)
Potassium	111.5 mg	(3% DV)	Beta Carotene	129.2 RE	

Ratings	Worst	Bad	Average	Good	Best
Weight Loss			4		
LowCal Density				6	
Filling		3			
Energizing			4		
Fiber		3			
Vitamins			5		
Minerals		3			
Overall			4		

THOUSAND ISLAND DRESSING

Serving: 1 tbsp (.56 oz)   **Fat & Oil**

Calories	59	(105 cal/oz)	Carbohydrate	2.37 g	(1% DV)
Fat Calories	51	(86% fat)	Dietary Fiber	.31 g	(1% DV)
Total Fat	5.62 g	(9% DV)	Protein	.16 g	(0% DV)
Saturated Fat	.94 g	(5% DV)	Vitamin A	49.9 IU	(1% DV)
Poly Fat	3.12 g		Vitamin C	0 mg	(0% DV)
Mono Fat	1.25 g		Calcium	1.7 mg	(0% DV)
Cholesterol	4.1 mg	(1% DV)	Iron	.1 mg	(0% DV)
Sodium	109.2 mg	(5% DV)	Folate	.2 mcg	(0% DV)
Potassium	17.6 mg	(1% DV)	Beta Carotene	0 RE	

Ratings	Worst	Bad	Average	Good	Best
Weight Loss		3			
LowCal Density	2				
Filling	1				
Energizing		3			
Fiber	2				
Vitamins	2				
Minerals	2				
Overall	2				

THOUSAND ISLAND DRESSING, LOW-CALORIE

Serving: 1 tbsp (.55 oz) **Fat & Oil**

Calories	24	(44.2 cal/oz)	Carbohydrate	2.48 g	(1% DV)
Fat Calories	15	(62% fat)	Dietary Fiber	.15 g	(1% DV)
Total Fat	1.68 g	(3% DV)	Protein	.15 g	(0% DV)
Saturated Fat	.31 g	(2% DV)	Vitamin A	49 IU	(1% DV)
Poly Fat	.92 g		Vitamin C	0 mg	(0% DV)
Mono Fat	.31 g		Calcium	1.7 mg	(0% DV)
Cholesterol	2.3 mg	(1% DV)	Iron	.1 mg	(0% DV)
Sodium	153 mg	(6% DV)	Folate	.2 mcg	(0% DV)
Potassium	17.3 mg	(0% DV)	Beta Carotene	0 RE	

Ratings	Worst	Bad	Average	Good	Best
Weight Loss			5		
LowCal Density			6		
Filling	2				
Energizing		3			
Fiber	2				
Vitamins	2				
Minerals	2				
Overall		4			

TOMATO & VEGETABLE JUICE, MOSTLY TOMATO

Serving: 1 cup (8.64 oz) **Beverage**

Calories	46	(5.3 cal/oz)	Carbohydrate	11.13 g	(4% DV)
Fat Calories	0	(0% fat)	Dietary Fiber	2.42 g	(10% DV)
Total Fat	0 g	(0% DV)	Protein	2.42 g	(5% DV)
Saturated Fat	0 g	(0% DV)	Vitamin A	2831.4 IU	(57% DV)
Poly Fat	0 g		Vitamin C	67.8 mg	(113% DV)
Mono Fat	0 g		Calcium	26.6 mg	(3% DV)
Cholesterol	0 mg	(0% DV)	Iron	1 mg	(6% DV)
Sodium	883.3 mg	(37% DV)	Folate	2.4 mcg	(13% DV)
Potassium	467.1 mg	(13% DV)	Beta Carotene	283.1 RE	

Ratings	Worst	Bad	Average	Good	Best
Weight Loss				9	
LowCal Density					10
Filling					10
Energizing			5		
Fiber			7		
Vitamins				9	
Minerals		4			
Overall				9	

TOMATO JUICE

Serving: 1 cup (8.68 oz)   **Beverage**

Calories	41	(4.8 cal/oz)	Carbohydrate	10.21 g	(3% DV)
Fat Calories	0	(0% fat)	Dietary Fiber	2.43 g	(10% DV)
Total Fat	0 g	(0% DV)	Protein	2.43 g	(5% DV)
Saturated Fat	0 g	(0% DV)	Vitamin A	1351.1 IU	(27% DV)
Poly Fat	0 g		Vitamin C	43.7 mg	(73% DV)
Mono Fat	0 g		Calcium	21.9 mg	(2% DV)
Cholesterol	0 mg	(0% DV)	Iron	1.4 mg	(8% DV)
Sodium	877.2 mg	(37% DV)	Folate	2.4 mcg	(12% DV)
Potassium	534.6 mg	(15% DV)	Beta Carotene	136.1 RE	

Ratings	Worst	Bad	Average	Good	Best
Weight Loss				9	
LowCal Density					10
Filling					10
Energizing		4			
Fiber				7	
Vitamins				8	
Minerals		4			
Overall				9	

TOMATO SOUP, PREPARED WITH WATER

Serving: 1 cup (8.71 oz)   **Soup**

Calories	85	(9.8 cal/oz)	Carbohydrate	16.59 g	(6% DV)
Fat Calories	22	(26% fat)	Dietary Fiber	0 g	(0% DV)
Total Fat	2.44 g	(4% DV)	Protein	2.44 g	(5% DV)
Saturated Fat	0 g	(0% DV)	Vitamin A	688.1 IU	(14% DV)
Poly Fat	0 g		Vitamin C	65.9 mg	(110% DV)
Mono Fat	0 g		Calcium	12.2 mg	(1% DV)
Cholesterol	0 mg	(0% DV)	Iron	1.8 mg	(10% DV)
Sodium	871.1 mg	(36% DV)	Folate	2.4 mcg	(4% DV)
Potassium	263.5 mg	(8% DV)	Beta Carotene	68.3 RE	

Ratings	Worst	Bad	Average	Good	Best
Weight Loss			7		
LowCal Density				9	
Filling				9	
Energizing			5		
Fiber	1				
Vitamins				8	
Minerals		4			
Overall			7		

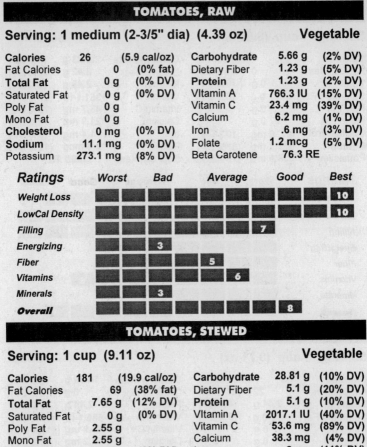

TOMATOES, RAW

Serving: 1 medium (2-3/5" dia) (4.39 oz)   **Vegetable**

Calories	26	(5.9 cal/oz)	Carbohydrate	5.66 g	(2% DV)
Fat Calories	0	(0% fat)	Dietary Fiber	1.23 g	(5% DV)
Total Fat	0 g	(0% DV)	Protein	1.23 g	(2% DV)
Saturated Fat	0 g	(0% DV)	Vitamin A	766.3 IU	(15% DV)
Poly Fat	0 g		Vitamin C	23.4 mg	(39% DV)
Mono Fat	0 g		Calcium	6.2 mg	(1% DV)
Cholesterol	0 mg	(0% DV)	Iron	.6 mg	(3% DV)
Sodium	11.1 mg	(0% DV)	Folate	1.2 mcg	(5% DV)
Potassium	273.1 mg	(8% DV)	Beta Carotene	76.3 RE	

Ratings	Worst	Bad	Average	Good	Best
Weight Loss					10
LowCal Density					10
Filling				7	
Energizing		3			
Fiber			5		
Vitamins			6		
Minerals		3			
Overall				8	

TOMATOES, STEWED

Serving: 1 cup (9.11 oz)   **Vegetable**

Calories	181	(19.9 cal/oz)	Carbohydrate	28.81 g	(10% DV)
Fat Calories	69	(38% fat)	Dietary Fiber	5.1 g	(20% DV)
Total Fat	7.65 g	(12% DV)	Protein	5.1 g	(10% DV)
Saturated Fat	0 g	(0% DV)	Vitamin A	2017.1 IU	(40% DV)
Poly Fat	2.55 g		Vitamin C	53.6 mg	(89% DV)
Mono Fat	2.55 g		Calcium	38.3 mg	(4% DV)
Cholesterol	0 mg	(0% DV)	Iron	2 mg	(11% DV)
Sodium	632.4 mg	(26% DV)	Folate	5.1 mcg	(8% DV)
Potassium	744.6 mg	(21% DV)	Beta Carotene	181.1 RE	

Ratings	Worst	Bad	Average	Good	Best
Weight Loss		3			
LowCal Density				8	
Filling					9
Energizing			7		
Fiber					9
Vitamins					9
Minerals			5		
Overall				7	

TORTELLINI, CHEESE-FILLED, MEATLESS, VEGETABLES

Serving: 1 Stouffer's meal (6.96 oz)   **Entree**

Calories	419	(60.2 cal/oz)	Carbohydrate	26.52 g	(9% DV)
Fat Calories	263	(63% fat)	Dietary Fiber	1.95 g	(8% DV)
Total Fat	29.25 g	(45% DV)	Protein	13.65 g	(27% DV)
Saturated Fat	7.8 g	(39% DV)	Vitamin A	3824 IU	(76% DV)
Poly Fat	13.65 g		Vitamin C	46.8 mg	(78% DV)
Mono Fat	7.8 g		Calcium	306.2 mg	(31% DV)
Cholesterol	23.4 mg	(8% DV)	Iron	1.8 mg	(10% DV)
Sodium	520.7 mg	(22% DV)	Folate	13.7 mcg	(8% DV)
Potassium	237.9 mg	(7% DV)	Beta Carotene	368.6 RE	

Ratings	Worst	Bad	Average	Good	Best
Weight Loss		3			
LowCal Density			5		
Filling			5		
Energizing				7	
Fiber			6		
Vitamins					9
Minerals				7	
Overall			5		

TORTELLINI, MEAT-FILLED, WITH TOMATO SAUCE

Serving: 1 cup (7.5 oz)   **Entree**

Calories	284	(37.8 cal/oz)	Carbohydrate	33.18 g	(11% DV)
Fat Calories	95	(33% fat)	Dietary Fiber	4.2 g	(17% DV)
Total Fat	10.5 g	(16% DV)	Protein	14.7 g	(29% DV)
Saturated Fat	4.2 g	(21% DV)	Vitamin A	703.5 IU	(14% DV)
Poly Fat	2.1 g		Vitamin C	6.3 mg	(10% DV)
Mono Fat	4.2 g		Calcium	111.3 mg	(11% DV)
Cholesterol	90.3 mg	(30% DV)	Iron	2.6 mg	(14% DV)
Sodium	1293.6 mg	(54% DV)	Folate	14.7 mcg	(4% DV)
Potassium	279.3 mg	(8% DV)	Beta Carotene	46.2 RE	

Ratings	Worst	Bad	Average	Good	Best
Weight Loss			6		
LowCal Density				7	
Filling			6		
Energizing				8	
Fiber					9
Vitamins			6		
Minerals				7	
Overall				7	

TORTILLA CHIPS SALTY SNACKS, CORN BASE

Serving: 10 chips (.64 oz)   **Snack**

Calories	90	(140.9 cal/oz)	Carbohydrate	11.32 g	(4% DV)
Fat Calories	42	(47% fat)	Dietary Fiber	1.26 g	(5% DV)
Total Fat	4.68 g	(7% DV)	Protein	1.26 g	(3% DV)
Saturated Fat	.9 g	(5% DV)	VItamin A	35.3 IU	(1% DV)
Poly Fat	.72 g		Vitamin C	0 mg	(0% DV)
Mono Fat	2.7 g		Calcium	27.7 mg	(3% DV)
Cholesterol	0 mg	(0% DV)	Iron	.3 mg	(2% DV)
Sodium	95 mg	(4% DV)	Folate	1.3 mcg	(0% DV)
Potassium	35.5 mg	(1% DV)	Beta Carotene	3.6 RE	

Ratings	Worst	Bad	Average	Good	Best
Weight Loss				6	
LowCal Density	1				
Filling	2				
Energizing			5		
Fiber			5		
Vitamins	2				
Minerals		3			
Overall		3			

TORTILLA, CORN

Serving: 1 tortilla (approx 5" dia) (.46 oz)   **Bakery**

Calories	29	(62.7 cal/oz)	Carbohydrate	6.06 g	(2% DV)
Fat Calories	4	(12% fat)	Dietary Fiber	.65 g	(3% DV)
Total Fat	.39 g	(1% DV)	Protein	.78 g	(2% DV)
Saturated Fat	0 g	(0% DV)	VItamin A	22.4 IU	(0% DV)
Poly Fat	.13 g		Vitamin C	0 mg	(0% DV)
Mono Fat	.13 g		Calcium	22.8 mg	(2% DV)
Cholesterol	0 mg	(0% DV)	Iron	.2 mg	(1% DV)
Sodium	11.2 mg	(0% DV)	Folate	.8 mcg	(0% DV)
Potassium	20 mg	(1% DV)	Beta Carotene	2.2 RE	

Ratings	Worst	Bad	Average	Good	Best
Weight Loss					9
LowCal Density			5		
Filling	2				
Energizing		4			
Fiber		3			
Vitamins	2				
Minerals		3			
Overall			5		

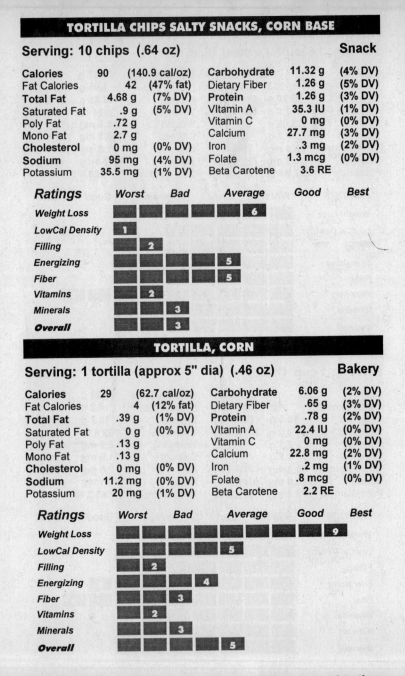

TORTILLA, FLOUR (WHEAT)

Serving: 1 medium (approx 8" dia) (1.86 oz)   **Bakery**

Calories	169	(90.9 cal/oz)	Carbohydrate	28.91 g	(10% DV)
Fat Calories	33	(19% fat)	Dietary Fiber	1.56 g	(6% DV)
Total Fat	3.64 g	(6% DV)	Protein	4.68 g	(9% DV)
Saturated Fat	.52 g	(3% DV)	VItamin A	0 IU	(0% DV)
Poly Fat	1.56 g		Vitamin C	0 mg	(0% DV)
Mono Fat	1.56 g		Calcium	42.6 mg	(4% DV)
Cholesterol	0 mg	(0% DV)	Iron	1.7 mg	(10% DV)
Sodium	248.6 mg	(10% DV)	Folate	4.7 mcg	(2% DV)
Potassium	68.1 mg	(2% DV)	Beta Carotene	0 RE	

Ratings	Worst	Bad	Average	Good	Best
Weight Loss			5		
LowCal Density	3				
Filling		4			
Energizing				7	
Fiber			5		
Vitamins		4			
Minerals		4			
Overall		4			

TOTAL

Serving: 1 cup (1.18 oz)   **Cereal**

Calories	116	(98.4 cal/oz)	Carbohydrate	26 g	(9% DV)
Fat Calories	6	(5% fat)	Dietary Fiber	2.97 g	(12% DV)
Total Fat	.66 g	(1% DV)	Protein	3.3 g	(7% DV)
Saturated Fat	0 g	(0% DV)	VItamin A	5820.2 IU	(116% DV)
Poly Fat	.33 g		Vitamin C	70 mg	(117% DV)
Mono Fat	0 g		Calcium	281.8 mg	(28% DV)
Cholesterol	0 mg	(0% DV)	Iron	21 mg	(116% DV)
Sodium	326 mg	(14% DV)	Folate	3.3 mcg	(116% DV)
Potassium	123.1 mg	(4% DV)	Beta Carotene	0 RE	

Ratings	Worst	Bad	Average	Good	Best
Weight Loss					9
LowCal Density	3				
Filling		4			
Energizing				7	
Fiber				8	
Vitamins					10
Minerals					10
Overall			7		

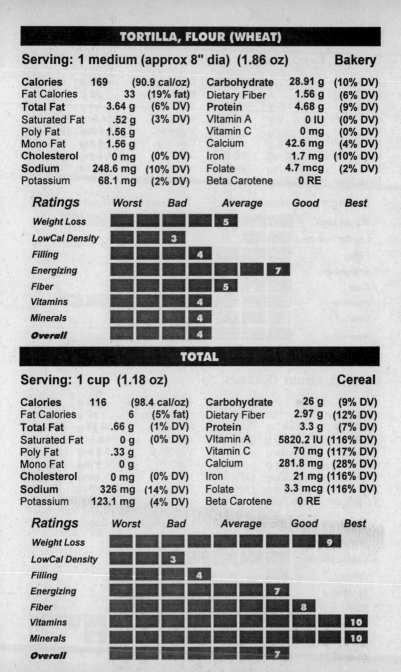

TRIX

Serving: 1 cup (1 oz)   Cereal

Calories	108	(107.8 cal/oz)	Carbohydrate	24.86 g	(8% DV)
Fat Calories	3	(2% fat)	Dietary Fiber	.28 g	(1% DV)
Total Fat	.28 g	(0% DV)	Protein	1.4 g	(3% DV)
Saturated Fat	0 g	(0% DV)	VItamin A	1234.5 IU	(25% DV)
Poly Fat	.28 g		Vitamin C	14.8 mg	(25% DV)
Mono Fat	0 g		Calcium	5.6 mg	(1% DV)
Cholesterol	0 mg	(0% DV)	Iron	4.5 mg	(25% DV)
Sodium	138.3 mg	(6% DV)	Folate	1.4 mcg	(25% DV)
Potassium	26.3 mg	(1% DV)	Beta Carotene	0 RE	

Ratings	Worst	Bad	Average	Good	Best
Weight Loss					9
LowCal Density	2				
Filling		4			
Energizing			6		
Fiber	2				
Vitamins					9
Minerals		4			
Overall			5		

TROUT, BAKED OR BROILED

Serving: 1 trout (5.82 oz)   Fish

Calories	306	(52.7 cal/oz)	Carbohydrate	.65 g	(0% DV)
Fat Calories	132	(43% fat)	Dietary Fiber	0 g	(0% DV)
Total Fat	14.67 g	(23% DV)	Protein	39.12 g	(78% DV)
Saturated Fat	3.26 g	(16% DV)	VItamin A	780.8 IU	(16% DV)
Poly Fat	4.89 g		Vitamin C	8.2 mg	(14% DV)
Mono Fat	4.89 g		Calcium	130.4 mg	(13% DV)
Cholesterol	112.5 mg	(37% DV)	Iron	.5 mg	(3% DV)
Sodium	570.5 mg	(24% DV)	Folate	39.1 mcg	(5% DV)
Potassium	868.8 mg	(25% DV)	Beta Carotene	4.9 RE	

Ratings	Worst	Bad	Average	Good	Best
Weight Loss	3				
LowCal Density			6		
Filling	1				
Energizing	2				
Fiber	1				
Vitamins					10
Minerals				8	
Overall		4			

TROUT, FLOURED OR BREADED, FRIED

Serving: 1 trout (6.96 oz)   **Fish**

Calories	521	(74.8 cal/oz)	Carbohydrate	18.52 g	(6% DV)
Fat Calories	263	(51% fat)	Dietary Fiber	1.95 g	(8% DV)
Total Fat	29.25 g	(45% DV)	Protein	44.85 g	(90% DV)
Saturated Fat	5.85 g	(29% DV)	VItamin A	177.5 IU	(4% DV)
Poly Fat	7.8 g		Vitamin C	0 mg	(0% DV)
Mono Fat	11.7 g		Calcium	124.8 mg	(12% DV)
Cholesterol	165.8 mg	(55% DV)	Iron	4.1 mg	(23% DV)
Sodium	826.8 mg	(34% DV)	Folate	44.9 mcg	(9% DV)
Potassium	754.7 mg	(22% DV)	Beta Carotene	0 RE	

Ratings	Worst	Bad	Average	Good	Best
Weight Loss	1				
LowCal Density			4		
Filling			4		
Energizing				6	
Fiber				6	
Vitamins				7	
Minerals					9
Overall			4		

TUNA NOODLE CASSEROLE, CREAM OR WHITE SAUCE

Serving: 1 cup (8 oz)   **Entree**

Calories	432	(54 cal/oz)	Carbohydrate	33.15 g	(11% DV)
Fat Calories	181	(42% fat)	Dietary Fiber	2.24 g	(9% DV)
Total Fat	20.16 g	(31% DV)	Protein	29.12 g	(58% DV)
Saturated Fat	4.48 g	(22% DV)	VItamin A	681 IU	(14% DV)
Poly Fat	6.72 g		Vitamin C	0 mg	(0% DV)
Mono Fat	6.72 g		Calcium	129.9 mg	(13% DV)
Cholesterol	47 mg	(16% DV)	Iron	2.6 mg	(15% DV)
Sodium	499.5 mg	(21% DV)	Folate	29.1 mcg	(4% DV)
Potassium	284.5 mg	(8% DV)	Beta Carotene	13.4 RE	

Ratings	Worst	Bad	Average	Good	Best
Weight Loss		3			
LowCal Density			6		
Filling			6		
Energizing				8	
Fiber			6		
Vitamins			7		
Minerals			7		
Overall		5			

TUNA SALAD

Serving: 1 cup (7.43 oz)   **Salad**

Calories	297	(40 cal/oz)	Carbohydrate	19.76 g	(7% DV)
Fat Calories	94	(31% fat)	Dietary Fiber	2.08 g	(8% DV)
Total Fat	**10.4 g**	**(16% DV)**	**Protein**	**29.12 g**	**(58% DV)**
Saturated Fat	2.08 g	(10% DV)	Vitamin A	178.9 IU	(4% DV)
Poly Fat	6.24 g		Vitamin C	4.2 mg	(7% DV)
Mono Fat	2.08 g		Calcium	33.3 mg	(3% DV)
Cholesterol	**41.6 mg**	**(14% DV)**	Iron	2.2 mg	(12% DV)
Sodium	**817.4 mg**	**(34% DV)**	Folate	29.1 mcg	(4% DV)
Potassium	405.6 mg	(12% DV)	Beta Carotene	4.2 RE	

Ratings	Worst	Bad	Average	Good	Best
Weight Loss		4			
LowCal Density			6		
Filling			5		
Energizing			6		
Fiber			6		
Vitamins				7	
Minerals			6		
Overall			5		

TUNA SALAD SANDWICH

Serving: 1 sandwich (5.43 oz)   **Sandwich**

Calories	325	(59.9 cal/oz)	Carbohydrate	31.31 g	(10% DV)
Fat Calories	123	(38% fat)	Dietary Fiber	1.52 g	(6% DV)
Total Fat	**13.68 g**	**(21% DV)**	**Protein**	**18 24 g**	**(36% DV)**
Saturated Fat	1.52 g	(8% DV)	Vitamin A	95.8 IU	(2% DV)
Poly Fat	6.08 g		Vitamin C	1.5 mg	(3% DV)
Mono Fat	4.56 g		Calcium	74.5 mg	(7% DV)
Cholesterol	**25.8 mg**	**(9% DV)**	Iron	2.6 mg	(14% DV)
Sodium	**656.6 mg**	**(27% DV)**	Folate	18.2 mcg	(6% DV)
Potassium	259.9 mg	(7% DV)	Beta Carotene	3 RE	

Ratings	Worst	Bad	Average	Good	Best
Weight Loss			5		
LowCal Density			5		
Filling			5		
Energizing				8	
Fiber			5		
Vitamins			6		
Minerals			6		
Overall			5		

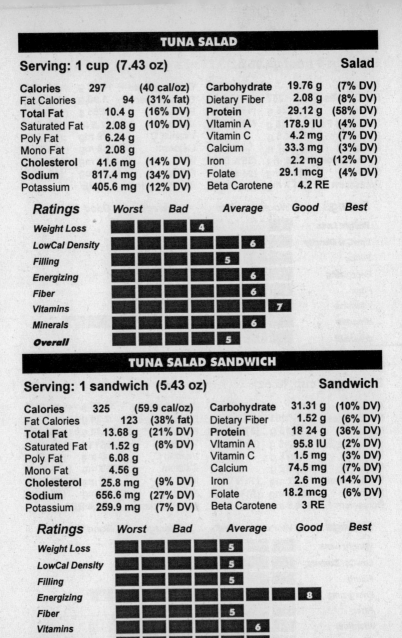

TUNA, CANNED, OIL PACK

Serving: 1 can, drained (5.71 oz) **Fish**

Calories	317	(55.5 cal/oz)	Carbohydrate	0 g	(0% DV)
Fat Calories	115	(36% fat)	Dietary Fiber	0 g	(0% DV)
Total Fat	12.8 g	(20% DV)	Protein	46.4 g	(93% DV)
Saturated Fat	3.2 g	(16% DV)	Vitamin A	124.8 IU	(2% DV)
Poly Fat	4.8 g		Vitamin C	0 mg	(0% DV)
Mono Fat	4.8 g		Calcium	20.8 mg	(2% DV)
Cholesterol	28.8 mg	(10% DV)	Iron	2.2 mg	(12% DV)
Sodium	566.4 mg	(24% DV)	Folate	46.4 mcg	(2% DV)
Potassium	331.2 mg	(9% DV)	Beta Carotene	0 RE	

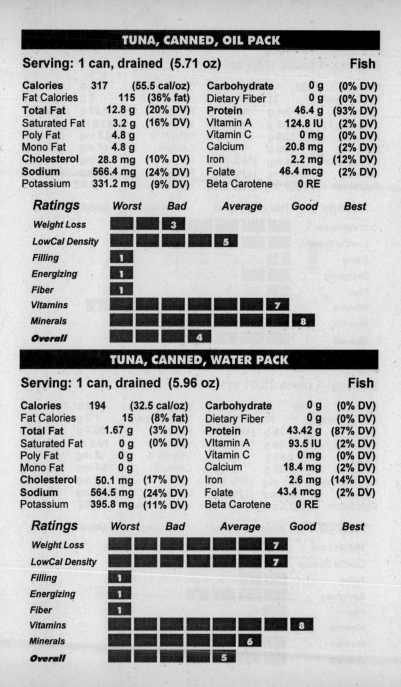

Ratings	Worst	Bad	Average	Good	Best
Weight Loss		3			
LowCal Density			5		
Filling	1				
Energizing	1				
Fiber	1				
Vitamins				7	
Minerals					8
Overall		4			

TUNA, CANNED, WATER PACK

Serving: 1 can, drained (5.96 oz) **Fish**

Calories	194	(32.5 cal/oz)	Carbohydrate	0 g	(0% DV)
Fat Calories	15	(8% fat)	Dietary Fiber	0 g	(0% DV)
Total Fat	1.67 g	(3% DV)	Protein	43.42 g	(87% DV)
Saturated Fat	0 g	(0% DV)	Vitamin A	93.5 IU	(2% DV)
Poly Fat	0 g		Vitamin C	0 mg	(0% DV)
Mono Fat	0 g		Calcium	18.4 mg	(2% DV)
Cholesterol	50.1 mg	(17% DV)	Iron	2.6 mg	(14% DV)
Sodium	564.5 mg	(24% DV)	Folate	43.4 mcg	(2% DV)
Potassium	395.8 mg	(11% DV)	Beta Carotene	0 RE	

Ratings	Worst	Bad	Average	Good	Best
Weight Loss				7	
LowCal Density				7	
Filling	1				
Energizing	1				
Fiber	1				
Vitamins				8	
Minerals			6		
Overall			5		

TUNA, FRESH, BAKED OR BROILED

Serving: 1 piece (3.04 oz)   **Fish**

Calories	130	(42.8 cal/oz)	Carbohydrate	.34 g	(0% DV)
Fat Calories	31	(24% fat)	Dietary Fiber	0 g	(0% DV)
Total Fat	3.4 g	(5% DV)	Protein	22.95 g	(46% DV)
Saturated Fat	.85 g	(4% DV)	Vltamin A	183.6 IU	(4% DV)
Poly Fat	.85 g		Vitamin C	2.6 mg	(4% DV)
Mono Fat	.85 g		Calcium	17 mg	(2% DV)
Cholesterol	45.1 mg	(15% DV)	Iron	.7 mg	(4% DV)
Sodium	299.2 mg	(12% DV)	Folate	23 mcg	(1% DV)
Potassium	446.3 mg	(13% DV)	Beta Carotene	2.6 RE	

Ratings	Worst	Bad	Average	Good	Best
Weight Loss				7	
LowCal Density				6	
Filling	1				
Energizing	2				
Fiber	1				
Vitamins					8
Minerals			5		
Overall			5		

TUNA, FRESH, FLOURED OR BREADED, FRIED

Serving: 1 piece (3.04 oz)   **Fish**

Calories	199	(65.4 cal/oz)	Carbohydrate	6.72 g	(2% DV)
Fat Calories	84	(42% fat)	Dietary Fiber	0 g	(0% DV)
Total Fat	9.35 g	(14% DV)	Protein	20.4 g	(41% DV)
Saturated Fat	2.55 g	(13% DV)	Vltamin A	70.6 IU	(1% DV)
Poly Fat	2.55 g		Vitamin C	.9 mg	(1% DV)
Mono Fat	4.25 g		Calcium	28.1 mg	(3% DV)
Cholesterol	56.1 mg	(19% DV)	Iron	1 mg	(6% DV)
Sodium	293.3 mg	(12% DV)	Folate	20.4 mcg	(1% DV)
Potassium	382.5 mg	(11% DV)	Beta Carotene	0 RE	

Ratings	Worst	Bad	Average	Good	Best
Weight Loss		4			
LowCal Density			5		
Filling	2				
Energizing		4			
Fiber	1				
Vitamins				7	
Minerals			5		
Overall		4			

TURBOT WITH VEGETABLES

Serving: 1 diet meal (8.61 oz)   Entree

Calories	330	(38.3 cal/oz)	Carbohydrate	18.8 g	(6% DV)
Fat Calories	174	(53% fat)	Dietary Fiber	4.82 g	(19% DV)
Total Fat	19.28 g	(30% DV)	Protein	21.69 g	(43% DV)
Saturated Fat	2.41 g	(12% DV)	Vltamin A	7572.2 IU	(151% DV)
Poly Fat	2.41 g		Vitamin C	7.2 mg	(12% DV)
Mono Fat	12.05 g		Calcium	41 mg	(4% DV)
Cholesterol	53 mg	(18% DV)	Iron	2.2 mg	(12% DV)
Sodium	1185.7 mg	(49% DV)	Folate	21.7 mcg	(8% DV)
Potassium	479.6 mg	(14% DV)	Beta Carotene	751.9 RE	

Ratings	Worst	Bad	Average	Good	Best
Weight Loss		4			
LowCal Density			7		
Filling		5			
Energizing			6		
Fiber					9
Vitamins					9
Minerals			6		
Overall			6		

TURKEY WITH GRAVY,DRESSING,POTATO,VEG,DESSERT

Serving: 1 Swanson meal (11.64 oz)   Entree

Calories	339	(29.1 cal/oz)	Carbohydrate	28.04 g	(9% DV)
Fat Calories	117	(35% fat)	Dietary Fiber	3.26 g	(13% DV)
Total Fat	13.04 g	(20% DV)	Protein	26.08 g	(52% DV)
Saturated Fat	3.26 g	(16% DV)	Vltamin A	612.9 IU	(12% DV)
Poly Fat	3.26 g		Vitamin C	13 mg	(22% DV)
Mono Fat	3.26 g		Calcium	71.7 mg	(7% DV)
Cholesterol	55.4 mg	(18% DV)	Iron	2.3 mg	(13% DV)
Sodium	1793 mg	(75% DV)	Folate	26.1 mcg	(11% DV)
Potassium	570.5 mg	(16% DV)	Beta Carotene	39.1 RE	

Ratings	Worst	Bad	Average	Good	Best
Weight Loss			5		
LowCal Density			7		
Filling			7		
Energizing			7		
Fiber			8		
Vitamins			7		
Minerals			7		
Overall			7		

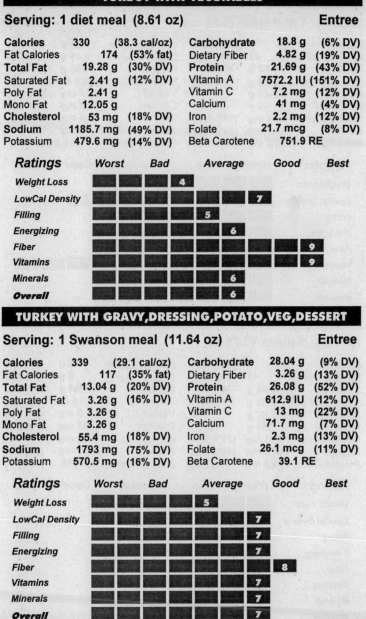

TURKEY WITH VEGETABLE, STUFFING

Serving: 1 diet meal (8.61 oz)　　　　　　　　　　**Entree**

Calories	198	(23 cal/oz)	Carbohydrate	17.11 g	(6% DV)
Fat Calories	43	(22% fat)	Dietary Fiber	2.41 g	(10% DV)
Total Fat	**4.82 g**	**(7% DV)**	**Protein**	**21.69 g**	**(43% DV)**
Saturated Fat	2.41 g	(12% DV)	VItamin A	11394.5 IU	(228% DV)
Poly Fat	2.41 g		Vitamin C	33.7 mg	(56% DV)
Mono Fat	0 g		Calcium	89.2 mg	(9% DV)
Cholesterol	**50.6 mg**	**(17% DV)**	Iron	2.4 mg	(13% DV)
Sodium	**826.6 mg**	**(34% DV)**	Folate	21.7 mcg	(10% DV)
Potassium	530.2 mg	(15% DV)	Beta Carotene	1139.9 RE	

Ratings	Worst	Bad	Average	Good	Best
Weight Loss				7	
LowCal Density				8	
Filling			6		
Energizing			6		
Fiber			7		
Vitamins					10
Minerals			7		
Overall			7		

TURKEY, DARK MEAT, ROASTED, SKIN NOT EATEN

Serving: 1 piece (2.79 oz)　　　　　　　　　　**Poultry**

Calories	145	(52 cal/oz)	Carbohydrate	0 g	(0% DV)
Fat Calories	49	(34% fat)	Dietary Fiber	0 g	(0% DV)
Total Fat	**5.46 g**	**(8% DV)**	**Protein**	**21.84 g**	**(44% DV)**
Saturated Fat	1.56 g	(8% DV)	VItamin A	0 IU	(0% DV)
Poly Fat	1.56 g		Vitamin C	0 mg	(0% DV)
Mono Fat	1.56 g		Calcium	25 mg	(2% DV)
Cholesterol	**65.5 mg**	**(22% DV)**	Iron	1.8 mg	(10% DV)
Sodium	**241.8 mg**	**(10% DV)**	Folate	21.8 mcg	(2% DV)
Potassium	224.6 mg	(6% DV)	Beta Carotene	0 RE	

Ratings	Worst	Bad	Average	Good	Best
Weight Loss			6		
LowCal Density			6		
Filling	1				
Energizing	1				
Fiber	1				
Vitamins			4		
Minerals			6		
Overall		4			

TURKEY, LIGHT MEAT, ROASTED, SKIN NOT EATEN

Serving: 1 piece (2.68 oz)   **Poultry**

Calories	117	(43.7 cal/oz)	Carbohydrate	0 g	(0% DV)
Fat Calories	20	(17% fat)	Dietary Fiber	0 g	(0% DV)
Total Fat	2.25 g	(3% DV)	Protein	22.5 g	(45% DV)
Saturated Fat	.75 g	(4% DV)	Vitamin A	0 IU	(0% DV)
Poly Fat	.75 g		Vitamin C	0 mg	(0% DV)
Mono Fat	.75 g		Calcium	14.3 mg	(1% DV)
Cholesterol	51.8 mg	(17% DV)	Iron	1 mg	(6% DV)
Sodium	221.3 mg	(9% DV)	Folate	22.5 mcg	(1% DV)
Potassium	227.3 mg	(6% DV)	Beta Carotene	0 RE	

Ratings	Worst	Bad	Average	Good	Best
Weight Loss				8	
LowCal Density			6		
Filling	1				
Energizing	1				
Fiber	1				
Vitamins			6		
Minerals			5		
Overall			5		

TURNIP, COOKED WITHOUT ADDED FAT

Serving: 1 cup, pieces (5.57 oz)   **Vegetable**

Calories	28	(5 cal/oz)	Carbohydrate	7.64 g	(3% DV)
Fat Calories	0	(0% fat)	Dietary Fiber	3.12 g	(12% DV)
Total Fat	0 g	(0% DV)	Protein	1.56 g	(3% DV)
Saturated Fat	0 g	(0% DV)	Vitamin A	0 IU	(0% DV)
Poly Fat	0 g		Vitamin C	18.7 mg	(31% DV)
Mono Fat	0 g		Calcium	34.3 mg	(3% DV)
Cholesterol	0 mg	(0% DV)	Iron	.3 mg	(2% DV)
Sodium	438.4 mg	(18% DV)	Folate	1.6 mcg	(4% DV)
Potassium	209 mg	(6% DV)	Beta Carotene	0 RE	

Ratings	Worst	Bad	Average	Good	Best
Weight Loss					10
LowCal Density					10
Filling					10
Energizing		4			
Fiber				8	
Vitamins			5		
Minerals	3				
Overall				9	

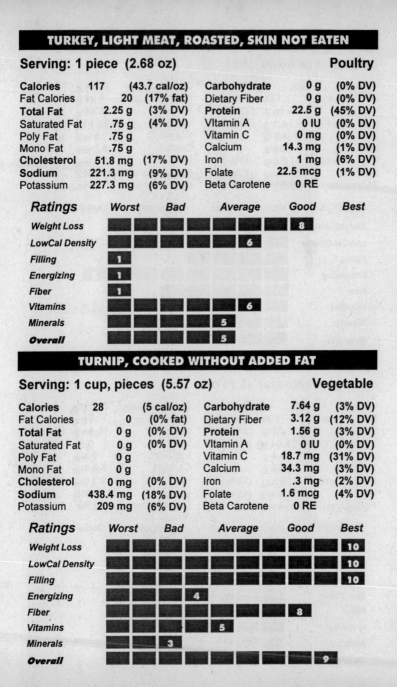

TURNOVER OR DUMPLING, APPLE

Serving: 1 turnover (2.93 oz)   **Dessert**

Calories	289	(98.8 cal/oz)	Carbohydrate	36.16 g	(12% DV)
Fat Calories	133	(46% fat)	Dietary Fiber	1.64 g	(7% DV)
Total Fat	14.76 g	(23% DV)	Protein	3.28 g	(7% DV)
Saturated Fat	4.1 g	(20% DV)	Vitamin A	22.1 IU	(0% DV)
Poly Fat	4.1 g		Vitamin C	.8 mg	(1% DV)
Mono Fat	6.56 g		Calcium	5.7 mg	(1% DV)
Cholesterol	0 mg	(0% DV)	Iron	1.3 mg	(7% DV)
Sodium	261.6 mg	(11% DV)	Folate	3.3 mcg	(1% DV)
Potassium	55.8 mg	(2% DV)	Beta Carotene	.8 RE	

Ratings	Worst	Bad	Average	Good	Best
Weight Loss		4			
LowCal Density	3				
Filling		4			
Energizing					8
Fiber			5		
Vitamins		4			
Minerals	3				
Overall		4			

TURNOVER, MEAT-FILLED, NO GRAVY

Serving: 1 turnover (3.14 oz)   **Entree**

Calories	334	(106.5 cal/oz)	Carbohydrate	21.91 g	(7% DV)
Fat Calories	198	(59% fat)	Dietary Fiber	.88 g	(4% DV)
Total Fat	22 g	(34% DV)	Protein	11.44 g	(23% DV)
Saturated Fat	7.04 g	(35% DV)	Vitamin A	0 IU	(0% DV)
Poly Fat	4.4 g		Vitamin C	0 mg	(0% DV)
Mono Fat	9.68 g		Calcium	8.8 mg	(1% DV)
Cholesterol	29 mg	(10% DV)	Iron	2.3 mg	(13% DV)
Sodium	369.6 mg	(15% DV)	Folate	11.4 mcg	(2% DV)
Potassium	110 mg	(3% DV)	Beta Carotene	0 RE	

Ratings	Worst	Bad	Average	Good	Best
Weight Loss		3			
LowCal Density	2				
Filling		3			
Energizing				6	
Fiber		4			
Vitamins		4			
Minerals			5		
Overall		3			

VEAL CHOP, LEAN ONLY EATEN

Serving: 1 chop (3.04 oz)   **Meat**

Calories	178	(58.4 cal/oz)	Carbohydrate	0 g	(0% DV)
Fat Calories	61	(34% fat)	Dietary Fiber	0 g	(0% DV)
Total Fat	6.8 g	(10% DV)	Protein	28.05 g	(56% DV)
Saturated Fat	2.55 g	(13% DV)	VItamin A	0 IU	(0% DV)
Poly Fat	0 g		Vitamin C	0 mg	(0% DV)
Mono Fat	2.55 g		Calcium	31.5 mg	(3% DV)
Cholesterol	143.7 mg	(48% DV)	Iron	1.1 mg	(6% DV)
Sodium	276.3 mg	(12% DV)	Folate	28.1 mcg	(3% DV)
Potassium	239.7 mg	(7% DV)	Beta Carotene	0 RE	

Ratings	Worst	Bad	Average	Good	Best
Weight Loss			5		
LowCal Density			5		
Filling	1				
Energizing	1				
Fiber	1				
Vitamins			5		
Minerals				6	
Overall		4			

VEAL CUTLET OR STEAK, LEAN ONLY

Serving: 1 piece (3.04 oz)   **Meat**

Calories	155	(50.9 cal/oz)	Carbohydrate	0 g	(0% DV)
Fat Calories	38	(25% fat)	Dietary Fiber	0 g	(0% DV)
Total Fat	4.25 g	(7% DV)	Protein	28.05 g	(56% DV)
Saturated Fat	.85 g	(4% DV)	VItamin A	0 IU	(0% DV)
Poly Fat	0 g		Vitamin C	0 mg	(0% DV)
Mono Fat	1.7 g		Calcium	6 mg	(1% DV)
Cholesterol	90.1 mg	(30% DV)	Iron	.7 mg	(4% DV)
Sodium	261.8 mg	(11% DV)	Folate	28.1 mcg	(3% DV)
Potassium	373.2 mg	(11% DV)	Beta Carotene	0 RE	

Ratings	Worst	Bad	Average	Good	Best
Weight Loss			6		
LowCal Density			6		
Filling	1				
Energizing	1				
Fiber	1				
Vitamins				7	
Minerals			6		
Overall			5		

VEAL PARMIGIANA, VEGETABLE, TORTELLINI IN BUTTER

Serving: 1 meal (12.14 oz)   Entree

Calories	707	(58.3 cal/oz)	Carbohydrate	54.74 g	(18% DV)
Fat Calories	337	(48% fat)	Dietary Fiber	3.4 g	(14% DV)
Total Fat	37.4 g	(58% DV)	Protein	37.4 g	(75% DV)
Saturated Fat	17 g	(85% DV)	Vitamin A	1788.4 IU	(36% DV)
Poly Fat	6.8 g		Vitamin C	10.2 mg	(17% DV)
Mono Fat	13.6 g		Calcium	414.8 mg	(41% DV)
Cholesterol	306 mg	(102% DV)	Iron	5.2 mg	(29% DV)
Sodium	1727.2 mg	(72% DV)	Folate	37.4 mcg	(14% DV)
Potassium	686.8 mg	(20% DV)	Beta Carotene	95.2 RE	

Ratings	Worst	Bad	Average	Good	Best
Weight Loss	2				
LowCal Density			5		
Filling			7		
Energizing					10
Fiber				8	
Vitamins				8	
Minerals					9
Overall			6		

VEAL PATTY, BREADED, COOKED

Serving: 1 patty (2.82 oz)   Meat

Calories	209	(74 cal/oz)	Carbohydrate	6.4 g	(2% DV)
Fat Calories	114	(55% fat)	Dietary Fiber	0 g	(0% DV)
Total Fat	12.64 g	(19% DV)	Protein	16.59 g	(33% DV)
Saturated Fat	4.74 g	(24% DV)	Vitamin A	27.7 IU	(1% DV)
Poly Fat	1.58 g		Vitamin C	0 mg	(0% DV)
Mono Fat	5.53 g		Calcium	24.5 mg	(2% DV)
Cholesterol	80.6 mg	(27% DV)	Iron	.9 mg	(5% DV)
Sodium	309.7 mg	(13% DV)	Folate	16.6 mcg	(3% DV)
Potassium	220.4 mg	(6% DV)	Beta Carotene	0 RE	

Ratings	Worst	Bad	Average	Good	Best
Weight Loss		3			
LowCal Density			4		
Filling	2				
Energizing			4		
Fiber	1				
Vitamins			5		
Minerals			5		
Overall		3			

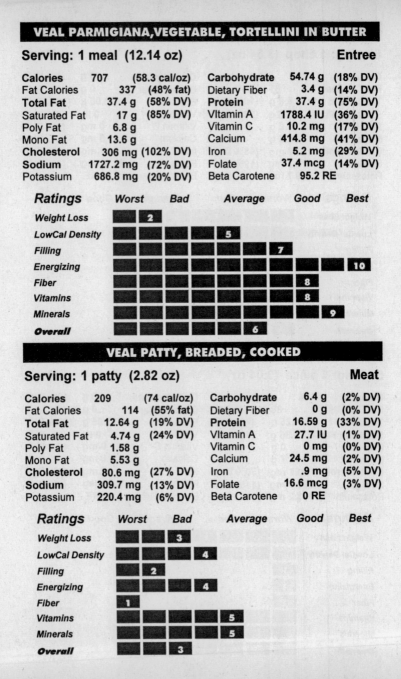

VEAL SCALLOPINI

Serving: 1 slice (3.43 oz)   **Entree**

Calories	257	(75 cal/oz)	Carbohydrate	1.06 g	(0% DV)
Fat Calories	173	(67% fat)	Dietary Fiber	0 g	(0% DV)
Total Fat	19.2 g	(30% DV)	Protein	17.28 g	(35% DV)
Saturated Fat	5.76 g	(29% DV)	Vitamin A	641.3 IU	(13% DV)
Poly Fat	3.84 g		Vitamin C	0 mg	(0% DV)
Mono Fat	8.64 g		Calcium	45.1 mg	(5% DV)
Cholesterol	62.4 mg	(21% DV)	Iron	.7 mg	(4% DV)
Sodium	381.1 mg	(16% DV)	Folate	17.3 mcg	(2% DV)
Potassium	227.5 mg	(7% DV)	Beta Carotene	14.4 RE	

Ratings	Worst	Bad	Average	Good	Best
Weight Loss		3			
LowCal Density			4		
Filling	1				
Energizing	2				
Fiber	1				
Vitamins				5	
Minerals				5	
Overall		3			

VEAL WITH PEPPERS, SAUCE, RICE (DIET MEAL)

Serving: 1 meal (13.18 oz)   **Entree**

Calories	306	(23.2 cal/oz)	Carbohydrate	32.47 g	(11% DV)
Fat Calories	66	(22% fat)	Dietary Fiber	3.69 g	(15% DV)
Total Fat	7.38 g	(11% DV)	Protein	25.83 g	(52% DV)
Saturated Fat	3.69 g	(18% DV)	Vitamin A	2745.4 IU	(55% DV)
Poly Fat	0 g		Vitamin C	73.8 mg	(123% DV)
Mono Fat	3.69 g		Calcium	55.4 mg	(6% DV)
Cholesterol	81.2 mg	(27% DV)	Iron	3.1 mg	(17% DV)
Sodium	885.6 mg	(37% DV)	Folate	25.8 mcg	(10% DV)
Potassium	848.7 mg	(24% DV)	Beta Carotene	273.1 RE	

Ratings	Worst	Bad	Average	Good	Best
Weight Loss			6		
LowCal Density				8	
Filling				8	
Energizing				8	
Fiber				8	
Vitamins					10
Minerals				8	
Overall				8	

VEAL, GROUND OR PATTY, COOKED

Serving: 1 patty (2.39 oz)　　　　　　　　**Meat**

Calories	156	(65.3 cal/oz)	Carbohydrate	0 g	(0% DV)
Fat Calories	78	(50% fat)	Dietary Fiber	0 g	(0% DV)
Total Fat	**8.71 g**	**(13% DV)**	**Protein**	**17.42 g**	**(35% DV)**
Saturated Fat	4.02 g	(20% DV)	Vitamin A	0 IU	(0% DV)
Poly Fat	.67 g		Vitamin C	0 mg	(0% DV)
Mono Fat	4.02 g		Calcium	7.4 mg	(1% DV)
Cholesterol	**67 mg**	**(22% DV)**	Iron	.7 mg	(4% DV)
Sodium	**197.7 mg**	**(8% DV)**	Folate	17.4 mcg	(2% DV)
Potassium	197 mg	(6% DV)	Beta Carotene	0 RE	

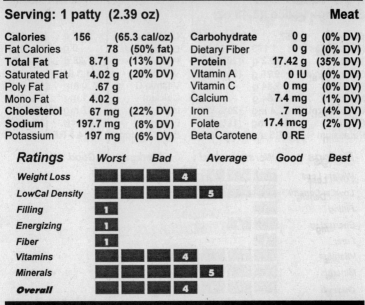

Ratings	Worst	Bad	Average	Good	Best
Weight Loss			4		
LowCal Density			5		
Filling	1				
Energizing	1				
Fiber	1				
Vitamins			4		
Minerals			5		
Overall			4		

VEAL, ROASTED, LEAN ONLY EATEN

Serving: 1 piece (3.04 oz)　　　　　　　　**Meat**

Calories	134	(44.2 cal/oz)	Carbohydrate	0 g	(0% DV)
Fat Calories	46	(34% fat)	Dietary Fiber	0 g	(0% DV)
Total Fat	**5.1 g**	**(8% DV)**	**Protein**	**21.25 g**	**(42% DV)**
Saturated Fat	1.7 g	(8% DV)	Vitamin A	0 IU	(0% DV)
Poly Fat	0 g		Vitamin C	0 mg	(0% DV)
Mono Fat	1.7 g		Calcium	17 mg	(2% DV)
Cholesterol	**113.9 mg**	**(38% DV)**	Iron	.8 mg	(5% DV)
Sodium	**288.2 mg**	**(12% DV)**	Folate	21.3 mcg	(3% DV)
Potassium	262.7 mg	(8% DV)	Beta Carotene	0 RE	

Ratings	Worst	Bad	Average	Good	Best
Weight Loss				6	
LowCal Density				6	
Filling	1				
Energizing	1				
Fiber	1				
Vitamins			5		
Minerals				6	
Overall			5		

VEGETABLE BEEF NOODLE SOUP, WITH WATER

Serving: 1 cup (8.71 oz)   **Soup**

Calories	81	(9.2 cal/oz)	Carbohydrate	9.52 g	(3% DV)
Fat Calories	22	(27% fat)	Dietary Fiber	0 g	(0% DV)
Total Fat	2.44 g	(4% DV)	Protein	4.88 g	(10% DV)
Saturated Fat	0 g	(0% DV)	VItamin A	1261.5 IU	(25% DV)
Poly Fat	0 g		Vitamin C	2.4 mg	(4% DV)
Mono Fat	0 g		Calcium	17.1 mg	(2% DV)
Cholesterol	4.9 mg	(2% DV)	Iron	1.1 mg	(6% DV)
Sodium	954 mg	(40% DV)	Folate	4.9 mcg	(2% DV)
Potassium	136.6 mg	(4% DV)	Beta Carotene	126.9 RE	

Ratings	Worst	Bad	Average	Good	Best
Weight Loss				7	
LowCal Density					9
Filling				7	
Energizing		4			
Fiber	1				
Vitamins			5		
Minerals		4			
Overall				7	

VEGETABLE CHICKEN OR TURKEY SOUP, WITH WATER

Serving: 1 cup (8.61 oz)   **Soup**

Calories	75	(8.7 cal/oz)	Carbohydrate	8.68 g	(3% DV)
Fat Calories	22	(29% fat)	Dietary Fiber	0 g	(0% DV)
Total Fat	2.41 g	(4% DV)	Protein	2.41 g	(5% DV)
Saturated Fat	0 g	(0% DV)	VItamin A	2549.8 IU	(51% DV)
Poly Fat	0 g		Vitamin C	0 mg	(0% DV)
Mono Fat	2.41 g		Calcium	16.9 mg	(2% DV)
Cholesterol	7.2 mg	(2% DV)	Iron	.8 mg	(5% DV)
Sodium	925.4 mg	(39% DV)	Folate	2.4 mcg	(1% DV)
Potassium	166.3 mg	(5% DV)	Beta Carotene	255.5 RE	

Ratings	Worst	Bad	Average	Good	Best
Weight Loss				7	
LowCal Density					9
Filling				7	
Energizing		4			
Fiber	1				
Vitamins			5		
Minerals		3			
Overall				7	

Serving: 1 cup (7.04 oz)　　　　　　**Vegetable**

Calories	179	(25.5 cal/oz)	Carbohydrate	25.81 g	(9% DV)
Fat Calories	53	(30% fat)	Dietary Fiber	3.94 g	(16% DV)
Total Fat	5.91 g	(9% DV)	Protein	5.91 g	(12% DV)
Saturated Fat	1.97 g	(10% DV)	Vitamin A	6900.9 IU	(138% DV)
Poly Fat	1.97 g		Vitamin C	33.5 mg	(56% DV)
Mono Fat	1.97 g		Calcium	43.3 mg	(4% DV)
Cholesterol	0 mg	(0% DV)	Iron	1.7 mg	(9% DV)
Sodium	862.9 mg	(36% DV)	Folate	5.9 mcg	(11% DV)
Potassium	287.6 mg	(8% DV)	Beta Carotene	665.9 RE	

Ratings	Worst	Bad	Average	Good	Best
Weight Loss	3				
LowCal Density				8	
Filling			7		
Energizing			6		
Fiber				9	
Vitamins					10
Minerals		5			
Overall			6		

Serving: 1 cup (4.54 oz)　　　　　　**Vegetable**

Calories	48	(10.6 cal/oz)	Carbohydrate	9.65 g	(3% DV)
Fat Calories	0	(0% fat)	Dietary Fiber	3.81 g	(15% DV)
Total Fat	0 g	(0% DV)	Protein	3.81 g	(8% DV)
Saturated Fat	0 g	(0% DV)	Vitamin A	1145.5 IU	(23% DV)
Poly Fat	0 g		Vitamin C	47 mg	(78% DV)
Mono Fat	0 g		Calcium	38.1 mg	(4% DV)
Cholesterol	0 mg	(0% DV)	Iron	1.2 mg	(7% DV)
Sodium	308.6 mg	(13% DV)	Folate	3.8 mcg	(10% DV)
Potassium	355.6 mg	(10% DV)	Beta Carotene	114.3 RE	

Ratings	Worst	Bad	Average	Good	Best
Weight Loss				9	
LowCal Density				9	
Filling			7		
Energizing		4			
Fiber				9	
Vitamins				8	
Minerals		4			
Overall				8	

VEGETABLE SOUP, PREPARED WITH WATER

Serving: 1 cup (8.61 oz)   Soup

Calories	82	(9.5 cal/oz)	Carbohydrate	13.01 g	(4% DV)
Fat Calories	22	(26% fat)	Dietary Fiber	0 g	(0% DV)
Total Fat	2.41 g	(4% DV)	Protein	2.41 g	(5% DV)
Saturated Fat	0 g	(0% DV)	Vitamin A	2089.5 IU	(42% DV)
Poly Fat	0 g		Vitamin C	2.4 mg	(4% DV)
Mono Fat	0 g		Calcium	16.9 mg	(2% DV)
Cholesterol	2.4 mg	(1% DV)	Iron	1 mg	(5% DV)
Sodium	809.8 mg	(34% DV)	Folate	2.4 mcg	(2% DV)
Potassium	192.8 mg	(6% DV)	Beta Carotene	209.7 RE	

Ratings	Worst	Bad	Average	Good	Best
Weight Loss				7	
LowCal Density					9
Filling				8	
Energizing			5		
Fiber	1				
Vitamins			5		
Minerals		4			
Overall				7	

WAFFLE, FRUIT

Serving: 1 round (4" dia) (1.39 oz)   Breakfast

Calories	97	(69.6 cal/oz)	Carbohydrate	15.83 g	(5% DV)
Fat Calories	21	(22% fat)	Dietary Fiber	.78 g	(3% DV)
Total Fat	2.34 g	(4% DV)	Protein	2.73 g	(5% DV)
Saturated Fat	.78 g	(4% DV)	Vitamin A	62 IU	(1% DV)
Poly Fat	.39 g		Vitamin C	1.2 mg	(2% DV)
Mono Fat	.78 g		Calcium	113.9 mg	(11% DV)
Cholesterol	17.6 mg	(6% DV)	Iron	.6 mg	(3% DV)
Sodium	271.8 mg	(11% DV)	Folate	2.7 mcg	(1% DV)
Potassium	80.3 mg	(2% DV)	Beta Carotene	1.6 RE	

Ratings	Worst	Bad	Average	Good	Best
Weight Loss				8	
LowCal Density		4			
Filling		4			
Energizing			5		
Fiber	3				
Vitamins	3				
Minerals			5		
Overall			5		

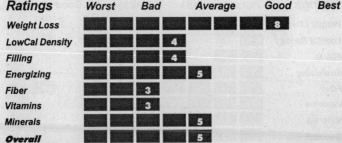

WAFFLE, PLAIN

Serving: 1 round (4" dia) (1.39 oz)   **Breakfast**

Calories	107	(77.2 cal/oz)	Carbohydrate	17.08 g	(6% DV)
Fat Calories	25	(23% fat)	Dietary Fiber	.39 g	(2% DV)
Total Fat	2.73 g	(4% DV)	Protein	3.12 g	(6% DV)
Saturated Fat	1.17 g	(6% DV)	Vitamin A	63.2 IU	(1% DV)
Poly Fat	.39 g		Vitamin C	.4 mg	(1% DV)
Mono Fat	.78 g		Calcium	131.8 mg	(13% DV)
Cholesterol	20.3 mg	(7% DV)	Iron	.7 mg	(4% DV)
Sodium	315.5 mg	(13% DV)	Folate	3.1 mcg	(1% DV)
Potassium	85 mg	(2% DV)	Beta Carotene	.8 RE	

Ratings	Worst	Bad	Average	Good	Best
Weight Loss				8	
LowCal Density		4			
Filling		3			
Energizing			6		
Fiber	2				
Vitamins		3			
Minerals			5		
Overall			5		

WALNUTS

Serving: 14 halves (1 oz)   **Snack**

Calories	180	(179.8 cal/oz)	Carbohydrate	5.12 g	(2% DV)
Fat Calories	156	(87% fat)	Dietary Fiber	1.4 g	(6% DV)
Total Fat	17.36 g	(27% DV)	Protein	3.92 g	(8% DV)
Saturated Fat	1.68 g	(8% DV)	Vitamin A	34.7 IU	(1% DV)
Poly Fat	10.92 g		Vitamin C	.8 mg	(1% DV)
Mono Fat	3.92 g		Calcium	26.3 mg	(3% DV)
Cholesterol	0 mg	(0% DV)	Iron	.7 mg	(4% DV)
Sodium	2.8 mg	(0% DV)	Folate	3.9 mcg	(5% DV)
Potassium	140.6 mg	(4% DV)	Beta Carotene	3.4 RE	

Ratings	Worst	Bad	Average	Good	Best
Weight Loss	2				
LowCal Density	1				
Filling	2				
Energizing		3			
Fiber			5		
Vitamins		4			
Minerals			5		
Overall	2				

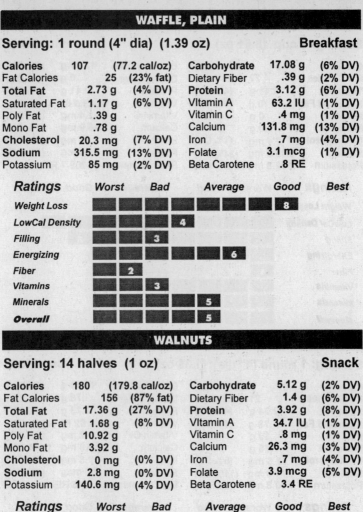

WATER CHESTNUT

Serving: 1 cup (5.64 oz)   Vegetable

Calories	79	(14 cal/oz)	Carbohydrate	19.59 g	(7% DV)
Fat Calories	0	(0% fat)	Dietary Fiber	3.16 g	(13% DV)
Total Fat	0 g	(0% DV)	Protein	1.58 g	(3% DV)
Saturated Fat	0 g	(0% DV)	Vitamin A	6.3 IU	(0% DV)
Poly Fat	0 g		Vitamin C	1.6 mg	(3% DV)
Mono Fat	0 g		Calcium	6.3 mg	(1% DV)
Cholesterol	0 mg	(0% DV)	Iron	1.4 mg	(8% DV)
Sodium	12.6 mg	(1% DV)	Folate	1.6 mcg	(2% DV)
Potassium	186.4 mg	(5% DV)	Beta Carotene	0 RE	

Ratings	Worst	Bad	Average	Good	Best
Weight Loss					9
LowCal Density					9
Filling					9
Energizing			6		
Fiber				8	
Vitamins		3			
Minerals			4		
Overall				8	

WATERMELON, RAW

Serving: 1 wedge (1/16 of melon) (10.21 oz)   Fruit

Calories	92	(9 cal/oz)	Carbohydrate	20.59 g	(7% DV)
Fat Calories	0	(0% fat)	Dietary Fiber	0 g	(0% DV)
Total Fat	0 g	(0% DV)	Protein	2.86 g	(6% DV)
Saturated Fat	0 g	(0% DV)	Vitamin A	1046.8 IU	(21% DV)
Poly Fat	0 g		Vitamin C	28.6 mg	(48% DV)
Mono Fat	0 g		Calcium	22.9 mg	(2% DV)
Cholesterol	0 mg	(0% DV)	Iron	.5 mg	(3% DV)
Sodium	5.7 mg	(0% DV)	Folate	2.9 mcg	(1% DV)
Potassium	331.8 mg	(9% DV)	Beta Carotene	105.8 RE	

Ratings	Worst	Bad	Average	Good	Best
Weight Loss					9
LowCal Density					9
Filling					10
Energizing			6		
Fiber	1				
Vitamins			6		
Minerals		4			
Overall				8	

WHEAT CEREAL, CHOCOLATE FLAVORED, COOKED

Serving: 1 cup (8.79 oz)   Cereal

Calories	207	(23.5 cal/oz)	Carbohydrate	32.47 g	(11% DV)
Fat Calories	44	(21% fat)	Dietary Fiber	2.46 g	(10% DV)
Total Fat	4.92 g	(8% DV)	Protein	9.84 g	(20% DV)
Saturated Fat	2.46 g	(12% DV)	Vitamin A	440.3 IU	(9% DV)
Poly Fat	0 g		Vitamin C	0 mg	(0% DV)
Mono Fat	2.46 g		Calcium	275.5 mg	(28% DV)
Cholesterol	17.2 mg	(6% DV)	Iron	1.5 mg	(8% DV)
Sodium	730.6 mg	(30% DV)	Folate	9.8 mcg	(6% DV)
Potassium	504.3 mg	(14% DV)	Beta Carotene	4.9 RE	

Ratings	Worst	Bad	Average	Good	Best
Weight Loss			5		
LowCal Density				8	
Filling				8	
Energizing				8	
Fiber				7	
Vitamins		4			
Minerals				8	
Overall				7	

WHEATIES

Serving: 1 cup (1.04 oz)   Cereal

Calories	101	(97.3 cal/oz)	Carbohydrate	23.05 g	(8% DV)
Fat Calories	5	(5% fat)	Dietary Fiber	2.61 g	(10% DV)
Total Fat	.58 g	(1% DV)	Protein	2.9 g	(6% DV)
Saturated Fat	0 g	(0% DV)	Vitamin A	1278.6 IU	(26% DV)
Poly Fat	.29 g		Vitamin C	15.4 mg	(26% DV)
Mono Fat	0 g		Calcium	43.8 mg	(4% DV)
Cholesterol	0 mg	(0% DV)	Iron	4.6 mg	(26% DV)
Sodium	276.1 mg	(12% DV)	Folate	2.9 mcg	(26% DV)
Potassium	108.5 mg	(3% DV)	Beta Carotene	0 RE	

Ratings	Worst	Bad	Average	Good	Best
Weight Loss				9	
LowCal Density	3				
Filling		4			
Energizing			6		
Fiber			7		
Vitamins				9	
Minerals			6		
Overall			6		

WHIPPED TOPPING, NONDAIRY, FROZEN

Serving: 1 cup (2.68 oz)　　　　　　　　**Fat & Oil**

Calories	239	(89 cal/oz)	Carbohydrate	17.33 g	(6% DV)
Fat Calories	169	(71% fat)	Dietary Fiber	0 g	(0% DV)
Total Fat	18.75 g	(29% DV)	Protein	.75 g	(2% DV)
Saturated Fat	16.5 g	(82% DV)	VItamin A	645.8 IU	(13% DV)
Poly Fat	.75 g		Vitamin C	0 mg	(0% DV)
Mono Fat	1.5 g		Calcium	4.5 mg	(0% DV)
Cholesterol	0 mg	(0% DV)	Iron	.1 mg	(0% DV)
Sodium	18.8 mg	(1% DV)	Folate	.8 mcg	(0% DV)
Potassium	13.5 mg	(0% DV)	Beta Carotene	64.5 RE	

Ratings	Worst	Bad	Average	Good	Best
Weight Loss	1				
LowCal Density		3			
Filling		3			
Energizing				6	
Fiber	1				
Vitamins		3			
Minerals	2				
Overall	2				

WHITING, BAKED OR BROILED

Serving: 1 piece (3.04 oz)　　　　　　　　**Fish**

Calories	112	(36.9 cal/oz)	Carbohydrate	.34 g	(0% DV)
Fat Calories	31	(27% fat)	Dietary Fiber	0 g	(0% DV)
Total Fat	3.4 g	(5% DV)	Protein	17.85 g	(36% DV)
Saturated Fat	.85 g	(4% DV)	VItamin A	219.3 IU	(4% DV)
Poly Fat	.85 g		Vitamin C	1.7 mg	(3% DV)
Mono Fat	1.7 g		Calcium	49.3 mg	(5% DV)
Cholesterol	66.3 mg	(22% DV)	Iron	.3 mg	(2% DV)
Sodium	334.1 mg	(14% DV)	Folate	17.9 mcg	(3% DV)
Potassium	252.5 mg	(7% DV)	Beta Carotene	2.6 RE	

Ratings	Worst	Bad	Average	Good	Best
Weight Loss				7	
LowCal Density				7	
Filling	1				
Energizing	2				
Fiber	1				
Vitamins			4		
Minerals			5		
Overall			5		

WHITING, FLOURED OR BREADED, FRIED

Serving: 1 fillet (3.11 oz)   **Fish**

Calories	189	(60.7 cal/oz)	Carbohydrate	6.87 g	(2% DV)
Fat Calories	86	(46% fat)	Dietary Fiber	0 g	(0% DV)
Total Fat	9.57 g	(15% DV)	Protein	17.4 g	(35% DV)
Saturated Fat	2.61 g	(13% DV)	Vitamin A	100.9 IU	(2% DV)
Poly Fat	2.61 g		Vitamin C	0 mg	(0% DV)
Mono Fat	4.35 g		Calcium	55.7 mg	(6% DV)
Cholesterol	75.7 mg	(25% DV)	Iron	.7 mg	(4% DV)
Sodium	329.7 mg	(14% DV)	Folate	17.4 mcg	(3% DV)
Potassium	228.8 mg	(7% DV)	Beta Carotene	0 RE	

Ratings	Worst	Bad	Average	Good	Best
Weight Loss			4		
LowCal Density			5		
Filling	2				
Energizing			4		
Fiber	1				
Vitamins			4		
Minerals			5		
Overall			4		

WONTON SOUP

Serving: 1 cup (8.61 oz)   **Soup**

Calories	188	(21.8 cal/oz)	Carbohydrate	15.91 g	(5% DV)
Fat Calories	65	(35% fat)	Dietary Fiber	0 g	(0% DV)
Total Fat	7.23 g	(11% DV)	Protein	14.46 g	(29% DV)
Saturated Fat	2.41 g	(12% DV)	Vitamin A	872.4 IU	(17% DV)
Poly Fat	0 g		Vitamin C	2.4 mg	(4% DV)
Mono Fat	2.41 g		Calcium	31.3 mg	(3% DV)
Cholesterol	53 mg	(18% DV)	Iron	1.9 mg	(10% DV)
Sodium	759.2 mg	(32% DV)	Folate	14.5 mcg	(5% DV)
Potassium	313.3 mg	(9% DV)	Beta Carotene	81.9 RE	

Ratings	Worst	Bad	Average	Good	Best
Weight Loss			4		
LowCal Density					8
Filling				6	
Energizing			5		
Fiber	1				
Vitamins				6	
Minerals			5		
Overall				6	

WONTON, FRIED, MEAT FILLED

Serving: 1 piece (1.07 oz)   **Entree**

Calories	97	(90.3 cal/oz)	Carbohydrate	6.48 g	(2% DV)
Fat Calories	54	(56% fat)	Dietary Fiber	.3 g	(1% DV)
Total Fat	**6 g**	**(9% DV)**	**Protein**	**3.9 g**	**(8% DV)**
Saturated Fat	1.2 g	(6% DV)	Vitamin A	302.4 IU	(6% DV)
Poly Fat	1.8 g		Vitamin C	.6 mg	(1% DV)
Mono Fat	2.7 g		Calcium	9 mg	(1% DV)
Cholesterol	**20.4 mg**	**(7% DV)**	Iron	.6 mg	(3% DV)
Sodium	**131.7 mg**	**(5% DV)**	Folate	3.9 mcg	(1% DV)
Potassium	60 mg	(2% DV)	Beta Carotene	28.2 RE	

Ratings	Worst	Bad	Average	Good	Best
Weight Loss				6	
LowCal Density	3				
Filling	2				
Energizing	4				
Fiber	2				
Vitamins	4				
Minerals	3				
Overall	4				

YAM, COOKED

Serving: 1 cup (5 oz)   **Vegetable**

Calories	162	(32.5 cal/oz)	Carbohydrate	38.5 g	(13% DV)
Fat Calories	0	(0% fat)	Dietary Fiber	5.6 g	(22% DV)
Total Fat	**0 g**	**(0% DV)**	**Protein**	**1.4 g**	**(3% DV)**
Saturated Fat	0 g	(0% DV)	Vitamin A	0 IU	(0% DV)
Poly Fat	0 g		Vitamin C	16.8 mg	(28% DV)
Mono Fat	0 g		Calcium	19.6 mg	(2% DV)
Cholesterol	**0 mg**	**(0% DV)**	Iron	.7 mg	(4% DV)
Sodium	**173.6 mg**	**(7% DV)**	Folate	1.4 mcg	(6% DV)
Potassium	935.2 mg	(27% DV)	Beta Carotene	0 RE	

Ratings	Worst	Bad	Average	Good	Best
Weight Loss			6		
LowCal Density			7		
Filling				8	
Energizing					9
Fiber					9
Vitamins			6		
Minerals		4			
Overall				7	

YELLOW BEANS, STRING, COOKED WITHOUT ADDED FAT

Serving: 1 cup (4.82 oz)　　　　　　　　　　**Vegetable**

Calories	47	(9.8 cal/oz)	Carbohydrate	10.53 g	(4% DV)
Fat Calories	0	(0% fat)	Dietary Fiber	1.35 g	(5% DV)
Total Fat	0 g	(0% DV)	Protein	2.7 g	(5% DV)
Saturated Fat	0 g	(0% DV)	Vitamin A	109.4 IU	(2% DV)
Poly Fat	0 g		Vitamin C	13.5 mg	(22% DV)
Mono Fat	0 g		Calcium	62.1 mg	(6% DV)
Cholesterol	0 mg	(0% DV)	Iron	1.7 mg	(10% DV)
Sodium	315.9 mg	(13% DV)	Folate	2.7 mcg	(11% DV)
Potassium	401 mg	(11% DV)	Beta Carotene	10.8 RE	

Ratings	Worst	Bad	Average	Good	Best
Weight Loss					9
LowCal Density					9
Filling				7	
Energizing		4			
Fiber			5		
Vitamins			5		
Minerals			5		
Overall				8	

YOGURT, FROZEN, LOWFAT MILK

Serving: 1 cup (6.89 oz)　　　　　　　　　　**Dessert**

Calories	207	(30 cal/oz)	Carbohydrate	37.83 g	(13% DV)
Fat Calories	17	(8% fat)	Dietary Fiber	0 g	(0% DV)
Total Fat	1.93 g	(3% DV)	Protein	9.65 g	(19% DV)
Saturated Fat	1.93 g	(10% DV)	Vitamin A	110 IU	(2% DV)
Poly Fat	0 g		Vitamin C	1.9 mg	(3% DV)
Mono Fat	0 g		Calcium	304.9 mg	(30% DV)
Cholesterol	9.7 mg	(3% DV)	Iron	.5 mg	(3% DV)
Sodium	117.7 mg	(5% DV)	Folate	9.7 mcg	(5% DV)
Potassium	438.1 mg	(13% DV)	Beta Carotene	3.9 RE	

Ratings	Worst	Bad	Average	Good	Best
Weight Loss				8	
LowCal Density				7	
Filling				7	
Energizing				8	
Fiber	1				
Vitamins		3			
Minerals				7	
Overall				7	

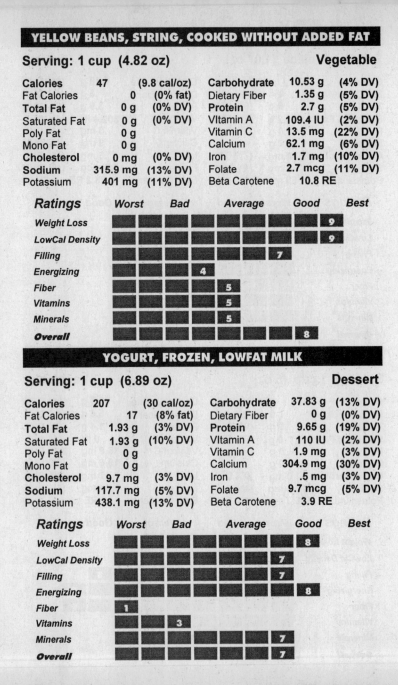

YOGURT, FRUIT VARIETY, LOWFAT MILK

Serving: 1 cup (8.11 oz)   **Dessert**

Calories	232	(28.6 cal/oz)	Carbohydrate	43.36 g	(14% DV)
Fat Calories	20	(9% fat)	Dietary Fiber	0 g	(0% DV)
Total Fat	2.27 g	(3% DV)	Protein	9.08 g	(18% DV)
Saturated Fat	2.27 g	(11% DV)	Vitamin A	104.4 IU	(2% DV)
Poly Fat	0 g		Vitamin C	2.3 mg	(4% DV)
Mono Fat	0 g		Calcium	345 mg	(35% DV)
Cholesterol	9.1 mg	(3% DV)	Iron	.2 mg	(1% DV)
Sodium	131.7 mg	(5% DV)	Folate	9.1 mcg	(5% DV)
Potassium	442.7 mg	(13% DV)	Beta Carotene	2.3 RE	

Ratings	Worst	Bad	Average	Good	Best
Weight Loss				8	
LowCal Density				8	
Filling				8	
Energizing					9
Fiber	1				
Vitamins		3			
Minerals				7	
Overall				7	

YOGURT, FRUIT VARIETY, NONFAT MILK

Serving: 1 cup (8.11 oz)   **Dessert**

Calories	213	(26.3 cal/oz)	Carbohydrate	43.13 g	(14% DV)
Fat Calories	0	(0% fat)	Dietary Fiber	0 g	(0% DV)
Total Fat	0 g	(0% DV)	Protein	9.08 g	(18% DV)
Saturated Fat	0 g	(0% DV)	Vitamin A	15.9 IU	(0% DV)
Poly Fat	0 g		Vitamin C	2.3 mg	(4% DV)
Mono Fat	0 g		Calcium	345 mg	(35% DV)
Cholesterol	4.5 mg	(2% DV)	Iron	.2 mg	(1% DV)
Sodium	131.7 mg	(5% DV)	Folate	9.1 mcg	(5% DV)
Potassium	440.4 mg	(13% DV)	Beta Carotene	0 RE	

Ratings	Worst	Bad	Average	Good	Best
Weight Loss				8	
LowCal Density				8	
Filling					9
Energizing					9
Fiber	1				
Vitamins		3			
Minerals				7	
Overall				7	

YOGURT, FRUIT, NONFAT MILK, LOW-CAL SWEETENER

Serving: 1 cup (8.61 oz)   **Dessert**

Calories	123	(14.3 cal/oz)	Carbohydrate	19.28 g	(6% DV)
Fat Calories	0	(0% fat)	Dietary Fiber	2.41 g	(10% DV)
Total Fat	0 g	(0% DV)	Protein	9.64 g	(19% DV)
Saturated Fat	0 g	(0% DV)	VItamin A	41 IU	(1% DV)
Poly Fat	0 g		Vitamin C	26.5 mg	(44% DV)
Mono Fat	0 g		Calcium	368.7 mg	(37% DV)
Cholesterol	2.4 mg	(1% DV)	Iron	.6 mg	(3% DV)
Sodium	139.8 mg	(6% DV)	Folate	9.6 mcg	(8% DV)
Potassium	549.5 mg	(16% DV)	Beta Carotene	2.4 RE	

Ratings	Worst	Bad	Average	Good	Best
Weight Loss				9	
LowCal Density				9	
Filling				8	
Energizing			6		
Fiber			7		
Vitamins			5		
Minerals				8	
Overall				8	

YOGURT, TOFU

Serving: 1 cup (9.36 oz)   **Dessert**

Calories	254	(27.2 cal/oz)	Carbohydrate	43.23 g	(14% DV)
Fat Calories	47	(19% fat)	Dietary Fiber	0 g	(0% DV)
Total Fat	5.24 g	(8% DV)	Protein	10.48 g	(21% DV)
Saturated Fat	0 g	(0% DV)	VItamin A	86.5 IU	(2% DV)
Poly Fat	2.62 g		Vitamin C	7.9 mg	(13% DV)
Mono Fat	0 g		Calcium	309.2 mg	(31% DV)
Cholesterol	0 mg	(0% DV)	Iron	2.8 mg	(15% DV)
Sodium	91.7 mg	(4% DV)	Folate	10.5 mcg	(4% DV)
Potassium	123.1 mg	(4% DV)	Beta Carotene	7.9 RE	

Ratings	Worst	Bad	Average	Good	Best
Weight Loss			6		
LowCal Density				8	
Filling					9
Energizing					9
Fiber	1				
Vitamins		4			
Minerals				8	
Overall				7	

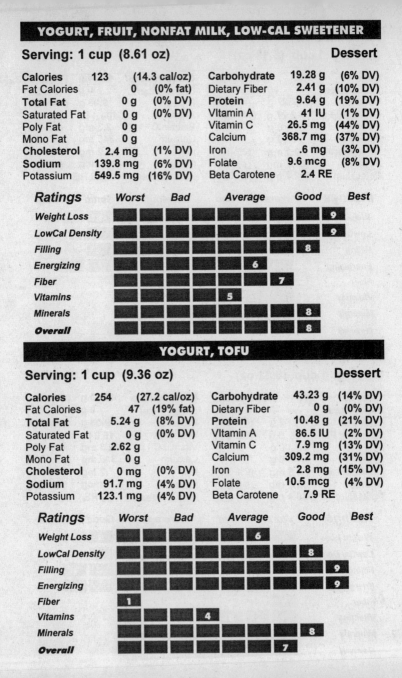

ZUCCHINI WITH TOMATO SAUCE, WITHOUT ADDED FAT

Serving: 1 cup (8.32 oz)   **Vegetable**

Calories	42	(5 cal/oz)	Carbohydrate	9.55 g	(3% DV)
Fat Calories	0	(0% fat)	Dietary Fiber	2.33 g	(9% DV)
Total Fat	0 g	(0% DV)	Protein	2.33 g	(5% DV)
Saturated Fat	0 g	(0% DV)	VItamin A	894.7 IU	(18% DV)
Poly Fat	0 g		Vitamin C	21 mg	(35% DV)
Mono Fat	0 g		Calcium	41.9 mg	(4% DV)
Cholesterol	0 mg	(0% DV)	Iron	1.1 mg	(6% DV)
Sodium	484.6 mg	(20% DV)	Folate	2.3 mcg	(8% DV)
Potassium	556.9 mg	(16% DV)	Beta Carotene	88.5 RE	

Ratings	Worst	Bad	Average	Good	Best
Weight Loss					9
LowCal Density					10
Filling					10
Energizing		4			
Fiber			6		
Vitamins			6		
Minerals			5		
Overall				8	

ZWIEBACK

Serving: 1 piece (.25 oz)   **Snack**

Calories	30	(119.3 cal/oz)	Carbohydrate	5.19 g	(2% DV)
Fat Calories	6	(21% fat)	Dietary Fiber	.21 g	(1% DV)
Total Fat	.7 g	(1% DV)	Protein	.7 g	(1% DV)
Saturated Fat	.28 g	(1% DV)	VItamin A	4.1 IU	(0% DV)
Poly Fat	.07 g		Vitamin C	.4 mg	(1% DV)
Mono Fat	.28 g		Calcium	1.4 mg	(0% DV)
Cholesterol	1.5 mg	(0% DV)	Iron	0 mg	(0% DV)
Sodium	16.2 mg	(1% DV)	Folate	.7 mcg	(0% DV)
Potassium	21.4 mg	(1% DV)	Beta Carotene	.4 RE	

Ratings	Worst	Bad	Average	Good	Best
Weight Loss					9
LowCal Density	2				
Filling	2				
Energizing		3			
Fiber	2				
Vitamins	2				
Minerals	2				
Overall		4			

Extraordinary Healthy Software Products!

Santé® CD-ROM Or Santé® Floppy Disk

PC users delight: **Santé®** CD-ROM (for good health), with tens of thousands of users world-wide is a must for anyone interested in cooking, health, and nutrition. This all-in-one cookbook, diet analysis, weight control and exercise package has complete information on over 18,000 foods (floppy version has 3,000) — famous brand-name foods from the USDA data banks, and from your favorite fast food restaurants. As a complete cookbook, **Santé®** offers fast, easy menu-planning, 415 delicious home recipes, shopping lists, meal costing, food buying, and storage tips. You can add all of your own recipes and resize them to fit your cooking needs. Santé ® also provides personalized plans for changing your weight and personalized nutrition guidelines and ratios. Dietician's advice on over 75 nutrition categories, RDA graphs, colorful calorie pie-charts and many nutritional analyses reports.

NutriStaR™ CD-ROM

Extraordinary food nutrient look-up reference. More than 40,000 foods and their nutritional values listing up to 100 nutrients each. The latest USDA data from Handbook Eight Standard Reference, Survey Database, Canadian reference in French and English, and over 20,000 of your favorite fast food and manufacturer's brand name foods. Full-text search finds the foods you want, fast and easy. If you have ever wondered what is in the foods you eat, this is a must-have reference tool.

Food/Analyst CD-ROM

A complete nutritional analysis software program that breaks down what you eat into specific nutrients, such as calories, fat, sugar, protein, cholesterol, vitamins, and much more. Direct access to over 80 nutrients and approximately 5,000 foods is provided. Track any number of meals, recipes, and people. Produces RDA graphs and multiple reports. Sorts foods from low to high by nutrient levels. Also includes user manual and context sensitive help. Very easy to use.

Special Discount Prices
For Edmund's Readers
See Order Form On Next Page

Food/Analyst Plus CD-ROM

Plan your meals and recipes and see what you are eating by specific nutrients such as calories, fat, sugar, protein, cholesterol, vitamins, and much more. Direct access to over 100 nutrients and approximately 23,000 foods is provided. Add your own foods and see what your meals/recipes cost per serving. Get a dietician's advice on over 75 nutrition subjects in an informative question/answer section. Track any number of meals, recipes, and people. Reference nutrient sorts (high to low of foods containing each nutrient). Export your person-data files for use by statistical or database programs. Produces RDA graphs, colorful pie charts and multiple reports. Includes user manual and context sensitive help. Very easy to use.

The Herbalist® Multimedia CD-ROM

David Hoffmann's encyclopedia of herbal medicine with full text search. See over 170 beautiful full-color herb photos. Hear David describe the herbs and their medicinal uses in a half-hour narration. Enjoy Jim Duke's herb music and verse. **The Herbalist® Multimedia CD-ROM** contains an extensive herbal glossary, medical and scientific citations, plant taxonomy and English to Latin cross references. It also includes extensive information on *Basic Principles of Herbalism,* such as how to choose the right herb, *Human Systems,* such as digestive, cardio-vascular, respiratory, nervous, and reproductive systems, *The Actions of Herbs,* such as anti-inflammatories, and diuretics, and *Medical Details* on over 180 herbs, such as chamomile, ginger, feverfew, and saw palmetto. Designed for all interested in health care, whether teacher, student, practitioner or patient. For Windows PCs or Macintosh.

Exercise*Break*®

Designed by a team of health care professionals, Exercise*Break*® automatically reminds you and shows you how to take a moment to stretch, relax, and perform a few simple exercises —right at your computer. Personalize the program to fit your needs. Focus on full-body relaxation, or give special attention to your fingers, wrists, shoulders, neck, back, or legs. Animated graphics for 50 exercise sequences. Avoid repetitive motion injuries, fatigue, and increase your productivity. Schedule as many or as few pop-up breaks as you want. Cancel your break with the touch of a button. Delivered on 3½" disks. Site licensing available.

Extraordinary Healthy
Software Products
Discount Order Form

	List Price	Edmund's Price
❑Santé® CD-ROM Or Santé® Floppy Disk	$59.95	$49.95
❑NutriStaR™ CD-ROM	$49.95	$39.95
❑Food/Analyst CD-ROM	$39.95	$29.95
❑Food/Analyst Plus CD-ROM	$199.95	$159.95
❑The Herbalist® Multimedia CD-ROM	$49.95	$39.95
❑Exercise*Break*® Windows/DOS	$29.95	$19.95
❑ Exercise*Break*® Macintosh	$39.95	$29.95

Free shipping and handling within US and Canada.   **Total** _____
Minnesota residents, please add 6.5% sales tax.

Money-Back Guarantee

Name _____

Address _____

City, State, Zip _____

Phone _____

Payment: ❑Mastercard   ❑VISA   ❑AMEX   ❑Check or Money Order

Make check or money order payable to:
Hopkins Technology LLC
421 Hazel Lane
Hopkins, MN 55343-7116

To Order, Please Call: 1-800-397-9211

Credit Card# _____   Expiration Date: _____

Cardholder Name: _____   Signature: _____

Bakery

#		Overall Rating	Page
1	Muffin, bran with fruit, low fat, no cholesterol	5.7	283
2	Muffin, fruit, reduced fat, no cholesterol	5.5	285
3	Corn pone, baked	5.4	170
4	Coffee cake, yeast type, low fat, no cholesterol	5.4	154
5	Tortilla, corn	5.2	432
6	Muffin, bran	5.0	283
7	Muffin, oatmeal	4.9	286
8	Danish pastry, cheese, low fat, no cholesterol	4.7	185
9	Popover	4.7	333
10	Cookie, brownie, with icing, dietetic	4.7	156
11	Cookie, fig bar	4.4	161
12	Muffin, fruit and/or nuts	4.4	285
13	Pannetone (Italian-style sweetbread)	4.4	301
14	Muffin, whole wheat	4.3	286
15	Sweet Roll, Mexican, Pan Dulce, no topping	4.3	417
16	Tortilla, flour (wheat)	4.3	433
17	Cookie, fortune	4.2	161
18	Cornbread muffin, stick, round	4.2	172
19	Coffee cake, yeast type	4.1	153
20	Biscuit, baking powder or buttermilk, from mix	4.0	44
21	Muffin, carrot	4.0	284
22	Cookie, Pfeffernusse	3.9	164
23	Sweet Roll, with fruit, frosted	3.9	418
24	Sweet Roll, cinnamon bun, frosted	3.9	417
25	Coffee cake, crumb or quick-bread type	3.8	153
26	Cookie, granola	3.8	162
27	Hush puppy	3.8	241
28	Cookie, carob	3.7	157
29	Cookie, butter or sugar cookie	3.7	157
30	Cookie, macaroon	3.7	162
31	Muffin, chocolate chip	3.7	284
32	Cookie, chocolate-covered marshmallow	3.6	158
33	Cookie, dietetic, oatmeal with raisins	3.6	159
34	Cookie, oatmeal, with raisins	3.6	163
35	Brioche	3.5	68
36	Cookie, vanilla wafer	3.5	167
37	Doughnut, cake type	3.4	188
38	Cookie, chocolate chip	3.3	158
39	Cookie, dietetic, sandwich type	3.3	160
40	Cookie, sandwich-type, not chocolate or vanilla	3.3	165
41	Cookie, sugar wafer	3.3	166
42	Cookie, dietetic, sugar or plain	3.2	160
43	Cookie, toffee bar	3.2	166
44	Cookie, peanut butter	3.2	164
45	Doughnut, jelly	3.2	188
46	Doughnut, raised or yeast	3.2	189
47	Cookie, brownie, with icing	3.1	156
48	Cookie, dietetic, chocolate chip	3.1	159
49	Cookie, short bread	3.1	165
50	Biscuit, cheese	3.0	44
51	Croissant	2.9	182
52	Danish pastry	2.9	184
53	Cookie, oatmeal, with chocolate chips	2.8	163
54	Danish pastry, with cheese	2.8	185

Beverage

		Overall Rating	Page
1	Tomato & vegetable juice, mostly tomato	8.7	428
2	Tomato juice	8.5	429
3	Cranberry juice drink, low calorie, with vitamin C	8.0	178
4	Tea	7.7	425
5	Tea, from powdered instant, low-cal sweetener	7.7	426
6	Cocoa, whey, & low calorie sweetener, fortified	7.6	151
7	Orange juice, frozen, unsweetened, + calcium	7.6	297
8	Coffee, made from ground, regular	7.5	155
9	Apricot nectar	7.4	17
10	Orange juice, frozen, unsweetened (reconstituted)	7.4	298
11	Tangerine juice	7.4	424
12	Fruit punch, fruit drink, or fruitade, vitamin C	7.4	217
13	Milk, chocolate, skim milk-based	7.4	277
14	Soft drink, sugar-free	7.3	393
15	Lemonade	7.2	258
16	Cranberry juice drink with vitamin C added	7.1	177
17	Milk, cow's, fluid, skim or nonfat	7.1	279
18	Pineapple juice, unsweetened	7.1	324
19	Tea, from powdered instant, presweetened	7.1	426
20	Apple juice	7.0	15
21	Prune juice	6.9	349
22	Soft drink	6.7	392
23	Cocoa, sugar, & dry milk mixture, water added	6.5	151
24	Grape juice, unsweetened	6.5	224
25	Milk, cow's, fluid, 1% fat	6.5	278
26	Coffee, from mix, whitener, low cal sweetener	6.1	154
27	Coffee, from mix, with whitener & sugar	6.0	155
28	Milk, cow's, fluid, 2% fat	5.8	278
29	Cappuccino	5.5	97
30	Milk shake, carry-out type	5.4	277
31	Milk, cow's, fluid, whole	5.2	279
32	Milk, malted, unfortified, made with milk	5.2	280
33	Eggnog, made with 2% lowfat milk	4.9	199

Bread

		Overall Rating	Page
1	Bread, wheat or cracked wheat, reduced calorie	6.4	64
2	Bread, rye, reduced calorie, high fiber	6.2	62
3	Bread, multigrain, reduced calorie, high fiber	6.0	57
4	English Muffin, wheat bran	5.7	204
5	Bread, reduced calorie, high fiber, white	5.7	61
6	English Muffin, 100% whole wheat	5.5	203
7	Bread, multigrain	5.3	56
8	Bread, pita, whole wheat, 100%	5.3	59
9	Bagel, whole wheat, 100%	5.2	23
10	English Muffin, with raisins	5.2	204
11	Bread, whole wheat, 100%	5.2	65
12	English Muffin, multigrain	5.2	203
13	Bagel, multigrain, with raisins	5.1	22
14	Bagel, wheat	5.1	23
15	Bread, pumpernickel	5.1	60
16	Roll, pumpernickel	5.1	369
17	Roll, whole wheat, 100%	5.1	370
18	Bagel, pumpernickel	5.0	22
19	Bread, French or Vienna, whole wheat, not 100%	5.0	54
20	Bread, rye	5.0	62

INDEX TO FOOD RANKINGS

Overall Rating | Page

Cereal

		Overall Rating	Page
1	Fiber One	7.4	206
2	Oatmeal, cooked	7.4	292
3	All-Bran	7.1	11
4	Grits, corn or hominy,regular,without added fat	7.0	229
5	Bran Buds	6.9	50
6	Wheat cereal, chocolate flavored, cooked	6.8	452
7	Bran Flakes 40%	6.5	50
8	Total	6.5	433
9	Just Rite	6.4	249
10	Fruit'N Fiber	6.3	218
11	Raisin bran	6.3	355
12	Mueslix Bran Muesli	6.0	282
13	Wheaties	6.0	452
14	Basic 4	5.9	25
15	Quaker Oat Squares	5.9	353
16	Product 19	5.9	349
17	Chex cereal	5.8	118
18	Cream of Rice, made with milk	5.8	179
19	Cream of Wheat, cooked, with milk & sugar	5.7	179
20	Froot Loops	5.5	214
21	Halfsies	5.5	232
22	Honey & Nut Toasty O's	5.5	238
23	Apple Jacks	5.4	15
24	Cheerios	5.4	105
25	Frosted Flakes, Kellogg	5.4	215
26	Life (plain & cinnamon)	5.4	260
27	Cocoa Puffs	5.4	150
28	King Vitamin	5.4	250
29	Lucky Charms	5.4	265
30	Apple Cinnamon Cheerios	5.3	14
31	Shredded Wheat, 100%	5.3	385
32	Alpha-Bits	5.2	13
33	Golden Grahams	5.2	222
34	Special K	5.2	400
35	Trix	5.2	434
36	Booberry	5.2	49
37	Grape-Nuts	5.2	224
38	Cap'n Crunch	5.1	96
39	Honeycomb, plain	5.1	239
40	Rice Krispies	5.1	361
41	Corn flakes	5.0	168
42	Kix	5.0	251
43	Cinnamon Toast Crunch	4.9	147
44	C.W. Post, with raisins	4.7	75
45	Donutz Cereal	4.7	187
46	Rice, puffed	4.2	364
47	Heartland Natural Cereal, plain	4.2	237
48	Granola	3.9	222
49	Sun Country 100% Natural Granola,with Almonds	3.6	412

Cheese

1	Cheese, cottage, lowfat (1-2% fat)	5.0	109
2	Cheese, Cheddar or Colby, lowfat	4.6	108
3	Cheese, processed, American, lowfat	4.6	112

Edmund's Food Ratings   466

Dessert

44	Cake, spice, with icing	4.8	91
45	Pie, blueberry, two crust	4.8	315
46	Pie, coconut cream	4.8	317
47	Cake, gingerbread, without icing	4.7	85
48	Cake, jelly roll	4.7	86
49	Cake, marble, with icing	4.7	88
50	Blintz, cheese-filled	4.7	46
51	Cake, yellow, standard-type mix	4.7	93
52	Pie, pudding, flavors other than chocolate	4.7	319
53	Cream puff, eclair, custard or cream filled, iced	4.6	180
54	Ice cream cone, chocolate covered or dipped	4.6	242
55	Ice cream, soft serve, other than chocolate	4.6	244
56	Pie, peach, two crust	4.6	318
57	Cake, lemon, lowfat, with icing	4.5	87
58	Cake, upside down (all fruits)	4.5	92
59	Pie, cherry, two crust	4.5	316
60	Pie, custard	4.5	317
61	Cake, applesauce, without icing	4.4	80
62	Cake, lemon, with icing	4.4	87
63	Pie, lemon meringue	4.4	318
64	Cake, ice cream & cake roll, chocolate	4.4	86
65	Cake, white, standard-type mix	4.4	93
66	Cake, chiffon, with icing	4.3	83
67	Ice cream, rich, flavors other than chocolate	4.3	244
68	Pie, black bottom	4.3	314
69	Pie, chiffon, not chocolate	4.3	316
70	Pie, apple, two crust	4.2	313
71	Cake, Boston cream pie	4.2	82
72	Sopaipilla with syrup or honey	4.2	394
73	Cake, chocolate, devil's food or fudge, home	4.1	83
74	Cake, German chocolate, with icing & filling	4.1	85
75	Cake, poppyseed, without icing	4.1	88
76	Cake, pound, without icing	4.1	89
77	Cake, torte	4.1	91
78	Cheesecake with fruit	4.1	116
79	Pie, cherry, fried	4.0	315
80	Turnover or dumpling, apple	4.0	442
81	Pie, sour cream, raisin	3.9	321
82	Cake, carrot, with icing	3.9	82
83	Cheesecake	3.8	116
84	Pie, pecan	3.7	319
85	Empanada, fruit-filled	3.7	201
86	Baklava	3.6	24
87	Pie, apple, fried	3.4	313
88	Ice cream bar or stick, chocolate covered	3.3	242
89	Fritter, apple	3.2	213

Entree

1	Shrimp & noodles in tomato-based sauce	8.3	386
2	Shrimp creole, rice, peppers	8.2	387
3	Rice with beans	8.1	362
4	Spanish rice	7.8	400
5	Potato, stuffed, baked, peel, brocolli & cheese	7.7	346
6	Beef stew, potatoes, vegetables & gravy	7.7	35
7	Spaghetti & meatballs, vegetable, dessert	7.7	399

Entree

		Overall Rating	Page
8	Rice, brown, cooked without added fat	7.6	363
9	Veal with peppers, sauce, rice (diet meal)	7.6	445
10	Beef, oriental style, vegetable, rice, & fruit	7.5	39
11	Lasagna with cheese & meat sauce	7.5	255
12	Stuffed green pepper	7.5	409
13	Chicken chow mein with rice	7.4	120
14	Chili, vegetarian (made with meat substitute)	7.3	145
15	Flounder with chopped broccoli	7.3	209
16	Turkey with vegetable, stuffing	7.3	440
17	Ham, glazed, sweet potato, vegetable	7.2	234
18	Rice, flavored, white & wild	7.2	363
19	Rice, wild, 100%, cooked without added fat	7.2	365
20	Sole with vegetables	7.2	394
21	Stuffed cabbage, meat & tomato sauce	7.2	409
22	Chicken cacciatore, noodles	7.1	120
23	Rice, white, regular, cooked without added fat	7.1	365
24	Seafood newburg, rice, vegetable	7.1	383
25	Beef shishkabob with vegetables (no potatoes)	7.0	33
26	Lasagna with cheese & meat sauce	7.0	255
27	Shrimp cocktail (with cocktail sauce)	7.0	387
28	Swedish Meatballs, sauce, noodles, vegetable	7.0	415
29	Beef, oriental style, vegetable, rice	6.9	39
30	Chicken fajitas	6.9	122
31	Couscous, plain, cooked without added fat	6.9	174
32	Macaroni & cheese, apples, vegetables	6.9	266
33	Rice pilaf	6.9	362
34	Gumbo with rice (New Orleans type)	6.9	230
35	Lamb or mutton stew, potatoes & vegetables	6.9	253
36	Ravioli, cheese-filled, with tomato sauce	6.9	357
37	Beef, noodles, & vegetables	6.8	38
38	Chicken teriyaki, rice, vegetable (frozen meal)	6.8	134
39	Sweet & sour pork with rice	6.8	415
40	Beef, rice, & vegetables	6.7	41
41	Chicken cordon bleu, vegetables	6.7	121
42	Chop suey, meatless	6.7	146
43	Tortellini, meat-filled, with tomato sauce	6.7	431
44	Beef, gravy, vegetable, dessert	6.7	37
45	Lasagna, meatless	6.7	256
46	Linguini with vegetables & seafood, wine sauce	6.7	262
47	Fajita with chicken & vegetables	6.6	205
48	Stew, vegetarian	6.6	407
49	Chili con carne with beans	6.5	143
50	Turkey with gravy,dressing,potato,veg,dessert	6.5	439
51	Burrito with beef & beans, refried beans, salsa	6.4	72
52	Chicken & vegetable entree with rice, Oriental	6.4	119
53	Corned beef, potatoes, & vegetables	6.4	173
54	Haddock with chopped spinach	6.4	231
55	Lasagna, vegetable	6.4	257
56	Lasagna, with chicken or turkey, & spinach	6.4	257
57	Macaroni & cheese	6.4	266
58	Swedish Meatballs, gravy, noodles	6.4	414
59	Almond chicken	6.4	12
60	Beans & franks, frozen meal	6.4	28
61	Manicotti, cheese-filled, tomato sauce	6.4	269
62	Potato, stuffed,baked,with peel,sour cream	6.4	347
63	Chicken with sauce, beans, vegetable, dessert	6.3	135

Entree

Entree

		Overall Rating	Page
120	Pizza, cheese	5.2	328
121	Calzone, with meat & cheese	5.2	94
122	Creamed dried beef on toast	5.2	180
123	Dim sum, meat filled (egg roll-type)	5.1	186
124	Tamale with meat	5.1	422
125	Tortellini, cheese-filled, meatless, vegetables	5.1	431
126	Chicken or turkey cacciatore	5.0	126
127	Chicken or turkey with dumplings	5.0	130
128	Chicken, fried, with potatoes	5.0	138
129	Chili dog (frankfurter,chili con carne, no bun)	5.0	144
130	Egg roll, meatless	5.0	193
131	Mexican casserole, ground beef, beans, tomato	5.0	276
132	Porcupine balls with tomato-based sauce	5.0	334
133	Beef curry	4.9	30
134	Corned beef hash	4.9	172
135	Egg roll, with beef and/or pork	4.9	193
136	Shrimp scampi	4.9	388
137	Chicken divan	4.8	122
138	Chicken or turkey pot pie	4.8	128
139	Egg foo yung	4.8	190
140	Eggplant & meat casserole	4.8	199
141	Crepes, filled with meat, fish, or poultry	4.7	181
142	Pizza with meat	4.7	327
143	Beef rolls, stuffed with vegetables or meat	4.7	32
144	Chicken kiev,rice-vegetable mix	4.7	124
145	Salisbury steak with gravy	4.7	374
146	Soft taco with beef, cheese, & lettuce	4.7	393
147	Steak teriyaki with sauce (mixture)	4.7	406
148	Nachos with beef, beans, cheese, sour cream	4.5	290
149	Pasta with pesto sauce	4.4	303
150	Spanakopitta	4.4	399
151	Chicken or turkey cordon bleu	4.3	127
152	Croissant, filled with ham & cheese	4.2	182
153	Pepper steak	4.2	310
154	Quesadilla with cheese, meatless	4.2	353
155	Puffs, fried, crabmeat & cream cheese filled	4.0	352
156	Knish, cheese	3.9	251
157	Kung Pao pork	3.9	252
158	Wonton, fried, meat filled	3.8	455
159	Flauta	3.6	208
160	Quiche with meat, poultry or fish	3.4	354
161	Nachos with cheese, meatless, no beans	3.3	290
162	Chicken wing with hot pepper sauce	3.2	134
163	Turnover, meat-filled, no gravy	3.2	442
164	Veal scallopini	3.1	445
165	Moo Shi Pork	2.9	282

Fat & Oil

1	Mayonnaise-type salad dressing, fat-free	5.5	273
2	Caesar dressing, low-calorie	5.2	79
3	French dressing, low-calorie	4.9	212
4	Russian dressing, low-calorie	4.9	371
5	Blue or roquefort cheese dressing, low-calorie	4.7	47
6	Thousand Island dressing, low-calorie	4.1	428
7	Butter replacement, fat-free powder	3.9	73

INDEX TO FOOD RANKINGS

Overall Rating   Page

Fish

29	Whiting, floured or breaded, fried	3.9	454
30	Catfish, baked or broiled	3.7	100
31	Flounder, floured or breaded, fried	3.7	210
32	Pike, battered, fried	3.7	324
33	Swordfish, floured or breaded, fried	3.7	420
34	Tuna, canned, oil pack	3.7	437
35	Pompano, battered, fried	3.3	331
36	Catfish, floured or breaded, fried	3.2	101
37	Mackerel, baked or broiled	3.2	268
38	Pompano, baked or broiled	3.2	331
39	Mackerel, floured or breaded, fried	2.9	268

Fruit

1	Papaya, raw	8.8	301
2	Strawberries, raw	8.4	408
3	Mango, raw	8.2	269
4	Raspberries, raw	8.1	356
5	Pear, raw	8.0	307
6	Orange, raw	7.9	298
7	Tangelo, raw	7.9	423
8	Blueberries, raw	7.8	47
9	Carambola (star fruit), raw	7.8	97
10	Grapefruit, raw	7.8	225
11	Watermelon, raw	7.8	451
12	Honeydew melon, raw	7.7	240
13	Nectarine, raw	7.7	291
14	Strawberries, frozen	7.7	407
15	Apple, raw	7.7	16
16	Kiwi fruit, raw	7.6	250
17	Peach, raw	7.6	304
18	Banana, raw	7.4	25
19	Fruit cocktail, cooked or canned	7.4	215
20	Tangerine, raw	7.4	424
21	Applesauce, stewed apples with sugar	7.4	17
22	Cantaloupe (muskmelon), raw	7.4	96
23	Pineapple, raw	7.3	325
24	Apple, baked with sugar	7.2	16
25	Grapes, raw	7.2	225
26	Plum, raw	6.9	330
27	Rhubarb, cooked or canned	6.9	360
28	Apricot, raw	6.9	18
29	Cherries, sweet, raw (Queen Anne, Bing)	6.8	117
30	Cranberries, cooked or canned	5.9	177
31	Prune, dried, uncooked	5.7	350
32	Avocado, raw	4.8	20
33	Guacamole	4.8	229
34	Raisins	4.7	355

Meat

1	Chicken liver, cooked	5.1	125
2	Beef liver, fried or broiled, no coating	4.9	31
3	Meatball, meatless, vegetarian	4.7	275
4	Ham, smoked or cured, cooked, lean only	4.7	235
5	Veal cutlet or steak, lean only	4.7	443

       Edmund's Food Ratings

Vegetable